Contact Lens Complications

SECOND EDITION

Nathan Efron
BScOptom PhD (Melbourne) DSc (Manchester) MCOptom
FAAO (Dip CL) FIACLE FCLSA FVCO ILTM
Professor of Clinical Optometry
Director, Eurolens Research
The University of Manchester
Manchester
United Kingdom

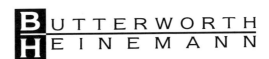

BUTTERWORTH
HEINEMANN

EDINBURGH LONDON NEW YORK OXFORD PHILADELPHIA ST LOUIS SYDNEY TORONTO 2004

This book is rededicated to
my wife, Suzanne,
my daughter, Zoe
and my son, Bruce

BUTTERWORTH-HEINEMANN
An imprint of Elsevier Limited

© 1994 Reed Educational and Professional Publishing Ltd
© 2004, Elsevier Limited. All rights reserved.
© Tear Film Classifications from J.P. Guillon
CD-ROM © 2004, Elsevier Limited; 2001 Reed Educational and Professional Publishing Ltd, Professor Nathan Efron &
Dr Philip Morgan

First published 1994
 Reprinted 2004, 2006

ISBN 0 7506 5534 8

British Library Cataloguing in Publication Data
A catalogue record for this book is available from the British Library

Library of Congress Cataloging in Publication Data
A catalog record for this book is available from the Library of Congress

Notice
Medical knowledge is constantly changing. Standard safety precautions must be followed, but as new research and clinical experience broaden our knowledge, changes in treatment and drug therapy may become necessary or appropriate. Readers are advised to check the most current product information provided by the manufacturer of each drug to be administered to verify the recommended dose, the method and duration of administration, and contraindications. It is the responsibility of the practitioner, relying on experience and knowledge of the patient, to determine dosages and the best treatment for each individual patient. Neither the Publisher nor the editors/contributor assumes any liability for any injury and/or damage to persons or property arising from this publication.

The Publisher

ELSEVIER
your source for books,
journals and multimedia
in the health sciences
www.elsevierhealth.com

Working together to grow
libraries in developing countries
www.elsevier.com | www.bookaid.org | www.sabre.org
ELSEVIER   BOOK AID International   Sabre Foundation

For Butterworth-Heinemann:
Publishing Director: Caroline Makepeace
Development Editor: Kim Benson
Production Manager: Yolanta Motylinska
Copy Editor/Project Manager: John Ormiston
Design/Layout: Judith Campbell

Printed in Spain

The
Publisher's
policy is to use
**paper manufactured
from sustainable forests**

CONTENTS

PREFACE

Shortly after the First Edition of this book was published in 1999, it became apparent to me that it would not be too long before I would need to prepare the Second Edition – and how right I was! There have been numerous advances in contact lens products and care systems, and in the knowledge base that underpins our understanding of contact lens practice. Preparing this book has been a great challenge, but at the same time it has been extremely rewarding, as it has forced me to confront the literature and come to terms with new concepts, approaches and theories concerning all aspects of contact lens complications. This book has not just been re-edited – it has been completely re-written and updated, with 11 new chapters and over 150 new illustrations and schematic diagrams added.

My basic approach to this topic remains unchanged – to deal with the ocular complications of contact lens wear in a systematic 'tissue by tissue' approach. I feel that this approach is intuitive to contact lens practitioners, because this is the way we think. We first identify the particular tissue in distress and then try and understand what is going wrong. The subject matter is divided into nine sections, seven of which relate to the primary anterior ocular structures that can affect, or be affected by, contact lenses (the other sections relate to slit-lamp biomicroscopy and grading systems). Within each section, various identifiable tissue pathologies or conditions are discussed in terms of the systematic consideration of signs, symptoms, pathology, etiology, management, prognosis and differential diagnosis. This systematic approach is reflected in the large 'Quick-find Index' on pages ix to xxxii, which is designed to assist practitioners to (a) gain a quick overview of a specific complication in a broader context, and (b) locate information on a particular complication in the main text.

I have deliberately placed heavy emphasis on the importance of understanding the various ocular complications that can occur. In particular, the development of an understanding of the etiology and pathology of a condition is critical to formulating a link between the presenting signs and symptoms, and the development of an appropriate management plan and formulation of an accurate prognosis.

In this Second Edition, I have expanded the grading scales to cover 16 of the most important contact lens complications; these are presented in Appendix A of this book, together with a comprehensive account of how they can be used (Chapter 29). In addition, all 16 grading scales have been converted into user-friendly movie morph sequences, which offer the possibility of computer-based grading. These grading morphs, and a self-help grading tutor, are available on the accompanying CD-ROM (details are given in Chapter 30). Also presented in this book is a system for classifying the various appearances of the tear film during contact lens wear.

In the preface to the First Edition of this book, I expressed the hope that contact lens tissue complications will eventually cease to occur, making this book redundant. Clearly, that time has not come yet. In the meantime, I hope that this book will assist contact lens practitioners to either prevent problems from occurring or identify problems at an early stage so that effective management strategies can be put in place for the ultimate benefit of our patients.

Nathan Efron

ACKNOWLEDGMENTS

Although I am the sole author of this book, I am not the sole illustrator. I am very fortunate to have been given open access to a number of extensive and outstanding slide libraries of contact lens complications, and in this regard I would like to thank Bausch & Lomb, the British Contact Lens Association, the International Association of Contact Lens Educators, and the Cornea and Contact Lens Research Unit. I salute the clinical excellence and skills of the many practitioners who took the photographs that belong to these magnificent collections; each of these clinicians is acknowledged by name in the Authorship copyright table on pages vi–viii. A special word of thanks to Brian Tompkins, who gave me access to his personal digital image collection. Brian's work is stunning – the evidence of this being that I have used no less than 39 of his images in this book.

It was an honour and a privilege to work with the renowned medical ophthalmic artist Terry Tarrant, who painted the grading scales that appear in Appendix A. Thanks also to CooperVision, who sponsor the production of handheld and poster-size versions of the grading scales and facilitate their world-wide distribution. Joe Tanner, who previously worked for Hydron UK (now CooperVision), provided great support for the grading scale project when it commenced in the mid-1990s; this support is now being continued through John Rogers of CooperVision. I thank Terry, Joe and John.

I am grateful to Dr Philip Morgan and Gordon Addison who assisted in the production of the grading morphs and grading tutor computer programs. Specifically, Gordon created the morph movie sequences and Phil created the interactive program in which the morphs are embedded. I am sure that the fruits of the labor of these two gentleman will be enjoyed by all who use these programs. I thank Phil and Gordon. I also thank Dr JP Guillon for giving me permission to publish his tear film classification system, which appears in Appendix B, and Jack Kanski for giving permission to use his phototgraph of the external hordeolum (stye) in the Quick-find Index.

I am most grateful to my publisher, Caroline Makepeace, for her constant support and encouragement over many years, and to her outstanding team at Elsevier for their tremendous technical support, with special thanks to Kim Benson (development editor), John Ormiston (copy editor) and Judith Campbell (designer),

My wife, Suzanne, has provided wonderful personal support throughout the writing of this book (and all my other books). Suzanne is an accomplished contact lens practitioner in her own right and has also provided material assistance by supplying some of the images used in the book, acting as a 'listening board' for ideas, and helping with proof reading of the manuscript. I am forever grateful. My children, Zoe and Bruce, are now old enough to appreciate the work that has to go into writing books, and through this understanding, and in other ways, have also provided their own form of support for this project, which is greatly appreciated.

And finally, I thank you, the reader, for showing faith in me by buying and/or using this book. I truly hope that my devotion and dedication to the subject has translated into an offering that will be of real clinical value, in the first instance to yourself, and ultimately to your patients, who deserve only the very best clinical care.

Nathan Efron

AUTHOR AND COPYRIGHT OWNER OF FIGURES

Every effort has been made to trace copyright holders of illustrations, but if any have been inadvertently overlooked or if any errors occur in the list below, the publishers will be pleased to make the necessary corrections at the first opportunity.

Key
- BCLA, British Contact Lens Association Slide Collection
- B-H, Butterworth–Heinemann
- B&L, Bausch & Lomb Slide Collection
- CCLRU, Cornea and Contact Lens Research Unit Slide Collection
- IOVS, Investigative Ophthalmology and Visual Science
- LWW, Lippincott Williams & Wilkins
- OAA, Optometrists Association Australia

Figure	Author	Copyright Owner	Figure	Author	Copyright Owner
Fig. 1.1	Patrick Caroline	Patrick Caroline	Fig. 5.6	Patrick Caroline	Patrick Caroline
Fig. 1.2	Nathan Efron	Nathan Efron	Fig. 5.7	Lourdes Llobet	B&L
Fig. 1.3	Nathan Efron	Nathan Efron	Fig. 5.8	Nathan Efron	Nathan Efron
Fig. 1.4	Nathan Efron	Nathan Efron	Fig. 5.9	Nathan Efron	Optician
Fig. 1.5	Patrick Caroline	B&L	Fig. 5.10	Nathan Efron	Optician
Fig. 1.6b	Adrian Bruce	B-H	Fig. 5.11	Patrick Caroline	B&L
Fig. 1.7b	Adrian Bruce	B-H	Fig. 5.12	Patrick Caroline	Patrick Caroline
Fig. 1.8b	Adrian Bruce	B-H	Fig. 5.13	Patrick Caroline	Patrick Caroline
Fig. 1.9b	Brian Tompkins	Brian Tompkins	Fig. 5.14	I DeSchepper	B&L
Fig. 1.10b	Sylvie Sulaiman	B&L	Fig. 5.15	J Prummel	B&L
Fig. 1.11b	Adrian Bruce	B-H	Fig. 5.16	Brian Tompkins	Brian Tompkins
Fig. 1.12b	Michael Hare	Michael Hare	Fig. 5.17	Brian Tompkins	Brian Tompkins
Fig. 2.1	Timothy Grant	B&L	Fig. 6.1	Nathan Efron	Optician
Fig. 2.2	Nathan Efron	Optician	Fig. 6.2	Nathan Efron	Optician
Fig. 2.3	Hilmar Bussaker	B&L	Fig. 6.3	Rolf Haberer	B&L
Fig. 2.4	Nathan Efron	Optician	Fig. 6.4	Timothy Golding	Timothy Golding
Fig. 2.5	Donna LaHood	B&L	Fig. 6.5	Timothy Golding	Timothy Golding
Fig. 2.6a	Brien Holden	CCLRU	Fig. 6.6	Hilmar Bussaker	Hilmar Bussaker
Fig. 2.6b	Brien Holden	CCLRU	Fig. 6.7	Hilmar Bussaker	Hilmar Bussaker
Fig. 2.6c	Brien Holden	CCLRU	Fig. 6.8	Hilmar Bussaker	Hilmar Bussaker
Fig. 2.7	Lucia McGrogan	Lucia McGrogan	Fig. 6.9	Hilmar Bussaker	Hilmar Bussaker
Fig. 2.8	Nathan Efron	Optician	Fig. 6.10	Xavier Llobet	B&L
Fig. 3.1	Desmond Fonn	B&L	Fig. 6.11	Arthur Back	B&L
Fig. 3.2	Nathan Efron	Optician	Fig. 6.12	Timothy Golding	Timothy Golding
Fig. 3.3	Meng Poey Soh	Meng Poey Soh	Fig. 6.13	Timothy Golding	Timothy Golding
Fig. 3.4	Desmond Fonn	B&L	Fig. 6.14	Donald Korb	LWW
Fig. 3.5	Frank Pettigrew	BCLA	Fig. 6.15	Donald Korb	LWW
Fig. 3.6	Jan Kok	B&L	Fig. 6.16	Patrick Caroline	B&L
Fig. 3.7	Robert Terry	CCLRU	Fig. 6.17	A Aan de Kerk	B&L
Fig. 3.8	Sylvie Sulaiman	B&L	Fig. 6.18	Arthur Back	B&L
Fig. 4.1	Brian Tompkins	Brian Tompkins	Fig. 6.19	Adrian Bruce	B&L
Fig. 4.2	Brian Tompkins	Brian Tompkins	Fig. 6.20	Timothy Golding	Timothy Golding
Fig. 4.3	Xavier Llobet	B&L	Fig. 6.21	Timothy Golding	Timothy Golding
Fig. 4.4	Brian Tompkins	Brian Tompkins	Fig. 6.22	Meng Poey Soh	Meng Poey Soh
Fig. 4.5	Brian Tompkins	Brian Tompkins	Fig. 6.23	Nathan Efron	Optician
Fig. 4.6	Lourdes Llobet	B&L	Fig. 6.24	Brian Tompkins	Brian Tompkins
Fig. 4.7	Brian Tompkins	Brian Tompkins	Fig. 7.1	Brian Tompkins	Brian Tompkins
Fig. 4.8	Brian Tompkins	Brian Tompkins	Fig. 7.2	Brian Tompkins	Brian Tompkins
Fig. 4.9	Brian Tompkins	Brian Tompkins	Fig. 7.3	Brian Tompkins	Brian Tompkins
Fig. 4.10	Arthur Back	B&L	Fig. 7.4	Kathy Dumbleton	Kathy Dumbleton
Fig. 4.11	Brian Tompkins	Brian Tompkins	Fig. 7.5	Nathan Efron	Nathan Efron
Fig. 4.12	Luigina Sorbara	B&L	Fig. 7.6a	Suzanne Efron	Suzanne Efron
Fig. 5.1	Brian Tompkins	Brian Tompkins	Fig. 7.6b	Suzanne Efron	Suzanne Efron
Fig. 5.2	Deborah Jones	BCLA	Fig. 7.7	Nathan Efron	Nathan Efron
Fig. 5.3	Brian Tompkins	Brian Tompkins	Fig. 7.8	Nathan Efron	Nathan Efron
Fig. 5.4	Deborah Jones	BCLA	Fig. 7.9	Brian Tompkins	Brian Tompkins
Fig. 5.5	Brian Tompkins	Brian Tompkins	Fig. 7.10	Brian Tompkins	Brian Tompkins

Figure	Author	Copyright Owner
Fig. 8.1	Lyndon Jones	B-H
Fig. 8.2	Timothy Golding	Timothy Golding
Fig. 8.3	Suzanne Efron	Suzanne Efron
Fig. 8.4	Brian Tompkins	Brian Tompkins
Fig. 8.5	Suzanne Efron	Suzanne Efron
Fig. 8.6	Suzanne Efron	Suzanne Efron
Fig. 8.7	Suzanne Efron	Suzanne Efron
Fig. 8.8	Timothy Golding	Timothy Golding
Fig. 8.9	Timothy Golding	Timothy Golding
Fig. 8.10	Shameem Amirbayat	Shameem Amirbayat
Fig. 8.11	Suzanne Efron	Suzanne Efron
Fig. 8.12	C Maldonado-Codina	C Maldonado-Codina
Fig. 8.13	C Maldonado-Codina	C Maldonado-Codina
Fig. 9.1	Brian Tompkins	Brian Tompkins
Fig. 9.2	Leon Davids	B&L
Fig. 9.3	MF Pettigrew	B&L
Fig. 9.4	Charline Gauthier	B&L
Fig. 9.5	Meng Poey Soh	Meng Poey Soh
Fig. 9.6	Brian Tompkins	Brian Tompkins
Fig. 9.7	HJ Rutten	B&L
Fig. 9.8	Nathan Efron	Optician
Fig. 9.9	Timothy Golding	Timothy Golding
Fig. 9.10	Nathan Efron	Optician
Fig. 9.11	Brian Tompkins	Brian Tompkins
Fig. 9.12	Suzanne Efron	Suzanne Efron
Fig. 10.1	Russell Lowe	B&L
Fig. 10.2	Brien Holden	CCLRU
Fig. 10.3	A Gustafsson	A Gustafsson
Fig. 10.4	Brian Tompkins	Brian Tompkins
Fig. 10.5	Robert Terry	B&L
Fig. 10.6	Brian Tompkins	Brian Tompkins
Fig. 10.7a	CD Euwijk	B&L
Fig. 10.7b	CD Euwijk	B&L
Fig. 10.8	Nathan Efron	Optician
Fig. 10.9	Nathan Efron	Optician
Fig. 10.10a	Eric Papas	B&L
Fig. 10.10b	Eric Papas	B&L
Fig. 10.11	Martina Alt	B&L
Fig. 10.12	Lyndon Jones	BCLA
Fig. 10.13	Nathan Efron	Optician
Fig. 10.14a	Maki Shiobara	B&L
Fig. 10.14b	Brien Holden	CCLRU
Fig. 10.15	VK Dada	B&L
Fig. 10.16	Desmond Fonn	B&L
Fig. 11.1	John Lawrenson	John Lawrenson
Fig. 11.2	Brien Holden	CCLRU
Fig. 11.3	Charles McMonnies	Charles McMonnies
Fig. 11.4	John Lawrenson	John Lawrenson
Fig. 11.5a	Eric Papas	B-H
Fig. 11.5b	Eric Papas	B-H
Fig. 11.6	Kathy Dumbleton	LWW
Fig. 11.7	John Lawrenson	John Lawrenson
Fig. 11.8	John Lawrenson	John Lawrenson
Fig. 11.9	Brian Tompkins	Brian Tompkins
Fig. 11.10	Author unknown	Origin unknown
Fig. 11.11	Nathan Efron	Optician
Fig. 11.12	John Lawrenson	John Lawrenson
Fig. 12.1	Robert Grohe	B-H
Fig. 12.2	Robert Grohe	B-H
Fig. 12.3	Robert Grohe	B-H
Fig. 12.4	Robert Grohe	B-H
Fig. 12.5	Robert Terry	B-H
Fig. 12.6	Robert Grohe	B-H
Fig. 12.7	Robert Grohe	B-H
Fig. 12.8	Robert Grohe	B-H
Fig. 12.9	Robert Grohe	B-H
Fig. 12.10	Robert Grohe	B-H
Fig. 12.11	Brian Tompkins	Brian Tompkins
Fig. 12.12	Brian Tompkins	Brian Tompkins
Fig. 12.13	Debbie Jones	Debbie Jones
Fig. 13.1	AJ Elder Smith	BCLA
Fig. 13.2	Mee Sing Chong	B&L
Fig. 13.3	Nathan Efron	Optician
Fig. 13.4	Brien Holden	CCLRU
Fig. 13.5	Nathan Efron	Optician
Fig. 13.6	Nathan Efron	Optician
Fig. 13.7	Padmaja Sankaridurg	B&L
Fig. 13.8	Brian Tompkins	Brian Tompkins
Fig. 13.9	Michael Hare	Michael Hare
Fig. 14.1	Gary Orsborn	B&L
Fig. 14.2	Brien Holden	CCLRU
Fig. 14.3	Brian Tompkins	Brian Tompkins
Fig. 14.4	Suzanne Efron	Suzanne Efron
Fig. 14.5	Luigina Sorbara	B&L
Fig. 14.6	Suzanne Efron	Suzanne Efron
Fig. 14.7	Kathy Dumbleton	B&L
Fig. 14.8	Lyndon Jones	B&L
Fig. 14.9	Arthur Back	B&L
Fig. 14.10	Richard Lindsay	B&L
Fig. 14.11	Michelle Madigan	CCLRU
Fig. 14.12	Nathan Efron	Optician
Fig. 14.13	Donna LaHood	B&L
Fig. 14.14	Deborah Jones	B&L
Fig. 14.15	W Vreugdenhil	B&L
Fig. 14.16	Mee Sing Chong	B&L
Fig. 15.1	Craig Woods	BCLA
Fig. 15.2	David Ruston	BCLA
Fig. 15.3	Steve Zantos	CCLRU
Fig. 15.4	Nathan Efron	Optician
Fig. 15.5	Des Fonn	OAA
Fig. 15.6	Tony Henriquez	Tony Henriquez
Fig. 15.7	Nathan Efron	Optician
Fig. 15.8	Nathan Efron	Optician
Fig. 15.9	Nathan Efron	Optician
Fig. 16.1	Suzanne Efron	Suzanne Efron
Fig. 16.2	Brian Tompkins	Brian Tompkins
Fig. 16.3	Suzanne Efron	Suzanne Efron
Fig. 16.4	Ian Cox	B-H
Fig. 16.5	Jan Bergmanson	B-H
Fig. 16.6	Jan Bergmanson	B-H
Fig. 16.7	Sylvie Sulaiman	B&L
Fig. 16.8	Ruth Cornish	Ruth Cornish
Fig. 17.1	Gary Osborne	B&L
Fig. 17.2	Russell Lowe	B&L
Fig. 17.3	Russell Lowe	B&L
Fig. 17.4	Nigel Burnett-Hodd	Nigel Burnett-Hodd
Fig. 17.5	Nigel Burnett-Hodd	Nigel Burnett-Hodd
Fig. 17.6	Nigel Burnett-Hodd	Nigel Burnett-Hodd
Fig. 17.7	C Euwijk	B&L
Fig. 17.8	Brien Holden	CCLRU
Fig. 17.9	Brien Holden	CCLRU
Fig. 17.10	Brien Holden	CCLRU
Fig. 17.11	Brien Holden	CCLRU
Fig. 17.12	Nathan Efron	Nathan Efron
Fig. 17.13	Meredith Reyes	B&L
Fig. 17.14	Sylvie Sulaiman	B&L
Fig. 18.1	Patrick Caroline	B&L
Fig. 18.2	Noel Brennan	B-H
Fig. 18.3	Noel Brennan	B-H
Fig. 18.4a	Desmond Fonn	Desmond Fonn
Fig. 18.4b	Brien Holden	CCLRU
Fig. 18.4c	Brien Holden	CCLRU
Fig. 18.5	Nathan Efron	Optician
Fig. 18.6	Steve Zantos	CCLRU
Fig. 18.7	Haliza Mutalib	Haliza Mutalib
Fig. 18.8	Nathan Efron	Optician
Fig. 18.9	Nathan Efron	Optician
Fig. 18.10	A Miller	CCLRU
Fig. 18.11	Patrick Caroline	B&L
Fig. 18.12a	Nathan Efron	Nathan Efron
Fig. 18.12b	Nathan Efron	Nathan Efron
Fig. 18.13	Nathan Efron	Optician

Figure	Author	Copyright Owner
Fig. 19.1	Ken Lebow	B-H
Fig. 19.2	Nathan Efron	Optician
Fig. 19.3	Jan Bergmanson	B-H
Fig. 19.4a	Haliza Mutalib	Haliza Mutalib
Fig. 19.4b	Haliza Mutalib	Haliza Mutalib
Fig. 19.5	Nathan Efron	OAA
Fig. 19.6	Nathan Efron	OAA
Fig. 19.7	Haliza Mutalib	Haliza Mutalib
Fig. 19.8	Albert Aandekerk	B&L
Fig. 19.9	Albert Aandekerk	B&L
Fig. 19.10a	Jan Kok	B&L
Fig. 19.10b	Jan Kok	B&L
Fig. 20.1	FE Ros	B&L
Fig. 20.2	FE Ros	B&L
Fig. 20.3	Ron Loveridge	B-H
Fig. 20.4a	Jan Kok	B&L
Fig. 20.4b	Sydney Bush	Sydney Bush
Fig. 20.5	Charline Gauthier	B&L
Fig. 20.6	Patricia Hyrnchak	B&L
Fig. 20.7	Meredith Reyes	B&L
Fig. 20.8	Patrick Caroline	B&L
Fig. 21.1	Rosemary Austin	B&L
Fig. 21.2	Barry Weissman	B-H
Fig. 21.3	Desmond Fonn	BCLA
Fig. 21.4	Michael Hare	Michael Hare
Fig. 21.5	Brien Holden	CCLRU
Fig. 21.6	Nathan Efron	Optician
Fig. 21.7	Patrick Caroline	B&L
Fig. 21.8	Nathan Efron	Optician
Fig. 21.9	Patrick Caroline	B&L
Fig. 21.10a	Michael Hare	Michael Hare
Fig. 21.10b	Michael Hare	Michael Hare
Fig. 21.11	Nathan Efron	Optician
Fig. 21.12	Brian Tompkins	Brian Tompkins
Fig. 21.13	Nathan Efron	Optician
Fig. 21.14	Nathan Efron	Optician
Fig. 21.15	Brian Tompkins	Brian Tompkins
Fig. 22.1	Luigina Sorbara	B&L
Fig. 22.2	Isabelle Jalbert	BCLA
Fig. 22.3	Nathan Efron	Nathan Efron
Fig. 22.4	Sarah Morgan	Sarah Morgan
Fig. 22.5	Brian Tompkins	Brian Tompkins
Fig. 22.6	Suzanne Efron	Suzanne Efron
Fig. 22.7	Brian Tompkins	Brian Tompkins
Fig. 22.8	Nathan Efron	Nathan Efron
Fig. 22.9a	Brien Holden	LWW
Fig. 22.9b	Brien Holden	LWW
Fig. 22.9c	Brien Holden	LWW
Fig. 22.10	Nathan Efron	Optician
Fig. 22.11	Nathan Efron	Optician
Fig. 22.12	Gisele Sachs	B&L
Fig. 22.13	Patrick Caroline	B&L
Fig. 22.14	Melanie Hingorani	Melanie Hingorani
Fig. 22.15a	Brian Tompkins	Brian Tompkins
Fig. 22.15b	Brian Tompkins	Brian Tompkins
Fig. 22.16	Suzanne Efron	Suzanne Efron
Fig. 22.17	Brian Tompkins	Brian Tompkins
Fig. 22.18	Miguel Lumeras	B&L
Fig. 23.1	Brien Holden	CCLRU
Fig. 23.2	Lyndon Jones	BCLA
Fig. 23.3	Lyndon Jones	BCLA
Fig. 23.4	Donna LaHood	CCLRU
Fig. 23.5	Meng Poey Soh	Meng Poey Soh
Fig. 23.6	Barry Weissman	B-H
Fig. 23.7	Barry Weissman	B-H
Fig. 23.8	Florence Mallet	B&L
Fig. 23.9	Suzanne Fleiszig	Suzanne Fleiszig
Fig. 23.10	Nathan Efron	Optician
Fig. 23.11	Andrew Tullo	Andrew Tullo
Fig. 23.12	Suzanne Fleiszig	Suzanne Fleiszig
Fig. 23.13a	Inma Perez-Gomez	Inma Perez-Gomez
Fig. 23.13b	Inma Perez-Gomez	Inma Perez-Gomez
Fig. 23.14	Andrew Tullo	Andrew Tullo
Fig. 23.15	FJ Palomar-Mascaro	B&L
Fig. 24.1	Russell Lowe	B&L
Fig. 24.2a	Stephen Klyce	Stephen Klyce
Fig. 24.2b	Stephen Klyce	Stephen Klyce
Fig. 24.3a	Donna LaHood	B&L
Fig. 24.3b	Craig Woods	B&L
Fig. 24.4	Robert Terry	B&L
Fig. 24.5	Helen Swarbrick	B&L
Fig. 24.6	Stephen Klyce	Stephen Klyce
Fig. 24.7a	Ruth Cornish	B&L
Fig. 24.7b	Ruth Cornish	B&L
Fig. 24.8	Suzanne Efron	Suzanne Efron
Fig. 24.9	Julia Mainstone	B-H
Fig. 25.1	Steve Zantos	CCLRU
Fig. 25.2	Charles McMonnies	Charles McMonnies
Fig. 25.3	Ronald Stevenson	BCLA
Fig. 25.4	Jan Bergmanson	B-H
Fig. 25.5	Nathan Efron	Optician
Fig. 25.6	Nathan Efron	Optician
Fig. 25.7	Steve Zantos	CCLRU
Fig. 26.1	Arthur Ho	CCLRU
Fig. 26.2	Nathan Efron	Optician
Fig. 26.3	Nathan Efron	Optician
Fig. 26.4	Haliza Mutalib	Haliza Mutalib
Fig. 26.5	Haliza Mutalib	Haliza Mutalib
Fig. 26.6	Nathan Efron	Nathan Efron
Fig. 26.7	Nathan Efron	Optician
Fig. 26.8a	Steve Zantos	CCLRU
Fig. 26.8b	Lewis Williams	CCLRU
Fig. 26.8c	Brien Holden	CCLRU
Fig. 26.9	Charline Gauthier	B&L
Fig. 27.1	C Maldonado-Codina	C Maldonado-Codina
Fig. 27.2a	Brien Holden	CCLRU
Fig. 27.2b	Brien Holden	CCLRU
Fig. 27.3	Nathan Efron	Nathan Efron
Fig. 27.4	Nathan Efron	Nathan Efron
Fig. 27.5	Nathan Efron	Optician
Fig. 27.6	Inma Perez-Gomez	Inma Perez-Gomez
Fig. 28.1	Rolf Haberer	B&L
Fig. 28.2	Brien Holden	IOVS
Fig. 28.3	Nathan Efron	Nathan Efron
Fig. 28.4a	Brien Holden	CCLRU
Fig. 28.4b	Brien Holden	CCLRU
Fig. 28.5	Nathan Efron	Optician
Fig. 28.6	Nathan Efron	Optician
Fig. 28.7	Nathan Efron	Optician
Fig. 28.8	Nathan Efron	Optician
Fig. 28.9	Nathan Efron	Optician
Fig. 28.10	Nathan Efron	Optician
Fig. 29.1	Nathan Efron	Nathan Efron
Fig. 29.2	Nathan Efron	B-H
Fig. 29.3	Nathan Efron	Nathan Efron
Fig. 29.4	Nathan Efron	Nathan Efron
Fig. 29.5	Nathan Efron	Nathan Efron
Fig. 29.6	Nathan Efron	Nathan Efron
Fig. 30.1	Nathan Efron	Nathan Efron
Fig. 30.2	Nathan Efron	Nathan Efron
Fig. 30.3	Nathan Efron	Nathan Efron
Fig. 30.4	Nathan Efron	Nathan Efron
Fig. 30.5	Nathan Efron	Nathan Efron
Fig. 30.6	Nathan Efron	Nathan Efron

CONTACT LENS COMPLICATIONS QUICK-FIND INDEX

Eyelids

Condition/appearance	Signs	Symptoms	Pathology

Blinking abnormalities	• Complete blink (80%)
	• Incomplete blink (17%)
	• Twitch blink (2%)
	• Forced blink (1%)
	
	p. 13
		• Dry eye if incomplete blink
		
		p. 14
			• Abnormal blinking can cause:
			  - lens surface drying
			  - deposition
			  - epithelial desiccation
			  - post-lens tear stagnation
			  - hypoxia
			  - hypercapnia
			  - 3 and 9 o'clock staining
			  - poor lens fitting
			p. 14

Ptosis	• Narrowing of palpebral aperture size
	  - no lens: 10.10 mm
	  - soft lens: 10.24 mm
	  - rigid lens: 9.76 mm
	• Large gap between upper skin fold and upper lid margin
	• Only seen in rigid lens wearers
	
	p. 19
		• Complaints of poor cosmesis when excessive
		
		p. 20
			• Trauma during insertion and removal caused by:
			  - forced lid squeezing
			  - lateral lid stretching
			• Rigid lens displacement of tarsus
			• Blink-induced lens rubbing
			• Blepharospasm
			• Papillary conjunctivitis
			p. 20

Meibomian gland dysfunction	• Cloudy, creamy yellow expression • Inspissated discharge • Poorly wetting lenses • Tear meniscus frothing • No secretion if blocked • Distended or distorted meibomian glands seen in retroillumination p. 28	• Smeary vision • Greasy lenses • Dry eye • Lens intolerance p. 28	• Blocked meibomian orifice • Increased keratinization of duct walls p. 29

External hordeolum (stye)	• Discrete inflamed swelling of anterior lid margin
	• Occurs singly or as multiple small abscesses
	
	p. 33
		• Mild discomfort
		• Extremely tender to touch
		• Mechanical effect of contact lenses:
		  - soft lens presses on stye and causes discomfort and increased lens movement
		  - rigid lens fitted interpalpebrally buffets lid margin
		p. 33
			• Inflammation of:
			  - tissue lining lash follicle, and/or
			  - associated gland of Zeis or Moll
			
			p. 33

Internal hordeolum (meibomian cyst)	• Enlarged swelling deep within tarsal plate • Lid swelling and distortion of lid margin • Overlying skin red p. 31	• Moderate discomfort • Mechanical effect of contact lenses: - soft lens presses on cyst to cause discomfort and increased lens movement p. 31	• Acute inflammation of: meibomian gland p. 31

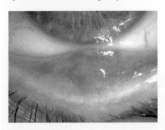

Etiology	Management	Prognosis	Differential diagnosis

• Tear break-up induces blinking
• Other unknown factors are involved
• Oral contraceptives reduce blink rate in females
	• Blink training
	• Alter lens fit
	  - less post-lens debris with rigid lenses
	  - interpalpebral rigid lens fit
	  - soft lenses solve 3 and 9 o'clock staining
		• Training can improve blinking
		• Altering lens design can improve blinking
			• Interruption to neural input
			• Interruption to muscular systems
			• Local eyelid pathology

p. 14	p. 17	p. 17	p. 18

• Lid edema
• Levator aponeurosis:
  - disinsertion
  - dehiscence
  - thinning
  - lengthening
	• Cease lens wear for 1–3 months
	• Cure papillary conjunctivitis
	• Refit with soft lenses
	• Lid surgery
	• Scleral lens ptosis crutch
	• Spectacle prop
	• Surgical tape
		• If edema: good
		• If aponeurogenic: poor
		• Surgery can yield good results
			• Soft lenses can alter palpebral aperture size
			• Embedded lens
			• Ectropion
			• Entropion
			• Lagophthalmos

p. 20	p. 21	p. 22	p. 23

• Increased turnover of ductal epidermis
• Abnormal meibomian oils
  - more keratin proteins
• Absence of lid rubbing
	• Warm compresses
	• Lid scrubs
	• Mechanical expression
	• Antibiotics
	• Artificial tears
	• Surfactant lens cleaning
	• Improved lid hygiene
		• Excellent if good control can be achieved	• External hordeolum
			  - localized swelling at lid margin
			• Internal hordeolum
			  - tender localized swelling
			• Chalazion
			  - chronic form of meibomian gland dysfunction

p. 29	p. 30	p. 31	p. 31

• typically acute staphylococcal infection
• Often occurs in patients with staphylococcal anterior blepharitis
	• Remove eyelash from affected follicle
	• Apply hot compress
	• May spontaneously discharge anteriorly
	• Cease lens wear during acute phase
		• Self limiting
		• Typical time course: 7 days
			• External hordeolum
			  - localized swelling at lid margin
			• Internal hordeolum
			  - tender localized swelling
			  - not at lid margin
			• Chalazion
			  - chronic form of meibomian gland dysfunction
			  - not at lid margin

p. 33	p. 33	p. 33	p. 31

• Typically acute staphylococcal infection
• Often occurs in patients with staphylococcal anterior blepharitis
	• Incision and curettage
	• Apply hot compress
	• Topical antibiotics following surgery
	• Cease lens wear during acute phase
		• Self-limiting
		• Typical time course: 7 days
			• External hordeolum
			  - localized swelling at lid margin
			• Internal hordeolum
			  - tender localized swelling
			  - not at lid margin
			• Chalazion
			  - chronic form of meibomian gland dysfunction
			  - not at lid margin

p. 31	p. 30	p. 31	p. 31

Eyelids *(cont.)*

Condition/appearance	Signs	Symptoms	Pathology

Staphylococcal anterior blepharitis	• Redness
	• Telangiectasis
	• Scaling of lid margins
	  - brittle, leaving bleeding ulcer
	    when removed
	• Lashes stuck together
	• Lash collarette
	• Madarosis
	• Poliosis
	• Tylosis
	p. 33
		• Burning
		• Itching
		• Mild photophobia
		• Foreign body sensation
		• Dry eye
		  - worse in morning
		• Lens intolerance
		
		p. 33
			• Staphylococcal endotoxin-
			  induced complications include:
			  - low grade conjunctivitis
			  - toxic punctate epitheliopathy
			
			p. 33

Seborrheic anterior blepharitis	• Redness
	• Telangiectasis
	• Scaling of lid margins
	  - shiny, waxy
	• Lashes stuck together
	• Madarosis
	• Poliosis
	
	p. 34
		• Burning
		• Itching
		• Mild photophobia
		• Foreign body sensation
		• Dry eye
		  - worse in morning
		• Lens intolerance
		• Symptoms less severe than
		  staphylococcal anterior
		  blepharitis
		p. 34
			• *Staphylococcal* endotoxin-
			  induced complications include:
			  - low grade conjunctivitis
			  - toxic punctate epitheliopathy
			
			p. 34

Mites	• Presence of mites
	• Erythema of lid margins
	• Lid hyperplasia
	• Madarosis
	• Conjunctival redness
	• Lash collarette
	• Follicular distension
	• Meibomian gland blockage
	• Lashes easily removed
	p. 34
		• Burning
		• Itching
		• Crusting
		• Swelling of lid margins
		• Loss of lashes
		• Lens intolerance
		
		p. 34
			• *Demodex folliculorum*
			  - resides in space between
			    follicle wall and lash
			  - eats epithelial lining of lash
			    follicle
			• *Demodex brevis*
			  - resides in gland of Zeis
			  - reproduces in oily
			    environment
			p. 35

Lice	• Presence of lice and nits
	• Erythema of lid margins
	• Conjunctival redness
	• Madarosis
	• Pre-auricular lymphadenopathy
	• Brown deposit at base of lashes
	  - blood from host
	  - feces from lice
	• Blue spots on lid margins
	  - secreted by lice
	
	p. 36
		• Burning
		• Itching
		• Crusting
		• Swelling of lid margins
		• Lens intolerance
		
		p. 36
			• Lice suck blood and serum from
			  lid margin via stylus
			• Secondary inflammation along
			  lid margins
			
			p. 37

Etiology	Management	Prognosis	Differential diagnosis
• Staphylococcal infection of eyelash follicle	• Antibiotic ointments • Promote lid hygiene • Corticosteroids • Artificial tears • May need to suspend lens wear during acute treatment phase	• Variable: expect periods of remission and exacerbation	• Need to differentiate from seborrheic anterior blepharitis (see below)
p. 33	p. 33	p. 33	p. 33
• Disorder of glands of Zeis or Moll	• Promote lid hygiene • Artificial tears	• Variable: expect periods of remission and exacerbation	• Need to differentiate from staphylococcal anterior blepharitis (see above)
p. 34	p. 34	p. 34	p. 34
• *Demodex folliculorum* • *Demodex brevis*	• Topical anesthetic and application of toxic substances • Vigorous lid scrubbing • Viscous ointment overnight • Heavy metal ointments • Pilocarpine gel • Avoid use of facial oils	• Good – if patient complies with treatment	• Lice - see below • Blepharitis - see both blepharitis entries above
p. 35	p. 37	p. 37	p. 37
• *Phthirus pubis*, also known as: - pubic louse - 'sucking louse' - 'crab louse'	• Mechanical removal • Cryotherapy (freezing) • Argon laser photoablation • 20% sodium fluorescein • Yellow mercuric oxide • Anticholinesterase agents • Vigorous lid scrubbing • Possibility of associated sexually transmitted disease • Heat application to clothing, bed clothing, sheets, towels, etc. • Soak combs, brushes, etc. • Isolate contaminated material for 2 weeks	• Good – if patient complies with treatment	• Mites - see above • Blepharitis - see both blepharitis entries above
p. 37	p. 38	p. 38	p. 38

Tear Film

Condition/appearance	Signs	Symptoms	Pathology
Dry eye	• Abnormalities in: - lipid layer viewed in specular reflection - tear volume - tear structure - tear film stability - post-lens tear film • Epithelial staining p. 43	• Primarily 'dryness' - use a dry eye questionnaire • Worse in females using oral contraceptives p. 48	• Lipid deficiency or excess • Aqueous deficiency • Rapid tear break up - caused by inter-mixing of lipid and mucus layers p. 48
Mucin balls	• Up to 200 small gray dots in direct illumination • Small transparent dots in indirect retroillumination • Display reversed illumination • Large mucin balls may collapse and take on a doughnut-like appearance with thick annular rim • Seen almost exclusively with silicone hydrogel lenses p. 55	• None • Vision can be compromised slightly in extreme cases p. 57	• Balls of collapsed mucin • Can indent epithelium to leave fluid-filled pits that display unreversed illumination • Deep mucin balls may affect underlying stromal keratocytes • Mucin ball formation may compromise corneal microbial defenses p. 57

Conjunctiva

Condition/appearance	Signs	Symptoms	Pathology
Conjunctival staining	• Normal eye: curved lines of staining in conjunctiva parallel to limbus (furrow staining) • Lens-wearing eye: - diffuse stain - coalescent stain - 'lens edge' stain p. 64	• Often none • 'Lens edge' stain may be associated with 'tight lens syndrome' p. 64	• Normal eye: fluorescein pools in natural conjunctival folds • Lens-wearing eye: - superficial epithelial cells traumatized or dislodged p. 65
Conjunctival redness	• Conjunctival redness • May be regional variation (specify) • Depends on lens type: - no lens: grade 0.78 - rigid lens: grade 0.96 - soft lens: grade 1.54 p. 69	• Often none • Itchiness • Congestion • Warm feeling • Cold feeling • Non-specific mild irritation p. 69	• Vasodilatation due to: - relaxation of smooth muscle - vessel blockage p. 70

Etiology	Management	Prognosis	Differential diagnosis

• Lens-induced changes in tear film:
 - tonicity
 - pH
 - composition
 - temperature profile
 - turnover
 - break up
	• Alter lens
	 • Alter solutions
	 • Rewetting drops
	 • Soft lens soaking
	 • Nutritional supplements
	 • Control of evaporation
	 • Reduce tear drainage
	    – punctal plugs
	 • Tear stimulants
	 • Management of associated disease
	 • Reduce or cease lens wear
		• Good if problem relates to lenses and/or solutions
		 • Poor if caused by underlying pathology
		    - e.g. keratoconjunctivitis sicca
			• Aqueous tear deficiency
			 • Lipid anomaly
			 • Lid surface anomalies
			 • Mucus deficiency
			 • Primary epitheliopathy
			 • Allergic dry eye

p. 48	p. 50	p. 52	p. 53
• Strong interfacial forces • Aqueous-deficient tears beneath silicone hydrogel lenses • Mucin-rich tears rolled up onto discrete balls • Balls enlarge and indent epithelium • Very large balls collapse to doughnut-like appearance	• Fit lenses flatter • Rewetting drops • More frequent lens removal • Refit with other lenses (not silicone hydrogels)	• Mucin balls and epithelial fluid-filled pits disappear within hours of lens removal • Mucin balls will recur	• Epithelial microcysts • Epithelial vacuoles • Epithelial bullae • Dimple veiling
p. 57	p. 59	p. 59	p. 59

Etiology	Management	Prognosis	Differential diagnosis
• 'Lens edge' stain caused by physical trauma of lens edge • Diffuse stain caused by other physical trauma: - deposits on back of lens - trauma induced by excessive movement of loose-fitting lens	• 'Lens edge' stain: - fit flatter lens • Lens trauma stain: - improve care regimen to alleviate deposit formation - improve lens fit	• Excellent: - recovery within 2–4 days	• Physiologic 'furrow staining' vs pathologic staining
p. 66	p. 67	p. 67	p. 67
• Hypoxia and hypercapnia • Mechanical irritation • Immunologic reactions • Infection • Inflammation - acute red eye • Solution toxicity • Change in tonicity • Change in pH • Neural control	• Remove cause - (see etiology) • Decongestants • If > grade 2 cease wear	• Excellent - recovery from acute redness within hours - recovery from chronic redness within 2 days	• Cease lens wear - rapid resolution implicates lens wear - slow resolution suggests other cause • 'Push test': - for conjunctival vs scleral involvement • Hemorrhage - redness between vessels
p. 71	p. 73	p. 74	p. 74

Conjunctiva (cont.)

Condition/appearance	Signs	Symptoms	Pathology

Papillary conjunctivitis
 	
	• Papillae on tarsal conjunctiva
	  - 'cobblestone' appearance
	  - giant papillae
	• Conjunctival redness
	• Conjunctival edema
	• Excess lens movement
	• Coated contact lens
	• Mucus discharge
	
	p. 77
		• Early (grades 1 and 2):
		  - lens awareness
		  - mild itching
		  - slight blur
		• Late (grades 3 and 4):
		  - lens discomfort
		  - intense itching
		  - blur
		  - reduced wearing time
		
		p. 77
			• Thickened conjunctiva
			• Distorted epithelial cells
			• Altered goblet cells
			• Inflammatory cells
			  - mast cells
			  - eosinophils
			  - basophils
			
			p. 78

Limbus

Condition/appearance	Signs	Symptoms	Pathology

Limbal redness
 	
	• Limbal redness
	• May be regional variation around limbus (specify)
	• Depends on lens type:
	  - absent with silicone hydrogel lenses
	
	p. 88
		• Often none
		• Associated pathology may cause discomfort or pain
		
		p. 88
			• Vasodilatation of terminal arcades and associated vascular forms:
			  - recurrent limbal vessels
			  - vessel spikes
			
			p. 90

Vascularized limbal keratitis
 	
	• Vascularized mass of tissue at the limbus
	• Conjunctival and limbal edema in late stages
	• Corneal infiltrates near limbus
	• Fluorescein staining of surrounding tissue
	• Appears at the 3 and/or 9 o'clock positions
	• Only seen in rigid lens wearers
	
	p. 94
		• Early (grades 1 and 2):
		  - lens awareness
		• Late (grades 3 and 4):
		  - discomfort
		  - photophobia
		
		p. 94
			• Epithelial cell hyperplasia
			• Vessel engorgement
			• Vessel encroachment
			• Tissue erosion
			• Tissue edema
			• Corneal infiltrates near limbus
			
			p. 95

Superior limbic keratoconjunctivitis
 	
	• Superior limbic redness
	• Infiltrates
	• Micropannus
	• Corneal staining
	• Conjunctival staining
	• Hazy epithelium
	• Papillary hypertrophy
	• Corneal filaments
	• Corneal warpage
	
	p. 99
		• Lens awareness
		• Burning
		• Itching
		• Photophobia
		• Slight vision loss
		  - with extensive pannus
		
		p. 99
			• Cornea
			  - epitheliopathy
			  - infiltrates
			• Conjunctiva
			  - epithelial keratinization
			  - epithelial edema
			  - inflammatory cells
			
			p. 100

Etiology	Management	Prognosis	Differential diagnosis

• Lens deposits
  - anterior lens surface
• Mechanical irritation
• Immunologic reaction
• Hypoxia under lid
• Solution toxicity:
  - thimerosal
• May be related to meibomian gland dysfunction
	• Cease lens wear until inflammation subsides
	• Reduce wearing time
	• Improve solutions
	• Ocular lubricant
	• Mast cell stabilizers
	• Non-steroidal anti-inflammatory agents
	• Change to a lens material that deposits differently
	• Increase frequency of lens replacement
	• Improve ocular hygiene
		• Papillae can remain for weeks, months or years
		• Lenses can still be worn
		• Treat according to symptoms
			• Follicle
			  - vessels on outside
			• Papilla
			  - central vascular tuft

p. 78	p. 81	p. 83	p. 83

Etiology	Management	Prognosis	Differential diagnosis

• Hypoxia and hypercapnia
• Mechanical irritation
• Immunologic reaction
• Infection
• Inflammation
  - acute red eye
• Solution toxicity
	• Remove cause
	  - (see Etiology)
	• Consider whether:
	  - acute local limbal redness
	  - chronic local limbal redness
	  - acute circumlimbal redness
	  - chronic circumlimbal redness
	• Fit silicone hydrogel lenses
		• Excellent
		  - recovery from acute redness within hours
		  - recovery from chronic redness within 2 days
			• Neovascularization
			• Vascularized limbal keratitis
			• Superior limbal keratoconjunctivitis

p. 91	p. 91	p. 92	p. 92

• Interruption to normal tear film dynamics around limbus
• Rigid lens with inappropriate edge design
• Severe sequel of 3 and 9 o'clock staining?
	• Early (grades 1 and 2):
	  - change from extended wear to daily wear
	  - reduce wearing time
	  - optimize lens edge design
	• Late (grades 3 and 4):
	  - cease lens wear for 5 days
	  - prescribe antibiotics and corticosteroids
	  - changes to soft lenses if intractable
		• Generally good
		• Recovery within days or weeks
		• 'Rebound' may occur
			• Neovascularization
			• Limbal redness
			• Phlyctenulosis
			• Peripheral corneal ulcer
			• Pterygium
			• Pseudopterygium
			• Pinguecula

p. 95	p. 95	p. 96	p. 97

• Lens deposits
  - posterior lens surface
• Mechanical irritation
• Immunologic reaction
• Hypoxia under lid
• Thimerosal
  - hypersensitivity
  - toxicity
	• Cease lens wear until inflammation subsides
	• Reduce wearing time
	• Improve solutions
	• Ocular lubricant
	• Mast cell stabilizers
	• Non-steroidal anti-inflammatory agents
	• Increase frequency of lens replacement
	• Surgery if severe
		• After ceasing lens wear:
		  - redness resolves rapidly
		  - epithelium resolves slowly
		  - can take from 3 weeks to 9 months to resolve
			• Superficial epithelial arcuate lesion
			  - conjunctiva not involved
			• Bacterial conjunctivitis
			• Infiltrative keratitis
			• Theodore's superior limbic keratoconjunctivitis

p. 101	p. 103	p. 104	p. 104

Corneal Epithelium

Condition/appearance	Signs	Symptoms	Pathology

3 and 9 o'clock corneal staining	• Punctate or diffuse staining at the 3 and 9 o'clock limbal locations
	• Triangular patters:
	  - apex away from central cornea
	  - 'base' corresponds to lens edge
	  - only seen in rigid lens wearers
	
	p. 109
		• Slight discomfort
		• Dryness
		
		p. 111
			• Epithelial disruption at limbus
			
			p. 111

Inferior epithelial arcuate lesion ('smile stain')	• Inferior arcuate stain parallel to limbus • Punctate form p. 110	• Slight discomfort p. 111	• Disruption to epithelium • Cells damaged or dislodged p. 111
Superior epithelial arcuate lesion (SEAL)	• Superior arcuate stain parallel to limbus • Full thickness lesion • Also known as 'epithelial splitting' p. 110	• Asymptomatic p. 111	• Full thickness splitting of epithelium p. 111
Epithelial plug	• Large area of full thickness epithelium missing • Usually circular pattern • Areas fills with fluorescein and fluoresces brightly p. 110	• Vision loss if plug is central • Can be asymptomatic or painful p. 111	• Epithelium completely removed with lens removal • Reduced number of hemidesmosomes compromises epithelial adhesion p. 111
Epithelial microcysts	• Minute scattered dots • Spherical or ovoid shape • 5–30 μm diameter • Reversed illumination p. 116	• Can cause slight discomfort • Can reduce vision slightly p. 116	• Intraepithelial sheets • Disorganized cell growth • Pockets of dead cells • Slowly pushed to surface p. 118

Etiology	Management	Prognosis	Differential diagnosis

• Rigid lens bridges lid away from ocular surface
• Ocular surface adjacent to lens edge not properly wetted
	• Alter lens design
	  - reduce thickness of lens edge
	  - smaller lens diameter
	• Blinking instructions
		• Following lens removal
		  - recovery, <24 hours
		• While wearing lenses
		  - slower recovery, 4–5 days
			• Vascularized limbal keratitis

p. 111	p. 113	p. 114	p. 114

• Metabolic
• Desiccation
  - insufficient post-lens tear film
  - lens adherence
  - lens dehydration
	• Alter lens fit
	  - more movement
	  - thicker lens
	• Alter lens type
	  - different material
		• Following lens removal
		  - rapid recovery, <24 hours
		• While wearing lenses
		  - slower recovery, 4–5 days
			• Lens edge stain
			• Lens insertion/removal trauma

p. 111	p. 113	p. 114	p. 114

• Mechanical chaffing of superior cornea
• Inward pressure of upper lid
• Contributing factors:
  - corneal topography
  - rigid lens modulus
  - mid-peripheral lens design
  - lens surface
	• Alter lens design
	  - less mid-peripheral bearing
	• Alter lens type
	  - lower modulus material
	  - better surface characteristics
		• Following lens removal
		  - recovery in 3 days
			• Lens edge stain
			• Lens insertion/removal trauma

p. 111	p. 113	p. 114	p. 114
• Severe metabolic compromise of epithelium • Chronic hypoxia	• Cease lens wear until epithelium has completely reformed • Refit with a high oxygen permeable lens material	• Following lens removal - recovery may take up to 1 week	• Lens insertion/removal trauma
p. 111	p. 113	p. 114	p. 114

• Possible factors
  - prolonged hypoxia
  - mechanical irritation
  - reduced oxygen uptake
  - reduced mitosis
  - typically hydrogel extended wear
	• If ≤ grade 2 microcysts
	  - no action
	  - monitor carefully
	• If ≥ grade 3 microcysts
	  - cease wear (1 month)
	  - reduce wearing time
	  - change to daily wear
	  - increase lens Dk/t
		• After ceasing wear
		  - increase during first 7 days
		  - decrease thereafter
		• Full recovery in 2 months
		• Microcysts will not recur with silicone hydrogel lenses
			• Tear film debris
			  - move on blink
			• Mucin balls
			• Vacuoles
			  - unreversed optics
			• Bullae
			• Bedewing
			  - endothelial
			• Dimple veiling
			  - very large

p. 119	p. 119	p. 120	p. 120

Corneal Epithelium (*cont.*)

Condition/appearance	Signs	Symptoms	Pathology
Epithelial edema	• Slight haziness of epithelium seen in optic section • Can occur during adaptation to rigid lens wear p. 122	• Asymptomatic • Appearance of haloes p. 122	• Disruption to epithelial cells • Extracellular edema around basal epithelial cells p. 123
Epithelial vacuoles	• Minute scattered dots • Spherical shape • 5–30 μm diameter • Unreversed illumination • Observed in corneal mid-periphery p. 122	• Asymptomatic • Do not affect vision p. 122	• Filled with gas or fluid p. 123
Epithelial bullae	• Minute scattered dots • Irregular shape (typically oval) • Indistinct edges • Flattened, pebble-like formations • 5–30 μm diameter • May coalesce into larger structures • Unreversed illumination • Observed in center of cornea p. 122	• Asymptomatic • Do not affect vision p. 122	• Filled with fluid p. 123
Epithelial wrinkling	• Linear wave patterns of epithelial pooling • Patterns intersect at about 70° • Discrete spots of staining appear at intersection of patterns • Similar pattern observed in keratograms p. 126	• Extremely painful • Extreme vision loss • Parallel time course of discomfort and vision loss p. 127	• Epithelium forms concertina-like folds • Anterior stroma may also be slightly folded p. 127

Etiology	Management	Prognosis	Differential diagnosis
• Hypotonic tears (as occurs during tearing) • Adaptation to rigid lens wear • Fluid enters epithelium • Fluid forms between basal epithelial cells	• Modify rigid lens adaptation wear regimen	• Rapid recovery upon ceasing of hypotonic stress (i.e., when tearing stops)	• Generalized epitheliopathy
p. 123	p. 124	p. 124	p. 124

• Related to excess edema?	• Generally innocuous
	• No management required
	• Note the number of vacuoles on record card
		• Rapid recovery upon ceasing lens wear	• Tear film debris
			  - move on blink
			• Microcysts
			  - reversed optics
			• Bullae
			• Bedewing
			  - endothelial
			• Dimple veiling
			  - very large

p. 123	p. 124	p. 124	p. 124

• Related to excess edema?	• Generally innocuous
	• No management required
	• Note the number of vacuoles on record card
		• Rapid recovery upon ceasing lens wear	• Tear film debris
			  - move on blink
			• Microcysts
			  - reversed optics
			• Vacuoles
			  - unreversed optics
			• Bedewing
			  - endothelial
			• Dimple veiling
			  - very large

p. 123	p. 124	p. 124	p. 124

• Mechanical etiology
• Critical lens factors
  - highly elastic hydrogel material
  - custom design
  - extremely thin
  - 50–55% water content
  - steep fitting
	• Remove lens immediately
	• Refit with lenses avoiding design features described in 'Etiology'
		• Good
		  - expect complete recovery
		  - can take up to a week to fully recover
		• Rate of recovery related to period of wear
			• Fischer–Schweitzer mosaic
			  - physiologic
			  - caused by excessive eye rubbing
			• Anterior crocodile shagreen of Vogt

p. 128	p. 129	p. 129	p. 129

Corneal Stroma

Condition/appearance	Signs	Symptoms	Pathology

Stromal edema	• <2% edema: undetectable
	  - 'safe'
	• >5% edema: vertical striae
	  - caution
	• >8% edema: posterior folds
	  - danger
	• >15% edema: loss of corneal transparency
	  - pathologic
	
	p. 134
		• <10% none
		• >10% discomfort
		
		p. 134
			• Edema
			  - increased fluid
			• Striae
			  - separated collagen fibrils
			• Folds
			  - physical buckling
			
			p. 135

Stromal thinning	• Only detected using pachometry after edema has resolved • True edema = apparent edema + stromal thinning • Stroma thins at about 2.1 μm per year p. 141	• None • Reduced vision if associated with corneal warpage p. 142	• Reduced stromal mass • Reduced keratocyte density • Stromal 'microdots' may represent keratocyte apoptosis p. 142

Deep stromal opacities (pseudo-dystrophy)	• Opacities in the deep stromal layers
	• Many appearances:
	  - whitish dots/opacities
	  - resembling cloudy dystrophy
	  - lattice-like pattern
	  - mottled cyan opacification
	• Possible associated endothelial changes
	
	p. 148
		• May be asymptomatic
		• Ocular discomfort and photophobia
		• May be some vision loss
		
		p. 149
			• Similar to pre-Descemet's dystrophy
			• Stromal 'microdots' may represent deep stromal opacities
			• Possible associated endothelial pathology
			
			p. 149

Superficial corneal neovascularization	• Superficial vessels
	  - from conjunctiva
	• 'Normal' responses:
	  - no lens: 0.2 mm
	  - Si–H lens: 0.2 mm
	  - daily wear rigid: 0.4 mm
	  - daily wear soft: 0.6 mm
	  - extended wear soft: 1.4 mm
	
	p. 154
		• No discomfort
		• Visual acuity loss if extreme
		
		p. 154
			• Sprouting or budding
			• Solid cord of vascular endothelial cells at growing tip
			• Thin vessel wall
			• Pericytes
			• Cell migration
			• Surrounding inflammatory cells
			• Disruption of stromal lamellae
			• Lipid material may surround vessels
			p. 155

Deep stromal neovascularization	• Fine, wildly tortuous branches • Vessels end in buds • Numerous small vessel anastomoses • Vessels 'stop' at limbus (tracing backward from cornea) • Often associated pathology p. 154	• No discomfort • VISUAL ACUITY loss if extreme p. 154	• Sprouting or budding • Solid cord of vascular endothelial cells at growing tip • Thin vessel wall • Pericytes • Cell migration • Surrounding inflammatory cells • Disruption of stromal lamellae p. 155

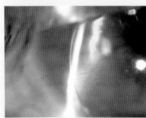

Etiology	Management	Prognosis	Differential diagnosis
• Primarily hypoxia (50%) - lactate theory • Other factors (50%): - tear hypotonicity - hypercapnia - increased temperature - increased humidity - mechanical	• Alleviate hypoxia - increase material Dk - reduce lens thickness - increase lens movement - increase edge lift • Alleviate hypercapnia - (as per hypoxia)	• Acute edema - resolves in 2–3 hours • Chronic edema - resolves in 7 days • Chronic edema thins stroma (see below)	• Striae - nerve fibers - ghost vessels • Folds - seen in diabetes • Haze - scarring - epithelial edema
p. 136	p. 137	p. 139	p. 139
• Chronic edema • Mechanical effect of lenses • Keratocyte dysfunction caused by: - hypoxia - tissue acidosis • Dissolution of mucopolysaccharide ground substance	• Alleviate chronic hypoxia - increase material Dk - reduce lens thickness - increase lens movement - increase edge lift • Alleviate hypercapnia - (as per hypoxia) • Alleviate mechanical effect of lenses	• Unknown time course - thought to be permanent	• Keratoconus - central corneal thinning • Pellucid marginal degeneration • Terrien's marginal corneal degeneration
p. 145	p. 145	p. 146	p. 146
• Numerous theories: - long-term contact lens wear - exposure to heavy metals - allergic reaction to thimerosal - exposure to chlorhexidine - chronic hypoxia - chronic hypercapnia - endothelial dysfunction - suction effects by the lens	• Alleviate chronic hypoxia - increase material Dk - reduce lens thickness - increase lens movement - increase edge lift • Avoid noxious preservatives	• Slow regression - many months/years	• Corneal dystrophies • Key differentiation: - deep stromal opacities occur deep in the stroma - deep stromal opacities are reversible
p. 150	p. 150	p. 150	p. 150
• Stromal softening - hypoxia-induced edema • Triggering agent - epithelial damage - solution toxicity - infection	• If severe: - cease lens wear permanently • If mild: - improve care system - increase Dk/t - reduce wearing time - monitor carefully	• On ceasing lens wear - vessels empty rapidly - ghost vessels remain - years to resolve • On reintroducing lens - ghost vessels rapidly refill	• Nerve fibres - any orientation - 'solid' • Striae - always vertical - white, whispy • Ghost vessels - start at limbus - relatively thick
p. 155	p. 158	p. 159	p. 160
• Often associated pathology: - graft - keratoconus - aphakia • Stromal softening - hypoxia-induced edema • Triggering agent: - epithelial damage - solution toxicity - infection	• Manage associated pathology • If severe - cease lens wear permanently • If mild - improve care system - increase Dk/t - reduce wearing time - monitor carefully	• On ceasing lens wear: - vessels empty rapidly - ghost vessels remain - years to resolve • On reintroducing lens: - ghost vessels rapidly refill	• Ghost vessels - start at limbus - relatively thick
p. 155	p. 158	p. 159	p. 160

Corneal Stroma (*cont.*)

Condition/appearance	Signs	Symptoms	Pathology

Corneal vascular pannus
 	
	• Plexus of parallel vessels from limbus on to peripheral cornea
	• Invading end:
	  - is even
	  - contains fibrotic tissue
	  - stains with rose bengal
	• Two types:
	  - active pannus: inflammatory
	  - fibrovascular pannus: degenerative
	
	p. 154
		• No discomfort
		• Visual acuity loss if extreme
		
		p. 154
			• Vessels penetrate between epithelium and Bowman's layer
			• Ingrowth of vessels
			• Ingrowth of collagen
			• Fatty plaques
			• Fibrotic tissue
			
			p. 155

Contact lens-induced peripheral ulcer (CLPU)
 	
	• Small, round peripheral ulcer
	  - 0.5–1.0 mm diameter
	• Slight surrounding infiltration
	• May be slight anterior chamber involvement
	• Ulcer and surround stains with fluorescein
	• Limbal and bulbar redness
	• Seen in extended wear patients
	
	p. 163
		• Eye redness
		• Excess tearing
		• Moderate-to-severe pain
		• Foreign body sensation
		• May be asymptomatic
		• Patient may report seeing white spot on eye
		• Noticed immediately upon waking
		
		p. 163
			• Focal excavation of epithelium
			• Infiltrates
			  - polymorphonuclear leukocytes
			• Necrosis of anterior stroma
			• Bowman's layer is intact
			
			p. 166

Contact lens-induced acute red eye (CLARE)
 	
	• Multiple small focal infiltrates
	  - up to 60
	• Diffuse infiltration in peripheral cornea
	• No staining
	• Rarely anterior chamber involvement
	• Conjunctival redness > grade 2
	• Seen in extended wear patients
	
	p. 164
		• Eye redness
		• Excess tearing
		• Irritation to moderate pain
		• Photophobia
		• Noticed immediately upon waking
		
		p. 164
			• Infiltrates
			  - subepithelium
			  - anterior stroma
			
			p. 166

Etiology	Management	Prognosis	Differential diagnosis

• Stromal softening
  - hypoxia-induced edema
• Triggering agent:
  - epithelial damage
  - solution toxicity
  - infection
	• If severe:
	  - cease lens wear permanently
	  - surgical removal
	• If mild:
	  - improve care system
	  - increase *Dk/t*
	  - reduce wearing time
	  - monitor carefully
		• On ceasing lens wear
		  - vessels empty rapidly
		  - ghost vessels remain
		  - years to resolve
		• On reintroducing lens:
		  - ghost vessels rapidly refill
			• Ghost vessels:
			  - start at limbus
			  - relatively thick

p. 155	p. 158	p. 159	p. 160

• Toxins from gram-positive bacteria
• Eye closure
• Hypoxia
	• Remove lens
	• Prescribe:
	  - fluoroquinolones
	  - antibiotic ointment
	• Unit dose saline
	• Cold compresses
	• Analgesics
	• Steroid eye drops
	• Fit disposable lenses
	• Alleviate trauma
	• Improve care system
	• Improve hygiene
	• Loosen lens fit
	• Change to daily wear
	• Fit rigid lenses
	• Fit low water lenses
	• Improve *Dk/t*
		• Excellent:
		  - 21% of cases resolve within 7 days
		  - all cases resolve within 2–3 weeks
			• Microbial keratitis
			• Epidemic keratoconjunctivitis
			  - typically bilateral
			• Stromal opacities
			• Stromal scars

p. 167	p. 169	p. 171	p. 172

• Toxins from gram-negative bacteria
• Eye closure
• Hypoxia
	• Remove lens
	• Prescribe:
	  - fluoroquinolones
	  - antibiotic ointment
	• Unit dose saline
	• Cold compresses
	• Fit disposable lenses
	• Alleviate trauma
	• Improve care system
	• Improve hygiene
	• Loosen lens fit
	• Change to daily wear
	• Fit rigid lenses
	• Fit low water lenses
	• Improve *Dk/t*
		• Excellent
		  - redness resolves in 3 days
		  - infiltrates resolve in 7–14 days
		  - vision (if affected) recovers in 2 days
		  - 70% of cases resolve within 2 weeks
		  - all cases resolve within 6 weeks
			• Keratoconjunctivitis
			  - typically bilateral
			• Conjunctivitis

p. 167	p. 169	p. 171	p. 172

Corneal Stroma (cont.)

Condition/appearance	Signs	Symptoms	Pathology

Infiltrative keratitis (IK)
 	
	• Small, multiple infiltrates
	  - mid-peripheral cornea
	  - irregular shape
	• Slight surrounding infiltration
	  - sectorial or circumferential
	• No anterior chamber involvement
	• Slight punctate staining
	• General bulbar redness
	• Seen in daily wear and extended wear patients
	
	p. 164
		• Eye redness
		• Excess tearing
		• Mild-to-moderate irritation
		• May be purulent discharge
		• Noticed any time of day
		
		p. 164
			• Anterior stromal infiltration
			  - subepithelium
			
			p. 166

Asymptomatic infiltrative keratitis (AIK)
 	
	• Small, focal, sometimes multiple infiltrates in peripheral cornea
	  - up to 0.4 mm diameter
	• Slight surrounding diffuse infiltration
	• Punctate staining with fluorescein
	• Seen in extended wear patients
	• Mild-to-moderate limbal and bulbar redness
	
	p. 164
		• Asymptomatic
		• Eye redness
		
		p. 164
			• Anterior stromal infiltration
			  - subepithelium
			
			p. 166

Asymptomatic infiltrates (AI)
 	
	• Small number (typically two), focal infiltrates in peripheral cornea
	  - <0.2 mm diameter
	• Slight surrounding diffuse infiltration
	• No staining with fluorescein
	• Seen in daily wear and extended wear patients
	
	p. 164
		• Asymptomatic
		
		p. 164
			• Anterior stromal infiltration
			  - subepithelium
			
			p. 166

***Pseudomonas* keratitis**
 	
	• Typically uniocular
	• Conjunctival redness
	• Lid swelling
	• Lacrimation
	• Photophobia
	• Mucopurulent discharge
	• Loss of vision
	• Culture positive
	• Deep ulcer can form
	  - haziness in stroma
	  - overlying epithelial defect
	• Hypopyon
	• Anterior chamber flare
	
	p. 176
		• Initial foreign body sensation
		• Worsening pain
		• Eye redness
		
		p. 176
			• Infiltrates could comprise:
			  - the offending micro-organisms
			  - inflammatory cells (polymorphonuclear leukocytes)
			  - bacterial endotoxins
			  - serum
			  - proteins
			• Bowman's layer destroyed
			
			p. 178

Etiology	Management	Prognosis	Differential diagnosis

• Toxins from bacteria	• Remove lens
	• Prescribe:
	  - fluoroquinolones
	  - antibiotic ointment
	• Unit dose saline
	• Cold compresses
	• Fit disposable lenses
	• Alleviate trauma
	• Improve care system
	• Improve hygiene
	• Loosen lens fit
	• Change to daily wear
	• Fit rigid lenses
	• Fit low water lenses
	• Improve Dk/t
		• Excellent
		  - resolves within 14 days
			• Microbial keratitis
			• Epidemic keratoconjunctivitis
			  - typically bilateral

p. 168	p. 169	p. 171	p. 172

• Toxins from gram-negative bacteria
• May be a normal protective cellular response of the cornea
	• Remove lens
	• Unit dose saline
	• Fit disposable lenses
	• Alleviate trauma
	• Improve care system
	• Improve hygiene
	• Loosen lens fit
	• Change to daily wear
	• Fit rigid lenses
	• Fit low water lenses
	• Improve Dk/t
		• Excellent
		  - resolves within 2 weeks
			• Epidemic keratoconjunctivitis
			  - typically bilateral

p. 168	p. 169	p. 171	p. 172

• Unknown
• May be a normal occurrence coincidental with lens wear
	• Remove lens
	• Fit disposable lenses
	• Alleviate trauma
	• Improve care system
	• Improve hygiene
	• Loosen lens fit
	• Change to daily wear
	• Fit rigid lenses
	• Fit low water lenses
	• Improve Dk/t
		• Excellent
		  - resolves within 2 weeks
			• Epidemic keratoconjunctivitis
			  - typically bilateral

p. 168	p. 169	p. 171	p. 172

• Bacterial infection
  - *Pseudomonas aeruginosa*
• Risk factors:
  - contaminated lenses
  - solution inefficacy
  - patient non-compliance
  - poor hygiene
  - hypoxia
  - swimming
  - continuous overnight use
  - overnight orthokeratology
  - mechanical trauma
  - smoking
  - diabetes
  - warm climates
  - gender
  - socio-economic class
	• Advise of risks
	• Antibiotics
	• Mydriatics
	• Non-steroidal anti-inflammatory agents
	• Analgesics
	• Tissue adhesives
	• Debridement
	• Alleviate trauma
	• Improve care system
	• Improve Dk/t
	• Improve hygiene
	• Avoid tap water
	• Revert to daily wear
	• Fit rigid lenses
		• Depends on speed of treatment
		  - excellent if rapid action is taken
		• Condition usually worsens during initial 24 hours, then improves
			• CLPU
			• *Acanthamoeba* keratitis

p. 179	p. 182	p. 183	p. 183

Corneal Stroma (cont.)

Condition/appearance	Signs	Symptoms	Pathology

Acanthamoeba keratitis 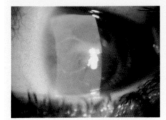	• Typically uniocular
	• Conjunctival redness
	• Lid swelling
	• Lacrimation
	• Photophobia
	• Loss of vision
	• Pseudodendrites
	• Radial keratoneuritis
	• Deep ulcer can form:
	  - haziness in stroma
	  - overlying epithelial defect
	• Hypopyon
	• Anterior chamber flare
	
	p. 176
		• Initial foreign body sensation
		• Excruciating pain
		• Eye redness
		
		p. 176
			• *Acanthamoeba* can be observed destroying stromal tissue
			  - confocal microscopy
			• Bowman's layer destroyed
			
			p. 179

Corneal warpage 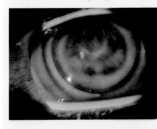	• Can manifest as change in corneal:
	  - curvature
	  - symmetry
	  - regularity
	• Corneal indentation
	  - may be associated with corneal binding
	
	p. 188
		• Spectacle blur
		• Haze
		  - if associated with excess edema
		
		p. 188
			• Surface Asymmetry Index
			  - more likely with rigid lenses
			  - decentered lens flattens cornea
			• Surface Regularity Index
			  - distortion may be symmetrical
			  - more likely with rigid lenses
			• Corneal indentation
			  - pressure from lens edge
			
			p. 190

Corneal Endothelium

Condition/appearance	Signs	Symptoms	Pathology

Endothelial bedewing 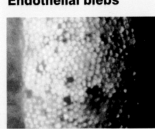	• Cluster of particles
	• 20–50 in number
	• Inferior cornea, near lower pupil margin
	• Display reversed illumination
	
	p. 200
		• Intolerance to lenses
		• Stinging sensation
		• Reduced vision
		
		p. 200
			• Inflammatory cells
			  - on endothelial surface
			  - may become entrapped within endothelium
			
			p. 201

Endothelial blebs	• Black non-reflecting areas • Apparent separation of cells p. 205	• None p. 205	• Edema of cell nucleus • Intracellular vacuoles • Extracellular vacuoles • Posterior surface bulging p. 206

Etiology	Management	Prognosis	Differential diagnosis

• Protozoan infection
  - *Acanthamoeba*
• Exists as:
  - trophozoite
  - cyst
• Risk factors:
  - contaminated lenses
  - solution inefficacy
  - patient non-compliance
  - poor hygiene
  - hypoxia
  - swimming
  - continuous overnight use
  - mechanical trauma
  - smoking
  - diabetes
  - warm climates
  - gender
  - socio-economic class
	• Advise of risks
	• Propamidine isethionate 0.1% (Brolene)
	• Polyhexamethylene biguanide 0.02%
	• Neomycin
	• Mydriatics
	• Topical steroids
	• Analgesics
	• Tissue adhesives
	• Debridement
	• Alleviate trauma
	• Improve care system
	• Improve *Dk/t*
	• Improve hygiene
	• Avoid tap water
	• Revert to daily wear
	• Fit rigid lenses
		• Slow time course of recovery
		  - may progress for many months despite aggressive therapy
		• Residual superficial nebula
		• Recurrence is common
		  - especially if treatment is stopped prematurely
			• *Pseudomonas* keratitis

p. 179	p. 182	p. 183	p. 183

•Edema
  - increased fluid
• Physical molding
  - pressure from rigid lenses
  - supplementary pressure from eyelids
• Associated pathology
  - e.g., keratoconus
	• Alleviate rigid lens bearing
	• Alleviate hypoxia
	• Corneal indentation
	  - patient-dependent
	  - likely to recur again in same patient
	• Keratoplasty for keratoconus
		• Rigid lens warpage
		  - full recovery in 5–8 months
		• Rigid lens binding
		  - full recovery in 24 hours
		• Soft lens warpage
		  - resolves in 7 days
			• Keratoconus
			  - other signs present such as stromal thinning, Vogt's striae and Fleischer's ring

p. 190	p. 192	p. 193	p. 194

Etiology	Management	Prognosis	Differential diagnosis

• Hypoxia
• Inflammatory mediators
  - prostaglandins?
• Inflammation of anterior uvea?
	• Reduce wearing time
	• Check for concurrent pathology
	• Check for raised intraocular pressure
		• Symptoms disappear in 3–5 days
		• Bedewing disappears in 3–5 months
		• Prolonged intolerance to lens wear
			• Microcysts
			  - epithelial
			• Guttae
			  - large dark spots
			• Bedewing
			  - on endothelium

p. 202	p. 202	p. 203	p. 203

• Acidic pH shift at endothelium caused by:
  - hypercapnia: carbonic acid
  - hypoxia: lactic acid
• Acute response
	• Not necessary	• After inserting lens:
		  - peak response in 10 minutes
		  - low level blebs continue
		• After removing lens
		  - disappear in 2 minutes
			• Guttae
			  - permanent
			• Bedewing
			  - lasts months
			• Blebs
			  - last minutes

p. 207	p. 208	p. 209	p. 209

Corneal Endothelium

Condition/appearance	Signs	Symptoms	Pathology

Endothelial cell loss	• Reduction in endothelial cell density (ECD) in central cornea
	• Apparent compensatory increase in cell size
	• ECD decreases with normal aging
	
	p. 212
		• None
		• Endothelial dysfunction leading to edema and discomfort if severe
		
		p. 212
			• Spreading out of cells toward periphery
			• Reduced ECD is therefore an artifact
			  - lower central ECD is compensated for by higher peripheral ECD
			  - no change in overall corneal ECD
			
			p. 212

Endothelial polymegethism	• Large variation in endothelial cell size
	• Small:large cell ratio:
	  - normal: 1:5
	  - polymegethism: 1:20
	
	p. 216
		• Corneal exhaustion syndrome:
		  - reduced wearing time
		  - discomfort
		
		p. 216
			• Altered lateral cell walls
			• Straightening of interdigitations
			• Cell volume unchanged
			• Cell organelles normal
			• Poor edema recovery
			
			p. 218

Etiology	Management	Prognosis	Differential diagnosis

• Possibly acidic pH shift at endothelium caused by:
  - hypercapnia: carbonic acid
  - hypoxia: lactic acid
• Chronic response
	• General strategy
	  - alleviate acidosis
	  - better materials
		• Possible long-term recovery (many years) after ceasing lens wear	• Effects of
			  - normal aging
			  - intraocular surgery
			  - eye disease
			  - systemic disease

p. 213	p. 214	p. 214	p. 214

• Acidic pH shift at endothelium caused by:
  - hypercapnia: carbonic acid
  - hypoxia: lactic acid
• Chronic response
	• General strategy
	  - alleviate acidosis
	  - better materials
	• Corneal exhaustion syndrome
	  - reduce wear time
	  - fit higher Dk/t lens
		• Possible long-term recovery (many years) after ceasing lens wear	• Guttae
			• Endothelial dystrophy

p. 219	p. 220	p. 221	p. 221

PART I EYE EXAMINATION

CHAPTER 1 **Slit-lamp biomicroscopy**

The instrument
Illumination and observation techniques
Slit-lamp examination procedure
Conclusion

SLIT-LAMP BIOMICROSCOPY

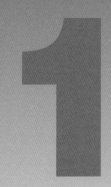

The slit-lamp biomicroscope (*Figure 1.1*) is a combined illumination and observation system that allows the eye to be examined from close distance at different magnifications. With the appropriate application of supplementary lenses and/or viewing techniques the instrument may be used to assess the condition of the vitreous, lens and retina from posterior pole to the ora serrata. Various ancillary instruments permit examination of the tear film, anterior chamber angle and retina, and measurement of the intraocular pressure, corneal sensitivity and corneal thickness. Since this book is concerned with the assessment of ocular complications of contact lens wear, the discussion that follows relates primarily to the use of the slit-lamp biomicroscope in examining the anterior ocular structures.

It has long been recognized that it is not possible to prescribe and fit contact lenses sensibly, or to provide ongoing care for contact lens patients, without constant access to a slit-lamp biomicroscope.[1] This instrument is undoubtedly the cornerstone of contact lens practice. It is used virtually every time a contact lens patient is seen, from the initial examination, through fitting to aftercare visits. Certainly, the vast majority of complications of contact lens wear cannot be detected or assessed without the aid of a slit-lamp biomicroscope. It is therefore imperative that contact lens practitioners have access to a slit-lamp biomicroscope and are fully versed in its mode of operation.

Almost all the discussions that relate to the assessment of contact lens complications throughout this book assume a thorough familiarity with the technique of slit-lamp biomicroscopy, and most of the clinical pictures have been taken through the microscope of this instrument. This chapter therefore outlines the design and construction of the slit-lamp biomicroscope, reviews key techniques of ocular illumination and examination (inasmuch as they relate to contact lens practice) and suggests a recommended examination procedure.

The Instrument

The general construct of a slit-lamp biomicroscope is indicated by its name; that is, the illumination system (the slit lamp) and viewing system (the biomicroscope). These two components are linked mechanically (*Figure 1.2*), so as to create a common focal point and centre of rotation; however, the mechanical linkage can be unlocked to allow the focal illumination to be directed away from the focal point of the viewing system, an essential requirement for some observation techniques, such as 'sclerotic scatter' (see below). The mechanically linked illumination and observation systems are always moved simultaneously – up and down with a height control, and focusing (in and out) and lateral (side to side) movements with a joystick. This linked control system facilitates rapid and accurate positioning of the slit beam on the area of interest on the eye and ensures that the microscope and illumination systems are simultaneously in focus.

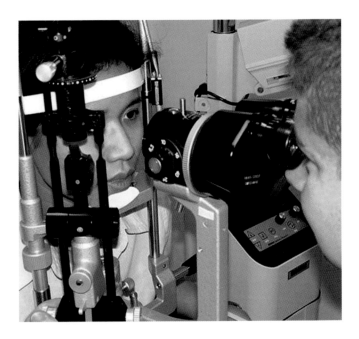

Figure 1.1
Slit-lamp
biomicroscope

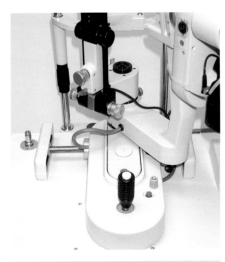

Figure 1.2
Mechanical system of a slit-lamp
biomicroscope

The patient is seated opposite the observer and the head of the patient is positioned in a conventional head mount that comprises a chin and brow rest. The linked illumination–observation system can be moved about independently of the head position, and a fixation target is provided to assist eye positioning and help the patient keep his or her eyes still. The entire head mount and linked illumination–observation system are contained on an instrument table, which can be adjusted in height (as can the practitioner and patient seats) to suit the examiner and patient.

The slit lamp

The illumination system is called the slit lamp – so-called because of its capacity to project a slit of light onto the ocular surface. The light source and optical elements of the slit lamp are classically contained in a vertically oriented housing (*Figure 1.3*). A bright light source (which generates approximately 600,000 lux) is a fundamental requirement for a slit lamp if subtle conditions are to be seen clearly. While halogen or xenon lamps are more expensive than tungsten lamps, they are the preferred illumination source as they provide a brighter light, last longer, render color better and generate less heat. The light is focused vertically into a slit configuration. It then reflects off a mirror mounted at 45° and is projected onto the eye.

Illumination brightness is controlled by a rheostat or multiposition switch, such that brightness can be adjusted to obtain the correct balance between patient comfort and optimal visibility of the area of interest. Generally, the broader the slit, the brighter the light and so the greater the patient discomfort, which means the illumination must be set lower.

The optical and aperture masking components within the illumination system are designed so that the emergent slit of light has sharp edges and an even spread of illumination. The slit width and height are continuously variable so that a section of light of any shape can be projected. The ability to vary the slit width has other practical applications, such as to form a reference for estimating the size of features of interest. Also, the slit can be rotated so that, for example, a horizontal rather than a vertical slit can be projected on to the eye. This facility can also be useful to measure the degree of rotation of soft toric lenses.

A number of filters, which serve to enhance the visibility of certain conditions, can be incorporated into the illumination system:[2]

- Green ('red-free') filter – enhances contrast when looking for corneal and iris neovascularization, since red vessels appear black if viewed through such a filter. A green filter may be used to increase the visibility of rose bengal staining on both the cornea and conjunctiva.
- Neutral density (ND) filter – reduces beam brightness and increases comfort for the patient.
- Polarizing filter – reduces unwanted specular reflections and can be useful to help enhance the visibility of subtle defects.
- Diffusing filter – diffuses the illumination source over a wide area and is used to provide broad, unfocused illumination for low magnification viewing of the general ocular surface.
- Cobalt blue filter – provides a suitable means of exciting sodium fluorescein to examine the ocular surface integrity. Illumination of fluorescein with cobalt blue light of 460–490 nm

produces a greenish light of maximum emission 520 nm. Any abraded area absorbs fluorescein and displays a fluorescent green area against a general blue background. The filter is occasionally used on its own to aid in the diagnosis of keratoconus. A frequent finding in this corneal ectasia is Fleischer's ring, which is formed by an annular iron deposition within the stroma at the base of the cone. The iron pigment is often difficult to see in white light, but usually appears in greater contrast when viewed through the cobalt blue filter.

- Yellow (Kodak Wratten No. 12) filter – this is not a filter contained within the illumination system, but is used as a supplementary barrier filter placed in front of the viewing system.[3] It significantly enhances the contrast of any fluorescent staining observed with the cobalt blue filter, as it allows transmission of the green, fluorescent light, but blocks the blue light reflected from the corneal surface. Custom-made barrier filters for certain slit lamps are available from some manufacturers. Inexpensive handheld versions may be constructed by using a cardboard mask and Lee filters No 101 Yellow.

The biomicroscope

A biomicroscope of high optical quality is essential if the observer is to achieve a comfortable, clear, focused binocular image of the eye (*Figure 1.4*). The optical system contains an objec-

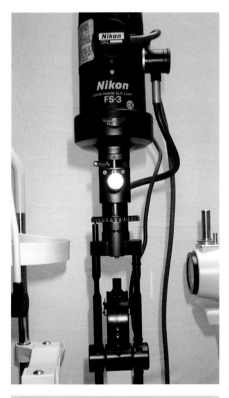

Figure 1.3

Illumination system of a slit-lamp biomicroscope

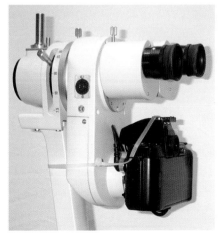

Figure 1.4

Observation system of a slit-lamp biomicroscope

tive, typically with ×3 to ×3.5 magnification, and an eyepiece with variable or interchangeable power. The normal range of total magnification is from ×6 to ×40. In some systems, magnification is continuously variable throughout this range. These systems have two key advantages:

- There is an uninterrupted view of the eye while the level of magnification is changed;
- The observer is not constrained to using discrete levels of magnification and can, in effect, choose any level of magnification within the available range.

However, such systems usually require additional optical elements to achieve the 'zoom' function, which may slightly compromise the optical quality of the image.

For the purposes of discussion throughout this book, the level of magnification used can be classified broadly as follows:

- Low: <×10 magnification;
- Medium: ×10 to ×25 magnification;
- High: >×25 magnification.

In most systems, magnification is changed in steps, with the typical progression being ×6, ×10, ×16, ×25 and ×40. These systems generally afford high optical quality, but there is the disadvantage of momentarily losing sight of the eye as the magnification is changed. Some systems require the eyepieces to be interchanged to obtain different levels of magnification. Needless to say, these systems are cumbersome and mitigate against a smooth examination procedure. Manufacturers of slit-lamp biomicroscopes could produce instruments with higher levels of magnification than ×40, but natural micronystagmoid eye movements make observation at such high magnification levels impractical.

The working distance of the biomicroscope (the distance from the eye to the front surface of the most anterior lens element of the biomicroscope) is typically set at about 11 cm, which is long enough to allow room to manipulate the eye, but not long enough to require an uncomfortable arm position during such manipulations.

Illumination and Observation Techniques

As it is a transparent structure, the cornea lends itself to examination using a wide variety of illumination and observational techniques. These are achieved by varying the illumination and observation conditions to optimize the visibility of the feature of interest in or on the cornea. There are essentially 13 illumination and/or observation techniques, which are discussed in turn with specific emphasis on those used more routinely in contact lens practice.

While the techniques discussed below may seem daunting and somewhat confusing to the novice, it is important to realize that many combinations of these illumination and observation conditions are visible within a single field of view, and are altered merely by the observer changing his or her direction of gaze. This is illustrated in *Figure 1.5*, in which five illumination and/or observation conditions are apparent simultaneously in a single field of view in a case of corneal neovascularization induced by contact lens wear.

Diffuse illumination

A ground-glass filter is placed in the focused light beam of the slit lamp. This defocuses and diffuses the light to give a broad, even illumination over the entire field of view. The angle of the illumination arm is not critical when the diffuser is in place, and can be anywhere from 10° to 70° in relation to the observation arm; it is simply convenient to place it at an angle of at least 45° so as to avoid partially obstructing the field of view. The slit is generally opened wide and high illumination usually does not cause too much patient discomfort in view of the diffuse nature of the light (*Figure 1.6*).

Diffuse illumination is generally used to provide low magnification views of the opaque tissues of the anterior segment, including the bulbar conjunctiva, sclera, iris, eyelid margins and the tarsal conjunctiva of the everted lids. Unusual signs in these tissues could include dilated blood vessels in the bulbar conjunctiva, pigmented areas in the conjunctiva or eyelids, roughness or opacity of the conjunctiva and abnormal eyelash position or orientation. Such signs could indicate conditions such as trichiasis, bulbar redness, pterygium or papillary conjunctivitis. In assessing the eyelid margins, consider the apposition of the lids and puncta against the globe. Also, look for clear glands near the base of the lashes and flaking or scaling of the eyelid skin. These may indicate the presence of ectropion, blepharitis or epiphora.

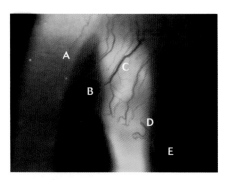

Figure 1.5
Slit-lamp photograph of neovascularization induced by a contact lens, whereby the vessels can be viewed using (A) direct focal illumination, (B) indirect focal illumination, (C) direct retroillumination, (D) marginal retroillumination and (E) indirect retroillumination

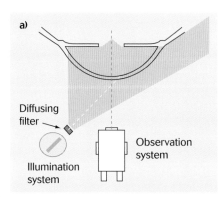
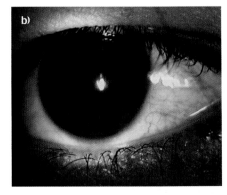

Figure 1.6
(a) Diffuse illumination slit-lamp technique (adapted from Jones and Jones[2]). (b) Diffuse illumination view of the cornea

Focal illumination – parallelepiped

Parallelepiped focal illumination is any illumination technique in which the slit beam and viewing system are focused coincidentally. The illumination is turned up to a reasonably high level of brightness (but not too high, to ensure that the patient remains comfortable) and the slit beam is placed at a separation of 40–60° on the side of the microscope that corresponds to the section of the cornea to be viewed. The beam is swept smoothly across the ocular surface and the illumination system moved across to the opposite side as the beam crosses the mid-point of the cornea. Typically, a beam width of 0.1–0.5 mm is chosen initially, which may be reduced to bring more contrast (with less light scatter) to the area of interest. The term 'parallelepiped' refers to the geometric shape of the illuminated optical section of the cornea under examination.

A slit width greater than 0.5 mm creates a condition known as 'broad beam' illumination, whereby the width of the beam is greater than the depth of the cornea (in effect, this creates a parallelepiped turned on its side). While scanning the external ocular surface, a low-to-medium magnification is chosen initially and the magnification is increased if any area of interest needs to be examined more closely.

Direct

With direct parallelepiped focal illumination, the section of the cornea *within* the illuminated beam is observed (*Figure 1.7*). This enables an assessment of the location, width and height of any object within the cornea or adjacent structures. The parallelepiped is the most commonly used direct illumination technique and is employed, for example, to assess corneal scarring, infiltrates and corneal staining.

Indirect

With indirect parallelepiped focal illumination, the section of the cornea *outside* the illuminated beam is observed. This is achieved by directing the gaze to either side of the illuminated beam. To achieve this configuration, the parallelepiped is positioned to one side of the feature of interest. Thus, the feature of interest is illuminated by side scattering of light from the parallelepiped. This technique may reveal the presence of subtle changes in corneal transparency, which may not have been visible using direct illumination.

Focal illumination – optic section

Focal illumination with an optic section is identical to parallelepiped focal illumination, except that a very thin beam of approximately 0.02–0.1 mm is used, essentially to create a 'cross-section' of the corneal tissue. The illumination beam is placed at a separation of 40–60° on the side of the microscope that corresponds to the section of the cornea to be viewed. Increasing the angle of the illumination arm increases the depth of the optic section in the cornea, but the same amount of light is spread over a greater depth of cornea, which reduces brightness and contrast and makes the deeper corneal layers, in particular, more difficult to visualize. As the light beam is so thin, the illumination must be turned up to maximum brightness.

Direct

In direct focal illumination with an optic section, the section of the cornea *within* the illuminated beam is observed (*Figure 1.8*). This provides the ability to assess accurately the depth of an object within the corneal layers (see *Figure 1.11*). Typical uses include assessment of the depth of a foreign body, location of a corneal scar and determining whether tissue within an area of staining is excavated, flat or raised.

Indirect

In indirect focal illumination with an optic section, the section of the cornea *outside* the illuminated beam is observed. This is achieved by directing the gaze to either side of the illuminated optic section. To achieve this configuration, the optic section is positioned to one side of the feature of interest. Thus, the feature of interest is illuminated by side scattering of light from the optic section.

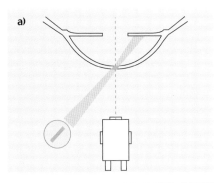
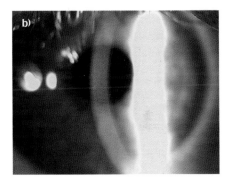

Figure 1.7
(a) Direct parallelepiped illumination technique (adapted from Jones and Jones[2]). (b) Direct parallelepiped view of the cornea

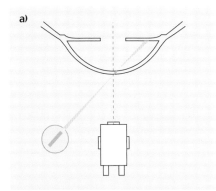
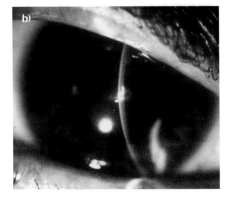

Figure 1.8
(a) Direct optic section illumination technique (adapted from Jones and Jones[2]). (b) Optic section view of a corneal foreign-body injury

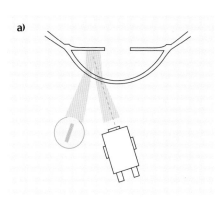

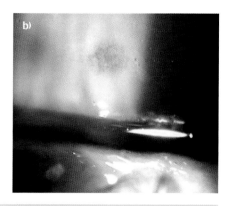

Figure 1.9

(a) Direct retroillumination technique (adapted from Jones and Jones[2]). (b) Corneal scar from a healed peripheral ulcer seen as a dull gray shadow in direct retroillumination

Indirect focal illumination from an optic section is, perhaps, only a theoretical consideration; a superior indirect view of a corneal anomaly is achieved with a wider beam (i.e., parallelepiped or broad beam).

Retroillumination

Retroillumination refers to any technique in which light is reflected from the iris, anterior lens surface or retina, and is used to back illuminate a section of the cornea that is positioned more anteriorly. The illumination and observation systems can be adjusted so that the feature of interest in the cornea is seen against a light background (such as a light-colored iris) or a dark background (such as a dark-colored iris, or the pupil in the case of indirect retroillumination).

This technique is particularly useful for examining neovascularization, scars, degenerations and dystrophies.

Direct

Direct retroillumination refers to the configuration whereby the retroillumination is directly behind the feature of interest in the cornea (*Figure 1.9*). Thus, for example, a corneal scar is viewed against an illuminated iris in the background. Using this technique, corneal opacities appear black against the bright field.

Indirect

Indirect retroillumination refers to the configuration whereby the retroillumination is not directly behind the feature of interest in the cornea, but is offset to one side (*Figure 1.10*). Thus,

the feature of interest is observed by virtue of backscattered light deflected away from the feature of interest in the cornea into the eye of the observer.

Marginal

Marginal retroillumination is a specific variant of indirect retroillumination, whereby the pupil margin is deliberately chosen as the background retroilluminated field against which the corneal feature is being observed (*Figure 1.10*). Simply put, the corneal feature of interest is viewed against a background of the illuminated pupil margin. This technique is typically used in association with high levels of magnification, and is used to assess the optical characteristics of transparent optical bodies in the

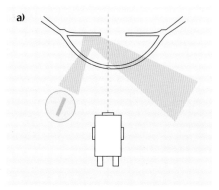

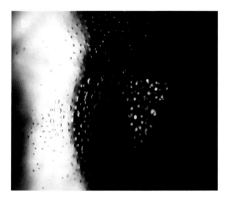

Figure 1.10

(a) Indirect and marginal retroillumination technique (adapted from Jones and Jones[2]). (b) Dimple veiling viewed by indirect retroillumination can be appreciated by observing the 'dimples' against both the dark pupil on the right and the illuminated iris on the left. Dimple veiling viewed by marginal retroillumination can be appreciated by observing the 'dimples' against the pupil margin; the dimples in this region clearly display unreversed illumination, which indicates that they contain a material of lower refractive index than the epithelium (i.e., fluid or air)

tear film or the cornea, such as mucin balls, epithelial microcysts, vacuoles and bullae.

Specular reflection

Specular reflection is a specific case of an optic section setup in which the angle of the incident slit beam is equal to the angle of the observation axis through one of the oculars (*Figure 1.11*). At this angle (typically 40–50°) the illumination beam is reflected from the smooth surfaces of the cornea and provides a mirror-like ('specular') reflection (see *Figure 1.12*). Such specular images occur at every interface between structures of different refractive indices, the most prominent of which are the anterior epithelial and posterior endothelial surfaces. The technique of specular reflection is typically used to view the endothelium.

To begin with, the lowest magnification setting is selected, and the illumination arm is set at an angle to the normal greater than the angle of the observation system to the normal. The illumination arm is then brought back toward the observation system while observing the corneal surface. At the point where specular reflection is achieved, a bright reflex fills one of the oculars (specular reflection cannot be achieved binocularly). The illumination–observation system should now remain in a fixed position, and the magnification is set to maximum so that the anterior and/or posterior corneal surface can be viewed in specular reflection. A very

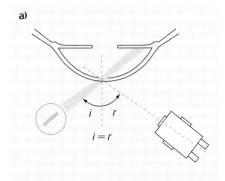

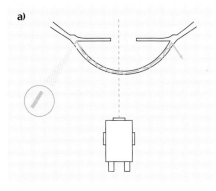

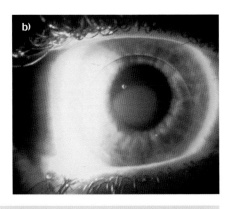

Figure 1.12

(a) Sclerotic scatter illumination technique (adapted from Jones and Jones[2]). (b) Central corneal edema viewed using sclerotic scatter

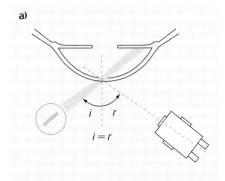

Figure 1.11

(a) Specular reflection illumination technique (adapted from Jones and Jones[2]); *i*, angle of incidence; *r*, angle of reflection. (b) Specular reflection view of the corneal endothelium.

bright reflection from the anterior surface constitutes a debilitating distraction when trying to observe the endothelium; this situation can be resolved by increasing the angle between the observation and illumination systems, although there is little room for maneuver before the specular reflection is lost.

The size of endothelial cells is such that, even at ×40 magnification, only gross anomalies of the endothelium can be detected, such as large guttae, blebs, bedewing, endothelial ruptures or deep folds. Subtle cellular characteristics of the endothelial mosaic, such as cell density or polymegethism, cannot be assessed. The tear film lipid layer and the inferior tear meniscus can also be examined readily using specular reflec-

tion, as well as the anterior surface of the crystalline lens. If a contact lens is being worn, front surface wetting can be assessed and the post-lens tear film may be observed using specular reflection.[4]

Sclerotic scatter

Sclerotic scatter is used to investigate subtle changes in corneal clarity that occur over a large area, such as central corneal edema. The slit lamp is set up for a wide-angle parallelepiped (45–60°) and the viewing system is focused centrally. The beam is manually offset ('uncoupled') and focused on the limbus. The slit beam is totally reflected internally across the cornea and a bright limbal glow is seen around the entire cornea (*Figure 1.12*). Any specific area of abnormality, such as a corneal scar, interrupts the beam in its passage and produces a light reflection in the otherwise clear cornea; abnormalities in the cornea are especially visible when viewed against a dark pupil in the background.

Tangential (oblique) illumination

Tangential (oblique) illumination is used infrequently in contact lens practice, but is nonetheless a useful technique. Oblique illumination is achieved by setting up a parallelepiped and then moving the illumination system away from the observation system until the angle between them is close to 90°. The observation system is positioned at 90° to the facial plane (i.e., straight ahead) and the illumination arm is adjusted until the light beam is almost tangential to the object of interest. Any raised areas

cast a shadow and this technique is particularly useful for viewing subtle irregularities on the surface of the iris, epithelium or contact lens *in situ*.

Conical beam

Conical beam is used specifically to examine the contents of the anterior chamber. A conical beam configuration is achieved by narrowing the slit beam down to about 1–2 mm in diameter and reducing the height of the beam to about the same dimensions. This effectively creates a circular beam of light. The illumination should be set to maximum and the room should be darkened. The arrangement of the illumination and observation system is essentially the same as that for tangential illumination. The observation system is positioned at 90° to the facial plane (i.e., straight ahead) and the illumination system is moved away from the observation system until the angle between them is close to 90°. Low-to-medium magnification should be used.

Static

The conical beam is projected sideways into the anterior chamber and left in a fixed position. Light from the conical beam must not strike the iris, because this scatters light and makes observation more difficult. Gaze is directed toward the black pupil. Any protein, debris or cellular matter floating in the aqueous reflects light toward the observer and is detected as a glint of light (flare) against the black background of the pupil. Numerous particles result in a glistening effect, as various particles slowly move and change orientation in the aqueous.

Oscillating

The positions of the observation and illumination systems are exactly the same as for a static conical beam examination, except that the observer must rapidly oscillate the illumination arm from side to side using the offset control. This oscillation technique increases the probability of detecting aqueous flare and glistening.

Slit-Lamp Examination Procedure

No single slit-lamp procedure is able to satisfy all observational requirements when a contact lens patient is examined. However, during an examination in which it is expected that no abnormalities will be detected (as in the case, for example, of an initial assessment of a prospective contact lens wearer), it is useful to develop a systematic procedure that ensures coverage of all aspects of the assessment in a logical and consistent manner. Usually, the examination starts with low magnification and diffuse illumination for general observation, with the magnification increasing and more specific illumination techniques being employed to view the structures in more detail as the examination progresses. A typical routine examination procedure using the slit-lamp biomicroscope is outlined below.

Overall view

The examination should begin with a number of sweeps across the anterior segment and adnexa, while using a broad beam and low magnification. The patient is first instructed to close his or her eyes and the skin on the eyelids, eyebrows and surrounding areas is examined. The patient is then requested to open his or her eyes and the lid margins and lashes are examined for signs of marginal blepharitis or hordeolum. The patency of the meibomian glands is assessed by gently squeezing the lids. The bulbar conjunctiva is then assessed for redness and the presence of any abnormalities, such as pinguecula or pterygia. The superior and inferior palpebral conjunctiva are examined to check for redness, follicles and papillae. The position and action of the eyes and eyelids are noted and the completeness of blinks can be assessed.

Cornea and limbus

The diffusing filter is removed and the corneal examination begins by uncoupling the slit-lamp illumination and observation systems and examining the cornea for gross opacification using the sclerotic scatter illumination technique. The slit lamp is then recoupled and a series of observation sweeps is carried out across the cornea, using medium magnification and a broad beam (2 mm wide). The limbal vasculature is examined to assess the degree of physiologic corneal vascularization (blood vessels that overlay clear cornea) and differentiate this from neovascularization (new blood vessels that grow into clear cornea). Blood vessels at the limbus are best observed using both direct illumination and indirect retroillumination. Once the limbus has been assessed, the cornea is examined with a parallelepiped to look for any abnormalities. During this procedure, a number of illumination techniques can be used sequentially. If a corneal anomaly is detected, the beam should be narrowed to form an optic section so that the depth and fine structure of the anomaly can be assessed. The endothelium should be viewed in specular reflection.

Staining examination

Fluorescein is instilled into the eye and a cobalt blue filter is interposed into the illumination system. A yellow (Kodak Wratten No. 12) barrier filter, if available, should also be interposed in the observation system. Gross epithelial surface irregularities are detected using diffuse illumination and low magnification. However, more subtle anomalies can be detected only with medium-to-high magnification, employing a parallelepiped and alternating between direct and indirect observation as the beam is swept slowly across the cornea. The illumination often needs to be set to a higher level of brightness to compensate for the loss of light through the excitation and barrier filters; however, if the illumination is too bright the fluorescence tends to be 'flooded out', which results in reduced contrast. Observation in white light, with or without the barrier filter, allows an alternative view of the corneal anomaly under observation.

Various features of the tear film can be assessed with the aid of fluorescein, such as lower tear meniscus height, degree of 'sluggishness' of the tear film upon blinking and tear break-up time.

Numerous other vital stains can be applied to the eye to highlight other anomalies, such as mucus accumulation, tissue devitalization or tissue necrosis. These are discussed in detail in Chapter 8.

Lid eversion

The final stage of the slit-lamp examination is lid eversion, to enable examination of the palpebral conjunctiva. This procedure is left to last for the following reasons:

- The procedure is slightly uncomfortable for the patient – no matter how carefully performed – and the patient may not wish to be subjected to any further ocular examination or eye manipulation thereafter;
- The procedure may slightly traumatize the cornea – no matter how carefully performed – which would confound interpretation of any corneal anomalies observed after lid eversion;
- Since the procedure is performed after fluorescein instillation, the opportunity exists to examine the tarsal conjunctiva both in white light and in cobalt blue light with a barrier filter. The latter procedure enhances the appearance of any papillae.

The procedure is conducted as follows. The illumination–observation system is pulled away from the patient and set in readiness to observe the tarsal conjunctiva. The best initial arrangement is low magnification and diffuse white light. The head of the patient is then positioned in the head-and-brow rest and the lid is everted by applying light pressure beneath the brow, grabbing and lightly pulling the eyelashes of the upper lid outward and upward so as to evert the lid. The thumb is then used to hold the lashes of the everted lid lightly against the upper orbital rim (resting the hand against the brow support and/or the patient's head). All other operations must therefore be conducted using the other (free) hand. A diffuse beam is directed at the tarsal conjunctiva, which is observed at low and then at medium magnification. Fluorescein is instilled if it has not already been instilled as part of the preceding examination, and excitation and barrier filters are interposed in the illumination and observation systems, respectively. The tarsal conjunctiva is re-examined, employing broad sweeps from side to side when using medium magnification.

When the examination has been completed, the eyelashes are pulled outward and the lid naturally reverts to its normal anatomic configuration. In view of the unavoidable discomfort for the patient, the whole procedure of lid eversion should not last longer than about 15 s.

Conclusion

As with any other clinical procedure, proficiency at using the slit-lamp biomicroscope only comes with clinical experience. All practitioners, whether experienced or novice, should invest time to study the features of an instrument that is being used for the first time, whether it be a newly acquired instrument or an existing instrument in a new and unfamiliar practice setting. The full diagnostic potential of a slit-lamp biomicroscope can be realized only if the location and mode of operation of all the controls, filters, mechanical adjustment mechanisms, etc., are known, understood and used creatively.

REFERENCES

1 Goldberg JB (1970). *Biomicroscopy for Contact Lens Practice: Clinical Procedures*. (Chicago: Professional Press).
2 Jones LW and Jones DA (2001). Slit lamp biomicroscopy. In: *The Cornea. Its Examination in Contact Lens Practice*, p. 1–49. Ed. Efron N. (Oxford: Butterworth–Heinemann).
3 Courtney RC and Lee JM (1982). Predicting ocular intolerance of a contact lens solution by use of a filter system enhancing fluorescein staining detection. *Int Contact Lens Clin.* **9**, 302–310.
4 Little SA and Bruce AS (1994). Postlens tear film morphology, lens movement and symptoms in hydrogel lens wearers. *Ophthalmic Physiol Opt.* **14**, 65–69.

PART II EYELIDS

BLINKING ABNORMALITIES

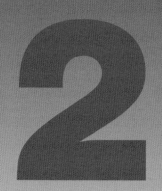

Blinking is a high-speed closure movement of the eyelids that is of short duration and has both reflex and spontaneous origins.[1] Reflex blinking can be elicited by a variety of external stimuli, such as strong lights, approaching objects, loud noises, and corneal, conjunctival or ciliary touch. Contact lenses elicit reflex blinking during lens insertion and removal, and during other instances of manual manipulation. Also, as a result of a reflex blink, contact lenses may mislocate or become dislodged from the eye. Aside from these phenomena, there is no reason to suppose that contact lens wear alters the essential nature of the reflex blink. For this reason, this chapter concentrates on spontaneous blinking activity associated with contact lens wear, and the term 'blink' should generally be taken to mean 'spontaneous blink'.

Blinking serves a number of useful functions, both with and without contact lenses. Although eyecare practitioners have long subscribed to the notion that their contact lens patients should execute full and regular blinks during lens wear, this topic has received little attention in the literature.

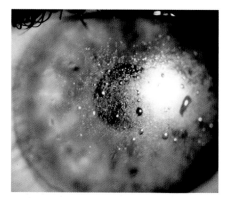

Figure 2.1
Non-wetting surface of a silicone elastomer lens

This chapter reviews the characteristics of the normal blink and examines how contact lens wear can affect, and be affected by, blinking behavior. Complications that arise from poor blinking behavior with contact lenses (such as lens surface drying, as shown in *Figure 2.1*) are reviewed, along with the question of clinical management of blinking abnormalities.

Normal Spontaneous Blinking

Mechanism of blinking

Eyelid closure during blinking is effected by the orbicularis oculi muscle, which is innervated by the seventh cranial nerve. The act of blinking is accomplished primarily by the upper lid. The lower lid remains virtually stationary. Closure is characterized by a progressive narrowing of the palpebral fissure in a zipper-like fashion, from the outer to inner canthus. This moving wave of closure serves to force aqueous in the inter-palpebral fissure toward the lacrimal puncta, and thus aids tear drainage.[2]

Spontaneous blinking occurs in all terrestrial vertebrates that possess eyelids, although the rate of blinking varies considerably between species. Large predatory cats execute less than one blink per minute, whereas some small species of monkey have blink rates as high as 45 times per minute. Infants have a very low spontaneous blink rate.[1]

Spontaneous blinking occurs in patients who have total congenital blindness, which indicates this is a phenomenon that is not learned and is not dependent upon visual input.[1] The rate of spontaneous blinking may alter in response to changes in the level of visual activity and in different emotional states. General environmental changes, such as the level of dryness or wind flow, may also alter the spontaneous blink rate. The frequency and completeness of blink is reduced

during intense concentration, such as when reading[2] or working on a visual display unit.

Types and patterns of blinking

Researchers must employ devious methods to monitor types and patterns of spontaneous blinking. This is necessary because of the methodological problem that subjects alter their blinking activity if they are aware that it is being measured.[2] Typically, subjects under such circumstances execute an increased proportion of voluntary forced blinks and a greater overall blink frequency. For this reason, hidden observers or video cameras are employed to record blinking activity while the subject, for example, is engaged in discussion or is asked to observe a silent movie.

Zaman and Doughty[3] highlighted other potential methodological pitfalls in quantifying blinking behavior. For example, simple averaging of blink rates may not always be appropriate because of the high chance of a non-Gaussian data distribution. These authors conclude that eye-blink monitoring over at least 3 minutes is required for valid data analysis. Fortunately, almost all blink researchers have used observation times in excess of this.

According to Abelson and Holly,[4] blinking can be classified into four basic types:
• Complete blink – the upper eyelid covers more than 67% of the cornea;
• Incomplete blink – the upper eyelid covers less than 67% of the cornea;
• Twitch blink – a small movement of the upper eyelid;
• Forced blink – lower lid raises to complete eye closure.
The percentage of all blinks that can be characterized by each of these four blink types, as determined by Abelson and Holly,[4] is illustrated in *Figure 2.2*. Subsequent research has confirmed these findings.[5,6]

Tsubota *et al.*[7] developed a computer-interfaced 'blink analyzer' to measure accurately the time course and pattern of blinking in 64 normal volunteers. They found that the average time taken to execute one complete blink (which they defined as the upper lid covering more that 85% of the cornea) was 0.20 ± 0.04 s, and that the average interblink period (IBP) was 4.0 ± 2.0 s. Taking one complete blink cycle as the sum of the blink time and IBP ($0.2 + 4.0 = 4.2$ s) gives an average blink frequency of 14.3 blinks/min (i.e., 60/4.2). This result is consistent with previous estimates of the spontaneous blink rate in humans.[5,8]

The small interruption to visual input during a blink is thought to be of practical significance only in occupations or tasks that require constant monitoring of rapidly changing visual images. (Paradoxically, blinking is problematic for researchers who monitor the blinking activity of experimental subjects, either directly or via video replays; in the latter case, viewing in slow motion solves this problem). Volkmann *et al.*[9] proposed that there is a suppression of the visual pathway associated with blinks so that the momentary interruption to visual input does not produce a conscious interruption to visual perception.

Various authors have suggested that there is a gender difference in blink rate. Hart[1] proposed that males blink more frequently than females, whereas Tsubota *et al.*[7] have suggested the converse; neither validated their claims statistically. Yolton *et al.*[8] has shed light on this issue by measuring the spontaneous blink rate in males, females not using oral contraceptives and females using oral contraceptives. The blink rates observed in these three groups were 14.5, 14.9 and 19.6 blinks per minute, respectively. This finding indicates that there is no intrinsic gender difference in blink rate, but the use of oral contraceptives induces a significantly greater blink rate, for reasons that are unclear.

Purpose of blinking

Spontaneous blinking in non-lens wearers serves the following functions:

- Maintenance of an intact pre-corneal tear film by constantly spreading the tear film evenly across the corneal surface;
- Removal of intrinsic and extrinsic particulate matter by forcing such debris into the lower lacrimal river;
- Facilitation of tear exchange by constantly swiping tears toward the puncta located at the inner canthus.

The importance of the first of the functions listed above (maintenance of an intact pre-corneal tear film) has been demonstrated in a number of studies that have examined blinking behavior in patients suffering from symptoms of dry eye.

Prause and Norn[10] advanced the theory that spontaneous blinking is, in part, a stimulus to rupture of the pre-corneal tear film. They tested this hypothesis by measuring tear break-up time (TBUT) and the IBP in a group of normal and dry eye patients. A statistically significant positive correlation between these two parameters was found in both groups (i.e., the more rapidly the tear film breaks up, the more frequently the patient blinks). The above finding was confirmed subsequently by Yap[11] in a group of normal subjects, although two other research groups found no such association.[8,12]

Prause and Norn[10] also demonstrated that, in general, the IBP was slightly less than the TBUT, which suggests that patients adopt a blink rate that prevents tear break up. Using quantitative videographic analysis, Tsubota *et al.*[7] found that the IBP in dry eye patients was 1.5 ± 0.9 s, compared with 4.0 ± 2.0 s in normal subjects.

Indirect evidence of the link between TBUT and IBP comes from the work of Tsubota and Nakamori,[13] who measured the tear evaporation rate from the ocular surface (TEROS) in 17 normal volunteers and found an increase in blink rate with increasing TEROS. This result is consistent with previous demonstrations of the positive correlation between IBP and TBUT, because tear break-up associated with more rapid blinking is expected to result in higher rates of tear evaporation.

Although the weight of evidence does suggest that blink rate is, in part, dependent upon the integrity of the tear film, other factors must be involved also. This was demonstrated by Collins *et al.*,[14] who found that blinking continued after instillation of a corneal topical anesthetic in a group of normal subjects. The blink rate did, however, drop from 24.8 to 17.2 blinks/min. If tear break-up is the sole determinant of blink rate, blinking would have stopped in the eyes with the anesthetized corneas.

Alterations to Blinking Caused by Contact Lenses

Blink rate

Hill and Carney[15] demonstrated, in a group of seven subjects, that blink rate increased from 15.5 blinks/min to 23.2 blinks/min after being fitted with polymethyl methacrylate (PMMA) contact lenses. A similar result was reported by York *et al.*,[16] although Brown *et al.*[17] did not confirm this result. It appears, however, that alterations to blink rate induced by PMMA lenses may be related more to reflex blinking than to spontaneous blinking; that is, the increased

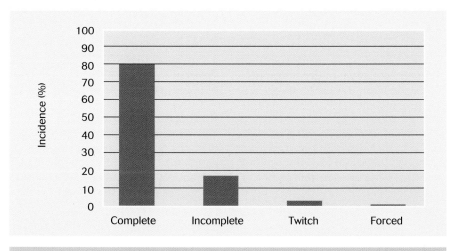

Figure 2.2
Frequency of occurrence of various blink types

blink rate may be a result of continual irritation caused by the lens edge buffeting against the lid margin.

In another group of seven subjects, Carney and Hill[18] demonstrated that blink rate increased from 12.1 blinks/min to 20.3 blinks/min after being fitted with soft contact lenses [presumably hydroxyethyl methacrylate (HEMA)]. The reason for this is less clear, as soft lenses are expected to be more comfortable and thus to induce less reflex blinking activity, although the earlier study of Brown et al.[17] found that blink rate was essentially unaffected by soft lens wear.

Although blink rate may be altered during contact lens wear, a supplementary consideration is whether or not any alteration to blinking activity is permanent. Yolton et al.[8] reported that the blink rate (16.2 ± 8.9 blinks/min) in a cohort of habitual contact lens wearers (the lens type was not specified) who had ceased lens wear at least 24 hours prior to blinking assessment was identical to that of a matched control group who had never worn contact lenses (16.2 ± 9.5 blinks/min), which suggests that alterations to blink rate induced by contact lenses are evident only during lens wear.

Blink type

Carney and Hill[15,18] examined the effects of hard and soft lens wear on the pattern of blinking. A decrease in the frequency of occurrence of long duration IBPs was observed in association with rigid lens wear, but not with soft lens wear. Neither rigid nor soft lens wear altered the proportion of complete, incomplete, twitch and forced blinks. An example of an incomplete blink in a soft lens wearer is shown in Figure 2.3.

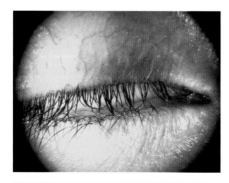

Figure 2.3
Incomplete blink in a soft lens wearer

Complications of Abnormal Blinking with Contact Lenses

Lens surface drying and deposition

The tear film on the front surface of both soft and rigid lenses has a different structure compared with that of the pre-ocular tear film (POTF); the lipid layer is thinner or absent, and the aqueous layer is of variable thickness, depending on the lens material and design.[19,20] Similarly, the tear film on the front surface of soft and rigid lenses is less stable than that of the POTF. Whereas the POTF in normal human subjects has a TBUT of at least 15 s,[21] the pre-lens tear film (PLTF) has a TBUT of between 3 and 10 s for soft lenses[21] and between 4 and 6 s for rigid lenses.[20] Given that the mean IBP in humans is 4.0 ± 2.0 s, and that contact lens wear has little effect on the IBP, it is clear that in some patients the IBP exceeds the PLTF TBUT, which leads to intermittent drying of the lens surface.

A case of severe drying of the surface of a silicone elastomer lens (which is naturally hydrophobic) is depicted in Figure 2.1. In view of the rapid TBUT of such a lens, an unsustainable interblink frequency of approximately 2 s is required to prevent the lens surface from drying.

It is generally recognized that a full and continuous tear film on the lens surface is important to maintain a clean surface with minimum deposition. The greater the discrepancy between the IBP and the PLTF TBUT, and the longer the tear disruption is maintained, the greater is the possibility for both extrinsic and intrinsic materials to adhere to the lens surface.

It also seems theoretically plausible that a discrepancy between the interblink period and the PLTF TBUT of soft lenses could result in a greater degree of lens dehydration, as water from the lens could evaporate directly into the atmosphere from a dry lens surface. This theory was tested by Young and Efron,[22] but no association could be demonstrated between PLTF TBUT and lens dehydration.

In general, therefore, lens surface characteristics can be optimized by ensuring that the IBP is shorter than the PLTF TBUT.

Visual degradation

Ridder and Tomlinson[23] found that vision with soft lenses degraded considerably when a target was presented less than 100 ms after the blink. They explained their finding in terms of blink suppression and prismatic shift of the retinal image induced by the movement of the contact lens produced by the blink. This explanation was reinforced by the observation that loose-fitting contact lenses caused an even greater decrement in immediate post-blink vision.

Blink-induced lens movement causes a reduction in visual performance that is potentially greater with toric than with spherical soft contact lenses because of the combination of vertical lens movement and rotation. Tomlinson et al.[24] found that prism ballasted lenses gave better overall visual performance than lenses of dynamic stabilization design at all times after the blink.

Prolonged lens settling

Golding et al.[25] postulated that the extent of lens settling and the degree of post-insertion lens movement are determined by the time-average pressure for post-lens tear film expulsion exerted on the lens by the eyelids. Specifically, they found that lens settling was prolonged (i.e., lens movement was significantly higher) for slower blink rates (10 blinks/min) compared with faster blink rates (30 blinks/min) or the eye closure condition.

Epithelial desiccation

Severe desiccation staining of the corneal epithelium is known to occur as a result of fitting extremely thin soft contact lenses of high water content.[26] This phenomenon relates primarily to the fitting of lenses of inappropriate design. However, Guillon et al.[27] demonstrated that epithelial desiccation can occur with lenses of high water content that have adequate thickness and good fit. They attribute this phenomenon to a break-up of the tear film at the inferior tear prism margin. This complication is theoretically avoidable if the blink rate is sufficient to prevent such PLTF TBUT.

Post-lens tear stagnation

The anterior ocular surface is host to a plethora of organic material, such as desquamated superficial epithelial and conjunctival cells, mucus, proteins, lipids, microorganisms and inflammatory cells. Environmental antigens (e.g., iron particles, dust, pollen, smoke, smog and other atmospheric pollutants) and particulate matter can also enter the tear film easily. The material listed above rarely poses a problem because it is washed away constantly by the tear film, primarily as a result of blinking. However, when such material locates behind the lens, problems can arise if the post-lens tear film is allowed to stagnate (*Figure 2.4*).

Infrequent and/or incomplete blinking during contact lens wear can be problematic theoretically, because the residency time of ocular pollutants in the post-lens tear film is increased, which thus heightens the potential for a traumatic, toxic, allergic or infectious insult of the cornea. Blinking serves to flush such debris out from beneath the lens, to be replaced by 'fresh' tears that contain a new set of pollutants. As long as there is this constant turnover of tears beneath the lens, which is referred to as 'tear exchange', long pollutant resident times can be avoided.

Daily wear of rigid contact lenses is known to be associated with a tear exchange of between 10 and 17% with each blink.[28] This contrasts with a tear exchange of only about 1% with each blink during hydrogel lens wear,[29] and a slightly greater amount with silicone hydrogel lenses.[30] These research findings, and accumulated clinical experience, have led practitioners to be aware of the importance of fitting soft lenses so that there is adequate movement of the contact lenses (in particular soft lenses) with each blink. Failure to ensure adequate lens movement may allow the stagnating post-lens tear film debris to induce an adverse reaction via a variety of different mechanisms, which leads to lens discomfort. Reducing the diameter of soft lenses can enhance tear

exchange;[31] however, smaller lenses tend to be less comfortable. Theoretical analyses suggest that fenestrations and channels can facilitate greater tear exchange in soft lenses by enhancing transverse (in–out) lens motion.[32]

Problems that relate to post-lens tear film tear stagnation are uncommon in daily wear because an awake, conscious patient can manipulate or remove an uncomfortable lens, and thus minimize any ocular trauma. As well, the lens is removed each day, which allows any sub-clinical insult that may have been developing to recover.

Post-lens tear stagnation is, however, of real concern in patients who sleep in lenses, and the problems manifest differently for rigid and soft lenses. In the case of rigid lenses, the aqueous phase is depleted overnight to leave a mucus-rich post-lens tear film that tends to create adhesion between the lens and cornea (*Figure 2.5*).[33] Blinking upon awakening in patients who have slept in rigid lenses is critical, because the blinking action tends to dislodge the adherent lens mechanically, so that a normal post-lens tear film can be re-established.

In the absence of blinking during overnight lens wear, material that was present in the post-lens tear film immediately prior to going to sleep, in addition to desquamated epithelial cells and inflammatory cells that accumulate throughout the night, is present beneath the lens upon waking in the morning.[34] Various forms of toxic, infectious, inflammatory or immunologic reactions may be initiated. If the patient continues to wear the lenses during the

waking hours, the rate of tear exchange, especially with soft lenses, may be insufficient to effect a rapid clearance of the post-lens tear film, which allows any adverse reactions that were initiated to continue.

A model can be constructed to illustrate the sequel of events that leads to corneal ulceration, in a patient who sleeps in soft contact lenses, as a result of inadequate blink-assisted clearance of debris from the post-lens tear film upon waking (*Figure 2.6*). Desquamated epithelial cells are trapped beneath a soft lens. These cells undergo lysis and irritate the underlying corneal epithelium, which causes corneal staining. The epithelium is unable to repair itself in the toxic post-lens tear film environment, and a sterile ulcer results.

Factors that govern the removal of debris from the post-lens tear film were investigated by McGrogan *et al.*,[35] who inserted soft lenses that contained polystyrene microspheres of various sizes and monitored the rate of removal of these microspheres from the post-lens tear film during blinking (*Figure 2.7*). The key determinant of microsphere removal was the size of the microspheres; larger microspheres were dislodged less easily from beneath the lens than were smaller microspheres. Lens modulus and lens fit had little effect on microsphere clearance.

Hypoxia and hypercapnia

The normal cornea constantly draws oxygen from the atmosphere to sustain its high levels of metabolic activity. At the same time, carbon dioxide – an

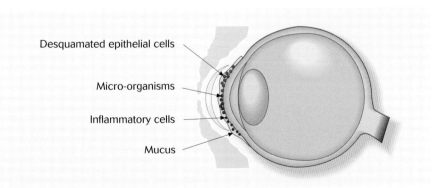

Figure 2.4
Various types of debris trapped beneath a soft lens

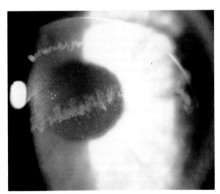

Figure 2.5
Mucus at the center and periphery of the cornea in the tear film beneath a rigid lens that was worn overnight

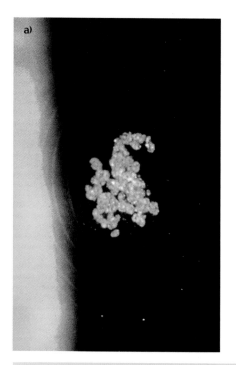
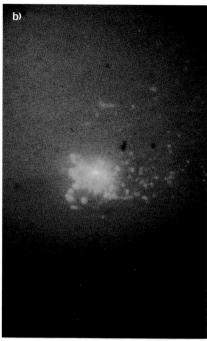
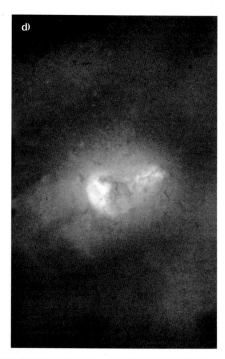

Figure 2.6

Complications caused by stagnating debris in the post-lens tear film. (a) Epithelial cells are trapped by the lens. (b) Cells lysis leads to epithelial disruption and staining. (c) A small sterile corneal ulcer forms

unwanted by-product of corneal metabolism – is released into the atmosphere from the corneal surface. Contact lenses form a potential barrier to both corneal oxygenation and carbon dioxide efflux, which results in reduced oxygenation (hypoxia) and increased levels of carbon dioxide (hypercapnia). Complications that arise from lens-induced hypoxia and hypercapnia are discussed throughout this book. A key goal of contact lens fitting is to minimize hypoxia and hypercapnia.

All contact lenses fitted today (aside from PMMA lenses) have some degree of gas transmissibility that allows oxygen to flow through the lens into the cornea and carbon dioxide to flow out of the lens into the atmosphere. This necessary gaseous exchange can be enhanced further by tear exchange, whereby the oxygen-depleted and carbon dioxide-rich tear film beneath the lens is replaced partially by freshly oxygenated and carbon dioxide-free tears from outside the lens. The higher the gas permeability of the fitted lens, the lower

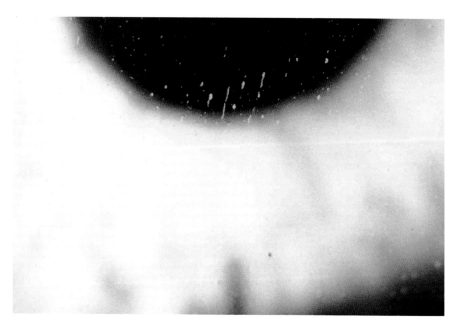

Figure 2.7

Polystyrene microspheres visible as single spheres and small 'tracks' (the latter as a result of a slow photographic shutter speed). The microspheres have a diameter of 10 μm (yellow) and 6 μm (pink).

is the reliance upon tear exchange to alleviate hypoxia and hypercapnia.

The effect of blinking on corneal hypoxia and hypercapnia beneath rigid and soft lenses has been studied extensively.[36,37] It has been demonstrated that blinking can partially alleviate corneal hypoxia and hypercapnia in both soft and rigid lenses.

Blinking also plays an important role in redistributing oxygenated tears evenly across the corneal surface beneath soft lenses, via a process known as 'tear mixing'.[38] This function is particularly important during the wearing of lenses of non-uniform thickness. For example, in the absence of effective tear mixing with a minus powered lens (thicker in the lens periphery than in the lens center), the corneal periphery suffers from greater levels of hypoxia than the central cornea, which can potentially result in pathology of the peripheral cornea and limbus. In this example, effective tear mixing allows highly oxygenated tears beneath the center of the lens to become interspersed with oxygen-deprived tears beneath the lens periphery, which results in an 'averaging' of available oxygen and less peripheral hypoxia.

3 and 9 o'clock staining

3 and 9 o'clock staining is a common problem with rigid lenses, and is thought to result from a lens-induced disturbance of the normal blink movement of the upper lid over the lens and cornea. A rigid lens tends to bridge the upper lid away from the cornea so that, during the downward movement of the upper lid in the course of a blink, the lid is unable to re-wet the 'bridged' regions of the cornea at the 3 and 9 o'clock locations. This leads to local drying and consequent staining of these 'bridged' corneal locations.

Poor lens design and fitting

With respect to the eyelids, rigid lenses can be fitted according to two basic philosophies – the intrapalpebral fit and the lid attachment fit. The intrapalpebral fit entails fitting a lens, typically of small diameter, so that it rests on the cornea between the upper and lower lid margins during primary gaze. The upper lid rides over the lens during the blink, which results in lens movement (essential for tear exchange) and lens re-positioning (essential for proper lens alignment with the optical axis of the eye).

Inappropriate lens design and fitting can result in an interference with proper blink-mediated lid–lens interaction. For example, an edge stand-off that is too great (caused by a peripheral lens curvature that is too flat or excessive edge lift) could lead to discomfort during the blink because of the constant buffeting of the lens edge against the lid margin. The lid may even gain leverage beneath the lens edge and cause the lens to be dislodged from the eye.

With a lid attachment fit, the upper lid lies over the lens periphery, into which may be designed a negative lens carrier. The purpose of this type of fit is to aid central lens positioning. The lens typically moves synchronously with each blink. A poorly designed lens carrier, or the use of a lens of inappropriate diameter, may result in a loss of synchrony of movement of the lid and lens, which leads to lens mislocation, discomfort and intermittent blur.

Management of Abnormal Blinking with Contact Lenses

Practitioners essentially have two options when faced with a clinical problem that relates to non-pathologic abnormalities of spontaneous blinking activity, such as infrequent or incomplete blinking. These options are either to train the patients to modify their blinking activity, or to make no attempt to modify the blinking activity, but instead to change the lens type or lens fit.

Early anecdotal reports proposed a variety of strategies to enhance blinking activity. These ranged from simple instructions and reminders,[39] to the employment of a small buzzer that sounded every 10 s, which acted as a prompt to execute a complete blink.[40] Although it was realized that such strategies only stimulate reflex rather than spontaneous blinks, the underlying assumption was that spontaneous blinking activity could be learned via training using reflex-stimulation techniques.

Collins et al.[6] tested the hypothesis that blinking could be trained by subjecting a group of unsuspecting volunteers who wore contact lenses to blink exercises (the volunteers were told that the purpose of the exercises was to improve vision). The exercise consisted of placing the index finger of each hand just lateral to the outer canthus to hold the lids taut while performing 10 complete forced blinks. This exercise was repeated three times daily for 2 weeks. Blinking exercises resulted in an increased frequency of complete blinks and a decreased frequency of incomplete and twitch blinks (*Figure 2.8*).

If blink training is thought to be impractical or inefficacious, the only alternative management strategy to alleviate blink-related contact lens problems is to alter the lens type, design or fit. By way of example, the following strategies are advocated.

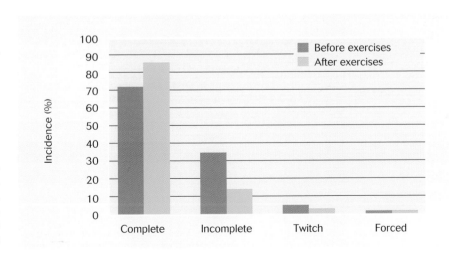

Figure 2.8

Percentage distribution of the various types of blink before and after blink training (adapted from Collins *et al.*[6])

Blink-associated problems that relate to debris removal, hypoxia and hypercapnia can be alleviated by:

- Changing from soft to rigid lenses;
- Changing a rigid lens design from aspheric to multicurve;
- Changing a rigid lens fit from lid attachment to intrapalpebral.

Blink-associated problems that relate to lens surface drying can be alleviated by changing from rigid to soft lenses. The same strategy solves 3 and 9 o'clock staining.

Sabau and Raad[41] conducted a theoretical analysis of the blink-induced dynamics of rigid lenses. They concluded that the motion of a rigid lens can be controlled by an appropriate choice of the lens material microstructure, and that lens motion can be enhanced by lowering the 'slip coefficient' and increasing lens material permeability. Thicker lenses, as well as thicker tear films, were predicted to cause the lens to squeeze faster and to slide slower.

Differential Diagnosis of Blinking Abnormalities

Practitioners should be alert to the possibility that apparent anomalies in the type or pattern of blinking activity in a contact lens wearer may be attributable to coincidental disease states. Interruptions to the neural input and/or muscular systems of the eyelids can adversely affect normal spontaneous blinking activity. For example, patients with Parkinson's disease exhibit a low blink rate. Increased mechanical resistance to eyelid movement, as in Grave's disease, can also reduce blink frequency. Local pathology of the eyelids (e.g., ptosis, chalazia, carcinomas, etc.) can alter eyelid function and movement, and hence interfere with normal blinking activity. It is therefore essential to rule out the possibility of concurrent pathology before blinking abnormalities can be ascribed to contact lens wear.

REFERENCES

1 Hart WM (1992). The eyelids. In: *Adler's Physiology of the Eye*, p. 1–17. Ed. Hart WM. (St Louis: Mosby Year Book).
2 Doane MG (1980), Interaction of the eyelids and tears in corneal wetting and the dynamics of normal human eyeblinks. *Am J Ophthalmol*. **89**, 507–510.

3 Zaman ML and Doughty MJ (1997). Some methodological issues in the assessment of the spontaneous eyeblink frequency in man. *Ophthalmic Physiol Opt*. **17**, 421–426.
4 Abelson MB and Holly FJ (1977). A tentative mechanism for inferior punctate keratopathy. *Am J Ophthalmol*. **83**, 866–870.
5 Carney LG and Hill RM (1982). The nature of normal blinking patterns. *Acta Ophthalmol (Copenh.)* **60**, 427–431.
6 Collins M, Heron H, Larsen R and Lindner R (1987). Blinking patterns in soft contact lens wearers can be altered with training. *Am J Optom Physiol Opt*. **64**, 100–103.
7 Tsubota K, Hata S and Okusawa Y (1996). Quantitative videographic analysis of blinking in normal subjects and patients with dry eye. *Arch Ophthalmol*. **114**, 715–720.
8 Yolton DP, Yolton RL, Lopez R, *et al.* (1994). The effects of gender and birth control pill use on spontaneous blink rates. *J Am Optom Assoc*. **65**, 763–770.
9 Volkmann F, Riggs L and Moore R (1980). Eyeblinks and visual suppression. *Science* **207**, 900–901.
10 Prause JU and Norn M (1987). Relation between blink frequency and break-up time? *Acta Ophthalmol (Copenh.)* **65**, 19–23.
11 Yap M (1991). Tear break-up time is related to blink frequency. *Acta Ophthalmol (Copenh.)* **69**, 92–97.
12 Bhatia RPS and Singh RK (1993). Tear film break-up time in contact lens wearers. *Ann Ophthalmol*. **25**, 334–338.
13 Tsubota K and Nakamori K (1995). Effects of ocular surface area and blink rate on tear dynamics. *Arch Ophthalmol*. **113**, 155–159.
14 Collins M, Seeto R and Campbell L (1989). Blinking and corneal sensitivity. *Acta Ophthalmol (Copenh.)* **67**, 525–530.
15 Hill RM and Carney LG (1984). The effects of hard lens wear on blinking behaviour. *Int Contact Lens Clin*. **11**, 242–246.
16 York M, Ong J and Robbins JC (1971). Variation in blink rate associated with contact lens wear and task difficulty. *Am J Optom Arch Am Acad Optom*. **48**, 461–469.
17 Brown M, Chinn S and Fatt I (1973). The effect of soft and hard contact lenses on blink rate, amplitude and length. *J Am Optom Assoc*. **44**, 254–258.
18 Carney LG and Hill RM (1984). Variation in blinking behaviour during soft lens wear. *Int Contact Lens Clin*. **11**, 250–254.
19 Guillon JP and Guillon M (1988). The status of the pre soft lens tear film during overnight wear. *Am J Optom Physiol Opt*. **65**, 40–45.
20 Guillon JP and Guillon M (1988). Pre-lens tear film characteristics of high *Dk* rigid gas permeable lenses. *Am J Optom Physiol Opt*. **65**, 73–77.
21 Holly FJ and Lemp MA (1977). Tear physiology and dry eyes. *Surv Ophthalmol*. **22**, 69–73.
22 Young G and Efron N (1991). Characteristics of the pre-lens tear film during hydrogel contact lens wear. *Ophthalmic Physiol Opt*. **11**, 53–58.

23 Ridder WH and Tomlinson A (1991). Blink-induced, temporal variations in contrast sensitivity. *Int Contact Lens Clin*. **18**, 231–237.
24 Tomlinson A, Ridder WH 3rd and Watanabe R (1994). Blink-induced variations in visual performance with toric soft contact lenses. *Optom Vis Sci*. **71**, 545–549.
25 Golding TR, Bruce AS, Gaterell LL, *et al.* (1995). Soft lens movement: Effect of blink rate on lens settling. *Acta Ophthalmol Scand*. **73**, 506–511.
26 Holden BA, Sweeney DF and Seger RG (1986). Epithelial erosions caused by thin high water contact lenses. *Clin Exp Optom*. **69**, 103–106.
27 Guillon JP, Guillon M and Malgouyres S (1990). Corneal desiccation staining with hydrogel lenses: Tear film and contact lens factors. *Ophthalmic Physiol Opt*. **10**, 343–348.
28 Cuklanz HD and Hill RM (1969). Oxygen requirements of corneal contact lens systems. *Am J Optom Arch Am Acad Optom*. **46**, 228–232.
29 Polse KA (1979). Tear flow under hydrogel contact lenses. *Invest Ophthalmol Vis Sci*. **18**, 409–413.
30 Paugh JR, Stapleton F, Keay L and Ho A (2001). Tear exchange under hydrogel contact lenses: Methodological considerations. *Invest Ophthalmol Vis Sci*. **42**, 2813–2820.
31 McNamara NA, Polse KA, Brand RJ, *et al.* (1999). Tear mixing under a soft contact lens: Effects of lens diameter. *Am J Ophthalmol*. **127**, 659–665.
32 Chauhan A and Radke CJ (2001). The role of fenestrations and channels on the transverse motion of a soft contact lens. *Optom Vis Sci*. **78**, 732–743.
33 Swarbrick HA and Holden BA (1987). Rigid gas permeable lens binding: Significance and contributing factors. *Am J Optom Physiol Opt*. **64**, 815–823.
34 Wilson G, O'Leary DJ and Holden BA (1989). Cell content of tears following overnight wear of a contact lens. *Curr Eye Res*. **8**, 329–335.
35 McGrogan L, Guillon M and Dilly N (1997). Post-lens particle exchange under hydrogel contact lenses – effect of contact lens characteristics. *Optom Vis Sci*. **74S**, 73.
36 Efron N and Carney LG (1981). Models of oxygen performance for the static, dynamic and closed lid wear of hydrogel contact lenses. *Aust J Optom*. **64**, 223–230.
37 Ang JH and Efron N (1990). Corneal hypoxia and hypercapnia during contact lens wear. *Optom Vis Sci*. **67**, 512–521.
38 Efron N and Fitzgerald JP (1996). Distribution of oxygen across the surface of the human cornea during soft contact lens wear. *Optom Vis Sci*. **73**, 659–665.
39 Korb D and Korb JE (1974). Fitting to achieve normal blinking and lid action. *Int Contact Lens Clin*. **1**, 57–61.
40 Jenkins MS, Rehkopf PG and Brown SI (1978). A simple device to improve blinking. *Am J Ophthalmol*. **85**, 869–872.
41 Sabau AS and Raad PE (1995). Blink-induced motion of a gas permeable contact lens. *Optom Vis Sci*. **72**, 378–386.

EYELID PTOSIS

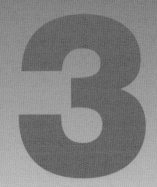

Contact lens practitioners routinely examine the tarsal conjunctiva and lid margins of their patients, but generally little attention is given to the overall integrity of the eyelids. Eyelid dysfunction, whether caused by contact lens wear or other factors, can pose a problem for contact lens wearers, because it could interfere with some of the important roles played by the eyelids.

This chapter concentrates on a condition that has received scant attention in the literature – contact lens induced ptosis (CLIP) of the eyelids. Ptosis is defined as "prolapse, abnormal depression, or falling down of an organ or part; applied especially to drooping of the upper eyelid".[1] Ptosis is not confined to the eyelids, so some authors prefer to use the more exact term 'blepharoptosis'. An assortment of other eyelid disorders that may be of relevance to contact lens wear is also considered here.

Perhaps CLIP is the only complication of contact lens wear for which surgical intervention is contemplated and occasionally executed (notwithstanding infectious keratitis associated with corneal ulceration, which sometimes requires hospitalization and can result in keratoplasty). It is for this reason that clinicians should have an appreciation of the typical manifestation of this condition, its likely causation, indications for surgery and other management options.

Signs

The classic appearance of ptosis is a narrowing of the palpebral fissure and a relatively large gap between the upper lid margin and the skin fold at the top of the eyelid (*Figure 3.1*). In a normal patient in the absence of ptosis, the skin fold at the top of the eyelid is only slightly higher than the upper eyelid margin. In some patients, these anatomic features can become virtually co-aligned toward the outer canthus.

It is possible to detect CLIP if:
- A patient reports that he or she detects a narrowing of the palpebral apertures;
- Palpebral aperture height is measured accurately on many occasions over time (to detect a trend);
- One eye is affected more than another.

As contact lenses are typically worn in both eyes, any narrowing of the palpebral apertures induced by contact lenses is expected to be bilateral. However, Kersten et al.[2] reported CLIP to be unilateral in 58% of a series of presenting patients. Unilateral CLIP can arise as a result of trauma related to lens handling, whereby the patient is more forceful with lens insertion and/or removal on either the right or left side. Unilateral CLIP can also result from uniocular lens wear, or the highly unusual scenario of wearing a different lens type in each eye

(i.e., rigid lens in one eye and a soft lens in the other eye).

Fonn and Holden[3,4] conducted a longitudinal trial designed to compare the ocular response to rigid and hydrogel contact lenses worn on an extended wear basis. The experimental protocol called for an interocular comparison; that is, a rigid lens was worn in one eye and a hydrogel lens in the other eye. It was observed that the palpebral aperture of the eye that wore the rigid lens was noticeably narrower than that in the eye fitted with the soft lens in 77% of the 40 subjects who participated in the trial[4] (*Figure 3.1*).

Severity

Various studies have quantified the extent of palpebral aperture closure that results from various modalities of contact lens wear. Fonn et al.[5] measured the palpebral aperture size (PAS) to be 10.10 ± 1.11 mm in non-wearers, 10.24 ± 0.94 mm in soft lens wearers and 9.76 ± 0.99 mm in rigid lens wearers. The difference in PAS between the rigid lens wearers and soft lens wearers (0.48 mm), and between the rigid lens wearers and non-lens wearers (0.34 mm), was statistically significant, but there was no significant difference in PAS between soft lens wearers and non-wearers (0.14 mm). The rigid lens wearers had been wearing lenses for 11.6 ± 8.4 years and the soft lens wearers for

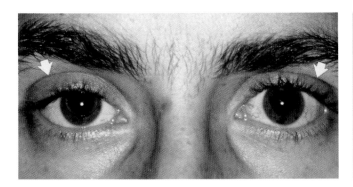

Figure 3.1
Unilateral right eye ptosis induced by rigid lens extended wear approximately 4 weeks after initiating wear. The left eye was wearing a soft lens as part of a research experiment. The skin folds, which are used as the reference point to assess the degree of ptosis, are indicated by the white arrows

8.2 ± 5.5 years. No gender difference in the development of CLIP was noted.

A similar study to that described above, by van den Bosch and Lemij,[6] found that the upper lid had lowered by 0.5 mm in a group of patients who had been wearing rigid lenses for an average of 16.3 years. The reason for a greater amount of ptosis in this study (versus that of Fonn *et al.*[5]) may be attributed to the greater lens wearing experience of the subjects examined (16.3 versus 11.6 years), although Fonn *et al.*[5] noted no such relationship within their own subject group. The position of the lower lid was unaltered by rigid lens wear.[6]

Time course of onset

Fonn and Holden[4] monitored the time course of onset of CLIP in 17 subjects who wore a soft lens in one eye and a rigid lens in the other. In the eye that wore the rigid lens, maximum ptosis (12% closure) was observed between 4 and 6 weeks after commencing lens wear; this was followed by a relative lessening of the ptosis to a point at which the PAS was 3% smaller compared with baseline after 13 weeks (*Figure 3.2*). The PAS remained fairly stable in the eye that wore the soft lens for the first 7 weeks, but paradoxically began to increase thereafter to be 7% wider compared with baseline after 13

weeks. (Apparent widening of the palpebral aperture as a result of soft lens wear is discussed later in this chapter.)

In the longer term, the pattern of onset can be variable. In one study,[6] all but two of 17 patients who presented to a clinic complaining of CLIP reported that the condition had developed gradually over the previous 12–24 months; most of these patients could illustrate this with photographs.[6] The other two patients in this study noted that the ptosis had existed for 6 and 16 years, respectively, and had gradually become worse.

Symptoms

Based on their observation of 17 patients who presented to a clinic complaining of advanced CLIP, van den Bosch and Lemij[6] demonstrated that this is a condition that generally is noticed by patients. No associated signs or symptoms were noted in any of these patients.

It is also interesting that, in prospective studies of palpebral aperture height in asymptomatic contact lens wearers,[5,6] none of the patients deemed to be suffering from CLIP were aware that they had this condition.

Prevalence

Ptosis is defined by van den Bosch and Lemij[6] as a situation in which the distance between the center of the pupil and the lower margin of the upper lid is less than 2.8 mm. Using this criterion, these authors determined that the prevalence of ptosis in a group of 46 rigid contact lens wearers who presented consecutively was 11%, versus 1% in a control group of non-lens wearers. Jupiter and Karesh[7] reported the prevalence of ptosis in a population of rigid lens wearers to be 4.7%. Kersten *et al.*[2] noted contact lens wear to be the only identifiable cause of acquired ptosis in 47% of a series of 91 patients between the ages of 15 and 50 years with this condition between April 1986 and May 1994.

Pathology

There is general agreement that the pathologic basis of CLIP is either edema that leads to lid swelling, or disinsertion, dehiscence (splitting), thinning or lengthening of the levator aponeurosis.[2,6,8] The relatively large gap between the upper lid margin and the skin fold at the top of the eyelid described above (also referred to as a 'high skin crease') develops because the posterior fibers of the levator aponeurosis on the tarsal plate disinsert, split or lengthen, while the anterior insertion of the levator aponeurosis into the orbicularis muscle and skin remains intact.[6] Thinning of the eyelid is also observed sometimes.

Etiology

A number of mechanisms have been advanced as possible causes of CLIP. These can be categorized broadly into aponeurogenic (i.e., involving some form of dysfunction of the aponeurosis) and non-aponeurogenic causes.

Aponeurogenic causes of ptosis induced by contact lenses

Forced lid squeezing
The unnatural 'forced blink' rigid lens removal technique places simultaneous, although antagonistic, forces on the orbucularis and levator muscles. Rigid lens wearers are instructed to open their eyes widely while executing a powerful blink, so both the levator and orbicularis

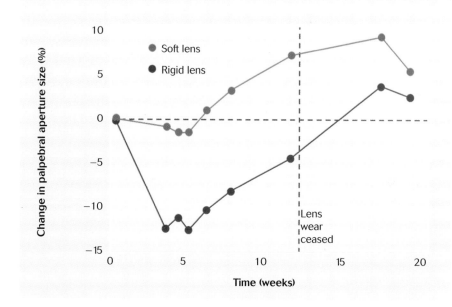

Figure 3.2
Changes in palpebral aperture size (%) over 13 weeks of extended wear of a rigid lens in one eye and a soft lens in the other eye, and 7 weeks recovery (adapted from Fonn and Holden[4])

muscles attempt to contract at the same time. The opposed actions of these two muscles might cause increased traction on the levator aponeurosis, which leads to disinsertion or dehiscence.[9]

Lateral eyelid stretching
To effect rigid lens removal, patients are often instructed to pull firmly on the outer canthus to create increased tension in the eyelids so that a greater leverage force is produced to enable the lens to be blinked out of the eye. Although this action primarily may lead (if anything) to a disinsertion or dehiscence of the lateral canthal ligament or the medial canthal tendon, it should not by itself lead to a disinsertion or dehiscence from the levator aponeurosis.[6] However, in combination with the antagonistic contraction of the orbucularis and levator muscles during forced blink removal described above, stretching or thinning of the levator aponeurosis cannot be discounted.

Consideration of the above two etiologic factors – forced lid squeezing and lateral eyelid stretching – leads to the disturbing conclusion that actions undertaken by both practitioners and patients may be responsible for CLIP in some cases. This conclusion is supported by the report of five cases of CLIP by Epstein and Putterman,[9] who observed that two of these cases developed directly after the patients were fitted with rigid lenses. The ptosis in these two patients did not resolve after cessation of lens wear.

Rigid lens displacement of tarsus
During repeated attempts to remove a rigid lens, the lid occasionally is pulled across the lens, which in turn exerts pressure on the palpebral conjunctiva. This unnatural pressure against the palpebral conjunctiva, effectively in an anterior direction against the posterior surface of the lid, could be directed against the levator aponeurosis, especially if the lens has migrated a little superiorly. This, in turn, could lead to disinsertion, dehiscence and/or thinning of the aponeurosis.[6]

Blink-induced lens rubbing
It has been argued by van den Bosch and Lemij[6] that every blink made during the regular wearing of a rigid lens causes the lens to rub against the eyelid structures, albeit less forcefully than during lens insertion and removal. This chronic rubbing and displacement of the lid away from the globe by the lens may cause a gradual thinning and stretching of the levator aponeurosis. Thus, the way in which the lens is fitted, and the size, thickness and positioning of the lens, may have a bearing on CLIP.

Non-aponeurogenic causes of ptosis induced by contact lenses

Edema
Constant physical irritation of any tissue in the body can result in a mild, subclinical inflammatory status and subsequent edema.[3–5] Thus, constant rubbing of a rigid lens against the tarsal conjunctiva is a possible cause of ptosis. Specifically, edema could lead to ptosis through a physical enlargement of the eyelid in all dimensions (including a downward displacement) as the lid absorbs increased levels of fluid. The increased mass of the edematous upper lid, combined with the effects of gravity, may cause a lowering of the lid (*Figure 3.3*).

Ptosis induced by a rigid lens in the right eye of a patient who also wore a soft lens in the left eye (as part of a research study) is shown in *Figure 3.3*. The region above and below the upper skin fold of the right eye appears slightly edematous, which suggests that edema from mechanical lens rubbing is the cause of the ptosis in this eye.

Blepharospasm
Rigid lenses are intrinsically uncomfortable, especially during the adaptation phase of lens wear. Discomfort is caused primarily by buffeting of the lens edge against the lid margins. Involuntary narrowing of the palpebral aperture (blepharospasm) is often adopted as a mechanism to stabilize the lens and prevent lens-lid buffeting. Blepharospasm is, therefore, another possible explanation of CLIP. Chronic involuntary blepharospasm may strain the levator muscle or cause, in turn, a higher tonus of the levator muscle. However, van den Bosch and Lemij[6] discount this mechanism as an important etiologic factor in CLIP because the lower lid – which is expected to adopt a slightly higher position as a result of blepharospasm – is unaffected by rigid lens wear.

Papillary conjunctivitis
Severe (grade 4) papillary conjunctivitis induced by a contact lens can be associated with excessive inflammation and edema of the eyelids, which can cause lid swelling and drooping.[10] Since papillary conjunctivitis typically manifests bilaterally, a bilateral CLIP results.[11] This situation is more prevalent in soft lens wearers. Papillary conjunctivitis also occurs in association with rigid lens wear, but it is rarely more severe than grade 2.

Patient Management

A key diagnostic criterion in deciding on an appropriate course of action to alleviate CLIP is to determine whether the CLIP is caused by:
- Aponeurogenic disorders, such as disinsertion, dehiscence or thinning of the aponeurosis;
- Non-aponeurogenic disorders, such as edema or involuntary blepharospasm;
- Papillary conjunctivitis induced by a contact lens.

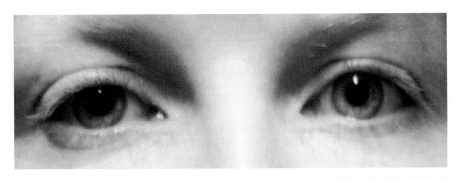

Figure 3.3
Apparent lid edema induced by a rigid lens in the region above and below the upper skin fold of the right eye, which led to ptosis. The left eye was wearing a soft lens as part of a research trial

To differentiate between these possible causes, patients who demonstrate CLIP should be required to cease lens wear for at least 1 month (to detect any trends toward recovery) and perhaps for as long as 3 months (to demonstrate complete resolution).

If the CLIP partially or completely resolves after ceasing lens wear for 1 month, the cause is lid edema and/or involuntary blepharospasm. The decision as to whether action needs to be taken is based largely on cosmetic considerations, although a severe ptosis can also interfere with vision if the lid wholly or partially covers the pupil. If the extent of ptosis is cosmetically unsightly, or it is more prominent in one eye with a noticeable asymmetry in PAS, the patient may need to be refitted with soft lenses (which do not induce ptosis).

The eyelids should also be inverted to determine if papillary conjunctivitis is involved and, if so, appropriate action should be taken to alleviate that condition. If the ptosis persists after resolution of the papillary conjunctivitis, it is likely that the aponeurosis has also been damaged by lens wear.

Surgical correction

If the CLIP does not resolve after ceasing lens wear for 1 month, the most likely cause is damage to the aponeurosis. Surgical correction is the preferred option in such cases.[12] The typical procedure is to reinsert the levator aponeurosis on the anterior surface of the tarsal plate under general anesthesia and reconstruct the skin crease. This procedure was carried out successfully by van den Bosch and Lemij[6] in a series of 10 patients who had developed ptosis as a result of rigid lens wear. After surgery, patients should not be refitted with rigid contact lenses – the obvious remaining alternatives being soft contact lenses, spectacles or refractive surgery.

A fascinating report by Levy and Stamper[13] reinforces the importance of observing the eyes after a prolonged period of cessation of lens wear to exclude non-aponeurogenic causes of CLIP. They reported the case of a rigid lens wearer who received extracapsular cataract surgery in the right eye. After surgery, the right eye was emmetropic and the patient continued to wear a rigid lens in the left eye. However, as a result of the surgery, the right eyelid was edematous and the palpebral aperture of that eye was the same as in the left

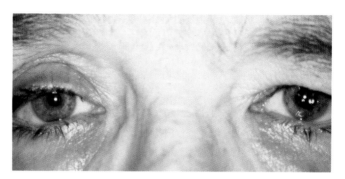

Figure 3.4
Ptosis in the right eye caused by rigid lens wear in that eye. The left eye was emmetropic (because of an intraocular lens) and did not require a contact lens

eye, which was also reduced because of the pre-existence of CLIP. At 8 weeks after surgery, the patient presented with an apparent ptosis of the lens-wearing (left) eye. The PAS was 12 mm in the right eye and 8 mm in the left eye.

Lid surgery was contemplated, but as a precaution the surgeon advised cessation of lens wear for a period to determine if the lens was the cause. The difference in PAS halved within 1 month and disappeared after 3 months. Surgery was therefore not performed.

Figure 3.4 illustrates the above point; it depicts the case of patient who was fitted with an intraocular lens to the left eye. The ametropic right eye was fitted with a rigid lens and displays an obvious ptosis.

Non-surgical management

Management strategies are available for patients with severe CLIP who do not wish to undergo lid surgery. The patient may be fitted with a 'ptosis crutch', 'ptosis prop' or 'ptosis lugs'.[14] This is a scleral lens that has either a cemented ledge or lugs fixed to the front surface, and/or a shelf cut into the front surface of the lens. In both cases, the lower border of the upper lid rests on the ledge or shelf, and thus keeps the eyelid open to the desired extent.

Figure 3.5 depicts the case of a blind eye with an inoperable ptosis that was fitted with an impression scleral prosthetic moulded shell with a superior shelf and ptosis crutch legs. In this picture, the lid appears to be supported more by the left lug, and the shelf (the white line that connects the two lugs) appears to be displaced from the upper lid margin. This appliance has been worn successfully for 10 years.

This approach in a patient with CLIP constitutes something of a paradox, because the patient is being fitted with a scleral lens – which can be considered to

be an extreme form of rigid lens – which was the likely cause of the problem in the first place. That is, the scleral lens with ptosis crutch may perpetuate or even exacerbate the very problem it is supposedly curing.

Other options for non-surgical correction of CLIP include:

- Instruct the patient to periodically raise the ptotic lid with his or her finger and rely on residual tone to keep the lid open for a period of time thereafter;
- Employ a spectacle frame-mounted lid prop;
- Attach one end of a small piece of surgical tape to the eyelid just above the lashes and the other end to the smooth skin below the eyebrow.

Prognosis

The prognosis for recovery from aponeurogenic CLIP is poor; the condition can be reversed only by surgical correction or other management options, as described above.

The prognosis for recovery from non-aponeurogenic CLIP is good. If the cause of ptosis is papillary conjunctivitis, the time course of resolution of the

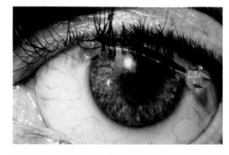

Figure 3.5
Scleral lens with ptosis lugs and shelf

ptosis parallels that for the recovery of the papillary conjunctivitis. A noticeable diminution of ptosis associated with a reduction of the severity of papillary conjunctivitis from grade 4 to grade 1 or 2 takes between 4 and 8 weeks.

According to Fonn and Holden,[4] complete resolution of non-aponeurogenic CLIP occurs within 6 weeks. In severe cases, resolution may take as long as 3 months.[13]

Differential Diagnosis

If a contact lens wearer presents with ptosis, other possible causes of this condition must be considered so that the appropriate course of management can be adopted.

Aponeurogenic ptosis

Any ptosis caused by disinsertion, dehiscence, thinning or lengthening of the levator aponeurosis can be referred to as aponeurogenic ptosis, of which there are two categories based on etiology – traumatic and involutional.

Surgery is the most common cause of traumatic aponeurogenic ptosis; specifically, damage to the levator aponeurosis can be caused by traction on the eyelids during surgery or by clumsy attempts of the patient to remove a patch over the eye after surgery. Trauma induced by forceful rigid lens removal and the chronic presence of a rigid lens are other possible causes of traumatic aponeurogenic ptosis.

Involutional aponeurogenic ptosis describes the process of damage to the levator aponeurosis caused by aging. Ocular inflammation and corticosteroid use can exacerbate this condition.[6]

The age profile of patients who presented with aponeurogenic ptosis induced by a contact lens was compared by van den Bosch and Lemij[6] with that of a patients who presented to the same clinic with involutional aponeurogenic ptosis. The age range was 18–56 years (mean 38.5 years) in the lens-wearing group and 48–88 years (mean 69 years) in the group with involutional aponeurogenic ptosis. Thus, patient age provides an important clue as to the cause of aponeurogenic ptosis. By measuring lid and vertical eye saccades with electromagnetic search coils, Wouters et al.[15] were able to differentiate between congenital ptosis and aponeurogenic ptosis (involutional or induced by a rigid lens).

Non-aponeurogenic ptosis

Non-aponeurogenic causes of ptosis include:

- Neurogenic disease, such as pathway interruption or palsy of the third cranial nerve that supplies the levator, Horner's syndrome or Marcus Gunn sign;
- Myogenic disease, which may be congenital or acquired – examples of the latter are muscular dystrophy or myasthenia gravis;
- Edema after lid surgery;
- Edema caused by traumatic eye injury;
- Edema that results from prolonged wear of a rigid contact lens (as described in detail in this chapter);
- Contact lens embedded in an upper eyelid (see below);
- Chalazion;
- Tumor;
- Dermatochalasis;
- Blepharospasm, possibly caused by photophobia secondary to other ocular diseases;
- Vernal and giant papillary conjunctivitis;
- Forms or nervous disposition that lead to idiosyncratic partial eye closure.

Other Eyelid Disorders Associated with Contact Lenses

Increase in palpebral aperture size

Hori-Komai et al.[16] reported the preoperative and post-operative palpebral fissure width in eyes that underwent laser in situ keratomileusis. In patients who had previously worn rigid lenses, PAS increased from 7.6 ± 1.6 mm before surgery to 8.7 ± 1.2 mm after surgery. In patients who had not worn lenses previously, PAS increased from 7.7 ± 1.9 mm before surgery to 8.9 ± 1.9 mm after surgery. The post-surgical increase in PAS in the rigid lens group could be attributed to a resolution of previous lens-induced ptosis; however, the reason for the increase in the control group is unclear.

Mutti and Seger[17] noted – in two unilateral soft lens wearers – a relative ptosis of 19% in the contralateral eyes that did not wear lenses. As these authors had no baseline data, they were unsure whether this appearance resulted from a widening of the palpebral aperture of the lens-wearing eye or a narrowing of the palpebral aperture of the eye that wore no lens.

Interestingly, Fonn and Holden[4] observed an 8% widening of the PAS in eyes that wore soft lenses, but failed to validate their data statistically. Fonn et al.[5] noted that the PAS of soft lens wearers was 1.4% greater than that of controls, but statistical analysis failed to reveal a significant difference.

Although widening of PAS induced by soft lenses can only be considered an anecdotal observation at the present time, it is interesting to speculate as to a possible cause. Mutti and Seger[17] tentatively attributed this phenomenon to neural feedback from stimulation of the lid by the lens edge and/or lens mass, which results in an increased reflex tonus of the levator or Müller's muscle, and thus causes a slight raising of the eyelid.

Embedded lens

Cases of rigid lenses becoming 'lost' and in some cases embedded in the upper palpebral conjunctiva were reported as early as 1963.[18,19] Since then, numerous accounts of similar occurrences have been published.[20–28] In the majority of these cases, the patient presents complaining of an otherwise 'quiet' lump in the upper lid, which can be misdiagnosed as a chalazion.[20–22] Jahn[20] reported the case of a 41-year-old female patient who had lost a rigid lens 12 months prior to noticing a lump in her left eye. She failed to associate the previously lost lens with the lid lump. The condition was diagnosed as chalazion and, to the great surprise of the surgeon a lens was extracted from the lump during surgical treatment of the 'chalazion'.

In two cases,[23,24] the embedded lens was inverted; that is, the convex surface of the lens faced the globe. Jones and Hassan[23] suggest that this inversion leads to greater mechanical irritation (compared with a non-inverted lens) and is a predominant factor in reducing the time taken for distressing symptoms to occur. They also suggest[23] that if the lens does not invert, deeper migration into a pretarsal or even orbital location[25] is more likely. Excessive lid swelling as a result of a lost[27] or embedded[26] lens can also give the appearance of ptosis in the affected eye.

Perhaps the most astonishing case of 'lost lenses' that re-appear later in the upper lid is that reported by Kelly.[28] A female patient reported that she had lost a lens and thought that it was still in her eye. A mucus-coated pellet was removed from beneath the upper eyelid, with a well-defined depression left on the upper globe. On further questioning, the patient reported she had lost, and subsequently re-ordered, a number of lenses over the previous 3 months, having reported to other clinicians that she thought a lens was in her eye (with nothing being found). The mucus-coated pellet removed from her eye was found to consist of eight PMMA lenses and one rigid gas permeable lens. The lessons to be learned from such a case are self-evident.

Ectropion

Ectropion is an outward turning of the eyelid from the globe, and is associated frequently with epiphora and chronic conjunctivitis. Four types of ectropion can be defined:[29]

- *Involutional* – senile change;
- *Cicatrical* – caused by scarring and contracture of the skin and underlying tissue, which pulls the eyelid away from the globe;
- *Congenital* – rare and typically associated with blepharophimosis syndrome;
- *Paralytic* – typically caused by a facial nerve palsy.[29]

The implications of ectropion in contact lens wearers is that the lower lid cannot be relied upon to help position the lens; that is, both rigid and soft lenses may mislocate inferiorly in an ectropic eye. An ectropic eyelid has a reduced effectiveness in cases where the lower lid is required for lid-assisted lens translation (e.g., alternating vision bifocals) or location (e.g., truncated toric lens). In addition, an eye with an ectropic eyelid may tend to be relatively dry because of an excessive rate of loss of tears.

Entropion

Entropion is an inversion of the eyelid toward the globe, and usually causes discomfort through rubbing of the eyelashes against the cornea. This phenomenon is known as pseudotrichiasis and should not be confused with 'true' trichiasis, which is an actual ingrowth of the lashes from an otherwise normal lid margin.

Four types of entropion can be defined:[29]

- *Involutional* – senile change;
- *Cicatrical* – caused by scarring and contracture of the palpebral conjunctiva, which pulls the eyelid toward the globe; this condition can

be caused by cicatrical pemphigoid, Stevens–Johnson syndrome, trachoma and chemical burns, and can involve the upper and lower lids;

- *Congenital* – rare, but can be dealt with surgically;
- *Acute spastic* – caused by spasm of the orbicularis that arises from ocular irritation; this condition typically resolves with removal of the irritation.[29]

An important implication of entropion in contact lens wearers is that the lower lid may interfere with correct lens positioning. An entropic eyelid with associated pseudotrichiasis can lead to corneal irritation; as an interim measure, soft contact lenses can be fitted to protect the cornea.

A pseudo-entropion can arise as a result of pressure on the eyelids from external forces. An example of such a case is shown in *Figure 3.6*; the lower lid has been temporarily folded inward because a scleral lens of insufficient diameter was fitted.

Lagophthalmos

Lagophthalmos refers to incomplete eyelid closure, and can result from a number of factors, such as facial nerve lesions, orbicularis weakness, ectropion or mechanical displacement caused by tumors. This condition can lead to corneal exposure and consequent keratitis. A soft lens provides protection, although lenses can fall out of the eye if the lagophthalmos is severe. In such cases, partial tarsorrhaphy or temporary taping together of the eyelids is indicated.

Rigid lenses are problematic because they do not completely cover the cornea. This can lead to corneal desiccation outside the lens edge, typically in the 3 and 9 o'clock positions.[29]

Nocturnal lagophthalmos (partial eye opening during sleep) is an anatomic variant in the normal human population; indeed, it occurs in 23% of the population.[30] Excessive 3 and 9 o'clock staining in some patients who sleep in rigid lenses could be explained by the presence of nocturnal lagophthalmos.

Rigid lens 'bridging'

Contact lenses act to displace the eyelids away from the globe. This action has been implicated in the etiology of traumatic aponeurogenic ptosis in rigid lens wear because of the greater displacement caused by such lenses. Rigid lenses also cause a 'bridging' of the tarsal conjunctiva away from the corneal surface at the lens edge, which is thought to be of etiologic significance in the development of 3 and 9 o'clock corneal staining. The areas of cornea immediately adjacent to the lens edge, especially at the 3 and 9 o'clock positions, are prone to dry out because these regions are not re-wetted by the passage of the eyelid against the eyeball.

Absence of eyelid

The destruction of an eyelid because of a tumor or other disease is a potentially blinding situation. The reason for one of the first recorded contact lens fittings (by a Dr Sämisch in Germany) was for a patient whose lower eyelid in one eye was destroyed completely as a result of carcinoma. The upper lid of this eye was partially missing, with the remaining portion thickened and entropic.[31] (Contact lens historians point out that, technically, a contact 'shell' was fitted, rather than a 'lens', because it had no power.[32]) The other eye was totally blind. The patient obtained useful vision with the aid of this prosthetic device,

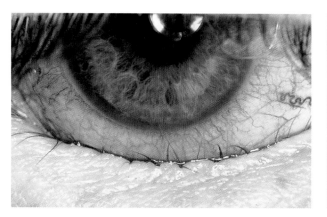

Figure 3.6

Pseudo-entropion caused by the fitting of a scleral lens of insufficient diameter which was worn continually day and night without ever removing it for over 20 years until he died.

Lids as a Lens-Positioning Tool

The eyelids are employed in a variety of ways to stabilize, position and translocate contact lenses to achieve various fitting and optical objectives. A detailed analysis of these strategies is beyond the scope of this book, but they are listed below so as to provide a clue to solving eyelid problems related to contact lenses that may have a direct bearing on lens performance.

Specifically, the eyelids are employed to:
- Move the lens with each blink so as to effect an exchange between the tears beneath the lens and the remaining tears on the ocular surface, which serves to remove particulate matter from beneath the lens, to facilitate corneal oxygenation and to prevent build-up of carbon dioxide beneath the lens;
- Continually re-wet the front surface of the lens with each blink;
- Position truncated rigid and soft toric lenses;
- Squeeze the 'thin zones' of toric lenses against the globe to provide correct lens orientation;
- Position rigid lenses by way of 'lid attachment' or 'interpalpebral' fitting philosophies;
- Translate alternating vision bifocals across the cornea so as to align the appropriate portion of the lens over the pupil.

Deformities or swelling of the eyelids, such as scarring of the lid margins (*Figure 3.7*) or swellings of the palpebral conjunctiva (*Figure 3.8*) can interfere with lid-mediated positioning of contact lenses.

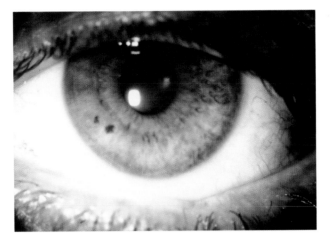

Figure 3.7
Distortion of the lower lid margin caused by scarring of the inferior palpebral conjunctiva, which may adversely affect lens positioning

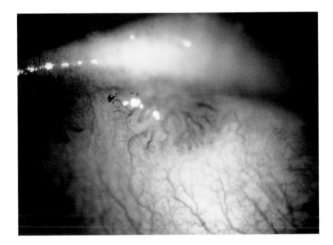

Figure 3.8
Mass of vascularized edematous tissue adjacent to the lid margin of a soft lens wearer, which could lead to lens mislocation

REFERENCES

1 Osol A (1973). *Blakiston's Pocket Medical Dictionary*. (New York: McGraw-Hill).
2 Kersten RC, de Conciliis C and Kulwin DR (1995). Acquired ptosis in the young and middle-aged adult population. *Ophthalmology* **102**, 924–928.
3 Fonn D and Holden BA (1986). Extended wear of hard gas permeable contact lenses can induce ptosis. *Contact Lens Assoc Ophthalmol J.* **12**, 93–97.
4 Fonn D and Holden BA (1988). Rigid gas-permeable vs. hydrogel contact lenses for extended wear. *Am J Optom Physiol Opt.* **65**, 536–542.

5 Fonn D, Pritchard N, Garnett B and Davids L (1996). Palpebral aperture sizes of rigid and soft contact lens wearers compared with nonwearers. *Optom Vis Sci.* **73**, 211–214.
6 van den Bosch WA and Lemij HG (1992). Blepharoptosis induced by prolonged hard contact lens wear. *Ophthalmology* **99**, 1759–1765.
7 Jupiter D and Karesh J (1999). Ptosis associated with PMMA/rigid gas permeable contact lens wear. *CLAO J.* **25**, 159–162.
8 Fujiwara T, Matsuo K, Kondoh S and Yuzuriha S (2001). Etiology and pathogenesis of aponeurotic blepharoptosis. *Ann Plast Surg.* **46**, 29–35.
9 Epstein G and Putterman AM (1981). Acquired blepharoptosis secondary to contact-lens wear. *Am J Ophthalmol.* **91**, 634–639.
10 Sheldon L, Biedner B, Geltman C and Sachs U (1979). Giant papillary conjunctivitis and ptosis in a contact lens wearer. *J Pediatr Ophthalmol Strabismus* **16**, 136–137.
11 Molinari JF (1983). Transient ptosis secondary to giant papillary conjunctivitis in a hydrogel lens patient. *J Am Optom Assoc.* **54**, 1007–1009.
12 Uchinuma E, Torikai K, Shioya N and Mukuno K (1983). Repair of ptosis possibly attributable to the long-term wearing of a contact lens. *Ann Plast Surg.* **11**, 252–254.

13 Levy B and Stamper RL (1992). Acute ptosis secondary to contact lens wear. *Optom Vis Sci.* **69**, 565–566.
14 Trodd TC (1971). Ptosis props in ocular myopathy. *Contact Lens Assoc Ophthalmol J.* **3**, 3–7.
15 Wouters RJ, van den Bosch WA, Mulder PG and Lemij HG (2001). Upper eyelid motility in blepharoptosis and in the aging eyelid. *Invest Ophthalmol Vis Sci.* **42**, 620–625.
16 Hori-Komai Y, Toda I and Tsubota K (2001). Laser *in situ* keratomileusis: Association with increased width of palpebral fissure. *Am J Ophthalmol.* **131**, 254–255.
17 Mutti DO and Seger RG (1988). Eyelid asymmetry in unilateral hydrogel contact lens wear. *Int Contact Lens Clin.* **15**, 252–253.
18 Green WR (1963). An embedded ('lost') contact lens. *Arch Ophthalmol.* **69**, 23–24.
19 Long JC (1963). Retention of contact lens in upper fornix. *Am J Ophthalmol.* **56**, 309–310.
20 Jahn D (1992). 'Pseudochalazion' due to a 'lost' contact lens. *Contactologia* **14**, 96–98.
21 Richter S, Sherman J and Horn D (1979). An embedded contact lens in the upper lid masquerading as a mass. *J Am Optom Assoc.* **50**, 372–373.
22 Jones D, Livesey S and Wilkins P (1987). Hard contact lens migration into the upper lid: An unexpected lid lump. *Br J Ophthalmol.* **71**, 368–370.

23 Jones D and Hassan HM (1987). Embedding of an inverted hard contact lens. *Am J Optom Physiol Opt.* **64**, 879–880.

24 Smalling OH (1971). Embedment of inverted corneal contact lens. *J Am Optom Assoc.* **42**, 755–758.

25 Nicolitz E and Flanagan JC (1978). Orbital mass as a complication of contact lens wear. *Arch Ophthalmol.* **96**, 2238–2239.

26 Yassin JG, White RH and Shannon GM (1970). Blepharoptosis as a complication of contact lens migration. *Am J Ophthalmol.* **70**, 536–537.

27 Patel NP, Savino PJ and Weinberg DA (1998). Unilateral eyelid ptosis and a red eye. *Surv Ophthalmol.* **43**, 182–187.

28 Kelly JM (1994). Contact lens build up (letter). *Optician* **207**(5437)**,** 13.

29 Kanski JJ (1999). *Clinical Ophthalmology*, Fourth Edition. (Oxford: Butterworth–Heinemann).

30 Howitt DA and Goldstein JH (1969). Physiologic lagophthalmos. *Am J Ophthalmol.* **68**, 355–356.

31 Müller FA and Müller AC (1910). *Das Künstliche Auge*. (Wiesbaden: JF Bergmann).

32 Efron N and Pearson RM (1988). Centenary celebration of Fick's Eine Contactbrille. *Arch Ophthalmol.* **106**, 1370–1377.

MEIBOMIAN GLAND DYSFUNCTION

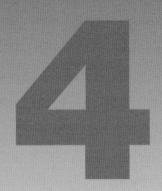

The meibomian glands in the upper and lower eyelids play a critical role in forming and maintaining a viable tear film. Specifically, these glands produce a clear, oily secretion that serves two main functions:

- To form a hydrophobic lining along the lid margins, which prevents epiphora;
- To form a thin lipid layer over the surface of the aqueous tear phase, which retards evaporative fluid loss.

There are approximately 25 meibomian glands in the upper eyelid and 20 meibomian glands in the lower eyelid, and the distribution of meibomian glands from inner to outer canthus is approximately uniform. The small orifices of the central canals of the meibomian glands open on the margin of the lid just in front of the mucocutaneous junction (*Figure 4.1*).

Meibomian gland dysfunction (MGD; *Figure 4.2*) may be defined as a bilateral non-inflammatory clinical condition in which there is a change in the lipid appearance from a normally clear state to a viscous and cloudy appearance, without any clinically observable meibomian gland abnormalities. However, some authors have adopted classification

systems and definitions that suggest an infectious and/or inflammatory etiology. For example, Bron *et al.*[1] offer the following definition of MGD: "... an infection of the meibomian gland without necessarily implying that inflammation is present". Wilhelmus[2] contends that MGD can also be termed 'posterior blepharitis'.

Although Wilhelmus[2] is correct in observing that meibomian gland secretions may be abnormal in posterior forms of seborrheic blepharitis, it is best to consider posterior blepharitis (an inflammatory condition) as a separate condition from MGD, which has a non-inflammatory etiology. This view is shared by Ong,[3] who notes that many patients with MGD seen in primary eye care clinics are free of signs or symptoms of lid margin inflammation.

The question as to whether the relationship between MGD and contact lens wear is causal or casual has been investigated by Ong.[3] The eyes of 81 contact lens wearers and 150 age- and sex-matched non-lens wearers were examined for evidence of MGD. The prevalence of MGD was 49% among the contact lens wearers and 39% among the

controls; this difference was not statistically significant, which suggests that contact lens wear is not a cause of MGD.

Although contact lens wear cannot be considered a cause of MGD, many problems that relate to contact lens wear can be traced to problems in tear film function; it is in this regard that MGD can be of etiologic significance. Such problems are considered under the heading 'contact lens-associated meibomian gland dysfunction' (CL-MGD). This chapter reviews the clinical ramifications of CL-MGD, and concludes with a brief examination of the implications for contact lens wear in association with other abnormalities of the meibomian gland.

Prevalence

According to Ong and Larke,[4] 20% of non-wearers of contact lenses show some loss of clarity of expressed meibomian oils, and opaque oils can be expressed from 6% of non-wearers of contact lenses. These figures rise to 30% and 11%, respectively, in contact lens wearers. Among contact lens wearers, about 10% of patients who complain of blurred vision and dryness can be demonstrated to have abnormal meibomian gland expressions.[4] The prevalence of MGD[5] and CL-MGD[4] is unrelated to gender.

Stanek[6] evaluated the lid and meibomian gland status of active-duty military forces (ADFs) and USA military veterans (USVs) to compare the prevalence of lid dysfunction and disease in each population. One examiner observed 113 consecutive patients in both groups during a 2 week period at two federal service optometry clinics. All eyes were graded with regard to negative findings (or normal), MGD and/or meibomitis from an established criterion. Stanek[6] reported that 90.3% of ADFs had normal lid findings, 5.3% had MGD (all contact lens patients) and 4.4% had

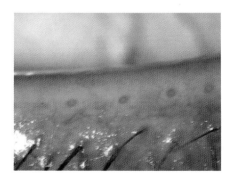

Figure 4.1
Normal meibomian gland orifices in the lower lid margin

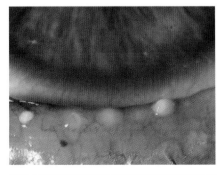

Figure 4.2
Inspissated secretion from meibomian glands in the lower lid of a contact lens wearer

meibomitis. In the USV group, 28.9% had normal findings and 71.1% had MGD or meibomitis (no patients wore

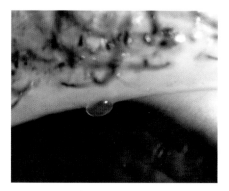

Figure 4.3
Clear secretion expressed from a normal meibomian gland in the upper lid

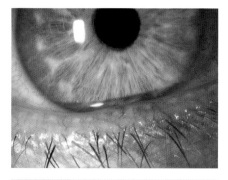

Figure 4.4
Enlargement and tortuosity of vessel and distortion of lid margin of a contact lens wearer. Blocked meibomian glands can be seen as intermittent, pale, slightly raised areas of tissue along the lid margin

contact lenses). These finding suggest an increased prevalence of MGD with age.

Hom *et al.*[5] conducted a survey of 398 normal patients who presented for a routine eye examination. Based on the principal clinical criterion of an absent or cloudy meibomian gland secretion upon expression, 39% were found to have MGD. The prevalence of MGD increased significantly with increasing age, in accordance with the finding of Stanek.[6] Hom *et al.*[5] reported that the prevalence of MGD was 41% among contact lens wearers and 38% among non-wearers. These figures broadly agree with those of Ong[3] of 49% and 39%, respectively, although Stanek[6] found a lower prevalence of MGD and/or meibomitis in young non-wearers (9.7%).

Signs and Symptoms

The oily secretion from the normal meibomian gland is generally clear (*Figure 4.3*). The key diagnostic feature of CL-MGD is a change in the appearance of the clear oil expressed from healthy meibomian glands to a cloudy creamy yellow oil (see *Figure 4.2*). This appearance is accompanied by symptoms of smeary vision, greasy lenses, dry eyes and reduced tolerance to lens wear. In severe cases, in which the meibomian orifices are blocked, gland secretion may be absent.

Long-standing cases of MGD may be associated with additional signs, such as irregularity, distortion and thickening of eyelid margins, slight distension of glands, mild to moderate papillary hypertrophy, vascular changes (*Figure 4.4*) and chronic

chalazia. The vascular changes have been described as neovascularization, but it is more likely in the majority of cases in which this change is observed that existing vessels have become distended and thus more visible

Of the 155 patients found to have MGD in the survey of Hom *et al.*,[5] 24 had blepharitis, four had chalazia and one meibomitis. None of the MGD-negative patients exhibited any of these conditions. Given that there is no difference in prevalence of MGD between contact lens wearers and non-wearers, these associated conditions are observed often in patients who wear contact lenses.

Examination of the lid margins using diffuse illumination at approximately ×20 magnification often reveals the presence of small oil globules at the orifices of the meibomian glands in patients who suffer from CL-MGD. The clarity of the secretion varies from a slight murkiness (*Figure 4.5*) to an almost opaque waxy milky yellow color (see *Figure 4.2*). Viewing the lid margins against the dark background of the pupil or against a dark-colored iris (see *Figure 4.3*) enhances the view of the expressed material.[7]

Frothing or foaming of the lower tear meniscus is sometimes observed in CL-MGD (*Figure 4.6*), especially toward the outer canthus.[4] This may arise from a lowering of the surface tension of the tear film because of an absent or abnormal lipid layer. The abnormal secretions may also result in the appearance of oily debris in the tear film (*Figure 4.7*).

The absence of oil globules at the meibomian gland orifices could indicate one of two extremes – normality or complete blockage. If oil globules are not

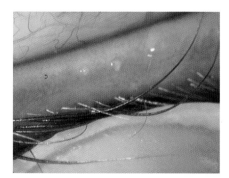

Figure 4.5
Slightly murky secretion expressed from a contact lens wearer with mild meibomian gland dysfunction

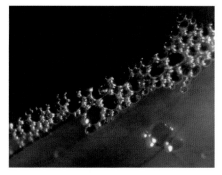

Figure 4.6
Frothing of the tear film

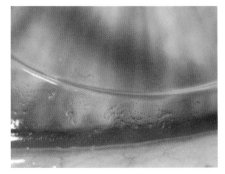

Figure 4.7
Oily debris in the tear film of a rigid contact lens wearer with meibomian gland dysfunction

observed on the lid margins of a symptomatic contact lens wearer, it may be necessary to conduct a provocative test to establish the state of health of the meibomian glands. This can be achieved by manual expression of the glands, so that the nature of the expressed oils can be assessed.

Meibomian gland expression is a simple and rapid provocative test that is only mildly uncomfortable for the patient. Anatomic considerations dictate that expression of the meibomian glands in the lower lid is the preferred procedure. The patient is instructed to gaze superiorly. In cases of mild meibomian orifice blockage, gentle pressure with the finger or thumb immediately below the lower lid margin, together with a slight rolling action of the finger or thumb toward the lid margin, generally results in the appearance of a small expression.

If nothing is expressed using the procedure described above, a more complete or even total meibomian blockage is indicated. In such cases, a support needs to be placed behind the lower lid margin so that increased pressure can be applied to force an expression of meibomian oils. This can be achieved by gently retracting the lower lid, placing a cotton-tipped bud behind the lid margin and firmly squeezing the lid margin between the cotton-tipped bud and thumb.

Sudden release of the blockage at high pressure can result in a copious expression in the form of a thick stream of apparently dehydrated material, akin to the result of forcefully squeezing a toothpaste tube; this is referred to as an 'inspissated' secretion. By careful observation and adopting the provocative tests described here, it is possible to grade the severity of CL-MGD using the grading scale for MGD presented in Appendix A.

Associated signs of CL-MGD include all those that arise from clinical diagnostic procedures designed to indicate the integrity or otherwise of the lipid layer. Specifically, patients who suffer from CL-MGD may display a reduced tear break-up time (measured either with fluorescein or non-invasively).[7] Examination of the tear layer in specular reflection using a tearscope may reveal a contaminated lipid pattern, which is exacerbated by the use of cosmetic eye make-up[8] (see Appendix B).

Tear ferning analysis is likely to reveal a disrupted pattern in the form of minimal ferning, which again indicates a

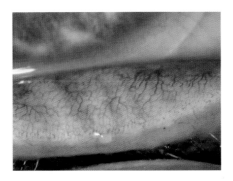

Figure 4.8

Distended meibomian glands in the lower lid

contaminated and poorly formed tear layer.[9] The presence of distended or distorted meibomian glands[10] confirms the diagnosis of CL-MGD (*Figure 4.8*); this appearance can be enhanced by transilluminating the lower lid during biomicroscopy.

Hope-Ross *et al.*[11] reported that in a series of 30 patients with recalcitrant recurrent corneal erosions, the prevalence of MGD was 100%. Marren[12] reported a statistically significant link between MGD, contact lens wear and corneal staining. These findings suggest that increased corneal staining (i.e., more than is typically observed in asymptomatic contact lens wearers) is associated with CL-MGD; however neither Hope-Ross *et al.*[11] nor Marren[12] could explain the basis for this link.

Pathology

Changes to both the ductal lining of the meibomian glands and the meibomian secretion in MGD have been reported in the literature. An increase in the turnover of epidermal epithelium around the orifices of the glands and an increase in the turnover of the epithelial lining of the ducts have been described; these changes can lead to mechanical clogging of the meibomian glands.[13,14] Blepharitis is frequently a secondary complication of MGD.[15]

Ong and Larke[4] failed to find any difference in the biochemical composition of meibomian secretions of contact lens wearers and non-wearers. They did, however, observe that abnormal meibomian oils began to melt at 35°C (versus 32°C for normal meibomian oils) and that the melting profile of abnormal meibomian oils comprised five or six

components (versus 5–12 components for normal meibomian oils). The results of this melting point analysis of meibomian secretions are consistent with the observation of a more free-flowing meibomian secretion in normals.

In a patient who wears contact lenses but does not suffer from MGD, the lipid layer is always separated from the lens surface by the aqueous phase of the tear layer. Some lipid can deposit on the lens surface – the magnitude and extent of this is determined in part by the polymeric nature of the lens material. Such lipid deposits are removed easily in practice using routine surfactant cleaning.

In CL-MGD, symptoms of blurred or greasy vision can probably be attributed to the adhesion of waxy dysfunctional meibomian oils to the surface of the contact lens, oils that are able to migrate more readily down to the lens surface as a result of the generally disrupted nature of the tear layer.[16]

As more lipid rapidly deposits on the lens, the surface becomes increasingly hydrophobic and is less able to sustain a continuous tear film. In addition, the abnormal and irregular lipid layer is less able to prevent evaporation of the aqueous tear fluid that covers the lens and the exposed anterior ocular structures. These factors combine to dehydrate the lens and to lead to a sensation of dryness; the association between hydrogel lens dehydration and dryness has been established by Efron and Brennan.[17]

Etiology

Some interesting, but largely unproved, theories have been advanced as to the cause of CL-MGD. Rengstorff[18] suggested that CL-MGD may be attributed to the fact that contact lens wearers rub their eyelids less frequently than non-wearers for fear of damaging or mechanically dislodging (and possibly losing) their lenses. This deprives the eyelid of the contact lens wearer of periodic rubbing, which (Rengstorff[18] claims) is essential to stimulate the meibomian glands mechanically so that they remain unblocked and free flowing.

This theory of Rengstorff[18] was tested by Marren,[12] who postulated that non-wearers of contact lenses who use eye make-up would be similarly reluctant to rub their eyes for fear of disrupting the make-up. However, no difference was found in the prevalence of MGD between those who wear eye make-up and those who do not.

An alternative 'eye rubbing' theory has been proposed to explain CL-MGD, but to the opposite effect. Various authors[19,20] have suggested an association between CL-MGD and contact lens induced papillary conjunctivitis (CLPC). Martin *et al.*[19] proposed that the itching created by CLPC stimulates eye rubbing which, rather than having a positive and stimulatory effect, as proposed by Rengstorff,[18] causes mechanical damage to the meibomian glands and consequent dysfunction.

Since there is no difference in the prevalence of MGD between contact lens wearers and non-wearers,[3,5] neither the meibomian stimulation theory of Rengstorff[18] nor the meibomian trauma theory of Martin *et al.*[19] can be supported.

From a tissue pathology standpoint, the cause of MGD is an increased keratinization of the epithelial walls of meibomian gland ducts.[13,14] This leads to the formation of keratinized epithelial plugs that form a physical blockage in meibomian ducts, which in turn restricts or prevents the outflow of meibomian oils (*Figure 4.9*). Increased levels of keratin proteins have been found in the meibomian oils of patients who suffer from MGD.[21] It is thought that the creamy yellow color of meibomian oils is a result of the presence of keratin proteins.

It is not known why some patients suffer from increased keratinization of the meibomian ducts, except to observe that it may be related to generalized systemic disorders; MGD is often observed in combination with seborrheic dermatitis and acne rosacea.

The increase in prevalence of MGD with age, as reported by Hom *et al.*,[5] may be because the overall gland width decreases with age,[22] presumably through a loss of gland acini. Other age-related factors that could lead to MGD include general morphologic changes[9] and orifice displacement[23] (*Figure 4.10*).

Patient Management

Although it is not possible to treat the underlying cause of MGD (epithelial keratinization of meibomian gland ducts and consequent contamination of meibomian oils with keratin proteins), it is possible to provide symptomatic relief by adopting one or more of the procedures described below, all of which should be undertaken with the contact lenses removed.

Warm compresses

Henriquez and Korb[24] advocated the use of warm compresses and lid scrubs to alleviate symptoms associated with CL-MGD. Cotton wool pads soaked in hot water (boiled water that has been allowed to cool for a few minutes) are massaged firmly against the closed eyelids. This procedure is intended to melt solidified lipids and thus unblock the meibomian orifices, to allow lipids to escape and reconstitute a trilaminate tear layer.

Lid scrubs

The maintenance of clean and healthy lid margins is likely to be of benefit by:
• Preventing additional debris from blocking the meibomian orifices;

• Lessening the probability of contamination of meibomian glands, which could result in infection.

The patient is advised to clean the lid margins each morning and evening by gently rubbing or 'scrubbing' with a clean facecloth pre-soaked in mildly soapy water.

Alternatively, a cotton-tipped bud pre-soaked in weak baby shampoo may allow a more controlled lid clean. Commercially available lid-hygiene kits are available. Proper attention to lid hygiene lessens the likelihood of MGD developing into a meibomian cyst (chalazion).

Paugh *et al.*[7] conducted a controlled, single-masked clinical trial that examined the symptomatic and therapeutic benefits of a combined treatment of warm compresses and lid scrubbing in patients who suffered from CL-MGD. These procedures were applied to one eye only, chosen at random, for 2 weeks, with the contralateral eye acting as a control.

After 2 weeks there was a significant improvement in the tear film quality of the treated eye, whereby the treated eye displayed a greater increase in tear break-up time (4.0 s greater than baseline) versus the non-treated eye (0.2 s greater than baseline). Improved comfort was also reported in the treated eye, but the experiment was single-masked (i.e., the patient knew which eye was being treated) and the possibility of subject bias in recording comfort levels cannot be discounted.

Mechanical expression

The patient can be instructed to express meibomian glands using the techniques described above. If this procedure is

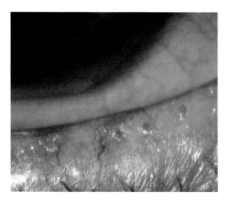

Figure 4.9

Plugs of keratinized epithelium and dried lipid secretions that block the meibomian gland orifices

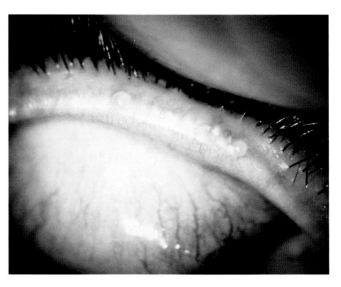

Figure 4.10

Meibomian blockage of the upper lid in a 50-year-old woman who reported contact lens intolerance. Increased visibility of vessels is apparent along the lid margin

adopted after the application of warm compresses, and lid hygiene procedures have been adopted, gentle pressure is usually all that is required to facilitate the expression of meibomian gland oils.

Antibiotics

Although CL-MGD is not an inflammatory condition, it is thought that systemic antibiotics, such as tetracycline, may act by killing bacteria that normally split neutral lipids into irritating fatty acids.

Artificial tears

Supplementing the tear film with artificial viscosity agents may help to increase tear volume and so prolong the formation of a tear layer over the lens and ocular surface. This should, at least, provide symptomatic relief and lessen the 'dryness' sensation.

Surfactant lens cleaning

Symptoms of blurred vision can be alleviated by ensuring that lenses are cleaned with an effective surfactant cleaning solution. Multipurpose lens-cleaning solutions, which are designed to be compatible with the eye, by necessity contain relatively weak surfactant agents. Although these solutions are perfectly adequate for the majority of contact lens wearers, patients who suffer from conditions that can result in excessive deposition of abnormal lipids (such as CL-MGD) are best advised to use a separate surfactant cleaning agent.

In severe cases of CL-MGD it may be necessary to advise the patient to use a surfactant cleaning agent every 4 hours. This should result in improved vision and comfort during lens wear. More frequent lens replacement is unlikely to have any impact, as lipid build-up occurs over minutes or hours (not days).

Prognosis

The underlying cause of MGD suggests that it is a chronic disorder with a poor prognosis for recovery. However, by adopting the procedures described above, CL-MGD can be kept under good control and adverse symptoms minimized. Intensive therapy over several weeks may be required to bring the condition under control, but once this has been achieved, good comfort and vision is possible if continued attention is paid to

lid hygiene and occasional strategies are adopted to alleviate acute problems (e.g., physical expression, warm compresses, etc.).

Differential Diagnosis

There are two aspects to the differentiation of CL-MGD from other disorders. First, it is important to be able to differentiate CL-MGD from other possible disorders of the meibomian gland and, indeed, of other glands at the lid margin.

An external hordeolum (stye) is a small swelling at the lid margin associated with a staphylococcal infection and inflammation of a lash follicle, and involves the glands of Zeis or Moll. An internal hordeolum is a small abscess associated with a staphylococcal infection and inflammation of a meibomian gland, and is observed as a tender swelling of the tarsal plate (*Figure 4.11*). Patients who suffer from these conditions complain of pain and tenderness; no such pain or tenderness is associated with MGD.

An internal hordeolum (also known as a meibomian cyst) is a chronic lipogranulomatous inflammation of a meibomian gland secondary to an obstruction to the gland orifice. Thus, MGD and meibomian cyst formation may be considered as acute and chronic manifestations, respectively, of the same disease process.

Bron and Mengher[25] reported the unusual case of 16-year-old girl who presented with contact lens intolerance. She was found to have a marked deficiency of meibomian glands in the

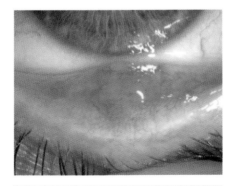

Figure 4.11
Internal hordeolum in a soft lens wearer, which was treated surgically

upper lids and almost total absence in the lower lids. Evidence of tear film instability was found and attributed to deficient lid-oil production. A daily wear soft contact lens was later fitted and tolerated.

Second, it is necessary to be able to differentiate the lipid irregularities and associated symptoms of dryness in patients with CL-MGD from other causes of tear film dysfunction in contact lens wearers. In general, this can be achieved by establishing the adequacy of the aqueous phase of the tear film by applying tests of tear volume (e.g., Schirmer's test or the cotton thread test) and of lacrimal gland function (e.g., the Lactoplate test). Symptoms of dryness and intermittent blurred vision in contact lens wearers in the presence of an adequate tear aqueous component should heighten suspicion of CL-MGD as the cause of the problem.

Other Meibomian Gland Disorders Associated with Contact Lenses

As discussed above under the heading of 'Differential diagnosis', other disorders of the meibomian gland may be encountered, such as chalazion and internal hordeolum. *Figure 4.12* is a facial thermogram of a soft lens wearer who suffered from an internal hordeolum of the right eye. The temperature distribution (red and yellow colors indicate warmer temperatures) confirms the increased temperature associated with the acute inflammation. In this case, lens wear was ceased until the condition resolved and the appearance of the tarsal plate returned to normal.

Contact lens wear should be suspended if a patient experiences a chalazion or internal hordeolum, and should not be resumed until the condition has resolved. As a prophylactic measure, greater attention to lid hygiene should be reinforced in patients who have suffered from meibomian gland disease; this advice could include the prescription of lid scrub kits.

Sebaceous gland carcinomas that involve the meibomian gland have also been described. These are the second most common form of malignancy of the eyelid, and account for 2–7 percent of all eyelid tumors and 1–5 percent of eyelid malignancies. Sebaceous gland

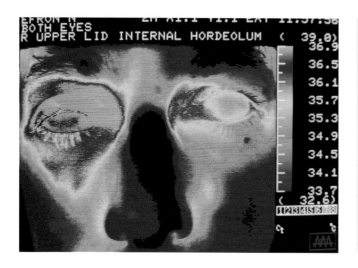

EFRON N
BOTH EYES
R UPPER LID INTERNAL HORDEOLUM
39.0)
36.9
36.5
36.1
35.7
35.3
34.9
34.5
34.1
33.7
32.6)

Figure 4.12
Facial thermogram of a soft lens wearer who suffered from an internal hordeolum of the right eye

carcinomas are observed most commonly in elderly women and in Asians. There is no reason to suppose that contact lens wear should be ceased in patients who suffer from such carcinomas, as long as the lenses are comfortable and the carcinoma remains under medical scrutiny.

REFERENCES

1 Bron AL, Benjamin L and Sibson GR (1991). Meibomian gland dysfunction: Classification and grading of lid changes. *Eye* **5**, 395–400.
2 Wilhelmus KR (1992). Inflammatory disorders of the eyelid margins and eyelashes. *Ophthalmol Clin North Am.* **10**, 187–192.
3 Ong BL (1996). Relation between contact lens wear and meibomian gland dysfunction. *Optom Vis Sci.* **73**, 208–210.
4 Ong BL and Larke JR (1990). Meibomian gland dysfunction: Some clinical, bio-chemical and physical observations. *Ophthalmic Physiol Opt.* **10**, 144–148.
5 Hom MM, Martinson JR, Knapp LL and Paugh JR (1990). Prevalence of meibomian gland dysfunction. *Optom Vis Sci.* **67**, 710–712.
6 Stanek S (2000). Meibomian gland status comparison between active duty personnel and U.S. veterans. *Mil Med.* **165**, 591–593.
7 Paugh JR, Knapp LL, Martinson JR and Hom MM (1990). Meibomian therapy in problematic contact lens wear. *Optom Vis Sci.* **67**, 803–806.
8 Guillon JP (1997). Dry eye in contact lens wear. *Optician* **214**(5622), 18–23.
9 Golding TR and Brennan NA (1989). The basis of tear ferning. *Clin Exp Optom.* **72**, 102–106.
10 Robin JB, Jester JV and Noble JR (1985). *In vivo* transillumination biomicroscopy and photography of meibomian gland dysfunction (a clinical study). *Ophthalmology* **92**, 1423–1426.
11 Hope-Ross MW, Chell PB and Kervick GN (1994). Recurrent corneal erosion: Clinical features. *Eye* **8**, 373–377.
12 Marren SE (1994). Contact lens wear, use of eye cosmetics, and Meibomian gland dysfunction. *Optom Vis Sci.* **71**, 60–62.
13 Korb DR and Henriquez AS (1980). Meibomian gland dysfunction and contact lens intolerance. *J Am Optom Assoc.* **51**, 243–251.
14 Gutgesell VJ, Stern GA and Hood CI (1982). Histopathology of meibomian gland dysfunction. *Am J Ophthalmol.* **94**, 383–389.
15 Driver PJ and Lemp MA (1996). Meibomian gland dysfunction. *Surv Ophthalmol.* **40**, 343–367.
16 Robin JB, Nobe JR, Suarez E, *et al.* (1986). Meibomian gland evaluation in patients with extended wear soft contact lens deposits. *CLAO J.* **12**, 95–98.
17 Efron N and Brennan NA (1988). A survey of wearers of low water content hydrogel contact lenses. *Clin Exp Optom.* **71**, 86–90.
18 Rengstorff RH (1980). Meibomian gland dysfunction in contact lens wearers. *Rev Optom.* **117**, 75–78.
19 Martin NF, Rubinfeld RS, Malley JD and Manzitti V (1992). Giant papillary conjunctivitis and meibomian gland dysfunction blepharitis. *CLAO J.* **18**, 165–169.
20 Mathers WD and Billborough M (1992). Meibomian gland function and giant papillary conjunctivitis. *Am J Ophthalmol.* **114**, 188–192.
21 Ong BL, Hodson SA and Wigham T (1991). Evidence of keratin proteins in normal and abnormal human meibomian fluids. *Curr Eye Res.* **10**, 1113–1117.
22 Pascucci SE, Lemp MA and Cavanagh HD (1988). An analysis of age-related morphologic changes in human meibomian glands. *Invest Ophthalmol Vis Sci.* **29S**, 213.
23 Norn M (1985). Meibomian orifices and Marx's line – studies by triple vital staining. *Acta Ophthalmol (Copenh.)* **63**, 698–702.
24 Henriquez AS and Korb DR (1981). Meibomian glands and contact lens wear. *Br J Ophthalmol.* **65**, 108–111.
25 Bron AJ and Mengher LS (1987). Congenital deficiency of meibomian glands. *Br J Ophthalmol.* **71**, 312–314.

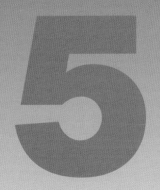

EYELASH DISORDERS

Disorders of the eyelashes (cilia) and of associated structures at the base of the eyelashes, such as the eyelash follicles, glands of Zeis and skin of the lid margin, have implications with respect to contact lens wear. Practitioners need to be aware of the possible existence of such conditions in contact lens wearers because these may explain ocular discomfort during lens wear, and in many instances contraindicate lens wear until the condition is resolved.

Eyelashes typically project from the anterior rounded border of the lid margin in two or three rows. They lie just anterior to the 'gray line' – an anatomic feature that indicates the position of the mucocutaneous junction. The superior eyelashes are longer and more numerous than those of the lower lid. As upper lashes normally curl up and lower lashes normally curl down, the lashes do not become tangled on eyelid closure. Eyelashes are typically darker than other hairs of the body, except in conditions such as alopecia areata.[1]

External Hordeolum (Stye)

An external hordeolum – commonly known as a 'stye' – presents as a discrete inflamed swelling of the anterior lid margin (*Figure 5.1*). It is extremely tender to touch, and may occur singly or as multiple small abscesses. A stye is an inflammation of the tissue that lines the lash follicle and/or an associated gland of Zeis or Moll. It is typically an acute staphylococcal infection, and as such commonly presents in patients with staphylococcal blepharitis.

Styes have a typical time course of about 7 days. Sometimes a stye discharges spontaneously in an anterior direction. If a patient is in particular discomfort, resolution can be facilitated by removing the eyelash from the infected follicle and applying hot compresses to the affected area.[2]

Contact lens wear may add to the discomfort of a stye because of the mechanical affect of the lens. In soft lens wearers, mechanical pressure against the lens between the stye and the globe may effectively grip the lens and result in excessive lens movement during blinking. With a rigid lens fitted interpalpebrally, the lens may buffer against the lid margin with each blink and so cause considerable discomfort. For these reasons, patients may prefer to cease lens wear during the acute phase of the formation of a stye.

Blepharitis

Blepharitis is typically classified as being either anterior or posterior. The condition is sometimes called 'marginal blepharitis' because it is observed along the lid margins. Anterior blepharitis is directly related to infections of the base of the eyelashes and manifests in two forms – staphylococcal blepharitis and seborrheic blepharitis. The severity of blepharitis can be quantified with reference to the grading scale for this condition given in Appendix A. Posterior blepharitis is a disorder of the meibomian glands and is considered in Chapter 4.

Staphylococcal anterior blepharitis

Staphylococcal anterior blepharitis is caused by a chronic staphylococcal infection of the eyelash follicles, and leads to secondary dermal and epidermal ulceration and tissue destruction. It is often observed in patients with atopic eczema and occurs more frequently in females and in younger patients.

Slit-lamp examination of patients who suffer from this condition reveals the presence of hyperemia, telangiectasis and scaling of the anterior lid margins. The scales are brittle (*Figure 5.2*) and when removed leave a small bleeding ulcer. The lashes may appear stuck together ,and in severe cases a yellow crust can form as a kind of sleeve that covers the base of the eyelash; these sleeves are called 'cuffs' or 'collarettes' (*Figure 5.3*).

In long-standing cases, there may be a loss of some eyelashes (madarosis), some eyelashes may turn white (poliosis) and the anterior lid margin may become scarred, notched, irregular or hypertrophic (tylosis).

Hypersensitivity to staphylococcal exotoxins may lead to secondary complications, such as low grade papillary and bulbar conjunctivitis, toxic punctate

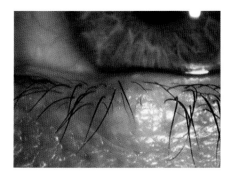

Figure 5.1
External hordeolum

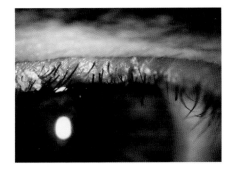

Figure 5.2
Staphylococcal anterior blepharitis with the lid margin covered in brittle scales

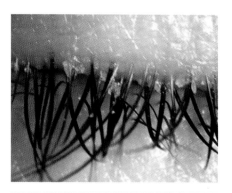

Figure 5.3
Collarettes surrounding the base of eyelashes in a patient with staphylococcal anterior blepharitis

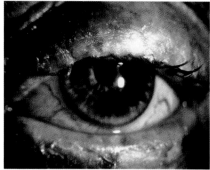

Figure 5.4
Seborrheic anterior blepharitis in which the eyelashes have become greasy and stuck together

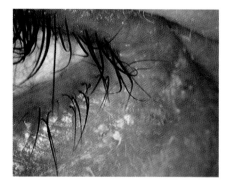

Figure 5.5
Yellow greasy scales along the lid margin in a patient with staphylococcal anterior blepharitis

epitheliopathy that involves the inferior third of the cornea and marginal corneal infiltrates.

Patients who suffer from staphylococcal anterior blepharitis may complain of burning, itching, foreign body sensations and mild photophobia. Associated tear film instability may also lead to symptoms of dryness. Symptoms are often worse in the morning.

The following management strategies may be employed:
- Antibiotic ointment – after removing crusts, antibiotic ointment is applied to the lid margins with a clean finger.
- Promote lid hygiene – crusts and toxic products can be removed by scrubbing the lids twice daily with a commercially available lid scrub. Alternatively, regular washing with a warm, moist face cloth and occasional rubbing with diluted baby shampoo should alleviate the condition.
- Corticosteroids – weak topical corticosteroids may be tried in more severe and protracted cases, especially if the strategies described above fail.
- Artificial tears – provide symptomatic relief if the blepharitis compromises the integrity of the tear film.

The treatment can be tailed off as appropriate as the condition improves. However, staphylococcal anterior blepharitis is difficult to treat and the pattern of recovery is characterized by periods of remission and exacerbation.[2]

Seborrheic anterior blepharitis

Seborrheic anterior blepharitis results from a disorder of the glands of Zeis and Moll, which connect with eyelash follicles. It is frequently associated with seborrheic dermatitis of the scalp, eyebrows, nasolabial folds, retro-auricular areas and sternum. The symptoms are similar to, but less severe than, those for staphylococcal anterior blepharitis.

The anterior lid margin displays a shiny, waxy appearance with mild erythema and telangiectasis (*Figure 5.4*). Soft, yellow greasy scales are observed along the lid margin (*Figure 5.5*); unlike staphylococcal anterior blepharitis, these scales do not leave a bleeding ulcer when removed. The eyelashes may also become greasy and stuck together.

As with the staphylococcal form, secondary complications of seborrheic anterior blepharitis include mild papillary conjunctivitis and punctate epitheliopathy. The main form of treatment is lid hygiene and artificial tears.[2]

Implications for contact lens wear

Contact lens wear is generally contraindicated during an acute phase of anterior blepharitis, especially if the cornea is compromised. If contact lenses are worn during mild cases of staphylococcal anterior blepharitis, attention to lens cleaning is critical to prevent continued recontamination of the eye. Faherty[3] suggests that contact lens wearers should be advised to be careful of cross-contamination between eyes, lenses, lens solutions and/or lens cases, and to use cosmetics properly and with care. Daily disposable contact lenses eliminate such problems of cross-contamination.

Keys[4] conducted a 4 month study on 20 contact lens wearers and six nonwearers who suffered from blepharitis, to test the efficacy of various treatment regimens:
- Eyelid cleaning with hypoallergenic soap;
- Lid scrubbing with dilute baby shampoo;
- Use of a commercial lid scrub.

It was concluded that all three regimens resulted in improvement, and that about 85% of patients preferred to use the commercial lid scrub.

Parasite Infestation of Eyelashes

Infestation of the eyelashes by mites or lice can lead to signs and symptoms that closely resemble blepharitis. Clinicians must therefore be aware of this possibility, and must be able to distinguish between the three species of parasite that most commonly infest human eyelashes and associated structures.[5] This is especially important in contact lens practice, as failure to identify parasitic eyelash infestation almost certainly leads to patient dropout.

Mites

Mite infestation is very common in humans, with a greater prevalence in older persons. In the USA, the prevalence of mites has been reported as 29% for 0–25 year olds, 53% for 26–50 year olds and 67% in 51–90 year olds.[6] Mite infestation in the eyelashes is ubiquitous and generally sub-clinical, but if present in excessive numbers, adverse signs and symptoms may develop. The mode of transmission of mites between humans is not clear, but may arise from intimate contact. Mites are also more abundant in diabetic and acquired immunodeficiency syndrome (AIDS) patients, and in patients on long-term corticosteroid therapy, which suggests that compromised immunity may also influence mite infestation.[7]

Two species of mite (*Demodex folliculorum* and *D. brevis*) are found in the human pilosebaceous gland complex; these are from the family Demodicidae, order Acarina (mites and ticks), class Arachnida (spiders, scorpions, ticks and mites) and phylum Arthropoda. Infestation with *Demodex* species is termed 'demodicosis'.[5]

Demodex folliculorum

D. folliculorum is a cigar-shaped mite with four evenly spaced stubby legs on the upper third of its body (*Figure 5.6*). It prefers to live in the space between the eyelash and the follicle wall, and in a single follicle typically exists in small colonies of 3–5 mites. This species of mite is always located above the level of the gland of Zeis, primarily because of its size.[7]

D. folliculorum is much smaller in diameter than the base of the eyelash; the mites bury themselves head first into the follicle and feed off the cytoplasm of follicular epithelium by clawing away at, and puncturing, the epithelial cell walls with sharp mouth parts. The shredded, hyperkeratinized cell material combines with lipids and sebum to form a clear collarette (*Figure 5.7*; in cases of staphylococcal anterior blepharitis, the collarettes have more of a creamy yellow appearance). Extensive mite activity can lead to an aggregation of cuffing material, such that the mites are trapped within the hair follicle. This can lead to follicle distension, granulomas, telangiectasis, hyperplasia, erythema, madarosis, hyperemia, burning and itching, which of course must be dealt with clinically.[5]

Demodex brevis

D. brevis is found in human skin rich in sebaceous glands and sebum production. It prefers to infest the gland of Zeis, and can reach this gland because of its very small size (0.18 mm long, whereas *D. folliculorum* is 0.38 mm long, *Figure 5.8*).[6] *D. brevis* has an almost identical structure to *D. folliculorum*, the former being shorter, but stubbier. *D. brevis* is often found alone in a single sebaceous gland. In a similar manner to the actions of *D. folliculorum*, *D. brevis* can block the

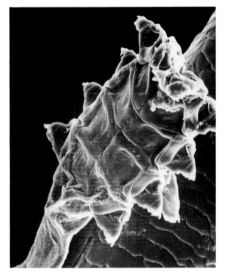

Figure 5.6
Electron micrograph of a follicle mite, *D. folliculorum*, lying on an epilated lash

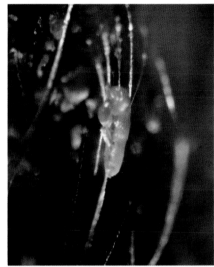

Figure 5.7
Collarette surrounding an eyelash of a contact lens wearer infested with mites

gland of Zeis and, indeed, can block meibomian glands, which leads to meibomian gland dysfunction and interference with lipid production, which in turn can result in dry eye symptoms.

D. brevis prefers to live in an oily, sebaceous environment, so it tends to thrive in the presence of oily cosmetics and facial preparations. This, in turn, can cause *D. brevis* to proliferate, and can lead to the following sequellae of events: meibomian glands, glands of Zeis and other facial sebaceous glands become blocked, the skin becomes dry,

the patient applies more oily facial creams, *D. brevis* again proliferates and the cycle continues.[8]

General characteristics

Demodex species are typically nocturnal, but even during the day a busy migration of organisms can be observed passing between eyelash follicles. Patient symptoms usually parallel the life cycle of the organisms. Nests of *D. folliculorum* are laid around the base of lashes, they hatch after about 2–3 days and the adult lives for 5–14 days.[9]

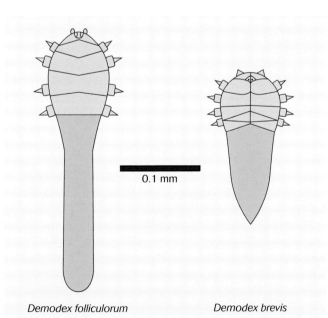

Figure 5.8
The two species of mite (*D. folliculorum* and *D. brevis*) are found in the human pilosebaceous gland complex

0.1 mm

Demodex folliculorum   *Demodex brevis*

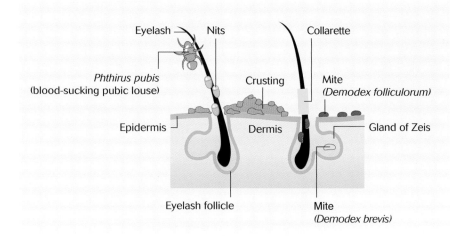

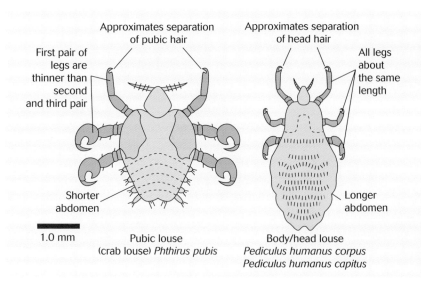

Figure 5.9
Preferred habitat of mites and lice that commonly infest the human pilosebaceous gland complex

Figure 5.10
Species of lice that infest the human body

Although they may be detected at high magnification (×40) on a slit-lamp biomicroscope, mites are difficult to observe because they are very small (much narrower than the width of an eyelash), they withdraw back into the follicle in bright light (being nocturnal in nature) and they are translucent. Diagnosis is confirmed by examination of epilated lashes under a light microscope; one or more mites observed on every two lashes is considered indicative of demodicosis.[10]

Additional signs of demodicosis include erythema of the lid margins, lid hyperplasia and madarosis (all of which give the impression of blepharitis), conjunctival injection, cuffing around lashes, follicular distension and meibomian gland blockage. Eyelashes are removed more easily during active infestation because of damage to the eyelash follicles. Typical symptoms of demodicosis are pruritus, burning, crusting, itching, swelling of the lid margins and loss of lashes. The itching often parallels the 10 day reproductive cycle.[5]

Figure 5.9 illustrates the preferred habitat of mites and lice that commonly infest the human pilosebaceous system.

Lice

Three species of lice infest the human body:
- Head louse (*Pediculus humanus capitis*);
- Body louse (*Pediculus humanus corpus*);
- Pubic louse (*Phthirus pubis*) or 'crab'.
These species are from the family Pediculidae, order Anoplura (the sucking lice), class Insecta and, like mites, they are classified as belonging to the phylum Arthropoda.[5]

P. capitis typically infests the scalp hair (especially the occipital region). During dense scalp infestation, *P. capitis* can be found in the eyelashes, but this is extremely rare. *P. corpus* inhabits seams and creases in clothing and feeds on the skin of patients. Infestation with these two species is termed pediculosis. The *Pediculus* species are typically 2.5–3.5 mm long (*Figure 5.10*), and are a vector in humans for serious diseases such as typhus, relapsing fever and trench fever.[11]

The crab louse, *Ph. pubis*, is most commonly found in pubic hair, but also in other coarsely spaced hair such as on the chest and thighs (*Figure 5.11*). Infestation with this species is termed phthiriasis. The crab louse is about 1.0–1.5 mm long, which is an ideal size for inhabitation among pubic hairs because these are spaced 2 mm apart, which corresponds to the anatomic grasping span of its legs. *Ph. pubis* can successfully infest eyelashes, which are also approximately 2 mm apart. Indeed,

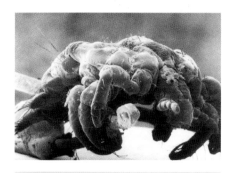

Figure 5.11
Electron micrograph of a crab louse, *Ph. pubis*

of the three species of louse discussed above, the crab louse is almost exclusively found among human eyelashes.[11] *Ph. pubis* has two pairs of strong grasping claws on the central and hind legs, which allow it to hold on to eyelashes with considerable tenacity.

Phthiriasis is considered to be a venereal disease because it is passed on by sexual contact. In adults, genital-to-eye transmission is the most probable cause of eyelash infestation, although infestation from contaminated bedding, towels and bed clothes is another possible mode of transfer. The eyelashes of children may be infested by eye-to-eye contact, and eyelashes of infants may be infested from contact with the chest hair of parents or siblings who themselves harbor the lice.[5]

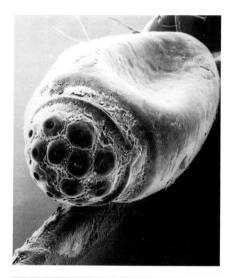

Figure 5.12
Electron micrograph of lice eggs, or 'nits', encapsulated in a characteristic cigar-shaped shell

The three species discussed above are known as 'sucking lice' because of their mode of feeding, which is to anchor mouth hooklets to the host skin and to extend a long hollow tube (stylus) into the dermis. Anticoagulants are secreted to facilitate unimpeded sucking of blood and serum.[5]

All of these lice have internal fertilization and lay eggs within 2 days of fertilization. The eggs, or 'nits', are encapsulated in a cigar-shaped shell (*Figure 5.12*). Nit shells are cemented to eyelashes about 1–2 mm from the base of the lash, and the nits hatch in 7–10 days. It takes lice about 1 month to reach adult stage, and the adult lives for a further month. Lice can survive for only 2 days if separated from the host.[5]

Signs of phthiriasis include pruritus of the lid margins, blepharitis, marked conjunctival injection and madarosis. Additional signs include pre-auricular lymphadenopathy and secondary infection along the lid margins at the site of lice bites. The most predominant symptom is intense itching, which is so severe that patients also report insomnia, irritability and mental depression.[11]

The most obvious sign of phthiriasis is the presence of oval, grayish-white nit shells attached to the base of lashes, which are easily identifiable using high magnification (×40) slit-lamp biomicroscopy (*Figure 5.13*). Adult lice can be difficult to detect because they are almost completely transparent. Reddish brown deposits at the base of lashes also indicate the presence of lice; these deposits are a combination of blood from the host and feces from the parasite. Blue spots may also be observed on

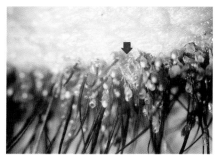

Figure 5.13
Slit-lamp photomicrograph of a nearly transparent louse at the lid margin (arrow) surrounded by a mass of nits encapsulated in shells, and some empty shells that have already hatched open

the lid margins; these are caused by enzymatic reactions from the digestive juices of the lice.[11]

Treatment of mite infestation

The main aim of treatment is to reduce the level of mite infestation to sub-clinical levels. In treating this condition, it should be assumed that there is a concurrent bacterial infection. The initial course of action is to attempt to remove as many mites and mite eggs as possible. This can be achieved by applying a topical anesthetic and swabbing the eyelid margins and eyelashes with a cotton-tipped applicator saturated in a contact lens cleaning solution, taking care to avoid contact with the cornea.[5]

Patients should be advised to engage in vigorous lid scrubbing twice daily (morning and evening) using commercially available preparations, diluted baby shampoo, non-allergenic soap or hot flannels. After the evening lid scrub, a viscous ointment should be applied to the upper and lower lid margins. This procedure:
- Traps mites in their follicles;
- Smothers and kills the trapped mites;
- Prevents mites from migrating and cross-contaminating adjacent follicles.

A lid scrub performed the following morning removes dead lice and associated debris trapped in the ointment. Heavy metal ointments, such as yellow mercuric oxide, are usually prescribed because of their supplementary antimicrobial efficacy. Pilocarpine gel has been suggested as a more potent alternative. Treatment should be continued for at least 3 weeks, even if early symptomatic relief is achieved.[5]

If the above measures are unsuccessful, more aggressive in-office therapy may need to be adopted. Vigorous scrubs with a cotton-tipped applicator soaked in alcohol or ether, performed weekly for 3 weeks, may bring the condition under control.[5]

Patients who experience symptoms of dryness because of demodectic infestation of the skin should be cautioned against the use of facial oils, and should be advised to wash the affected areas daily with soap.[5]

Practitioners should be alert to the possibility of alarming patients about the existence of 'spider-like' parasites on their body. It should be explained that this is a chronic condition that can be kept under control if the patient complies with the treatment protocol.

Treatment of lice infestation

The initial course of action is to remove the lice mechanically from the lashes with forceps, while visualizing the process using medium-to-high power on a slit-lamp biomicroscope. This may be difficult because the lice typically maintain a tight grasp on the lashes. Heavy infestations are best removed using cryotherapy (freezing) or argon laser photoablation. The latter technique effectively slices through the lashes; the result is initially unsightly, but the patient should be reassured that the lashes quickly grow to full length. Lice and nits are also killed by the application of 20% sodium fluorescein.[11]

The patient should be advised to apply yellow mercuric oxide ophthalmic ointment twice daily to the lid margins to smother and kill adult lice. This therapy should be continued for 2 weeks to cover at least one complete lice life cycle. Anticholinesterase agents may also be tried. More potent insecticides are seldom used today because of the potential for serious corneal injury. Patients should be warned that symptoms may persist beyond the effective eradication of lice because of residual lice-induced hypersensitivity reactions.[11]

Patients should be referred for treatment of pubic infestation and other possible sexually transmitted diseases. Sexual partners and family members should also be examined for eyelash infestation and counseled about the possibility of the concurrent infestation of pubic hair. More potent pediculicidal ointment can be applied to regions of the body away from the eyes, and so offer the possibility of rapid and effective treatment.[11]

The home environment should also be sanitized to eradicate lice, for which heat application is the most effective course of action. Lice are killed if bed clothing, towels, sheets and clothes are washed in boiling water for 30 minutes. Combs, brushes and hair accessories should be soaked in lice-killing products or in boiling water for 10 minutes. Isolation of blankets and other large items from the host for 2 weeks ensures the death of all lice and nits.[11]

Management in contact lens wearers

In general, contact lens wearers who present with parasitic infestation of the eyelids should be treated in the same way as similarly infested non-wearers.

Paradoxically, contact lenses (soft lenses in particular) serve a protective function during parasitic eyelash infestation because they prevent the cornea from the mechanical effects of altered lid margins and lashes, and prevent toxins and debris from coming into contact with the cornea.[12]

It is advisable to cease lens wear during the treatment period, which in severe cases may last up to 1 month. Contact lenses can theoretically serve as a vector for the transmission of mites, lice, nits or other potentially toxic or allergenic by-products of the infestation process. The probability of such vectoral transmission increases if patients are partially non-compliant by, for example, failing to surfactant clean and/or manually rub their lenses after lens removal. An intense cleaning regimen is indicated for patients with eyelash infestations. The best modality of lens wear for patients with recurrent parasitic eyelash infestation is daily disposable contact lenses.

Caroline et al.[13] highlighted the sensitive nature of managing crab lice infestation in that it is primarily a sexually transmitted disease. They caution that loss to follow-up is to be expected in a significant number of patients who may be too embarrassed to return to their eyecare practitioner for further care of the eyelash infestation or, indeed, for further contact lens management.

Other Eyelash Disorders Associated with Contact Lenses

Insects trapped in eyelashes

Dead flying insects are observed occasionally on the lid margins, just posterior to the base of the eyelashes. These insects perhaps land on the lid margin quite accidentally, realize that they have found a soft, moist and succulent environment (the conjunctiva and meibomian secretions) and take measures to anchor themselves in position. Another possibility is that they quickly become stuck in the oily lipid secretions of the lid margin. A strong reflex blink or eye rub by the host may then kill or incapacitate the insect, which remains in place until physically dislodged.

Figure 5.14 shows an insect trapped on the upper lid margin of a soft contact lens wearer who noticed discomfort in her left eye during a holiday in Spain.

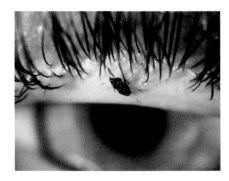

Figure 5.14
Insect stuck on the upper lid margin, just posterior to the row of lashes

The patient attributed the consequent irritation to a split in her contact lens; she returned to her practitioner who detected the insect on slit-lamp examination. Figure 5.15 shows a flying insect trapped on the lower lid margin of a rigid contact lens patient.

These cases highlight the importance of a thorough examination of the lid margins when trying to find a cause of discomfort apparently related to contact lens wear.

Shedded eyelash that enters the eye

The life cycle of an eyelash is about 5 months, and it takes about 2 months for a new eyelash to become fully grown.[1] Thus, there are frequent opportunities for a shedded eyelash to enter the eye. In non-wearers of contact lenses, an eyelash that enters the eye typically elicits an intense foreign body discomfort sensation, which causes increased lacrimation and results in the lash being flushed out. In contact lens wearers, the lash

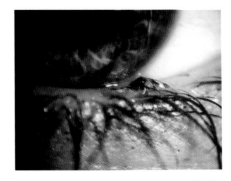

Figure 5.15
Insect stuck on the lower lid margin, just posterior to the row of lashes

may become lodged beneath the lens, which is generally very uncomfortable. The patient removes the lens and often attempts to remove the eyelash as well, if it can be located. Examination of the eye after such an incident may reveal evidence of corneal epithelial trauma; if severe, lens wear should be ceased until the epithelium has recovered.

Trichiasis

Trichiasis is a condition in which the eyelashes curl inward toward the globe (*Figure 5.16*). This can manifest as a primary condition or be secondary to entropion (*Figure 5.17*). Whatever the cause, the result can be discomfort and persistent abrasion of the cornea by the eyelashes, and in those who do not wear contact lenses this can lead to significant corneal decompensation, in the form of a vascular pannus, if left untreated for a significant length of time.[2]

Contact lenses can act as a protective buffer against corneal damage – soft lenses offer more protection than rigid lenses because of their greater corneal coverage. However, the cornea can be damaged when the lenses are not worn, and subsequent lens wear in the presence of an epithelial trauma is problematic because the epithelial breach may render the eye more susceptible to microbial infection. Inward growing eyelashes should therefore be treated by one of the following techniques:

- Epilation – eyelashes are mechanically removed with the aid of forceps;
- Electrolysis – the eyelash follicle is destroyed by passing an electrical current through a fine needle inserted into the lash root;
- Cryotherapy – the lash follicle is frozen with a nitrous oxide cryoprobe at –20°C.[2]

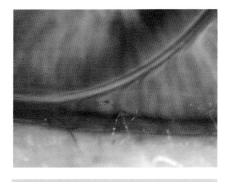

Figure 5.16
Ingrowing eyelash from the lower lid that irritates the ocular surface of a rigid lens wearer

Distichiasis

Distichiasis is a condition whereby eyelashes emerge from regions of the lid margin other than the their typical location. For example, eyelashes may emerge from between or even from within meibomian gland orifices. Distichiasis can be congenital or acquired, and typically causes the same problems of irritation

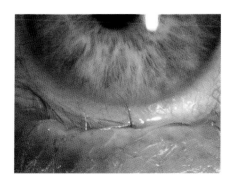

Figure 5.17
Trichiasis that resulted from entropion

and corneal trauma as occur in trichiasis.[2] The implications with respect to contact lens wear are also similar; the condition is usually treated using cryotherapy.

REFERENCES

1 Bron AJ, Tripathi RC and Tripathi BJ (1997). *Wolff's Anatomy of the Eye and Orbit*, Eighth Edition. (London: Chapman & Hall Medical).

2 Kanski JJ (2003). *Clinical Ophthalmology*, Fifth Edition. (Oxford: Butterworth–Heinemann).

3 Faherty B (1992). Chronic blepharitis: Easy nursing interventions for a common problem. *J Ophthalmic Nurs Technol*. **11**, 20–22.

4 Keys JE (1996). A comparative study of eyelid cleaning regimens in chronic blepharitis. *CLAO J*. **22**, 209–215.

5 Edmondson W and Christenson MT (1992). Lid parasites. In: *Clinical Optometric Pharmacology and Therapeutics*, p. 42.1–42.9, Ed. Onefrey B. (Philadelphia: Lippincott–Raven).

6 Sengbusch HG and Hauswirth JW (1986). Prevalence of hair follicle mites, *Demodex folliculorum* and *D. brevis* (Acari: Demodicidae), in a selected human population in western New York, USA. *J Med Entomol*. **23**, 384–389.

7 English FP and Nutting WB (1981). Demodicosis of ophthalmic concern. *Am J Ophthalmol*. **91**, 362–366.

8 Heacock CE (1986). Clinical manifestations of demodicosis. *J Am Optom Assoc*. **57**, 914–916.

9 Anderson PH and Jones WL (1988). A recalcitrant case of *Demodex* blepharitis. *Clin Eye Vis Care* **1**, 39–41.

10 Fulk GW and Clifford C (1990). A case report of demodicosis. *J Am Optom Assoc*. **61**, 637–639.

11 Couch JM, Green WR and Hirst LW (1982). Diagnosing and treating *Phthirus pubis* palpebrarum. *Surv Ophthalmol*. **26**, 219–226.

12 Holland BJ and Siderov J (1998). Phthiriasis and pediculosis palpebrarum. *Clin Exp Optom*. **80**, 8–13.

13 Caroline PJ, Kame RT and Hatashida JK (1991). Pediculosis parasitic infestation in a contact lens wearer. *Clin Eye Vis Care* **3**, 82–85.

PART III TEAR FILM

DRY EYE

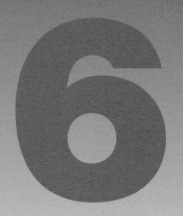

The integrity of the tear film is critical for safe and comfortable contact lens wear. If the tear film is of insufficient quantity or quality, the patient generally complains of having a 'dry eye'. Thus, in the contact lens field, the term 'dry eye' is taken as an all-encompassing phrase that encapsulates various aspects of tear film dysfunction relating to contact lens wear. These aspects include, but are not restricted to, patient symptomatology, alterations to tear chemistry, lens deposition, effects on tissue integrity and vision, infection and lens performance.

The tear film in contact lens wear differs in many ways from the normal, undisturbed tear film. The most obvious difference from a clinical perspective is a necessary structural reorganization, whereby the tears are compartmentalized into the pre-lens tear film and post-lens tear film. In addition, the integrity of the tear film remains altered for a short period after ceasing lens wear.

This chapter considers the key clinically relevant features of the tear film by contrasting the nature of the tear film in the presence and absence of contact lens wear. In the course of this discussion, important clinical tests of tear film integrity are reviewed. Also, consideration is given to the way in which the results of such tests can be interpreted and applied clinically to solve problems of tear film dysfunction that are invariably reported as 'dry eye'.

The Normal Tear Film

Structure
Appreciation of the structure of the tear film in both the undisturbed eye and the eye that wears a contact lens is confounded by the ongoing uncertainty as to its normal structure. The description of the tear film originally proposed by Wolff,[1] although perhaps somewhat simplistic, is regarded as providing the most

useful, clinically relevant model of tear film structure (*Figure 6.1*). According to this model, the tear film is about 7 μm thick and is composed of an outer lipid layer (approximately 0.1 μm thick), an intermediate aqueous phase (7 μm), and an inner mucus layer (0.05 μm).

Subsequent research suggested refinements of the original Wolff model and provided important insights into the fine structure of the component layers of the tear film. Tiffany[2] accepts the basic structure as outlined by Wolff, but argues that the interfaces between the air, lipid, aqueous, mucus and epithelium have their own peculiar physicochemical properties; he thus concludes that the tear film should technically be considered as composed of six layers. Prydal and Campbell[3] suggest that the Wolff model does not take into account the true thickness of the mucus layer and argue that the tear film should be thought of as being 34–45 μm thick, but with the same trilaminate structure as proposed originally. King-Smith *et al.*[4] measured

reflectance spectra from the human cornea and claimed that these results indicated the tear film to be 3 μm thick.

More radical theories have been proposed by others. Baier and Thomas[5] argue from a theoretical standpoint (based upon the appearance of oil slicks on the ocean as viewed from space) that the structure of the tear film is the reverse of that proposed by Wolff; that is, the outer layer of the tear film is a mucinous glycoprotein gel, and an inner lipid layer lines the epithelium. Hodson and Earlam[6] suggest that the tear film has no defined structure, but instead is composed of a loose fibronectin gel in which the lipid, mucus and aqueous components are intermixed. Alternative models of tear film structure are illustrated in *Figure 6.2*.

Function
In the normal eye (lenses not worn), the tear film serves six important functions:
- Optical – the tear film maintains an optically uniform interface between the air and cornea;
- Mechanical – the tear film acts as a vehicle for the continual blink-mediated removal of intrinsic and extrinsic debris and particulate matter that constantly enters the eye;
- Lubricant – the tear film ensures a smooth movement of the eyelids over the globe during blinking
- Bactericidal – the tear film contains defense mechanisms in the form of proteins, antibodies, phagocytotic cells and other immunodefense mechanisms that prevent ocular infection;
- Nutritional – the tear film provides the corneal epithelium with the necessary supplies of oxygen, glucose amino acids and vitamins;
- Waste removal – the tear film acts as an intermediate reservoir for the removal of by-products of metabolism from the cornea, such as carbon dioxide and lactate.

Figure 6.1
Structure of the pre-corneal tear film

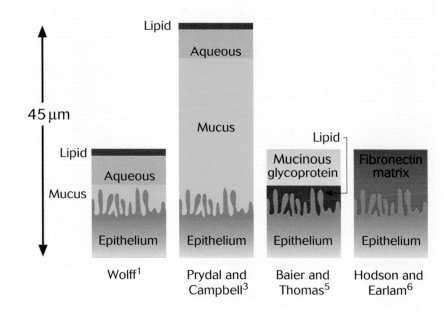

Figure 6.2

Alternative theories of tear film structure

The functions of the tear film during uncomplicated contact lens wear essentially fall into the same categories as those above for the normal tear film, but can be re-stated with subtle differences:

- Optical – the tear film maintains an optically uniform interface between the air and the anterior surface of the lens;
- Mechanical – the tear film acts as a vehicle for the continual blink-mediated removal of intrinsic and extrinsic debris and particulate matter from the front of the lens and from beneath the lens;
- Lubricant – the tear film ensures a smooth movement of the eyelids over the front surface of the lens, and of the lens over the globe, during blinking;
- Bactericidal – the tear film contains defense mechanisms in the form of proteins, antibodies, phagocytotic cells and other immunodefense mechanisms that prevent ocular infection;
- Nutritional – the tear film provides the corneal epithelium with the necessary supplies of oxygen, glucose amino acids and vitamins, via the lid-activated tear pump;
- Waste removal – the tear film acts as an intermediate reservoir for the removal of by-products of metabolism from the cornea, such as carbon dioxide and lactate, that are flushed out from beneath the lens via the lid-activated tear pump.

Signs of Tear Film Dysfunction in Dry Eye Related to Contact Lenses

General observation

The most fundamental test that a clinician can apply when investigating tear film dysfunction in a contact lens wearer is to observe the tears using the slit-lamp biomicroscope. Similar techniques as employed to examine the eye in which no lenses are worn can also be applied to the lens-wearing eye. The overall integrity of the tears during lens wear can be assessed by observing the general flow of the tear film over the lens surface after a blink, as indicated by the movement of tear debris. A 'sluggish' movement may indicate an aqueous-deficient, mucus-rich and/or lipid-rich tear film, and the amount of debris provides an indication of the level of contamination of the tears – perhaps, for example, from overuse of cosmetics. A sluggish and/or contaminated tear film is potentially problematic, and could result in increased deposit formation, intermittent blurred vision and discomfort.

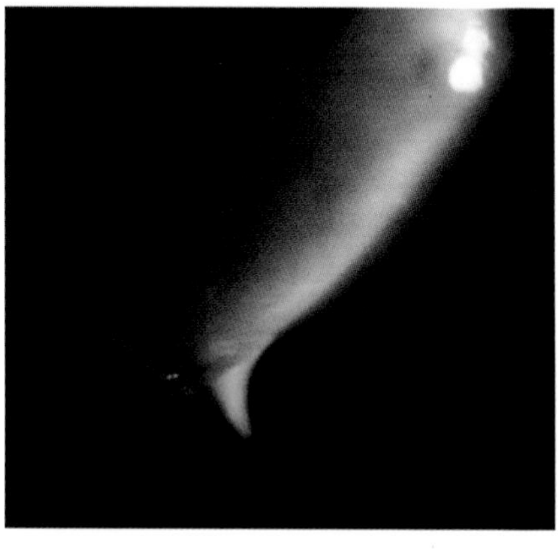

Tear volume

The volume of tears in prospective and current contact lens wearers can be assessed by observing the height of the lower lacrimal tear prism (*Figure 6.3*). Mainstone *et al.*[7] found that measurements of the radius of curvature and height of the tear meniscus correlated well with cotton thread test results, non-invasive tear break-up time (NITBUT) and scores for ocular surface staining, which demonstrates the value of such an assessment in diagnosing dry eye conditions.

Tear-film volume can be measured in the eye (no lens worn) using the Schirmer test, or the preferred and less invasive cotton thread tear test. The Schirmer test involves the placement of one end of a strip of filter paper into the lower fornix and measuring the length of paper that becomes wet over a given time period (*Figure 6.4*). The greater the length of wetting, the greater the tear volume (assuming that there has been no reflex stimulation).

Figure 6.3

Full inferior tear meniscus stained with fluorescein

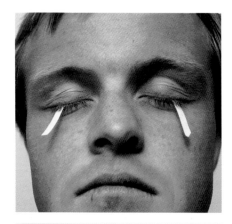

Figure 6.4

Schirmer test

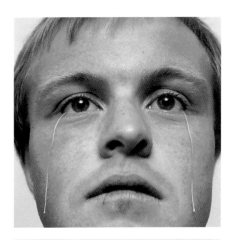

Figure 6.5
Cotton thread tear test

The cotton thread test, as adapted by Hamano *et al.*,[8] involves impregnating fine cotton threads with the pH-reactive dye phenolsulfophthalein, which turns the thread yellow in air. A cotton thread is looped over the lower lid margin, one end hangs down over the cheek and the other end rests in the lower lid cul-de-sac (*Figure 6.5*). As a result of a tear-induced shift in pH, the yellow thread turns red as it soaks up the tears. The greater the passage of redness down the thread, the greater the tear volume (again assuming that there has been no reflex stimulation).

Hamano *et al.*[8] applied this test to 1600 asymptomatic polymethyl methacrylate (PMMA), rigid and soft (hydroxyethyl methacrylate, HEMA) lens wearers, and observed a mean wetting length of 16.9 mm over 15 s. This result was no different from that of normal subjects (no lenses worn), which suggests that, from a clinical perspective, contact lenses do not alter tear production in normal subjects.

Tear film structure and quality

It was established in 1921 that certain structural aspects of the tear film can be assessed clinically by observing the corneal surface in specular reflection.[9] This can be achieved using the slit-lamp biomicroscope by setting the angle of the illumination arm equal to the angle of the microscope arm (say, 30° to the normal) and observing a thin vertical beam at ×30–40 magnification. The limitations of this approach – such as the need to use a narrow beam and the generation of heat from the light source – can be overcome by using a wide-field,

cold cathode light source, which is available as a handheld instrument known as a tearscope.[10]

As discussed above, the component layers of the tear film are extremely thin. The refractive index differences between the air–lipid and lipid–aqueous boundaries cause destructive interference within the lipid layer, which results in the appearance of colored fringes, from which the thickness of the lipid layer can be inferred. The aqueous layer of the pre-corneal tear film cannot be observed using this technique because of an insufficient refractive index difference between the aqueous–mucus and mucus–epithelium interfaces.

These colored fringe patterns, coupled with the general morphologic appearance and dynamic characteristics of the lipid layer when viewed in specular reflection, led Guillon and Guillon[11] to devise the following six-category lipid layer classification scheme, with the various appearances below ranked in order of increasing lipid layer thickness:

- Open marmorial ('marble-like', 15–30 nm thickness, observed in 21% of the population) – a static, gray, marble-like appearance with a sparse open meshwork pattern, which may represent a contraindication for contact lens wear in some patients because the thin lipid layer may lead to rapid evaporative tear loss (*Figure 6.6*);
- Closed marmorial (30–50 nm, 10%) – a static gray, marble-like appearance with a more compact meshwork pattern, which is thought to represent a stable lipid layer satisfactory for contact lens wear;

- Flow pattern (50–80 nm, 23%) – also termed 'wave pattern', a dynamic marmorial appearance, but constantly flowing and changing between blinks, and is thought to represent a full lipid layer that is generally satisfactory for contact lens wear, although there may be a tendency for excess lipid to accumulate (*Figure 6.7*);
- Amorphous pattern (80–90 nm, 24%) – a more-or-less even pattern with a pale blue appearance, which (as for flow pattern) is thought to represent a full lipid layer that is generally satisfactory for contact lens wear, although there may be a tendency for excess lipid to accumulate;
- First-order color fringe pattern (90–140 nm, 10%) – discrete fringes of brown and blue, superimposed on an amorphous gray background, which is thought to represent a full lipid layer that may be problematic for contact lens wear (*Figure 6.8*);
- Second-order color fringe pattern (140–180 nm, 5%) – discrete fringes of green and red, superimposed on an amorphous gray background, which is thought to represent a full lipid layer that is problematic for contact lens wear, because an excess lipid coating on the lens can reduce wettability (*Figure 6.9*);
- 'Other' (>180 nm, 7%) – highly variable colored patterns, which sometimes form as globules or pockets of intense fringe formation (*Figure 6.10*), that do not fall comfortably into any of the other categories, and probably represent heavy lipid contamination and thus may contraindicate contact lens wear.

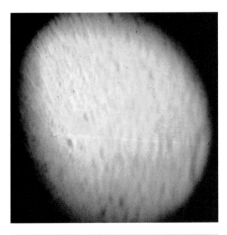

Figure 6.6
Open marmorial lipid formation viewed in specular reflection

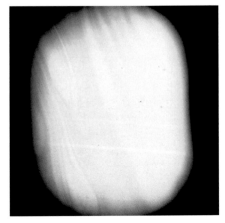

Figure 6.7
Flow pattern lipid formation viewed in specular reflection

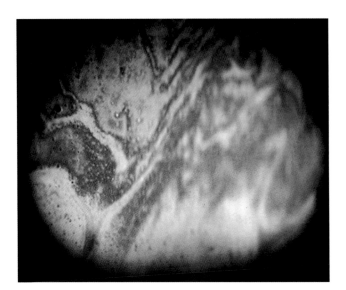

Figure 6.8
First-order color-fringe lipid pattern viewed in specular reflection

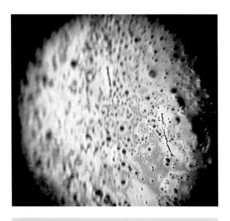

Figure 6.9
Second-order color fringe lipid pattern viewed in specular reflection

The Guillon tear film classification system in Appendix B illustrates the appearance of the pre-corneal tear film lipid layer in patients with dark- and light-colored irides.

Although the aqueous phase of the pre-corneal tear film cannot be observed using a tearscope, it is often visible on the front surface of a contact lens because the pre-lens lipid layer is generally poorly formed or absent. The thicker the pre-lens lipid layer, the less visible are the aqueous fringes. When aqueous fringes can be observed, it is possible to estimate the thickness of this layer by counting the number of fringes across the field of a tearscope. Less than five fringes indicates an aqueous layer thickness of <1 µm, and more than 10 fringes indicates an aqueous layer thickness of 2 µm. An aqueous without fringes is probably more than 3.5 µm thick.

Using a tearscope, Young and Efron[12] evaluated the structure of the tear films on the surfaces of a range of hydrogel lenses of various water contents. They observed that the lipid layer was either absent or very thin on all the lenses, although there was a tendency for lenses with higher water content to support a thin lipid layer. The aqueous phase was generally found to be thicker on lenses of higher water content.

As with hydrogel lenses, the lipid layer is extremely thin or absent on the surface of rigid lenses.[13] The aqueous phase over such lenses is also somewhat thin, typically 2–3 µm thick; this variation in thickness is thought to be patient dependent. A poorly wetting hydrophobic surface of a rigid lens takes on a hazy appearance if the surface is allowed to dry (*Figure 6.11*). The haziness is thought to result from a rapidly drying mucoprotein coating.

The appearance of the tear film on the surface of soft and rigid lenses is shown in Appendix B.

Tear film stability

The structural integrity of the pre-lens tear film can be assessed by measuring the elapsed time from the execution of a normal blink until the tear film breaks up; this is known as the tear break-up time (TBUT). The classic method used to measure TBUT, of instilling fluorescein into the eye and observing the break-up of the fluorescein pattern, cannot be applied to the eye wearing a contact lens because fluorescein is absorbed into the lens material, and thus discolors (and perhaps destroys) the lens and confounds the estimated time of break-up. In addition, fluorescein is known to destabilize the tear film.

Non-invasive techniques are preferred to measure the break-up of the pre-ocular and pre-lens tear film.[14] A black-and-white grid in an illuminated hemispherical dome can be projected optically onto the

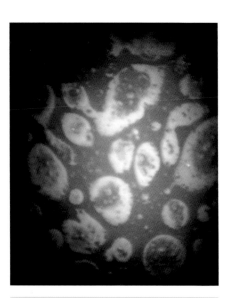

Figure 6.10
Discrete islands of color fringes, in the form of lipid globules, viewed in specular reflection

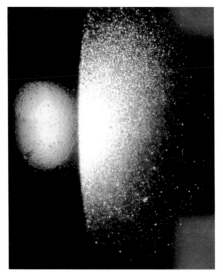

Figure 6.11
Haze on the surface of a high *Dk* rigid lens, observed 4 s after a blink

that longer PLTF NITBUTs are generally associated with lenses of higher water content. This latter finding is consistent with the thicker aqueous layer present on lenses of higher water content observed by Young and Efron[12] in the same study. The PLTF NITBUT of rigid lenses typically ranges from 4 to 6 s.[15]

Optical aberrations created by break-up of the tear film contribute to the decline in image quality observed objectively and psychophysically. Tutt et al.[16] suggest that the decline in image quality that accompanies pre-lens tear break-up may be a direct cause of the blurry vision complaints commonly encountered in patients with lens-induced dry eye.

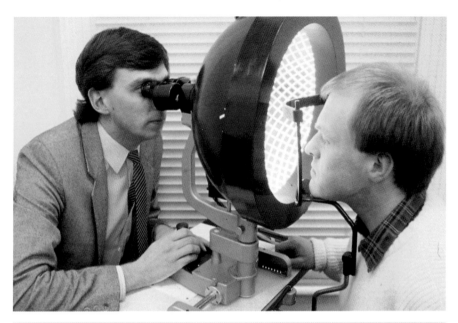

Figure 6.12
System for projecting a grid onto the eye to measure NITBUT

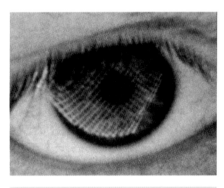

Figure 6.13
Reflection of the grid (*Figure 6.12*) on the ocular surface

eye and observed (*Figure 6.12*); the time taken for the reflected grid to begin breaking up is the NITBUT (*Figure 6.13*). When contact lenses are being worn, the pre-lens tear film non-invasive break-up time (PLTF NITBUT) is recorded.

In an eye not wearing a lens, the tear film remains stable for at least 30 s. In many patients NITBUT may be considerably greater than this, but such measurements are not possible because few patients can voluntarily refrain from blinking for periods longer than 30 s. Young and Efron[12] demonstrated that tear break-up occurs within 3–10 s on the front surface of hydrogel lenses, and

Ocular surface staining

Tissue disruption to the surface of the cornea[17] and conjunctiva[18] can occur during contact lens wear as a consequence of disruption of the tear layer. This can be detected readily by instilling fluorescein into the eye and observing the eye in cobalt blue light on a slit-lamp biomicroscope. Perhaps the most common manifestation of this problem in patients who wear rigid lenses is 3 and 9 o'clock staining. This is a form of desiccation staining that may also be observed in association with soft lens wear, particularly in regions where the cornea has become intermittently exposed, or in regions of the cornea where the overlying lens has become dehydrated.

Fluorescein staining indicates the presence of disrupted and/or missing superficial cells. In advanced cases, staining with rose bengal also reveals the presence of devitalized or dead superficial cells. Itoh et al.[19] reported that tear film instability induced by rigid lenses is associated with damage to the ocular surface epithelium and mucus layer. The topic of ocular surface staining is dealt with in more detail in Chapter 8.

Lid wiper epitheliopathy

Only a small portion of the marginal conjunctiva of the upper lid acts as a wiping surface to spread the tear film over the ocular surface or over the surface of a contact lens.[20] This is because the palpebral surface of the upped lid arches away from the ocular surface, and so creates a space ('Kessing's space'[21]). This contacting surface at the lid margin has been termed the 'lid wiper'[20] (*Figure 6.14*). According to Korb et al.,[20] 80% of contact lens wearers who suffer from dry eye display fluorescein staining of the lid

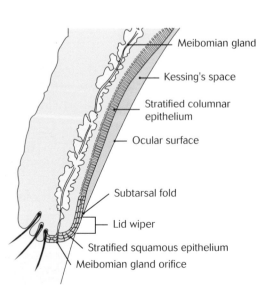

Meibomian gland

Kessing's space

Stratified columnar epithelium

Ocular surface

Subtarsal fold

Lid wiper

Stratified squamous epithelium

Meibomian gland orifice

Figure 6.14
Areas of contact and non-contact with the ocular surface. The area of the lid wiper starts posterior to the meibomian glands, where the stratified squamous epithelium changes from keratinized to non-keratinized tissue, and extends superiorly to the tarsal fold. Adapted with permission from Korb et al.[20]

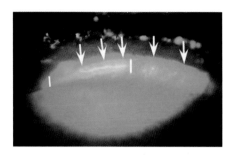

Figure 6.15
Lid wiper epitheliopathy appears as an area of linear fluorescein staining between the two white lines. The arrows indicate the path of the mucocutaneous junction

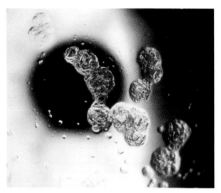

Figure 6.16
'Jelly bumps' on a soft lens

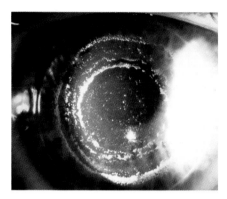

Figure 6.17
Calcium ring deposits on a soft lens

wiper (*Figure 6.15*), versus only 13% of asymptomatic lens wearers.

Lens deposits

Numerous factors, many of which are interactive, are involved in the formation of deposits on the front or back surface of contact lenses. These factors include:

- Lens wear modality;
- Lens replacement frequency;
- Bulk chemical composition of the lens material;
- Lens water content;
- Physicochemical nature of the lens surface (such as ionicity);
- Chemical composition of lens maintenance solutions;
- Adequacy of lens maintenance procedures (a measure of patient compliance);
- Hand contamination;
- Proximity to environmental pollutants; and
- Intrinsic properties of the tears of the patient.

The most common tear-derived components of lens deposits are proteins, lipids and calcium.

Visible lens deposits take months or years to form, and thus are encountered rarely in modern contact lens practice because lenses (in particular soft lenses) are disposed of and replaced regularly. The most common form of visible deposition derived from the tear film is known as 'jelly bumps' or 'mulberry deposits', which consist of various layered combinations of mucus, lipid, protein and sometimes calcium (*Figure 6.16*). Barnacle-like calcium carbonate deposits, which are also derived from the tear film, can project anteriorly and

can be a source of discomfort (*Figure 6.17*). Iron deposits, which are derived from exogenous sources, appear as small red–orange spots or rings and form when iron particles become embedded in the lens and oxidize to form ferrous salts (*Figure 6.18*).

It is clear that proteins and lipids from the tears can deposit on contact lenses within minutes of insertion. Although these rapidly forming deposits cannot be seen and do not generally compromise vision or comfort, they can reduce lens surface wettability.[22]

Both tear quality and composition have a bearing on deposit formation. An excess of a particular tear component coupled with a compromised structural integrity of the tears, which leads to rapid tear break-up and excessive surface drying, are intrinsic factors thought to be conducive to deposit formation. Indeed, some clinical evidence supports the notion that lens deposition is a particular problem in dry eye patients who wear contact lenses.[23]

Post-lens tear film

The tear film between a contact lens and the cornea can also be viewed by specular reflection using the slit-lamp biomicroscope.[24] As for the pre-lens tear film, the thickness of the post-lens tear film can be inferred from the appearance of the specular reflection; an amorphous appearance indicates a relatively thick, aqueous film, and colored patterns and striated formations (texture without color) indicate thinner tear films (*Figure 6.19*). Patterned appearances occur in 25% of soft lens wearers, irrespective of lens type. Although patterned appearances are associated with

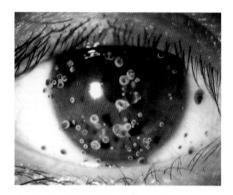

Figure 6.18
Iron deposits on a soft lens

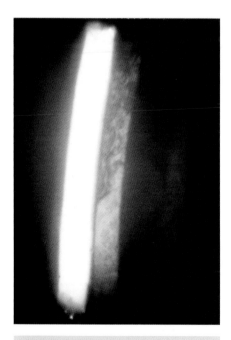

Figure 6.19
Color fringe patterns in the post-lens tear film observed in specular reflection

reduced lens movement, they are unrelated to dryness symptoms.[24]

There are conflicting reports in the literature as to the true thickness of the post-lens tear film. Lin *et al.*[25] used pachometry to determine the thickness of a 58% water-content hydrogel lens; they reported this to be 11–12 μm. Using a reflection spectra technique, Nichols and King-Smith[26] reported a post-lens tear film thickness of 2–3 μm beneath 'traditional' hydrogel lenses and 1–2 μm beneath silicone hydrogel lenses. Brennan *et al.*[27] demonstrated that thinner post-lens tear films are associated with a lower post-lens tear exchange.

Symptoms

Of all the symptoms experienced by contact lens wearers, that of 'dryness' is reported most frequently;[28,29] indeed, in one survey of over 100 contact lens wearers,[29] only 25% of patients stated that they had not experienced this symptom. Brennan and Efron[29] reported that, in a group of contact lens wearers, all the females who used oral contraceptives reported experiencing 'dryness' at times, versus 63% of females who were not using oral contraceptives and 76% of males; these differences were statistically significant.

A major difficulty in assessing the symptom of 'dryness' is that many stimuli may elicit this sensation; that is, it cannot be assumed that the cause of a patient symptom of 'dryness' is necessarily because the eye is dry. A case in point is the study described above, which reported an increased prevalence in the symptom of dryness for females who used oral contraceptives.[29] Tomlinson *et al.*[30] found no effect on tear physiology of serum hormone changes induced by oral contraceptive use or by normal cyclic variations in healthy young females.

As there are no specific 'dryness receptors' in human tissue, ocular dryness must be a response to specific coding of afferent neural inputs. Aside from an actual dry eye, reports of 'dryness' may arise from the neural misinterpretation of stimuli that are unrelated to dry eye, such as vasodilation induced by the mechanical irritation of ocular tissues by the lens. Lowther[31] reported a more rapid tear break-up (lower TBUT) in a group of contact lens wearers with dry eye symptoms versus a group of contact lens wearers without dry eye symptoms,

but Bruce *et al.*[32] failed to demonstrate such an association in a similar experiment. Little and Bruce[24] found no relationship between post-lens tear film morphology and hydrogel lens comfort.

A prudent approach in dealing with a tentative diagnosis of dry eye induced by contact lenses is to apply a comprehensive questionnaire[28,33,34] that draws in other systemic correlates of dryness, such as dryness of other mucous membranes of the body, use of medications, effect of different challenging environments and times when dryness is noted. Such questionnaires are somewhat time-consuming, although they can be conducted by ancillary staff. Dry eye questionnaires can help identify a true dry eye situation in prospective or current contact lens wearers and thus form a clinical rationale for a more detailed assessment.

Pathology and Etiology

Alterations to tear chemistry, composition and structure may be responsible for various adverse signs and symptoms during contact lens wear. Certain aspects of tear physiology during contact lens wear have been explored through the development and application of existing and experimental methodologies. The results of some of these tests that have more immediate clinical relevance are reviewed here. In cases where our understanding of the basis of tear film dysfunction during contact lens wear is poorly understood, various theories have been developed; these are also reviewed.

Tonicity

Immediately after the insertion of either rigid[35] or soft[36] lenses, reflex tearing creates a hypo-osmotic tear film that returns to normal or to slightly hyperosmotic levels once adaptation is complete. Martin[36] observed symmetrical binocular changes in tear osmolarity during monocular lens wear, which suggests that that bilateral reflex lacrimation is responsible for changes in tear tonicity after lens insertion.

In adapted patients, daily rigid lens wear and extended soft lens wear are associated with elevated levels of tear osmolarity, whereas tear osmolarity is normal in adapted daily soft lens wear.[37] Three mechanisms could explain these hyperosmotic shifts:

- Reduced tear stimulation caused by reduced corneal sensitivity;
- Increased lens-induced tear evaporation; or
- Leaching of deposits from the lens into the tears.

Acid–base balance (pH)

Theoretically, an acidic shift in tear pH with contact lens wear might be expected because of a retardation by the lens of the normal carbon dioxide efflux into the atmosphere; the carbon dioxide would then dissolve in the tears and reduce to carbonic acid, and so induce an acidic pH shift.

Although Norn[38] reported that all lens types do induce an acidic pH shift during lens wear, other studies failed to arrive at a consensus on the direction of the pH shift (if any) that resulted from contact lens wear. Tapasztó *et al.*[39] reported an acidic shift during rigid lens wear, but Carney and Hill[40] found no such change. With soft lenses, various authors have reported acidic shifts,[41] alkaline shifts[42] and no shifts in pH.[39] Carney *et al.*[43] reported that the buffering capacity of tears (i.e., the intrinsic capacity of tears to dampen down pH change) is unaffected by lens wear.

Composition

Contact lenses only appear to alter the composition of tears during the adaptation phase of lens wear. When contact lenses are worn for the first time, the increased reflex lacrimation tends to dilute the concentration of those components of the tears that are not secreted from the lacrimal gland (i.e., serum-derived components). This phenomenon is particularly evident during adaptation to rigid lenses, which induce a more intense lacrimation response. Tear components that display increased levels during adaptation, but not during subsequent adapted lens wear, include serum-derived proteins (such as albumin, IgG and transferrin), sodium, chloride, potassium and cholesterol.

Certain components of tears do alter during inflammation, metabolic stress and mechanical trauma, and in many cases these changes are linked to contact lens wear. For example, Vinding *et al.*[44] reported decreased tear concentrations of secretory IgA in long-tern wearers of daily wear and extended wear soft contact lenses, a finding thought to indicate a higher prevalence of sub-clinical corneal and conjunctival inflammation in such patients. Schultz and Kunert[45] reported increased levels of interleukin-6 in basal tears of contact lens wearers versus non wearers of lenses. Fullard and Carney[46] noted an increase in the ratio of lactate dehydrogenase (LDH) to malate dehydrogenase (MDH) during soft lens wear, and Imayasu et al.[47] observed increased LDH levels in the tears of rabbits fitted with contact lenses of low oxygen transmissibility; these findings are consistent with the known anaerobic shift in the corneal epithelium caused by hypoxia during lens wear.

When a small sample of tears is taken from the eye and allowed to dry on a microscope slide, fern-like crystallization patterns may form; these indicate certain characteristics of the tear film, including the salt-to-macromolecule ratio, lipid contamination of mucus and altered tear rheology.[48] A well-structured ferning pattern (*Figure 6.20*) represents a good or even excessive supply of mucus, whereas a disrupted pattern with very few or absent ferns (*Figure 6.21*) may indicate mucus deficiency. Kogbe and Liotet[49] recommend that the tear ferning test be used in contact lens practice to diagnose marginal dry eye as the cause of contact lens intolerance. Ravazzoni et al.[50] reported that the tear ferning test showed sensitivity of 100%, specificity of 87% and diagnostic precision of 97% when performed after 1 month of contact lens wear, which indicates that this test may be useful for predicting contact lens tolerance in a clinical setting.

Temperature

Morgan et al.[51] demonstrated how infrared ocular thermography can provide a measure of the thickness of the tear film that overlies the cornea. Soh[52] adapted this technique to explore the apparent temperature of the tear film on the surface of rigid contact lenses. *Figure 6.22* is a thermogram of an eye wearing a rigid lens. Warmer colors appear red and cooler colors blue. Lower temperatures (blue) are thought to indicate a thinner tear film.[51] Thinning is evident toward the inferior of the lens, which is where tear break-up is expected to occur first. Martin and Fatt[53] demonstrated that contact lens wear induces a very small increase in the temperature of the post-lens tear film.

Tear film turnover

The turnover rate of the tear film is about 16% of the total tear volume per minute.[54] The main determinants of tear turnover are aqueous tear production – primarily from the main lacrimal gland – and tear loss via drainage and/or evaporation. Tear turnover rate can be determined by measuring the decay over time of the fluorescence of tears stained with fluorescein. Such studies have failed to detect any change in tear production induced by contact lenses, except during the initial adaptation

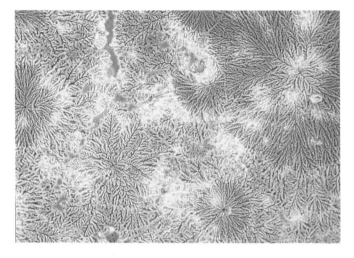

Figure 6.20
Well-structured tear-ferning pattern

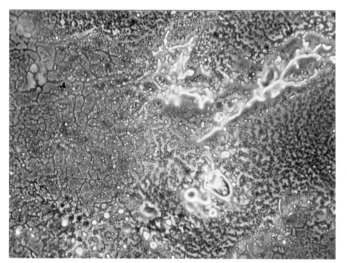

Figure 6.21
Tear sample that displays an absence of ferning

Figure 6.22
Ocular thermogram presumably showing tear thinning on the inferior portion of a rigid contact lens

phase, in which increased lacrimation is observed. Tomlinson and Cederstaff[55] found that tear evaporation increases during wear of all contact lens types, which is presumably because the integrity of the lipid layer of the tear film is compromised during lens wear.

Chang and Chang[56] demonstrated that tear clearance is delayed in patients who have papillary conjunctivitis associated with contact lens wear. They propose that delayed tear clearance might increase the protein and inflammatory mediator concentrations in the tear film and contribute to the pathogenesis or aggravate the severity of papillary conjunctivitis associated with contact lens wear.

Tear break-up

The precise mechanism that leads to tear film break-up is not known. The most popular theory is that advanced by Holly.[57] According to this theory, tear break-up occurs when lipid, which is hydrophobic in nature, migrates down to the mucus layer and compromises the hydrophilicity of the epithelial surface. Tears recede from this region of poor wettability and a dry spot forms. As the tears continue to recede, further intermixing of lipid and mucus occurs at the receding edge, and the field of hydrophobicity increases, which thus increases the dry area – and the process continues. Alternative theories propose

that tear break-up is caused by rupture of the mucus layer[41] or disturbance of the superficial epithelial glycocalyx.[58]

Figure 6.23 is an illustration of the clinical appearance of the thinning and breaking up of the tear film using a projected grid, together with a schematic representation of the process of disruption of the tear film according to the model of Holly.[57]

Gorla and Gorla[59] adopted a theoretical approach in an attempt to determine the reason for pre-corneal tear film break-up. They analyzed nonlinear thin film rupture by investigating the stability of tear films in response to finite amplitude disturbances. The dynamics of the liquid film was formulated using Navier–Stokes equations, which include a body-force term attributable to van der Waals attractions. They managed to solve the governing equation using the finite difference method as part of an initial value problem for spatial periodic boundary conditions.

The mechanism of tear break-up on the surface of contact lenses must be different from that on the surface of the eye because of the absence of properly formed lipid or mucus layers on the lens surface. Rapid pre-lens TBUTs[12] suggest that tear thinning occurs as a result of both evaporation[60] and lateral surface tension forces that draw tear fluid from the lens surface into the surrounding

tear meniscus at the lens edge. Tear break-up is likely to be expedited by the presence of surface deposition.

Feedback model

A 'feedback model' has been proposed to explain the pathogenesis of dry eye.[61,62] This theory suggests a link between ocular surface damage and lacrimal gland function. Specifically, it has been proposed that damage to the ocular surface creates a negative feedback loop, which results in damage to the lacrimal gland. One may further surmise that the chronic sub-clinical ocular surface damage caused by contact lens wear sends negative feedback signals to the lacrimal gland, which in turn induces or exacerbates dry eye pathology and symptomatology.

Management

Most of the strategies applied to alleviating signs and symptoms of dryness in the normal eye (no lens worn) can also be applied to the eye during contact lens wear. This section reviews these strategies, with particular emphasis on their application in contact lens wear.

Choice of lens and solution

The most fundamental choice to make when attempting to solve a dry eye problem related to contact lenses is whether to fit soft or rigid lenses. This choice depends on a number of factors, such as the precise nature of the problem. For example, 3 and 9 o'clock staining induced by a rigid lens can be solved by changing the patient from rigid to soft lenses, to prevent epithelial drying at the 3 and 9 o'clock corneal positions. Problems related to surface drying with a soft lens of low water content can be solved by fitting a lens of higher water content, which has a longer TBUT.[12]

Efron and Brennan[63] reported that patients who wear soft lenses are more likely to complain of 'dryness' the more the lens has dehydrated; however, other studies[64,65] found that such associations were weak or absent. Notwithstanding these equivocal findings – and uncertainty as to the pathophysiologic meaning of the subjective complaint of dryness, as discussed above – it is possible that some patients are most comfortable when they wear a lens that dehydrates the least. Research to date has failed to reveal the material characteristics that determine

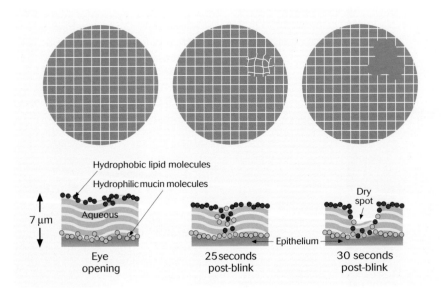

Figure 6.23

The intact tear film observed at eye opening (left), followed by tear thinning at 25 s (middle) and tear break-up at 30 s (right). The top row illustrates this sequence as observed using a projected grid (NITBUT measurement). The bottom row illustrates how a dry spot forms

lens dehydration in the eye, so practitioners must rely on comparative data published in the literature.[66] Frequent lens replacement is also desirable because the pre-lens tear film breaks up more readily in the presence of lens surface contamination.

As a general rule, the characteristics of the contact lens most suited to a patient who experiences dry eye problems are:
- Soft lens – for full corneal coverage;
- Lens with a high water content – to maximize the volume of water in front of the lens;
- Lens that displays minimal in-eye dehydration[67] – to prevent ocular surface desiccation;
- Lens that is replaced frequently[68] – for optimal, deposit-free surface characteristics.

Discomfort and symptoms of dryness are usually associated with the use of solutions that contain first-generation preservatives, such as thimerosal and chlorhexidine. Changing to a solution system that contains current-generation preservatives of large molecular weight, or one that contains no preservatives, typically solves solution-related problems. The use of solutions that contain re-wetting or lubrication agents also helps to alleviate dry eye symptoms.

Re-wetting drops

A strategy commonly used in the management of dry eye related to contact lenses is to supplement the tear film with viscous substitutes and gels. The most popular form of delivery of these agents is via the periodic instillation of re-wetting drops; alternative delivery systems include ointments and inserts (solid pellets that dissolve slowly over time). Golding et al.[69] found that re-wetting drops improve pre-lens tear film stability for a period of only 5 minutes after instillation, and that saline performs no differently from specially formulated products that contain viscoelastic lubrication agents. The same authors[70] also found that saline drops provide short-term symptomatic relief indistinguishable from that of re-wetting drops. None of these solutions were found to reduce lens dehydration. From these studies it can be surmised that there is a psychologic rather than a physical or physiologic basis for the perception of long-term symptomatic relief (i.e., enhanced comfort for longer than 5 minutes) provided by saline or re-wetting drops.

Caffery and Josephson[71] evaluated the performance of 10 different commercially available re-wetting drops and found little difference between them, except that non-preserved solutions were preferred to those that contained preservatives.

Soft lens soaking

Based upon the observation of Efron and Brennan[63] that lens dehydration leads to complaints of dryness, it would seem reasonable that removal of the lens from the eye and rehydration in saline solution can redress the problem. Although such a procedure has yet to be validated experimentally, Lowther[72] has advocated that patients be advised to adopt the following soaking procedure if lens-related symptoms of dryness occur:
- Remove the lens;
- Soak in unit-dose preservative-free saline in the palm of the hand for 10–20 s, and reinsert the lens.

Nutritional supplements

Some researchers[73,74] have suggested that systemic malnutrition, and consequent malnutrition of the tear film and ocular surface, can be the source of dry eye problems. While it is clear that gross vitamin A deficiency can cause serious disease of the ocular surface, there is no evidence that vitamin A drops or, indeed, other such nutritional supplements, can alleviate dry eye problems related to contact lenses. Of interest, however, is the claim of Patel et al.[74] that pre-corneal tear film stability can be enhanced by the systemic ingestion of vitamin and trace element dietary supplements.

Control of evaporation

Various approaches to reducing tear evaporation in patients who suffer from dry eye symptoms related to contact lenses can be adopted. One strategy is to modify the local environment around the eye. This can be achieved by having the patient wear spectacles with a tightly fitting side-shield. The use of tightly fitting swimming goggles represents a more extreme treatment. Clearly, such approaches will be rejected by most contact lens wearers because the very reason they are wearing contact lenses is to avoid wearing spectacles or goggles. Alternatively, the use of a room humidifier may provide some relief.

Patients can be offered the following advice about the environment in which they may spend a significant amount of time:
- Air conditioners tend to have a dehumidifying effect on the local atmosphere;
- The environment in airplanes is generally of low humidity;
- Certain regions of the world have a temperature–humidity relationship that results in a low atmospheric water-vapor pressure, which in turn is conducive to rapid lens dehydration. To help practitioners offer the appropriate advice in this regard, Fatt and Rocher[75] tabulated the time of year, in various cities throughout the world, when patients can expect to experience dryness problems related to lens dehydration.

Reduction of tear drainage

Tear volume can be preserved by blocking the puncta with punctal plugs (*Figure 6.24*). Lowther and Semes[76] inserted temporary dissolvable collagen plugs into one eye of 32 patients with soft lens and dry eye problems, and conducted a 'sham' procedure in the other eye. They found improvement in both the plugged eye and the control eye, which demonstrated a powerful placebo effect, and suggested that dissolvable implants were not effective as a provocative test of the efficacy of permanent punctal plugs.

Giovagnoli and Graham[77] reported that symptomatic patients with soft lenses enjoyed a 35% increase in comfortable wearing time after the insertion of permanent punctal plugs into the lower puncta. This finding suggests that punctal plugs are a viable alternative for contact lens patients who suffer from discomfort through tear insufficiency.

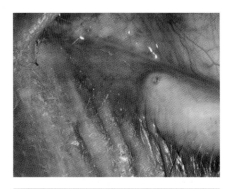

Figure 6.24
Punctal plug in the lower punctum

Tear stimulants

Pharmacological stimulation of residual tear function is a relatively new approach to treating problems related to dry eye. A variety of agents that can enhance basal lacrimal secretion, such as pilocarpine, 3-isobutyl-1-methylxanthine, eledoisin, bromhexine and ciclosporin, have been investigated for possible commercial development.[78] Some of these substances are administered topically, and some systemically. Further research is required to determine whether such an approach:

• Can be applied clinically to dry eye patients who do not wear lenses; and
• Will be of benefit to symptomatic contact lens wearers.

Management of associated disease

It is beyond the scope of this chapter to review all of the possible disease states that can affect the tear film adversely, except to say that practitioners need to be alert to the various possibilities. Perhaps the most common ocular disease state in contact lens wearers associated with lens dryness is meibomian gland dysfunction. Severe blockage of the meibomian gland orifices can result in a lipid deficiency in the tear film, which leads to a more rapid tear loss. Abnormal lipid may also be secreted from diseased meibomian glands, which leads to lipid deposition on the lenses that can result in intermittent blurred vision and discomfort. Treatment strategies, such as warm compresses, lid scrubs and mechanical expression, can be applied to alleviate this condition (see Chapter 4).

Tear secretion is depressed after laser-assisted in-situ keratomileusis[79] and photorefractive keratectomy (PRK)[79,80] during the first 6 months after surgery. Ozdamar *et al.*[81] reported that PRK causes a decrease in tear flow and tear film stability, which is probably caused by decreased corneal sensation after PRK. Post-operative dry eye problems are therefore to be expected in patients who need to be fitted with contact lenses after refractive surgery.

Bandage lenses

It may seem paradoxical to be considering the prescription of soft contact lenses for patients with intractable dry eye problems in a review of the problems associated with, or induced by, contact lenses as outlined in this chap-ter. However, it is clear that patients with severe aqueous deficiency can benefit from bandage lenses. The best type of lens is one with the characteristics described above as being the most suitable for contact lens patients with dry eye problems. It may also be necessary for patients who wear bandage lenses to use re-wetting drops. Rigorous aftercare monitoring of patients who wear bandage lenses is essential in view of the known increase in susceptibility to corneal ulceration in such patients because of the underlying disease state.[82]

Reduced wearing time or cessation of lens wear

Symptoms of dryness typically become worse throughout the daytime wearing period,[33] to the point where the lenses are so uncomfortable that they are removed; indeed, discomfort from dryness is often the limiting factor in determining maximum lens-wearing time. If all other strategies to alleviate extreme dryness fail, the only advice, albeit unsatisfactory, that can be offered to patients is that the strategy that they have already been forced to adopt – that of reducing lens-wearing time – is both the problem itself and the solution to the problem.

The ultimate sanction in the management of intractable tear film dysfunction related to contact lenses is to advise the patient to cease lens wear. In such cases, refractive surgery[83] or overnight orthokeratology[84] may provide a suitable solution.

Prognosis

The prognosis for recovery from tear film dysfunction related to contact lens wear depends on the specific cause of the problem. If the symptoms relate to the wearing of inappropriate lenses or the use of unsuitable solutions, the prognosis may be good if the right lens and/or solution can be found. Similarly, a good prognosis can be advised if the problem is caused by an associated disease state that can be managed successfully – such as meibomian gland dysfunction. In cases for which the underlying cause is difficult to treat – such as aqueous deficiency because of keratoconjunctivitis sicca – the prognosis is poor, although further research into new strategies such as the clinical application of tear-stimulating agents[78] do hold future promise of a better prognosis for some patients.

An additional consideration of prognostic interest is whether the tear film is disrupted after lens removal and, if so, how long it takes for the tear film to return to normal. This question was addressed by Kline and DeLuca,[85] who documented a 54% decrease in TBUT measured within 10 minutes of removal of a hydrogel lens (compared with pre-fitting estimates of TBUT). Faber *et al.*[86] made a similar observation, and noted that the TBUT had largely returned to normal within 25 minutes of lens removal. Thus, lens-induced disruption to the pre-corneal tear film is short-lived after lens removal.

Differential Diagnosis

As already discussed, practitioners need to be alert to the myriad of associated disease states that can occur concurrently with contact lens wear so that these can be differentiated from conditions caused by the contact lens alone. Differential diagnosis between tear film dysfunction associated with contact lenses versus tear film dysfunction caused by associated disease can be effected by ceasing lens wear for 1 month; if problematic signs and symptoms persist for this period, it is unlikely that contact lenses are the cause of the problem.

Albietz and Golding[87] classified the various dry eye subtypes not related to contact lenses, as listed below, together with the common causes and prevalence (shown in parentheses):

• Aqueous tear deficiency caused by lacrimal gland dysfunction (0.5–3.0%);
• Lipid anomaly caused by meibomian gland dysfunction (39.8%);
• Lid surfacing anomalies caused by eyelid or blinking dysfunction (1.4–3.0%);
• Mucus deficiency caused by conjunctival goblet cell disorder (rare);
• Primary epitheliopathy caused by epithelial disorder (rare);
• Allergic dry eye caused by non-goblet epithelial cell disorder (unknown).

Attempts should, of course, be made to treat associated ocular pathology identified as a possible cause of dry eye symptoms in a contact lens wearer. Whether or not the associated pathology is cured completely, the practitioner will be in a much better position to devise a viable management plan and to formulate an accurate prognosis of ongoing contact lens wear success.

REFERENCES

1 Wolff E (1946). The muco-cutaneous junction of the lid margin and the distribution of the tear fluid. *Trans Ophthalmol Soc UK* **66**, 291–305.

2 Tiffany JM (1988). Tear film stability and contact lens wear. *J Br Contact Lens Assoc.* **11**, 35–38.

3 Prydal JI and Campbell FW (1992). Study of precorneal tear film thickness and structure by interferometry and confocal microscopy. *Invest Ophthalmol Vis Sci.* **33**, 1996–2005.

4 King-Smith PE, Fink BA, Fogt N, *et al.* (2000). The thickness of the human pre-corneal tear film: Evidence from reflection spectra. *Invest Ophthalmol Vis Sci.* **41**, 3348–3359.

5 Baier RE and Thomas EB (1996). The ocean: The eye of earth. *Contact Lens Spectrum* **11**, 37–38.

6 Hodson S and Earlam R (1994). Of an extracellular matrix in human pre-corneal tear film. *J Theor Biol.* **168**, 395–398.

7 Mainstone JC, Bruce AS and Golding TR (1996). Tear meniscus measurements in the diagnosis of dry eye. *Curr Eye Res.* **15**, 653–657.

8 Hamano H, Hori M and Hamano T (1983). A new method for measuring tears. *CLAO J.* **9**, 281–287.

9 Koby ES (1924). *Microscopie de l'Oeil vivant.* (Paris: Mason et Cie).

10 Guillon JP (1998). Use of the Tearscope Plus and attachments in the routine examination of the marginal dry eye contact lens patient. *Adv Exp Med Biol.* **438**, 859–867.

11 Guillon JP and Guillon M (1988). Tear film examination in the contact lens patient. *Contax* **3**: 14–20.

12 Young G and Efron N (1991). Characteristics of the pre-lens tear film during hydrogel contact lens wear. *Ophthalmic Physiol Opt.* **11**, 53–58.

13 Guillon M, Guillon JP and Mapstone V (1989). Rigid gas permeable lenses *in vivo* wettability. *Trans Br Contact Lens Assoc.* Conference Proceedings, 24.

14 Mengher LS, Bron AJ, Tonge SR and Gilbert DJ (1985). A non-invasive instrument for clinical assessment of the pre-corneal tear film stability. *Curr Eye Res.* **4**, 1–7.

15 Guillon M and Guillon JP (1988). Pre-lens tear film characteristics of high *Dk* rigid gas permeable lenses. *Am J Optom Physiol Opt.* **65**, 73–78.

16 Tutt R, Bradley A, Begley C and Thibos LN (2000). Optical and visual impact of tear break-up in human eyes. *Invest Ophthalmol Vis Sci.* **41**, 4117–4123.

17 Wilson G and Laurent J (1998). The size of corneal epithelial cells collected by contact lens cytology from dry eyes. *Adv Exp Med Biol.* **438**, 831–834.

18 Albietz JM (2001). Conjunctival histologic findings of dry eye and non-dry eye contact lens wearing subjects. *CLAO J.* **27**, 35–40.

19 Itoh R, Yokoi N and Kinoshita S (1999). Tear film instability induced by rigid contact lenses. *Cornea* **18**, 440–443.

20 Korb DR, Greiner JV, Herman JP, *et al.* (2002). Lid-wiper epitheliopathy and dry-eye symptoms in contact lens wearers. *CLAO J.* **28**, 211–216.

21 Kessing SV (1967). A new division of the conjunctiva on the basis of x-ray examination. *Acta Ophthalmol (Copenh.)* **45**, 680–683.

22 Jones L, Franklin V, Evans K, *et al.* (1996). Spoilation and clinical performance of monthly vs. three monthly Group II disposable contact lenses. *Optom Vis Sci.* **73**, 16–21.

23 Doughman DJ (1975). The nature of 'spots' on soft lenses. *Ann Ophthalmol.* **7**, 345–348.

24 Little SA and Bruce AS (1994). Postlens tear film morphology, lens movement and symptoms in hydrogel lens wearers. *Ophthalmic Physiol Opt.* **14**, 65–68.

25 Lin MC, Graham AD, Polse KA, *et al.* (1999). Measurement of post-lens tear thickness. *Invest Ophthalmol Vis Sci.* **40**, 2833–2838.

26 Nichols J and King-Smith E (2001). *In-vivo* thickness of the pre- and post-lens tear film and silicone hydrogel contact lenses measured by interferometry. *Optom Vis Sci.* **78**, 51S.

27 Brennan NA, Jaworski A, Shuley V, *et al.* (2001). Studies of the post-lens tear film. *Optom Vis Sci.* **78**, 51S.

28 McMonnies CW and Ho A (1986). Marginal dry eye diagnosis: History versus biomicroscopy. In: *The Pre-ocular Tear Film in Health, Disease and Contact Lens Wear*, Ed. Holly FJ, p. 32–40. (Dry Eye Institute: Lubbock).

29 Brennan NA and Efron N (1989). Symptomatology of HEMA contact lens wear. *Optom Vis Sci.* **66**, 834–838.

30 Tomlinson A, Pearce EI, Simmons PA and Blades K (2001). Effect of oral contraceptives on tear physiology. *Ophthalmic Physiol Opt.* **21**, 9–16.

31 Lowther GE (1993). Comparison of hydrogel contact lens patients with and without the symptoms of dryness. *Int Contact Lens Clin.* **20**, 191–196.

32 Bruce AS, Golding TR and Au SWM (1995). Mechanisms of dryness in soft lens wear. *Clin Exp Optom.* **78**, 168–173.

33 Begley CG, Caffery B, Nichols KK and Chalmers R (2000). Responses of contact lens wearers to a dry eye survey. *Optom Vis Sci.* **77**, 40–46.

34 Begley CG, Chalmers RL, Mitchell GL, *et al.* (2001). Characterization of ocular surface symptoms from optometric practices in North America. *Cornea* **20**, 610–618.

35 Terry JE and Hill RM (1977). Osmotic adaptation to rigid contact lenses. *Arch Ophthalmol.* **37**, 785–788.

36 Martin DK (1987). Osmolality of the tear fluid in the contralateral eye during monocular contact lens wear. *Acta Ophthalmol (Copenh.)* **65**, 551–555.

37 Farris RL, Stuchell RN and Mandel ID (1981). Basal and reflex human tear analysis. I. Physical measurements: Osmolarity, basal volumes, and reflex flow rate. *Ophthalmology* **88**, 852–857.

38 Norn MS (1988). Tear fluid pH in normals, contact lens wearers, and pathological cases. *Acta Ophthalmol (Copenh.)* **66**, 485–488.

39 Tapasztó I, Koller A and Tapasztó Z (1988). Biochemical changes in the human tears of hard and soft contact lens wearers. II. The pH variations in the human tears of hard and soft contact lens wearers. *Contact Lens J.* **16**, 265–271.

40 Carney LG and Hill RM (1976). Tear pH and the hard contact lens patient. *Int Contact Lens Clin.* **3**, 27–32.

41 Hill RM and Carney LG (1977). Tear pH and the soft contact lens patient. *Int Contact Lens Clin.* **4**, 68–72.

42 Andres S, Garcia ML, Espina M, *et al.* (1988). Tear pH, air pollution, and contact lenses. *Am J Optom Physiol Opt.* **65**, 627–631.

43 Carney LG, Mauger TF and Hill RM (1990). Tear buffering in contact lens wearers. *Acta Ophthalmol (Copenh.)* **68**, 75–78.

44 Vinding T, Eriksen JS and Nielsen NV (1987). The concentration of lysozyme and secretory IgA in tears from healthy persons with and without contact lens use. *Acta Ophthalmol (Copenh.)* **65**, 23–26.

45 Schultz CL and Kunert KS (2000). Interleukin-6 levels in tears of contact lens wearers. *J Interferon Cytokine Res.* **20**, 309–310.

46 Fullard RJ and Carney LG (1986). Use of tear enzyme activities to assess the corneal response to contact lens wear. *Acta Ophthalmol (Copenh.)* **64**, 216–220.

47 Imayasu M, Petroll WM, Jester JV, *et al.* (1994), The relation between contact lens oxygen transmissibility and binding of *Pseudomonas aeruginosa* to the cornea after overnight wear. *Ophthalmology* **101**, 371–388.

48 Golding TR and Brennan NA (1989). The basis of tear ferning. *Clin Exp Optom.* **72**, 102–106.

49 Kogbe O and Liotet S (1987). An interesting use of the study of tear ferning patterns in contactology. *Ophthalmologica* **194**, 150–153.

50 Ravazzoni L, Ghini C, Macri A and Rolando M (1998). Forecasting of hydrophilic contact lens tolerance by means of tear ferning test. *Graefes Arch Clin Exp Ophthalmol.* **236**, 354–358.

51 Morgan PB, Tullo AB and Efron N (1995). Infrared thermography of the tear film in dry eye. *Eye* **9**, 615–618.

52 Soh MP (1994). *Infrared Thermography of the Anterior Eye during Contact Lens Wear*, PhD Thesis (Manchester: University of Manchester).

53 Martin DK and Fatt I (1986). The presence of a contact lens induces a very small increase in the anterior corneal surface temperature. *Acta Ophthalmol (Copenh.)* **64**, 512–518.

54 Puffer MJ, Neault RW and Brubaker RF (1980). Basal precorneal tear turnover in the human eye. *Am J Ophthalmol.* **89**, 369–376.

55 Tomlinson A and Cedarstaff TH (1982). Tear evaporation from the human eye: The effects of contact lens wear. *J Br Contact Lens Assoc.* **5**, 141–147.

56 Chang SW and Chang CJ (2001). Delayed tear clearance in contact lens associated papillary conjunctivitis. *Curr Eye Res.* **22**, 253–257.

57 Holly FJ (1973). Formation and stability of the tear film. *Int Ophthalmol Clin.* **13**, 73–86.

58 Liotet S, Van Bijsterveld OP, Kogbe O and Laroche L (1987). A new hypothesis on tear film stability. *Ophthalmologica* **195**, 119–124.

59 Gorla MS and Gorla RS (2000). Nonlinear theory of tear film rupture. *J Biomech Eng.* **122**, 498–503.

60 Craig JP, Singh I, Tomlinson A, *et al.* (2000). The role of tear physiology in ocular surface temperature. *Eye* **14**, 635–641.

61 Stern ME, Beuerman RW, Fox RI, *et al.* (1998). The pathology of dry eye: The interaction between the ocular surface and lacrimal glands. *Cornea* **17**, 584–588.

62 Mathers WD (2000). Why the eye becomes dry: A cornea and lacrimal gland feedback model. *CLAO J.* **26**, 159–165.

63 Efron N and Brennan NA (1988). A survey of wearers of low water content hydrogel contact lenses. *Clin Exp Optom.* **71**, 86–80.

64 Pritchard N and Fonn D (1995). Dehydration, lens movement and dryness ratings of hydrogel contact lenses. *Ophthalmic Physiol Opt.* **15**, 281–286.

65 Fonn D, Situ P and Simpson T (1999). Hydrogel lens dehydration and subjective comfort and dryness ratings in symptomatic and asymptomatic contact lens wearers. *Optom Vis Sci.* **76**, 700–704.

66 Brennan NA and Efron N (1987). Hydrogel lens dehydration: A material dependent phenomenon? *Contact Lens Forum* **12**, 28–28.

67 Lemp MA, Caffery B, Lebow K, *et al.* (1999). Omafilcon A (Proclear) soft contact lenses in a dry eye population. *CLAO J.* **25**, 40–47.

68 Jurkus JM and Gurkaynak D (1994). Disposable lenses and the marginal dry eye patient. *J Am Optom Assoc.* **65**, 756–758.

69 Golding TR, Efron N and Brennan NA (1990). Soft lens lubricants and prelens tear film stability. *Optom Vis Sci.* **67**, 461–465.

70 Efron N, Golding TR and Brennan NA (1991). The effect of soft lens lubricants on symptoms and lens dehydration. *CLAO J.* **17**, 114–118.

71 Caffery BE and Josephson JE (1990). Is there a better 'comfort drop'? *J Am Optom Assoc.* **61**, 178–182.

72 Lowther GE (1997). *Dryness, Tears and Contact Lens Wear*. (Boston: Butterworth–Heinemann).

73 Caffery BE (1991). Influence of diet on tear function. *Optom Vis Sci.* **68**, 58–62.

74 Patel S, Ferrier C and Plaskow J (1994). Effect of systemic ingestion of vitamin and trace element dietary supplements on the stability of the pre-corneal tear film in normal subjects. In: *Lacrimal Gland, Tear Film and Dry Eye Syndromes*, Ed. Sullivan DA, p. 285–287. (New York: Plenum Press).

75 Fatt I and Rocher P (1994). Contact lens performance in different climates. *Optom Today* **34**, 26–28.

76 Lowther GE and Semes L (1995). Effect of absorbable intracanalicular collagen implants in hydrogel contact lens patients with drying symptoms. *Int Contact Lens Clin.* **22**, 238–243.

77 Giovagnoli D and Graham SJ (1992). Inferior punctal occlusion with removable silicone punctal plugs in the treatment of dry-eye related contact lens discomfort. *J Am Optom Assoc.* **63**, 481–485.

78 Bron A, Hornby S and Tiffany J (1997). The management of dry eye. *Optician* **214**(5613), 13–17.

79 Benitez-del-Castillo JM, del Rio T, Iradier T, *et al.* (2001). Decrease in tear secretion and corneal sensitivity after laser *in situ* keratomileusis. *Cornea* **20**, 30–32.

80 Lee JB, Ryu CH, Kim J, *et al.* (2000). Comparison of tear secretion and tear film instability after photorefractive keratectomy and laser *in situ* keratomileusis. *J Cataract Refract Surg.* **26**, 1326–1331.

81 Ozdamar A, Aras C, Karakas N, *et al.* (1999). Changes in tear flow and tear film stability after photorefractive keratectomy. *Cornea* **18**, 437–438.

82 Dohlman C, Bouchoff SA and Mobilia EE (1973). Complications in use of soft contact lenses in corneal disease. *Arch Ophthalmol.* **90**, 367–375.

83 Toda I, Yagi Y, Hata S, *et al.* (1996). Excimer laser photorefractive keratectomy for patients with contact lens intolerance caused by dry eye. *Br J Ophthalmol.* **80**, 604–608.

84 Nichols JJ, Marsich MM, Nguyen M, *et al.* (2000). Overnight orthokeratology. *Optom Vis Sci.* **77**, 252–259.

85 Kline LN and DeLuca TJ (1975). Effect of gel lens wear on the precorneal tear film. *Int Contact Lens Clin.* **2**, 56–62.

86 Faber E, Golding TR, Lowe R and Brennan NA (1991). Effect of hydrogel lens wear on tear film stability. *Optom Vis Sci.* **68**, 380–384.

87 Albietz JM and Golding TR (1994). Differential diagnosis and management of common dry eye subtypes. *Clin Exp Optom.* **77**, 244–248.

MUCIN BALLS

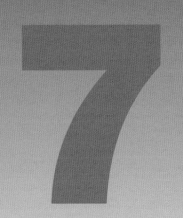

Various forms of organic and inorganic matter can accumulate in the post-lens tear film. These include intrinsic matter such as desquamated epithelial cells, inflammatory cells and microorganisms, and extrinsic matter such as dust particles that may have entered the eye from the atmosphere. Most of this matter is flushed away during daily lens wear as a result of the blink-activated tear pump. The accumulation of such debris during extended lens wear is potentially more problematic because it can be retained at the corneal surface for longer periods – such as overnight during sleep. An important requirement of extended wear lenses is that such matter is flushed out from beneath the lens as soon as the patient begins to blink upon awakening in the morning.

A characteristic form of debris known as 'mucin balls' has been observed in patients who wear high oxygen performance silicone hydrogel contact lenses. Although the appearance of mucin balls was first formally reported in the literature in 2000[1,2] – corresponding with the market release of silicone hydrogel lenses – earlier anecdotal reports suggested that this phenomenon had been observed previously. Other descriptive terms used include lipid plugs,[3] tear microspheres,[4] microdeposits[5] and spherical post-lens debris.[2] Some authors[6,7] suggest that a small number of mucin balls can be observed in some patients who use conventional hydrogel lenses on an extended wear basis.

Signs

Mucin balls are observed within minutes of lens insertion between the posterior lens surface and the corneal epithelium. Under direct white light at low illumination they appear as a mass of discrete gray dots that seem to be fixed in position; that is, they do not move in synchrony with the contact lens after a blink. At higher magnification under direct white light illumination, mucin balls appear as cream–gray, round or ovoid inclusions that may be near spherical or somewhat flattened (*Figure 7.1*). When viewed using indirect retro-illumination, mucin balls display reversed illumination, which indicates that the material from which the mucin ball is composed (presumably mucin, see later) is of a higher refractive index than the surrounding medium (tear aqueous). Under these illumination conditions, some mucin balls take on a distinct doughnut-like appearance with a thick annular rim and membrane across the center (*Figure 7.2*).

Tan *et al.*[4] and Craig *et al.*[8] suggest that mucin balls are observed more commonly in the superior cornea, although this characteristic has not been reported by other authors.[1,2,9] Mucin balls can also become embedded in the conjunctival epithelium close to the limbus (see 'Differential diagnosis' in Chapter 8). Estimates of the size (diameter) of individual mucin balls vary: Fonn *et al.*[1] and Dumbleton *et al.*[2] reported 20–200 μm and Craig *et al.*[8] made a similar estimate of 10–200 μm, whereas Bourassa and Benjamin[5] and Tan *et al.*[4] reported 40–120 μm. Sweeney *et al.*[7] suggested that mucin balls fall into two size categories: small (10–20 μm) and large (20–50 μm). Ladage *et al.*[10] measured the size of mucin balls in three patients using corneal confocal microscopy, and reported a size range from 33.9 to 78.8 μm (mean 57.9 ± 14 μm). These estimates are quite large in comparison with the thickness of the tear film beneath silicone hydrogel lenses (1–2 μm)[11] and the corneal epithelium (about 50–70 μm).[12]

Various factors govern the number of mucin balls present at any given time. In their respective case reports, Bourassa and Benjamin[5] observed 20–30 mucin balls and Fonn *et al.*[1] observed up to 50 mucin balls over a number of visits. In clinical trials of patients who wore silicone hydrogel lenses, Fonn *et al.*[1] reported that 95% of the patients displayed less than 50 mucin balls over a 3 month period, and Sweeney *et al.*[7] and Tan *et al.*[6] reported

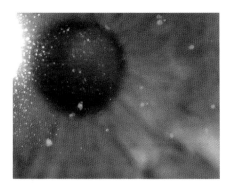

Figure 7.1
Mucin balls observed under direct illumination at high magnification

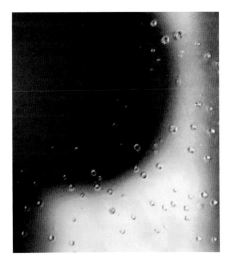

Figure 7.2
Mucin balls observed using indirect marginal retro-illumination display a flattened doughnut appearance. The mucin balls at the inferior pupil margin display reversed illumination

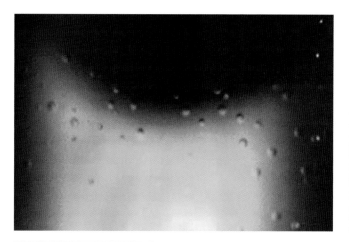

Figure 7.3

Fluid-filled pits in the epithelium caused by depressions created by large mucin balls that have since become dislodged. The pits display unreversed illumination

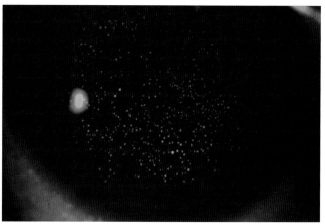

Figure 7.4

A combination of mucin balls and aqueous-filled epithelial depressions that stain with fluorescein (it is not possible to distinguish between these two features when the staining pattern is viewed under fluorescent light)

that the mean number of mucin balls over a 12 month period did not exceed an average of 20. All seven patients who wore silicone hydrogel lenses in the clinical trial of Craig et al.[8] demonstrated between 60 and 100 mucin balls within 22 days of commencing lens wear. Sometimes in excess of 100 mucin balls may be observed.[1,6] Craig et al.[8] reported 230 mucin balls in one subject.

After lens removal, the majority of mucin balls are blinked away to leave depressions (also termed 'imprints' or 'pits') in the epithelial surface. These depressions fill with tear aqueous and appear as transparent spherical inclusions that display unreversed illumination when viewed at high magnification with a slit-lamp biomicroscope using retro-illumination (*Figure 7.3*). Some mucin balls appear to remain lodged in the surface of the epithelium; these continue to display reversed illumination, which thus allows these two entities to be differentiated. Upon instillation of fluorescein into the eye, both the remaining mucin balls and the aqueous in the epithelial depressions stain with fluorescein, which results in a pattern of punctate spots over the cornea. It is virtually impossible to distinguish between mucin balls and the aqueous-filled epithelial depressions; both appear as discrete, solid, fluorescent-green spots of similar size when viewed under fluorescent light (*Figure 7.4*). Mucin balls do not stain with rose bengal, which suggests that there is no co-existing disturbance of corneal surface integrity.[7]

Time course

Sweeney et al.[7] and Tan et al.[6] reported that mucin balls increase in number and size over the initial few months of silicone hydrogel lens extended wear. Morgan and Efron[9] conducted a randomized, crossover clinical trial in which 30 subjects each wore a pair of PureVision (Bausch & Lomb) and Focus Night & Day (CIBA Vision) silicone hydrogel contact lenses for 8 weeks on an extended wear basis. The percentage of patients who presented with mucin balls increased to 37% and 54% of patients for PureVision and Focus

Night & Day, respectively, after 4 weeks, and began to decline thereafter (*Figure 7.5*). Dumbleton et al.[2] did not detect a change in the mean grade of mucin ball appearance over a 6 month period among 92 patients who wore Focus Night & Day lenses.

Prevalence

As stated above, Morgan and Efron[9] reported that between 37% and 54% of patients who wear silicone hydrogel lenses display mucin balls after about 4 weeks. Tan et al.[6] observed that the per-

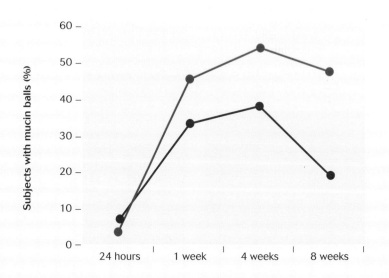

Figure 7.5

Incidence and time course of mucin-ball formation with two types of silicone hydrogel lenses. Red circles, Focus Night & Day; blue circles, PureVision

centage of all subjects who wear silicone hydrogel lenses and have mucin balls varied from 37% to 82% during the year. Dumbleton et al.[2] reported that mucin balls were observed in 70% of patients at one or more visits of their clinical trial, and in 29% of subjects at all three visits, while wearing Focus Night & Day lenses.

Associated observations

Morgan and Efron[9] analyzed the results of their clinical trial to see if the presence of mucin balls was related to any other clinical results. Paradoxically, high-contrast visual acuity was demonstrated to be about one letter better in the presence of mucin balls;[9] this is consistent with the report of Dumbleton et al.,[2] who showed that the subjective appreciation of vision was superior in the presence of mucin balls after 6 months of wear. There was no difference for low-contrast visual acuity.[9] It is not clear why vision should be better in the presence of mucin balls.

Some biomicroscopic signs appear to be related to mucin balls.[9] An unexpected finding in the study of Morgan and Efron[9] was that conjunctival and limbal redness were both reduced and the number of microcysts appeared to increase in subjects who exhibited mucin balls. The apparent association between the appearance of mucin balls and epithelial microcysts, also observed by Tan et al.,[6] may be an artefact that relates to the difficulty in differentiating mucin balls from microcysts.

An association was revealed between the presence of mucin balls and increased corneal fluorescein staining;[9] this is probably because the remaining mucin balls and fluid-filled epithelial pits stain with fluorescein. The above associations concerning mucin balls contrast with those of other authors,[2,4,7] who found no relationship between biomicroscopic signs and mucin balls.

Naduvilath[13] demonstrated an association between the appearance of mucin balls and the development of contact lens induced peripheral ulcer (CLPU; see Chapter 22). Specifically, patients who display mucin balls have a ×1.6 probability of developing CLPU compared with patients who do not display mucin balls.

Symptoms

Dumbleton et al.[2] found no association between the appearance of mucin balls

and overall comfort, waking comfort, waking dryness or day-end dryness, although the process of lens removal was reported as being slightly less comfortable in the presence of mucin balls. Other authors[4,7,9] reported that subjective comfort is unaffected by the presence of mucin balls.

Etiology

The reasons for the formation of mucin balls are unclear and likely to be complex. The prevailing hypothesis is that the low deposition rate of silicone hydrogel materials prevents any significant uptake of deposits (protein, lipid and mucins) onto or into the lens matrix during lens wear. The depletion of aqueous during overnight wear of silicone hydrogel lenses – as evidenced by the very thin post-lens tear film – results in a viscous, mucin–lipid layer between the lens and epithelial surface. This layer is likely to contain much more mucin than lipid, which reflects the respective proportions of these two entities in the tear film. Silicone hydrogel lenses are thought to induce high interfacial forces, which, when coupled with the high modulus of elasticity (greater stiffness) of such lenses, creates a sheering of this viscous, mucin-rich post-lens layer in the course of lens movement induced by normal blinking (daytime wear) and rapid eye movements (during sleep). These sheering forces have the effect of rolling the mucin-rich post-lens layers into spheres, which are observed as mucin balls.

The difference in mucin-ball response between the PureVision (Bausch & Lomb) and Focus Night & Day (CIBA Vision) silicone hydrogel contact lenses reported by Morgan and Efron[9] may be related to differences in interfacial shear forces as a result of the different types of surface treatments applied to each lens. A classic plasma surface modification is used to render the surface of the PureVision lens hydrophilic, whereas a plasma coating is applied to the Focus Night & Day lens to enhance surface wettability. Certainly, the chemical composition and nature of the lens mold used in the manufacture of silicone hydrogel lenses can affect mucin ball formation; for example, Lai and Friends[14] found that the use of polar plastic molds minimized mucin ball formation.

Dumbleton et al.[2] further postulated that a greater mismatch in shape between

the back surface of the lens and the epithelial surface may increase the degree of lens movement over the ocular surface and thus create more sheering and, consequently, more mucin balls. In support of this theory, they demonstrated that subjects who exhibited mucin balls had significantly steeper keratometry readings along the flatter meridian than those who did not (bearing in mind that all lenses in their experiment had the same back optic zone radius, BOZR);[2] that is, those with relatively flatter, looser lens fits exhibited a greater number of mucin balls. No such association between corneal curvature and mucin formation was found by other authors who fitted single-BOZR lenses.[4,9]

Pathology

Structure and composition of mucin balls

Using a corneal confocal microscope, Craig et al.[8] reported that mucin balls display a highly reflective core with a more poorly reflective, apparently translucent, outer layer. The diameter of the central core relative to the outer coating varied among mucin balls. This bilayered appearance was confirmed by the same authors[8] using phase-contrast microscopy of mucin balls obtained from the back surface of lenses removed from the eye.

The name 'mucin balls' infers that these entities are composed primarily of tear mucins (mucins are the glycoprotein components of mucus and vary greatly in molecular size). Millar et al.[15] analyzed mucin balls using light microscopic histochemistry, scanning electron microscopy, electron microscopic elemental analysis and confocal microscopy. They demonstrated that mucin balls are PAS positive, which indicates that glycoproteins are a major component. Lipids and bacteria were not detected. Millar et al.[15] concluded that mucin balls were made exclusively of collapsed mucin.

Pathogenesis of mucin ball formation

Within minutes of lens insertion, mucin ball formation begins at the interface of the posterior lens surface and the precorneal tear film. Sweeney et al.[7] suggest that mucin balls are more prominent in the superior quadrant of the cornea beneath the resting position of the upper eyelid. The mucinous layer of the tear film, along with some lipid components,

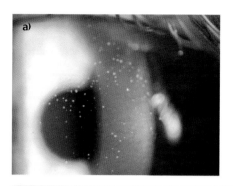
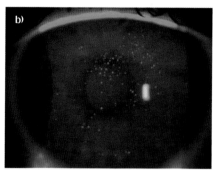

Figure 7.6

Evidence of staining caused by mucin balls and fluid-filled pits. (a) Mucin balls and fluid-filled pits observed behind the lens in white light. (b) After lens removal, most of the mucin balls are washed away and some remain. Fluorescein stains the remaining mucin balls, and fills epithelial pits created by the mucin balls that subsequently were washed away. Upon careful inspection, the concordance between the position of the mucin balls and fluid-filled pits observed in white light (a) versus the appearance of the same entities stained with fluorescein (b) can be seen

is apparently 'rolled up' into discrete elements. At first, the resultant mucin balls are small in size and appear as an assortment of scattered debris in the form of individual deposits or small clumps of material. They remain fixed in position after a blink, which suggests that mucin balls are somehow fixed to, or partially embedded in, the epithelium (*Figure 7.6*).

With continuing lens wear, the mucin balls increase in size and some become deeply embedded in the epithelium, probably because of the force of the lens (*Figure 7.7*). At this point, slit-lamp examination using indirect retro-illumination reveals two forms of refractile elements. Those that display reversed illumination are the mucin balls that lie in the aqueous phase of the tear film. Those that display unreversed illumination are a either mucin balls buried deeper in the epithelial surface or fluid-filled pits created by mucin balls that subsequently became dislodged through blinking. These illumination effects are observed both with and without (*Figure 7.8*) the lens on the eye. As stated previously, both mucin balls and fluid-filled pits stain with fluorescein and their appearance under fluorescent light is identical.

After prolonged periods of lens wear, some of the mucin balls become so large that they cannot maintain their spherical shape and collapse inwardly. This results in a doughnut appearance, with a flat center and tire-like annulus around the rim.[1] A small circular island of material can sometimes be observed in the center of the collapsed mucin ball (*Figure 7.9*).

It is unclear why mucin balls should collapse in this way, rather than the more intuitive scenario of the near-spherical mucin balls simply becoming flattened into a disciform shape.

Consequential pathology

Ladage *et al.*[10] were able to replicate the formation of mucin balls in a rabbit model, and observed Ki-67-positive stromal cells immediately beneath indentations that reached the epithelial basement membrane. This indicates that active pro-

liferation of stromal cells was stimulated focally. These authors also noted a local increase in keratocyte density immediately beneath deep mucin balls. Stromal keratocytes do not divide unless stimulated to do so, which led Ladage *et al.*[10] to conclude that the Ki-67-positive stromal cells represent either dividing keratocytes or activated fibroblasts.

From a theoretical standpoint, clinicians ought to be concerned about the formation of mucin balls inasmuch as they represent a compromise of the mucus phase of the pre-corneal tear film. For example, Fleiszig *et al.*[16] demonstrated the critical importance of the mucus phase in preventing the attachment of potentially pathogenic bacteria to the corneal surface. In the absence of a properly formed mucus layer, which may occur as a result of extensive mucin ball formation, bacteria are more likely to attach to the cornea and establish an infection.

Aside from the protective function of mucus, potentially pathogenic organisms are more likely to establish an infectious process if there is a breach of the corneal epithelium. Fonn *et al.*[1] and Pritchard *et al.*[17] observed that fluorescein does not generally penetrate into the epithelium, which they suggest indicates that this corneal layer is not breached as a result of mucin ball formation. However, inspection of images of fluorescein staining in patients who have extensive mucin ball formation (*Figure 7.10*) reveals a diffuse

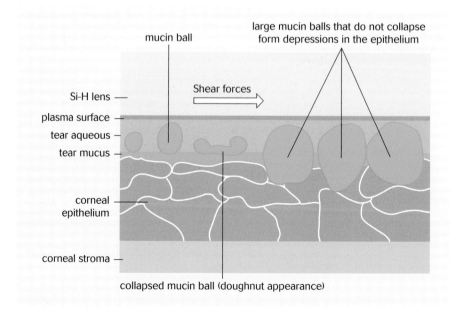

Figure 7.7

The formation of mucin balls and epithelial depressions

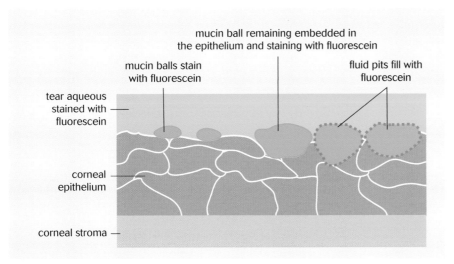

tear aqueous
stained with
fluorescein

mucin balls stain
with fluorescein

mucin ball remaining embedded in
the epithelium and staining with fluorescein

fluid pits fill with
fluorescein

corneal
epithelium

corneal stroma

Figure 7.8
The way in which mucin balls lead to the formation of fluid-filled pits

halo of staining around some mucin balls, suggestive of a corneal breach.

Concerns that the above factors could lead to an increased occurrence of infectious keratitis among silicone hydrogel contact lens wearers can be allayed because early indications are that the incidence of sight-threatening corneal ulceration with silicone hydrogel lenses is low.

Fonn *et al.*[1] and Pritchard *et al.*[17] reported the case of a patient who demonstrated extensive mucin ball formation. This patient, who was using silicone hydrogel lenses on an extended wear basis, also presented with an acute red eye reaction, an asymptomatic epithelial defect (with rapid diffusion of fluorescein into the stroma), two further instances of asymptomatic infiltrates and symptoms of dryness

over an 18 month period. These adverse events may have been coincidental to the appearance of mucin balls in this patient.

Mucin balls may cause a slight, though temporary, irregularity in the corneal surface that could reduce its wettability if present as a chronic condition.[2] Aside from this, mucin balls do not seem to compromise ocular integrity. As discussed previously, mucin balls are not associated with increased corneal inflammation, corneal staining (apart from that staining directly attributable to the mucin balls) or conjunctival redness,[2,7,9] and patients who display mucin balls do not experience discomfort or reduced vision.[2,7,9]

Management

The obvious strategy to prevent mucin ball formation, should this be the aim of the clinician, is to refit the patient with a lens type that is not made from silicone hydrogel materials. However, patients are likely to be highly motivated to wear silicone hydrogel lenses because of their comfort and convenience when used for continuous wear.

In patients who wear silicone hydrogel lenses, mucin ball formation can be minimized by:
- Optimizing lens fit – flat-fitting lenses are thought to exacerbate mucin ball formation;[2,6,9]
- Advising the patient to use lubricating drops after waking and before sleep;[2,6]

- Advising the patient to adopt a shorter wearing schedule (such as removing the lenses once every six nights instead of 30 nights).[2]

Prognosis

After lens removal, those mucin balls not embedded in the epithelium are blinked away rapidly. The residual 'embedded' mucin balls, and the fluid-filled pits, generally resolve in a matter of hours.[2] In severe cases, embedded mucin balls may remain in the epithelium for up to 7 days.[1] Mucin balls reform again if silicone hydrogel lens wear is recommended.

Differential Diagnosis

Clinicians need to be able to differentiate mucin balls – and the fluid-filled epithelial pits they cause – from other phenomena induced by contact lenses that occur at or near the ocular surface, such as epithelial microcysts, epithelial vacuoles, epithelial bullae and dimple veiling.

Microcysts and mucin balls are similar in size. As explained in Chapter 15, microcysts can be observed, using optic section illumination with a slit-lamp biomicroscope, to be within the epithelium and to display reversed illumination. Therefore, unlike mucin balls, microcysts do not stain with fluorescein. However, microcysts that are breaking through the epithelial surface do stain

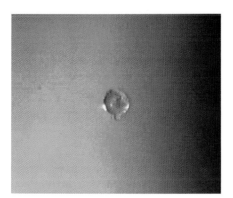

Figure 7.9
Large single mucin ball that has collapsed into the form of a doughnut, showing a thin surrounding annulus and a small central island

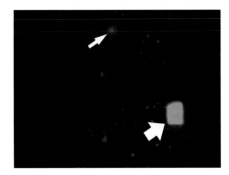

Figure 7.10
Fluorescein staining caused by mucin balls. Fluorescein diffusion into the surrounding epithelium and possibly also the stroma is evidenced by the diffuse fluorescent haze around one of the punctate stains (thin arrow). The thick arrow indicates the square slit-lamp light reflex

Table 7.1
Differential diagnosis of intraepithelial and epithelial surface phenomena

	Size (μm)	Shape	Colour (seen in direct illumination)	Distribution	Refractive index relative to surround	Optical appearance	Staining with fluorescein	Associated contact lenses
Mucin balls	10–200	Spherical or doughnut-shaped	Gray	More in superior cornea	Higher	Reversed illumination	Yes	Silicone hydrogel lenses
Epithelial pits (induced by mucin balls)	10–200	Spherical	Clear	More in superior cornea	Lower	Unreversed illumination	Yes	Silicone hydrogel lenses
Epithelial microcysts	5–30	Spherical or irregular	Gray	Pan-corneal	Higher	Reversed illumination	No*	Low oxygen performance lenses
Epithelial vacuoles	5–30	Spherical	Clear	Mid-peripheral cornea	Lower	Unreversed illumination	No	Low oxygen performance lenses
Epithelial bullae	5–30	Irregular (roughly oval)	Clear	Pan-corneal or central	Lower	Unreversed illumination	No	Rigid lenses
Dimple veiling	10–200	Spherical	Clear	Corresponding to large post-lens tear space	Lower	Unreversed illumination	Yes	Flat fitting rigid (or soft) lenses

*Except when breaking through the epithelial surface.

with fluorescein and may be indistinguishable from mucin balls.

Epithelial vacuoles reside within the epithelium, display unreversed illumination and do not stain with fluorescein (see Chapter 16). Epithelial bullae are similar to vacuoles, but are more oval in shape, and have an irregular and indistinct border. Fluid-filled epithelial pits induced by mucin balls also display unreversed illumination, but unlike fluid vacuoles, they do stain with fluorescein.

Dimple veiling induced by contact lenses refers to the formation of fluid-filled pits in the epithelial surface as a result of pressure from individual air bubbles trapped beneath rigid contact lenses (and to a lesser extent in soft lenses). The epithelial depressions ('dimples') fill with the aqueous phase of the tear film, stain with fluorescein and display unreversed illumination; as such, they may be indistinguishable in appearance from fluid-filled epithelial pits induced by mucin balls. Dimple veiling tends to occur in clustered regions, which correspond to areas of loose lens fitting that can support the existence of large air bubbles. Thus, the type of lens (i.e., a poorly fitting rigid lens versus a silicone hydrogel lens) is likely to be a key factor in differentiating these otherwise similar phenomena.

A summary of the features that differentiate the conditions described above is given in *Table 7.1*.

REFERENCES

1 Fonn D, Pritchard N and Dumbleton K (2000). Factors affecting the success of silicone hydrogels. In: *Silicone Hydrogels. The Rebirth of Continuous Wear Contact Lenses*, Ed. Sweeney DF, p. 214–234. (Oxford: Butterworth–Heinemann).
2 Dumbleton K, Jones L, Chalmers R, *et al.* (2000). Clinical characterization of spherical post-lens debris associated with Lotrafilcon high-*Dk* silicone lenses. *CLAO J.* **26**, 186–92.
3 Fleming C, Austen R and Davies S (1994). Pre-corneal deposits during soft contact lens wear. *Optom Vis Sci.* **71**, 152S–153S.
4 Tan J, Keay L and Jalbert I (1999). Tear microspheres (TMSS) with high *Dk* lenses. *Optom Vis Sci.* **76S**, 226.
5 Bourassa S and Benjamin WJ (1988). Transient corneal surface 'microdeposits' and associated epithelial surface pits occurring with gel contact lens extended wear. *Int Contact Lens Clin.* **15**, 338–340.
6 Tan J, Keay L, Jalbert I, *et al.* (2003). Mucin balls with wear of conventional and silicone hydrogel contact lenses. *Optom Vis Sci.* **80**, 291–297.
7 Sweeney DF, Keay L, Jalbert I, *et al.* (2000). Clinical performance of silicone hydrogel lenses. In: *Silicone Hydrogels. The Rebirth of Continuous Wear Contact Lenses*, Ed. Sweeney DF, p. 90–149. (Oxford: Butterworth–Heinemann).
8 Craig JP, Sherwin T, Grupcheva CN and McGhee CN (2002). An evaluation of mucin balls associated with high-*Dk* silicone hydrogel contact lens wear. *Adv Exp Med Biol.* **506**, 917–923.
9 Morgan PB and Efron N (2002). Comparative clinical performance of two silicone hydrogel contact lenses for continuous wear. *Clin Exp Optom.* **85**, 183–192.
10 Ladage PM, Petroll WM, Jester JV, *et al.* (2002). Spherical indentations of human and rabbit corneal epithelium following extended contact lens wear. *CLAO J.* **28**, 177–180.
11 Nichols J and King-Smith E (2001). In-vivo thickness of the pre- and post-lens tear film and silicone hydrogel contact lenses measured by interferometry. *Optom Vis Sci.* **78**, 51S.
12 Bron AJ, Tripathi RC and Tripathi BJ (1997). *Wolff's Anatomy of the Eye and Orbit*, Eighth Edition. (London: Chapman & Hall Medical).
13 Naduvilath TJ (2003). *Statistical Modelling of Risk Factors Associated with Soft Contact Lens-Related Corneal Infiltrative Events*. PhD Thesis (Newcastle: University of Newcastle).
14 Lai YC and Friends GD (1997). Surface wettability enhancement of silicone hydrogel lenses by processing with polar plastic molds. *J Biomed Mater Res.* **35**, 349–356.
15 Millar TJ, Papas EB, Ozkan J, *et al.* (2003). Clinical appearance and microscopic analysis of mucin balls associated with contact lens wear. *Cornea* **22**, 740–745.
16 Fleiszig SM, Zaidi TS, Ramphal R and Pier GB (1994). Modulation of *Pseudomonas aeruginosa* adherence to the corneal surface by mucus. *Infect Immunol.* **62**, 1799–1804.
17 Pritchard N, Jones L, Dumbleton K and Fonn D (2000). Epithelial inclusions in association with mucin ball development in high-oxygen permeability hydrogel lenses. *Optom Vis Sci.* **77**, 68–72.

PART IV CONJUNCTIVA

CONJUNCTIVAL STAINING

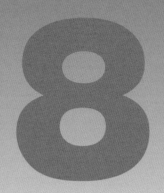

In the open eye, contact lenses are primarily in physical apposition with the cornea. Well-fitted rigid lenses generally reside almost exclusively on the cornea, and only occasionally impinge upon the limbus. The situation is different with soft lenses. If the surface area of the cornea[1] is taken to be 132 mm^2, and the surface area of a soft lens – with typical dimensions of 14.5 mm diameter and 8.7 mm back optic zone radius – is 213 mm^2, then 38% of the surface area of a soft lens lies in apposition with the bulbar conjunctiva. It is therefore apparent that changes in the conjunctiva caused by the physical presence of soft lenses might be observed.

Contact lenses can also affect the conjunctiva via mechanisms that do not involve direct physical contact. Thick rigid lenses can 'bridge' the upper lid away from the conjunctiva, which prevents blink-activated wetting and causes drying of the region of corneal and conjunctival tissue adjacent to the lens. Contact lens solutions can cause toxic or immunologic reactions of the conjunctiva. Lens-induced changes in the volume and composition of the pre-ocular tear film may also lead indirectly to changes in the conjunctiva.

For the reasons outlined above, careful inspection of the bulbar conjunctiva constitutes an essential part of the external ocular examination of contact lens wearers. An important technique that can be employed to reveal conjunctival tissue damage is to use vital dyes. This chapter reviews the various conjunctival staining techniques that have been proposed, and considers normal and abnormal appearances of the stained conjunctiva in response to contact lens wear.

Appropriate Staining Agents

Fluorescein sodium (more commonly referred to as 'fluorescein') is generally adopted as the stain of first choice in ophthalmic diagnosis. It is assumed that fluorescein provides information about the surface quality of the conjunctiva by pooling in natural creases, folds and ridges in the conjunctiva, and entering interepithelial spaces where an abrasion has occurred.[2] To optimize visualization of conjunctival staining, a cobalt blue 'excitation' filter, incorporated into the illumination system of the slit-lamp biomicroscope, is required to limit illumination to wavelengths of light that maximally absorb fluorescein. When viewing the conjunctiva illuminated in this way, the sclera scatters the incident blue light and desaturates the fluorescent light. (This problem is not encountered when fluorescent staining is viewed over a transparent cornea). A yellow 'barrier' filter (*Figure 8.1*) interposed within the observation system is therefore essential to limit light transmission back through the eyepieces and maximize contrast between the stained and unstained areas of conjunctiva.

Even with the use of excitation and barrier filters, the blue incident light excites a natural greenish fluorescence in the conjunctiva and sclera, which

Figure 8.1
A yellow barrier filter fitted to the front of the observation system of a slit-lamp biomicroscope

causes a general background glow that may diminish the contrast of any additional fluorescence present.[3] A similar problem is encountered whereby the contrast of subtle corneal staining can be diminished because the background fluorescent glow emanates from the crystalline lens. An added difficulty with respect to the observation of fluorescein staining of the conjunctiva is that fluorescein is slightly lipid soluble and stains the entire conjunctiva to some extent, which further reduces contrast.[3] In view of these limitations of fluorescein, researchers have investigated the utility of other staining agents to stain the conjunctiva. Sulphorhodamine B, which has an orange fluorescence that can be separated from the green natural fluorescence of the ocular tissues, gives a greater contrast than fluorescein.[3]

Norn[4] reported that rose bengal stains degenerated epithelial cells and mucus; however, Tseng[5] subsequently disputed this long-held belief by demonstrating that rose bengal also rapidly stains healthy epithelial cells when there is insufficient surface mucus. Contrast between rose-bengal stained and unstained areas is usually poor, although the appearance can be enhanced by viewing the stained region in 'red free' light by interposing a green filter in the illumination system. Patients find this staining agent to be uncomfortable.[6] Lissamine green has similar properties to rose bengal in that it stains degenerate and dead epithelial cells and mucus. Manning *et al.*[6] reported that lissamine green is better tolerated by patients than is rose bengal, and is equally as effective as rose bengal in evaluating the ocular surface. However, Emran and Sommer[7] believe that lissamine green is an inadequately sensitive test for practical use.

Numerous other stains have been investigated, including Congo red,[8] neutral red,[9] trypan blue,[10] bromothymol blue[11] and fluorexon.[12] Foster[13] cites 34 different chemical substances that have been used for ocular surface staining. In addition, the possible benefits of using various mixtures of staining agents have been examined, such as fluorescein–rose bengal[14] and tetrazolium–alcian blue.[15] The key characteristics of various staining agents applied clinically are outlined in *Table 8.1*.

While useful properties of some of the alternative staining agents described above have been demonstrated, the general utility, safety, broad acceptance and ready availability of fluorescein means that it is the staining agent of first choice for investigating ocular surface compromise. Rose bengal may be used as a supplementary stain to check for degenerate epithelial cells and mucus. Thus,

throughout the remainder of this textbook, reference is made only to the use of fluorescein and rose bengal, which can be considered to be the two primary ocular surface staining agents.

Staining Technique

Fluorescein can be administered in liquid form from an eye dropper, but this method is seldom used today because of the propensity of *Pseudomonas aeruginosa* to flourish in liquid fluorescein sodium and hence the high risk of *Pseudomonas* corneal infection. This problem can be overcome by using sterile single-dose units; however, the standard method of introducing fluorescein dye into the eye is via sterile, single-use fluorescein-impregnated paper strips (*Figure 8.2*).

The preferred technique is to introduce a small drop of sterile unpreserved saline onto the fluorescein-impregnated tip of the paper strip, and then to lightly apply the end of the strip to the surface of the eye. Although the strip should not be applied directly onto the cornea, it can be applied to any part of the bulbar or palpebral conjunctiva. If conjunctival staining is to be assessed, the strip should be applied to a region of the conjunctiva of 'least interest', such as the lower palpebral conjunctiva. This is because a very high fluorescein concentration is usually deposited at the point of contact of the fluorescein strip (irrespective of how delicately the fluorescein is applied), which leaves an intense discrete region of iatrogenic 'pseudo-staining' (*Figure 8.3*).

To instil fluorescein into the lower lid, have the patient look up, gently retract the lower lid by a small amount and allow the moistened fluorescein strip to

Table 8.1
Ocular surface staining agents

Stain	Features revealed/highlighted
Fluorescein sodium	'Colors' the tear film Fills gaps, and thus reveals 'missing' cells Enters and stains damaged epithelial cells Enters and reversibly stains hydrogel lenses
Fluorexon	Essentially fluorescein with a high molecular weight 'Colors' the tear film Fills gaps, and thus reveals 'missing' cells Enters and stains damaged epithelial cells Does not fluoresce as brightly as fluorescein Cannot enter and stain hydrogel lenses
Sulphorhodamine B	Essentially fluorescein with different fluorescent characteristics 'Colors' the tear film Fills gaps, and thus reveals 'missing' cells Enters and stains damaged epithelial cells Does not fluoresce as brightly as fluorescein
Lissamine green	Stains degenerate and dead cells Stains mucus (e.g., mucus threads) Similar to rose bengal, but better tolerated
Rose bengal	Stains dead cells Stains mucus (e.g., mucus threads) Reveals absence of surface mucus by staining normal surface tissue unprotected by mucus
Neutral red	Stains epithelial inclusion bodies and granulocytes Essentially a less efficient version of rose bengal
Congo red	Stains dead and degenerate cells Stains mucus (e.g., mucus threads) Similar staining effect as rose bengal and lissamine green, but less effective and less intense
Alcian blue	Only stains mucus (e.g., mucus threads) Used as a counter-stain to rose bengal to help differentiate between dead cells and mucus
Trypan blue	Stains dead cells Stains mucus (e.g., mucus threads)
Bromothymol blue	Stains dead cells Stains degenerate cells Stains mucus (e.g., mucus threads)
Methylene blue	Stains nerve tissue Clearly outlines areas of corneal ulceration
Tetrazolium	Stains degenerate cells, but not live or dead cells The red stain coloration only appears about 4 minutes after the stain has entered the cell
Iodonitrotetrazolium	Stains degenerate cells, but not live or dead cells The red stain coloration only appears about 4 minutes after the stain has entered the cell

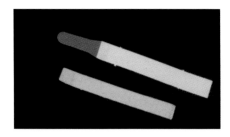

Figure 8.2
Single-use paper strips with the tips impregnated with sodium fluorescein (top) and rose bengal (bottom)

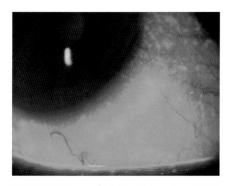

Figure 8.3
Bright patch of fluorescent 'pseudo-staining' on the conjunctiva that corresponds to the location of the physical application of a fluorescein-impregnated paper strip to the globe

lightly touch the inner surface (palpebral conjunctiva) of the lower lid. Physical touch may not be required if a sufficient amount of fluorescein, in the form of a 'hanging drop', remains suspended from the moistened strip.

The amount of fluorescein that enters the eye using the above technique usually provides the correct balance between there being enough fluorescein to effect useful staining, but insufficient to 'flood' the eye, which could reduce contrast and possibly induce false staining. Abdul-Fattah et al.[16] have demonstrated that the amount of fluorescein entering the eye can be controlled by using paper strips in which the fluorescein-impregnated portion varies in area, whereby a smaller area results in less fluorescein entering the eye. Only reduced amounts of fluorescein are usually required to assess the tear film in suspected dry eye patients; Korb et al.[17] reported that a specially modified fluorescein strip with a substantially reduced area of fluorescein impregnation (the 'Dry Eye Test') provided a significant reduction in sensation upon application, improved single measurement reliability and enhanced measurement precision, compared with a conventional fluorescent strip.

Signs and Symptoms

The normal eye

When fluorescein is instilled into a normal eye, patterns of small, thin, curved lines of staining can be observed on the bulbar conjunctiva (*Figure 8.4*). The curved lines of staining in regions of

conjunctiva close to the cornea are generally concentric with the limbus, whereas they tend to run parallel to the lid margins in regions of the bulbar conjunctiva further away from the cornea. Although the term 'staining' is used to describe these patterns, it is not true staining in that there is no tissue disruption. This appearance is best described as 'normal furrow staining'. What is being observed is pooling of fluorescein in the normal concertina folding or furrows of the conjunctiva.[18] The conjunctiva is essentially fixed to the globe at the region of the limbus, as well as to the eyelids, so this normal pattern of 'staining' varies at different gaze directions, as the conjunctiva stretches and folds up in a concertina-like manner to accommodate the position of the globe.

Schwallie et al.[19] characterized the day-to-day variability in normal conjunctival staining by instilling fluorescein into the eyes of 16 subjects who were monitored for 1 week. All eyes showed some degree of normal conjunctival staining over the week of observation. In total, normal conjunctival staining was noted in 71% of ocular evaluations. Overall, staining ranged from grade 0 to 3, with a mean of 0.5. There was a significant variation in the average grade of staining between subjects. Also, a significant variation in the range of grading was observed between subjects; the day-to-day range of conjunctival staining varied by 0.5 grading scale units in six subject, by 1.0 grading scale units in six subjects and by 1.5 grading scale units in four subjects.

A high correlation of staining grade was observed between the two eyes. This finding has important clinical implications in the evaluation of uniocular 'abnormal' conjunctival staining, in that the contralateral (unaffected) eye can be used for comparison against the appearance of the eye suspected to have suffered conjunctival compromise.

Contact lens wear

Lakkis and Brennan[18] assessed the extent of conjunctival staining in 48 hydrogel lens wearers and 50 control subjects not wearing lenses. Ignoring the 'normal conjunctival staining' described above, these authors observed that only 12% of the controls displayed conjunctival staining greater than grade 1.0, whereas 62% of lens wearers had staining above this level. The mean difference in the grade of staining varied between 0.12 and 0.15 for overall conjunctival staining, and contact lens wearers displayed most staining temporally.

Various forms of lens-induced conjunctival staining can be observed. A diffuse punctate region of staining (or 'stipple staining') may be observed near the limbus, which corresponds to the region of conjunctiva covered by a soft lens (*Figure 8.5*). In some areas, the punctate spots can tend to coalesce. However, confluent areas of staining that represent total coalescence, which can sometimes be observed in the cornea, are rarely caused by contact lens wear. This form of conjunctival staining is usually observed only in soft lens wearers. Lakkis and Brennan[18] reported that temporal conjunctival staining in

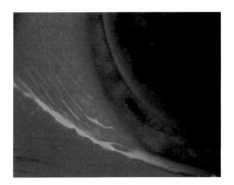

Figure 8.4
Normal conjunctival furrow staining in a rigid lens wearer. The fine arcuate lines of 'staining' result from pooling of fluorescein in normal conjunctival folds and are unrelated to lens wear

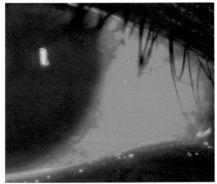

Figure 8.5
Stipple staining in the region of conjunctiva covered by a silicone hydrogel lens (the lens has been removed). The staining is more intense in the proximity of the lens edge

soft lens wearers was related to the symptom of dryness and superior conjunctival staining was more related to the symptom of itchiness.

An arcuate band of staining that corresponds to the lens edge may be seen 2–3 mm from the limbus. This may form as a continuous band or as a broken line, and can vary from being just visible to being an intense ring of fluorescence up to about 0.5 mm wide. Arcuate conjunctival staining is usually observed in soft lens wearers (*Figure 8.6*), but is sometimes observed after overnight wear of rigid lenses that have become decentered during sleep (*Figure 8.7*). Covey et al.[20] reported that high levels of conjunctival edge staining occur with silicone hydrogel lenses (see *Figure 8.5*); specifically, they reported a mean grade of conjunctival staining of 2.4 ± 0.6 in silicone hydrogel lens wearers versus 0.9 ± 0.7 in controls not wearing lenses (the latter being 'normal furrow staining').

Rigid lenses can indirectly affect the conjunctiva near the limbus by bridging the upper lid away from the ocular surface. This causes corneal and conjunctival desiccation in the 'bridged' zone (through inadequate lid-mediated ocular surface rewetting), which can manifest as staining of both of these tissues. Indeed, this is thought to be the mechanism responsible for 3 and 9 o'clock staining.

Pathology

Fluorescein staining is observed when fluorescein fills gaps or enters damaged cells. Putting aside the 'normal conjunctival staining' that results from pooling within conjunctival folds, lens-induced fluorescein staining indicates missing or damaged epithelial cells (because of physical insult or desiccation), or gaps created by compression of the lens edge (see 'Etiology' below). Conjunctival epithelial cells may become damaged or dislodged if there is insufficient lubrication between the lens and conjunctiva, as could occur in a patient with a pre-existing or lens-induced dry eye. Deposits on the back surface of a lens could physically traumatize or dislodge conjunctival cells.

The integrity of the conjunctiva during contact lens wear has been studied using impression cytology. This is a mildly invasive technique whereby a small disc of filter paper is pressed momentarily onto the anesthetized conjunctiva and removed. Superficial conjunctival epithelial and goblet cells adhere to the filter paper, which is fixed to a glass slide, stained and examined under a microscope. Using this technique, Adar et al.[21] reported alterations to conjunctival epithelial cell morphology (*Figure 8.8*), a reduction in goblet cell density (*Figure 8.9*) and the appearance of snake-like chromatin in a group of contact lens wearers, especially those who were symptomatic. Albietz[22] also reported a significant reduction in goblet cell density, as well as a greater expression of ocular surface antigens to the conjunctival inflammatory markers HLA DR and CD 23, in contact lens wearers versus

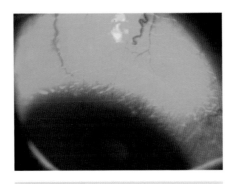

Figure 8.6
Arcuate band of fluorescein staining that corresponds to the edge of a soft lens. Normal conjunctival furrow staining is also clearly evident

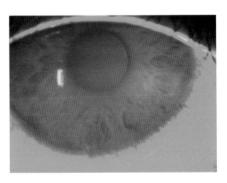

Figure 8.7
Arcuate band of fluorescein staining that corresponds to the edge of a rigid lens which was bound to the eye upon awakening after overnight lens wear

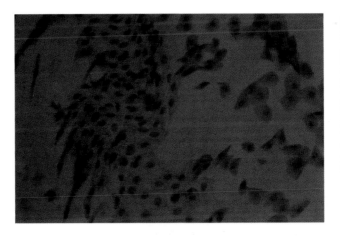

Figure 8.8
Confluent sheet (left of frame) and smaller clump (right of frame) of conjunctival cells collected using impression cytology. The cell borders, cytoplasm and nuclei are clearly visible

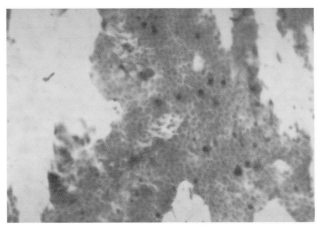

Figure 8.9
Conjunctival goblet and epithelial cells collected using impression cytology. The goblet cells are the large dark pink bodies and the fainter, light pink array of smaller bodies in the background are the conjunctival cells

controls. There was an even greater level of conjunctival inflammatory markers in symptomatic lens wearers (who complained of 'dry eye' principally).

In contrast to the results of other researchers using impression cytology, Connor et al.[23] reported an *increase* in goblet cell count in patients who wore biweekly replacement lenses, and attributed this to be a beneficial adaptive response to the mechanical insult caused by the lens. These authors subsequently reported that daily disposable lens wear does not result in a reduction of goblet cell density, which suggests that this modality of lens wear is less irritating to the ocular surface than lenses which are not replaced daily.[24]

Other techniques have been used to examine the integrity of the conjunctiva, but these produce less satisfactory information. The corneal irrigation chamber[25] is used primarily to collect tear fluid that overlies the cornea; however, the irrigation procedure also results in the collection of loose conjunctival cells (*Figure 8.10*). Norn[26] described a method that involved the cytologic examination of conjunctival cells collected in tear fluid from the inferior conjunctival fornix. Scraping the anesthetized conjunctiva with a surgical blade[27] or swabbing with a cotton-tipped applicator[28] is somewhat invasive and cells are prone to being lost or damaged during transfer. Conjunctival biopsy (excision of a small tissue sample) preserves the three-dimensional structure of the tissue sample, but this is highly invasive and not suitable for repeated scientific investigations.[29]

Etiology

In their analysis of conjunctival staining induced by contact lenses, Lakkis and Brennan[18] were unable to identify any link between the appearance of conjunctival staining and subject age, gender, experience of wearing contact lens, wearing time per week, wearing time on the day of examination, lens water content, lens age, lens movement, lens decentration, lens lag in upgaze or lens maintenance system. The only associations found, as described above, was with the symptoms of dryness and itchiness. Robboy and Cox[30] suggested that reduced tear film quality in soft lens wearers may be the cause of conjunctival staining, whereby a lack of tear fluid leads to conjunctival desiccation and associated tissue disruption.

It is likely that significant arcuate staining corresponding to the edge of a lens is related to the physical presence of the lens edge. The staining could be attributed to compression into the conjunctiva by a tightly fitting lens, which results in an indentation in which fluorescein pools. Indirect support for this theory comes from the finding of Robboy and Cox[30] of a significant inverse relationship between conjunctival staining and lens movement; that is, the edge of a static, tightly fitting soft lens is more likely to compress the conjunctiva than is a free-moving lens. Lenses with a high modulus of elasticity (i.e., more stiff), such as silicone hydrogel lenses, are also prone to cause conjunctival indentation and subsequent staining.[20] This probably results because the edge profile of the lens fails to yield sufficiently enough

to conform to the surface topography of the globe, and instead retains its edge form and presses into the conjunctiva. Hydrogel lenses of lower modulus are more likely to conform to the surface anatomy of the eye.

Lens-edge staining may also be attributed to physical abrasion of the lens edge rubbing against the conjunctiva; certainly, such a mechanism was likely to have occurred with the imperfect and/or unpolished lens edges used in the early days of disposable soft contact lenses.[31-34]

Punctate staining close to the limbus could result from either the mechanical irritation of a loosely fitted soft lens (moving to such an extent that the lens edge impinges upon the limbus) or some other property of the peripheral zone of the lens. Deposits on the back surface of a soft lens, near to the lens edge, could theoretically result in abrasion of the conjunctiva. As described previously, rigid lenses can cause limbal tissue desiccation by bridging the upper lid away from the surface of the eye, which prevents proper wetting.

It is unlikely that conjunctival staining is attributed to lens-induced hypoxia because conjunctiva at the limbal region is supplied with an oxygen-rich vascular supply. Nor does there appear to be any relationship between conjunctival staining and infection. Norn[2] observed that the conjunctiva did not stain with infectious keratitis, and Lakkis and Brennan[18] demonstrated that most individuals have conjunctival staining in the absence of infection. Albietz[22] noted that conjunctival staining observed in lens wearers in her study could not be attributed to toxic reactions to contact lens solutions because all of the subjects in her study used modern cold-chemical systems, which are known to be minimally toxic to the ocular surface.

The general consensus of impression cytology researchers[21,22] is that the available data support a mechanical theory for the pathogenesis of conjunctival surface damage induced by contact lenses. For example, Albietz[22] points out that there was no difference in the degree of conjunctival cell metaplasia, goblet cell loss or appearance of snake-like chromatin between symptomatic (dry eye) and asymptomatic contact lens wearers, although the former group displayed greater levels of ocular surface inflammation. Also, contact lens wear-

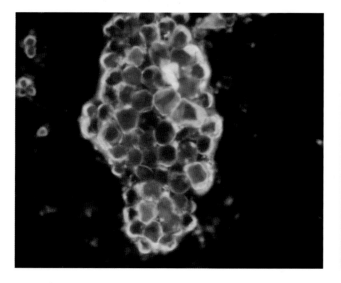

Figure 8.10

A clump of cuboidal conjunctival cells collected using the irrigation chamber

ers suffered an overall loss of goblet cells compared with controls not wearing lenses. Thus, the changes in conjunctival morphology observed – especially goblet cell loss – cannot be attributed to inflammation and is thus more likely to be of mechanical origin. The dry eye symptoms of contact lens wearers who display conjunctival decompensation are more likely to be associated with allergic and immune-mediated inflammatory processes.[22]

Management

Since mechanical factors are the most likely cause of conjunctival staining, it follows that removal of the mechanical insult should solve the problem. Of course, action only needs to be taken if the severity of staining is deemed to be of clinical significance. A grading scale for conjunctival staining is given in Appendix A. As a general rule, conjunctival staining of less than grade 3 may not require clinical action,[18] although the patient should be monitored carefully. Clinical intervention is required when the conjunctival staining is greater than grade 3 (*Figure 8.11*) and/or when there is associated pathology, such as venous stasis distal to lens-edge compression or excessive conjunctival or limbal redness in the region of conjunctival insult. The key clinical intervention in such cases is the immediate cessation of lens wear.

In the case of soft lenses, edge staining can be alleviated by changing the lens fit so that the lens edge does not compress the conjunctiva. Two key strategies are indicated. First, the lens

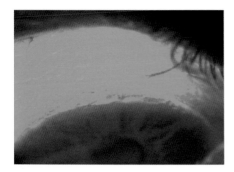

Figure 8.11
Heavy conjunctival staining of about grade 3.5 that has formed beneath the peripheral zone of a soft lens. Such an appearance warrants immediate cessation of lens wear

should be fitted so as to create a looser fit. This should result in greater lens movement and thus prevent the lens edge from bearing on a fixed location. Second, a lens with greater back optic zone radius (flatter fit) should be fitted so that less inward force is brought to bear by the lens edge against the conjunctiva. Of course, fitting a flatter lens also generally creates a looser fit, which allows both strategies to be invoked simultaneously.

The solution to lens-edge staining with silicone hydrogel lenses is more problematic. Such staining is attributed to the high modulus of the lens material, which is a parameter beyond the control of the practitioner (and, apparently, the manufacturers). If a given lens brand is available in a different base curve, change to a flatter base curve. If this does not solve the problem, change to a different lens brand, even if it has the same nominal base curve as the offending lens (because the overall lens design is different, which may alleviate the problem). If the staining still persists and its severity is judged to be clinically significant, the patient may have to change to hydrogel or rigid lenses.

If the conjunctival staining is thought to result from lens-edge imperfections, lens replacement should solve the problem. If such conjunctival staining persists despite frequent lens replacements, the problem may be related to an inferior product rather than a 'one-off' problematic lens; in such circumstances, a change to a product of superior edge quality is indicated. Conjunctival staining attributed to direct mechanical abrasion from deposits on the posterior lens surface can be alleviated by tackling the deposit problem with one or more of the following strategies:

• Improving the lens cleaning regimen;
• Changing to a lens material that is less prone to deposition;
• Prescribing a lens that is to be replaced more regularly.

As noted earlier, rigid lenses generally do not impinge physically upon the conjunctiva, but may affect the limbal conjunctiva adversely by preventing proper wetting of the ocular surface adjacent to the lens edge. The latter case may represent a precursor to 3 and 9 o'clock corneal staining; the various strategies advocated to resolve this problem are outlined in Chapter 14. Lens-edge conjunctival staining after overnight wear of rigid lenses is usually associated with overnight lens

binding, even though the lens may not appear to be bound when the patient is examined later the same day following overnight wear. Strategies to alleviate overnight rigid lens binding necessarily also resolve conjunctival staining that arises from the bound edge of the lens; such strategies are reviewed in Chapter 24.

Prognosis

The prognosis for recovery from corneal staining induced by contact lenses is good; Knop and Brewitt[35] reported that mechanical damage induced by contact lenses to the conjunctiva reverses after ceasing lens wear. According to Schwallie *et al.*,[19] the average duration of an episode of conjunctival staining in non-lens wearers is 2.0 ± 2.4 days. From this information they concluded that most forms of conjunctival staining should resolve within about 4 days of ceasing lens wear; if it does not, alternative causes of staining need to be investigated. The prognosis for recovery from conjunctival staining induced by contact lenses has not been investigated, but is also likely to recovery within 4 days of cessation of lens wear. Further research is required to confirm this. As a general guide, contact lens wear that has been ceased because of excessive conjunctival staining should not be recommended until the severity of staining has subsided to below Grade 1.0.

Differential Diagnosis

The primary exercise in the differential diagnosis of conjunctival staining is to be able to discern physiologic from pathologic staining. As highlighted by Lakkis and Brennan,[18] the arcuate conjunctival folds or furrows described under the heading 'The normal eye' (above) are normal and are observed in all lens wearers and non-lens wearers. The diagnosis of deep continuous arcs or rings of conjunctival staining that correspond to the lens edge is self evident, although the cause of punctate conjunctival staining is less obvious. A bright patch of conjunctival staining may well be iatrogenic, and correspond to the location of an overzealous application of a fluorescein strip to the eye. As stated previously, conjunctival fluorescein staining is unlikely to be associated with ocular infection or metabolic distress.

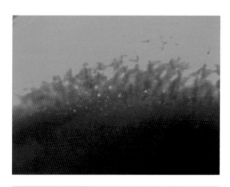

Figure 8.12
Bright spots of conjunctival staining, which indicate the presence of mucin balls

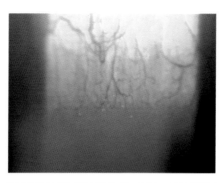

Figure 8.13
Mucin balls embedded in the conjunctiva, seen here in white light

Small, round intense spots of conjunctival staining observed near the limbus may be conjunctival mucin balls (*Figure 8.12*). These are balls of mucin embedded in the conjunctival epithelium, and they occur almost exclusively with silicone hydrogel lenses (see Chapter 7). In white light, the mucin balls are clearly visible as spherical refractile elements (like small spherical beads of glass), and they exhibit a pattern of distribution that corresponds with the staining pattern (*Figure 8.13*). Thus, silicone hydrogel lens wear is a key factor in differentially diagnosing conjunctival mucin balls from other causes of conjunctival stipple staining.

REFERENCES

1 Kwok LS (1984). Calculation and application of the anterior surface area of a model human cornea. *J Theor Biol.* **108**, 295–313.
2 Norn MS (1964). Fluorescein vital staining of the cornea and conjunctiva. *Acta Ophthalmol (Copenh.)* **42**, 1038–1045.
3 Eliason JA and Maurice DM (1990). Staining of the conjunctiva and conjunctival tear film. *Br J Ophthalmol.* **74**, 519–522.
4 Norn MS (1970). Rose bengal vital staining. Staining of cornea and conjunctiva by 10 percent rose bengal, compared with 1 percent. *Acta Ophthalmol (Copenh.)* **48**, 546–559.
5 Tseng SC (1994). Evaluation of the ocular surface in dry-eye conditions. *Int Ophthalmol Clin.* **34**, 57–69.
6 Manning FJ, Wehrly SR and Foulks GN (1995). Patient tolerance and ocular surface staining characteristics of lissamine green versus rose bengal. *Ophthalmology* **102**, 1953–1957.
7 Emran N and Sommer A (1979). Lissamine green staining in the clinical diagnosis of xerophthalmia. *Arch Ophthalmol.* **97**, 2333–2335.
8 Norn MS (1976). Congo red vital staining of cornea and conjunctiva. *Acta Ophthalmol (Copenh.)* **54**, 601–610.
9 Marner K and Norn MS (1978). Vital staining properties of neutral red. Vital staining of cornea and conjunctiva. *Acta Ophthalmol (Copenh.)* **56**, 742–750.
10 Norn MS (1967). Trypan blue. Vital staining of cornea and conjunctiva. *Acta Ophthalmol (Copenh.)* **45**, 380–389.
11 Norn MS (1968). Bromothymol blue. Vital staining of conjuctiva and cornea. *Acta Ophthalmol (Copenh.)* **46**, 231–242.
12 Norn MS (1973). Fluorexon vital staining of cornea and conjunctiva. *Acta Ophthalmol (Copenh.)* **51**, 670–678.
13 Foster J (1980). The spectrum of topical diagnosis. *Suid-Afrikaanse Argief Oftalmol.* **7**, 23–31.
14 Norn MS (1967). Vital staining of the cornea and conjunctiva with a mixture of fluorescein and rose bengal. *Am J Ophthalmol.* **64**, 1078–1080.
15 Norn MS (1972). Tetrazolium–alcian blue mixture. I. Vital staining of cornea and conjunctiva. *Acta Ophthalmol (Copenh.)* **50**, 277–285.
16 Abdul-Fattah AM, Bhargava HN, Korb DR, *et al.* (2002). Quantitative *in vitro* comparison of fluorescein delivery to the eye via impregnated paper strip and volumetric techniques. *Optom Vis Sci.* **79**, 435–438.
17 Korb DR, Greiner JV and Herman J (2001). Comparison of fluorescein break-up time measurement reproducibility using standard fluorescein strips versus the Dry Eye Test (DET) method. *Cornea* **20**, 811–815.
18 Lakkis C and Brennan NA (1996). Bulbar conjunctival fluorescein staining in hydrogel contact lens wearers. *CLAO J.* **22**, 189–194.
19 Schwallie JD, Long WD Jr and McKenney CD (1998). Day to day variations in ocular surface staining of the bulbar conjunctiva. *Optom Vis Sci.* **75**, 55–61.
20 Covey M, Sweeney DF, Terry R, *et al.* (2001). Hypoxic effects on the anterior eye of high-*Dk* soft contact lens wearers are negligible. *Optom Vis Sci.* **78**, 95–99.
21 Adar S, Kanpolat A, Surucu S and Ucakhan OO (1997). Conjunctival impression cytology in patients wearing contact lenses. *Cornea* **16**, 289–294.
22 Albietz JM (2001). Conjunctival histologic findings of dry eye and non-dry eye contact lens wearing subjects. *CLAO J.* **27**, 35–40.
23 Connor CG, Campbell JB, Steel SA and Burke JH (1994). The effects of daily wear contact lenses on goblet cell density. *J Am Optom Assoc.* **65**, 792–794.
24 Connor CG, Campbell JB and Steel SA (1997). The effects of disposable daily wear contact lenses on goblet cell count. *CLAO J.* **23**, 37–39.
25 Fullard RJ and Wilson GS (1986). Investigation of sloughed corneal epithelial cells collected by non-invasive irrigation of the corneal surface. *Curr Eye Res.* **5**, 847–856.
26 Norn M (1987). Ferning in conjunctival–cytologic preparations. Crystallisation in stained semiquantitative pipette samples of conjunctival fluid. *Acta Ophthalmol (Copenh.)* **65**, 118–123.
27 Whitcher JP (1987). Clinical diagnosis of the dry eye. *Int Ophthalmol Clin.* **27**, 7–24.
28 Duszynski L (1954). Cytology of the conjunctival sac. *Am J Ophthalmol.* **37**, 576–578.
29 Abdel-Khalek LM, Williamson J and Lee WR (1978). Morphological changes in the human conjunctival epithelium. II. In keratoconjunctivitis sicca. *Br J Ophthalmol.* **62**, 800–806.
30 Robboy MW and Cox IG (1991). Patient factors influencing conjunctival staining with soft contact lens wearers. *Optom Vis Sci.* **68S**, 163.
31 Seger RG and Mutti DO (1988). Conjunctival staining and single-use contact lenses with unpolished edges. *Contact Lens Spectrum* **3**, 36–37.
32 Devries DK, Lingel NJ, Patrick TC and Spitzer LJ (1989). A clinical evaluation of edge induced conjunctival staining with Acuvue and SeeQuence disposable lenses. *Optom Vis Sci.* **66S**, 115S.
33 Lingel NJ, Patrick TC, Hagen BN and Vizina BA (1990). A clinical evaluation of edge induced conjunctival staining with SeeQuence and NewVues disposable lenses. *Optom Vis Sci.* **67S**, 100.
34 Efron N and Veys J (1992). Defects in disposable contact lenses can compromise ocular integrity. *Int Contact Lens Clin.* **19**, 8–18.
35 Knop E and Brewitt H (1992). Conjunctival cytology in asymptomatic wearers of soft contact lenses. *Graefes Arch Clin Exp Ophthalmol.* **230**, 340–347.

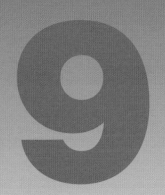

CONJUNCTIVAL REDNESS

Increased conjunctival redness in response to contact lens wear is recognized so easily that it serves as a fundamental indicator to clinicians of the physiologic status of the eye wearing contact lens. It is not surprising that the first two clinical reports of contact lens wearing trials on humans – conducted independently in the late 1880s by Adolf Fick[1] and August Müller[2] – used conjunctival redness as a measure of the severity of reaction to, and time course of recovery from, the impact of lens wear.

Conjunctival redness is so obvious and easily recognizable that it is perhaps the only tissue reaction to contact lens wear that is also reported as a symptom by patients (*Figure 9.1*). Indeed, excessive eye redness is cosmetically unsightly and is often perceived as a potential disadvantage of wearing contact lenses.

It is generally recognized in eye care that the clinical presentation of a 'red eye' can be one of the most difficult cases to solve because of the numerous possible known causes. This problem may be even more complex in a contact lens wearer because there are many other causes of red eye related to contact lenses.

Definitions

Throughout the literature, the terms hyperemia, engorgement, injection, erythema, vascularity and redness are often used as synonyms. These terms are defined as follows:
- Hyperemia – an increase of blood in a part;[3]
- Engorgement – excessive fullness of a vessel caused by accumulation of blood;[3]
- Erythema – redness of the skin produced by congestion of the capillaries;[3]
- Injection – the act of forcing a liquid into a part;[3]
- Vascularity – the condition of being vascular;[3]

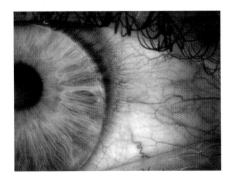

Figure 9.1
Conjunctival redness (grade 2.7)

- Redness – of a color at the end of the spectrum next to orange and opposite to violet, as of blood.[4]

Strictly speaking, *hyperemia*, *engorgement* or *injection* is the cause and *redness* is the effect. That is, an increased volume of blood in the conjunctival vessels (*hyperemia*, *engorgement* or *injection*) causes an increased appearance of redness. The term *erythema* refers to redness of the skin; thus, the use of this term to describe conjunctival redness is acceptable in the broad context of considering the conjunctiva to be a specially adapted form of skin (technically, it is a mucus membrane). The term vascularity is somewhat ambiguous and could represent both the cause and effect. Since this book is structured primarily in terms of considering clinical signs, the expression 'conjunctival redness' is used here.

Prevalence

Most contact lens wearers experience an episode of eye redness, no matter how mild, that may or may not be related to lens wear. Conjunctival redness is such a common sign that few studies have documented its prevalence. According to Stapleton *et al.*,[5] 37 of 1104 contact lens wearers (3.4%) who attended the acci-

dent and emergency department at Moorfields Eye Hospital were diagnosed primarily as having 'red eye related to contact lenses'. However, this figure underestimates the true prevalence of red eye as a presenting symptom because many of the other patients in that study were diagnosed as having conditions that would certainly have been associated with eye redness, such as toxic disorders, keratitis, conjunctival abrasion, etc. That is, eye redness would be a secondary sign in these cases. Virtually all patients who present to their eye care practitioner with complaints of ocular discomfort have associated eye redness.

Signs and Symptoms

The term 'conjunctival redness' is potentially confusing because it may not be clear whether this refers to redness of the bulbar, limbal or tarsal conjunctiva. Indeed, in his 1888 thesis on contact lenses, Müller[2] clearly differentiated between the extent of bulbar conjunctival redness, bulbar episcleral redness and limbal redness and he used the degree of redness in these three tissue types as the basis of his analysis of the likely pathophysiologic effects of lens wear. This chapter concentrates on bulbar conjunctival redness. Tarsal conjunctival redness is considered in Chapter 10 and limbal redness is the topic of Chapter 11.

As with all adverse responses that can involve a wide expanse of tissue, there may be significant regional variations in the extent of redness with respect to a given conjunctival structure. *Figure 9.2* illustrates severe bulbar conjunctival redness limited to the 3 and 9 o'clock position, associated with circumlimbal redness, in a patient wearing rigid lenses. The limbal engorgement suggests corneal involvement, which is consistent with the fact that this patient also displayed 3 and 9 o'clock staining.

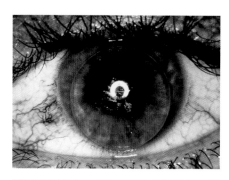

Figure 9.2

Localized 3 and 9 o'clock bulbar conjunctival redness and circumlimbal redness in a rigid contact lens wearer

There is also considerable variation in the magnitude of a hyperemic response between individuals, as noted by Fick[1] in his 1888 paper. He observed, "The degree of injection … varies greatly." Fick[1] also used the conjunctival hyperemic response to discover that the eye adapts to lens wear; he observed, "The degree of injection … is apt to be absent entirely in those … eyes … which have already been utilized in a long series of experiments. Apparently, therefore, a sort of toleration is established very soon." Interestingly, Papas[6] suggests that subjective judgments of erythema made by human observers do not rely primarily on color, but can be approximated closely by a univariate, linear model that involves only the proportion of the scene occupied by vessels (i.e., erythema can be judged equally well from black-and-white versus color images).

Conjunctival redness is generally asymptomatic, but patients may complain of itchiness, congestion, non-specific mild irritation or a warm or cold feeling. The existence of pain usually indicates corneal involvement (e.g., keratitis) or other tissue pathology (e.g., uveitis or scleritis).

Inferior bulbar conjunctival redness was assessed in asymptomatic contact lens wearers by McMonnies and Chapman-Davies.[7,8] The mean grading of redness was as follows:

- No lenses – 0.8;
- Rigid lenses – 1.0;
- Hydrogel lenses used in the absence of preservative-based care systems – 1.5;
- Hydrogel lenses used in conjunction with preservative-based care systems – 2.1.

Silicone hydrogel lenses seem to induce much lower levels of conjunctival redness.

Fonn et al.[9] reported that silicone hydrogel lenses worn on an extended wear basis induced significantly lower grades of conjunctival redness compared with those observed with hydrogel extended wear lenses. Morgan and Efron[10] also demonstrated that silicone hydrogel lenses worn on an extended wear basis induce relatively low grades of conjunctival redness (between 0.4 and 0.6). Covey et al.[11] were unable to detect any difference in the grades of conjunctival redness between patients wearing silicone hydrogel lenses on an extended wear basis (2.4 ± 0.4) versus those in patients who did not wear lenses (2.3 ± 0.4).

As well as being statistically significant, these differences are undoubtedly clinically significant. Greater redness with hydrogel lenses, compared with no lens wear or rigid lens wear, is plausible because hydrogel lenses impinge upon the limbus and conjunctiva, whereas rigid lenses generally do not. The study of McMonnies and Chapman-Davies[7,8] was conducted in the mid-1980s – at a time when relatively unsophisticated and potentially toxic preservatives (thimerosal and chlorhexidine) were included in contact lens solutions. The use of current-generation preservatives is less likely to be associated with increased conjunctival redness.[12]

The increasing availability of video-capture technology that can be interfaced with sophisticated computer-based image analysis systems has led a number of researchers to develop objective techniques for measuring the level of conjunctival redness in response to contact lens wear.[13–16] Owen et al.[15] used such a system to demonstrate that, over a 4-month period, rigid lens wear was associated with an increase in conjunctival redness, whereas soft lens wear was not associated with increased redness. These results do not necessarily conflict with those of McMonnies and Chapman-Davies,[7,8] who examined the conjunctivae of adapted lens wearers. The data of Owen et al.[15] probably reflect the general ocular irritation experienced during the initial adaptive phase of rigid lens wear.

Holden et al.[17] measured the extent of general conjunctival redness and limbal redness in a group of patients who had worn a hydrogel lens of high water content on an extended wear basis for an average of 5 years. General conjunctival redness was graded as 0.9 (versus 0.7 in control eyes not wearing lenses) and limbal redness was graded as 1.1 (versus 0.3 in control eyes not wearing lenses). From these data it can be inferred that extended wear soft lenses have a much greater impact on limbal redness than general conjunctival redness.

Guillon and Shah[16] used a computer-based video-capture system to monitor objectively diurnal changes in conjunctival redness in patients wearing soft lenses on a daily and extended wear basis. Non-lens wearers displayed similar levels of redness in the morning and evening, but less redness during the day. With daily wear lenses, conjunctival redness was greatest in the evening, whereas extended wear of soft lenses was associated with greatest levels or redness upon waking.

Pathology

The bulbar conjunctiva contains a rich plexus of arterioles. Unlike arteries, arteriolar walls contain little elastic connective tissue. They do, however, contain a thick layer of smooth muscle that is richly enervated with sympathetic nerve fibres. The smooth muscle, as well as being under central autonomic control, can be influenced by numerous local changes.

Vasodilation refers to enlargement in the circumference of a vessel through relaxation of its smooth muscle layer, which leads to decreased resistance and increased blood flow through the vessel.[18] This is known as active hyperemia. Since blood vessels can be observed directly through the transparent conjunctiva, this leads to an appearance of increased redness (less white sclera is visible).

Vasodilation can also occur as a result of passive mechanisms, such as vessel blockages. *Figure 9.3* shows a distended arteriole possibly caused by a blockage near the limbus.

Arteriolar muscle normally displays a state of constriction known as vascular tone. This ongoing tonic activity is attributed to two factors:

- Intrinsic myogenic activity caused by fluctuating membrane potentials;
- Norepinephrine (noradrenaline) release from sympathetic fibres that enervate the arterioles.

Vessel circumference can thus be either increased or decreased by altering one or both of the above mechanisms.[18] This can be achieved by local control mechanisms or intrinsic controls; the latter mechanism relates more to blood-pressure regulation and has relatively little influence on conjunctival redness.

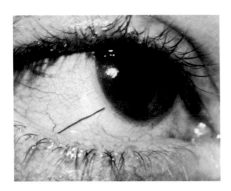

Figure 9.3
Single distended conjunctival vessel presumed to be caused by a blockage at the limbus

Etiology

Eye redness to various degrees is a sign and symptom of virtually every adverse response to contact lens wear. As a physical entity that comes into direct contact with the conjunctiva, a contact lens can have a local mechanical effect on the conjunctiva that results in increased redness. As a device that can interfere with the normal metabolic processes of the cornea and conjunctiva and is used in association with various solutions, a contact lens can also affect the level of conjunctival redness via a local chemical or toxic effect. Local infection and inflammation can also cause eye redness. Each of these influences is considered in turn.

Metabolic influences

Conjunctival arterioles are exposed to the various chemical components of the interstitial fluid in the tissue. During metabolic activity, the concentration of these chemical components can change, which leads to vessel dilation and an increase in blood flow. The following metabolic influences relax arteriolar smooth muscle:

- Hypoxia is caused by the lens – lenses of lower oxygen transmissibility (Dk/t) induce greater levels of hypoxia;[11]
- Hypercapnia is caused by the lens – lenses of lower carbon dioxide transmissibility (Dk/t) induce greater levels of hypercapnia;
- Acidic shift – through the accumulation of lactic and carbonic acid as a consequence of hypoxia and hypercapnia, respectively;
- Increased osmolarity – from an increased metabolic production of osmotically active particles;
- Increased potassium – caused by repeated action potentials, which cause a flood of potassium that cannot be removed by the sodium–potassium pump.

Chemical influences

Non-toxic chemicals introduced into the eye either directly or indirectly (with contact lens insertion) can lead to conjunctival redness for the following reasons:

- Acidic shift – caused by the introduction into the eye of a solution of different pH to that of conjunctival tissue;
- increased osmolarity – caused by the introduction into the eye of a hypertonic contact lens solution.

Toxic reaction

A toxic reaction can occur through exposure to noxious preservatives, buffers, enzymes, chelating agents or other chemical agents incorporated into contact lens solutions.[19] Paugh *et al.*[20] demonstrated an association between the concentration of hydrogen peroxide solution introduced into the eye and the degree conjunctival redness, and found a concentration of 800 ppm (the highest concentration tested) caused a degree of redness of grade 2.7. *Figure 9.4* displays an acute circumlimbal toxic response to an experimental disinfecting solution for contact lenses; note the associated conjunctival hemorrhaging.

Allergic reaction

That the conjunctiva supports and reflects immunologic activity is evidenced clinically by atopic patients who display variations in conjunctival redness that coincide with seasonal fluctuations in the concentration of airborne antigens such as pollen. Allergic reactions may also be triggered by chemicals in contact lens solutions or deposits on contact lenses.[19]

Neural control

The rich sympathetic enervation of conjunctival arterioles can exert an overall influence on conjunctival redness. Thus, pharmacologic agents that modulate sympathetic enervation affect eye redness. Such agents generally are not used in conjunction with contact lens care systems. The arteriolar system of the body in general is under sympathetic control for the regulation of blood pressure, but variations in conjunctival redness as a result of this central control mechanism are likely to be minimal.

Inflammation

Inflammation is the reaction of tissue to injury, and is characterized by heat, swelling, redness, pain and loss of function. In the conjunctiva, the association between heat and redness has been demonstrated by Efron *et al.*,[21] who showed that a change of one grade of conjunctival redness corresponds to a change in conjunctival temperature of 0.15°C. *Figure 9.5* is a graphic example

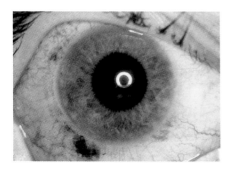

Figure 9.4
Circumlimbal toxic response to an experimental disinfecting solution for contact lenses

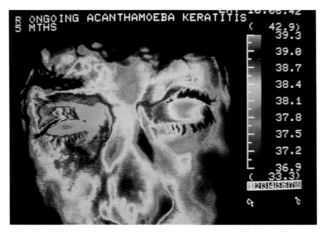

Figure 9.5
Ocular thermogram, (of a patient who suffered from acanthamoeba keratitis) that indicates an increased temperature of the inflamed right eye

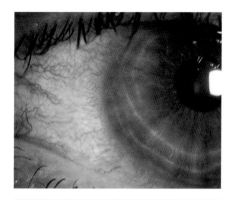

Figure 9.6
Contact lens acute red eye (CLARE)

of the association between ocular inflammation (primarily involving the cornea and conjunctiva, but also the surrounding facial tissues) and ocular temperature in a patient who suffered from acanthamoeba keratitis. This image, obtained using ocular thermography,[22,23] demonstrates how this technique can be used to monitor ocular inflammation related to contact lenses in terms of the heat generated from a hyperemic eye.

Contact lens acute red eye syndrome

A syndrome known as the 'contact lens acute red eye' (CLARE) is observed from time to time in patients with extended wear contact lenses.[24] This is an inflammatory response in which the patient wakes in the morning with unilateral bulbar conjunctival and limbal redness, discomfort, lacrimation and photophobia (*Figure 9.6*). The severity

of these signs and symptoms can vary from being mild to severe. On slit-lamp examination, anterior stromal infiltrates are usually observed near the limbus, but by definition there is no overlying epithelial staining or underlying erosion of stromal tissue (ulceration).

This syndrome is generally attributed to the pathologic effects of proteases released by Gram-negative bacteria,[25,26] which may be adherent to the contact lens or may enter the eye via lens solutions during lens insertion and removal. Other factors that may be of significance in the etiology of CLARE include:

- An immobile lens;
- Direct or indirect effects of hypoxia and/or hypercapnia (e.g., respiratory distress) in lenses of low *Dk/t*;
- Toxicity or inflammation caused by trapped post-lens debris;
- Mechanical effect of the lens;
- Toxic, inflammatory, immunologic or mechanical effect of lens deposits;
- Tear film thinning;
- Hypersensitivity or toxicity to preservatives re-released back into the eye from content lenses of high water;[24]
- Increased temperature beneath the lens.

Mechanical influences

Contact lenses can come into direct contact with the conjunctiva and cause mechanical damage.[27] Trauma is known to cause mast cell degranulation, which results in histamine release. Histamine is the major cause of vasodilation in an injured area, and can also lead to conjunctival chemosis (swelling). Young and Coleman[28] demonstrated that physical irritation from a loosely fitting lens can induce significant conjunctival redness.

Figure 9.7 shows the eye of a 35-year-old woman who suffered a traumatic injury to this eye while wearing a rigid lens. The lens broke into many pieces and a small fragment became embedded in her conjunctiva (arrow), and caused mild redness. The patient was asymptomatic and refused surgical treatment to remove the lens fragment. This case illustrates that chronic mechanical irritation, albeit asymptomatic, can induce conjunctival redness.

Many of the reactions described above are mediated by intrinsic substances in the body, such as prostaglandins, which are described as 'local hormones' in that they are synthesized locally, they have short half-lives, they exert a rapid and often profound effect and they finally metabolize to a biologically inactive form. *Figure 9.8* illustrates a possible mechanism of prostaglandin-mediated vasodilation caused by lens-induced hypoxia, as proposed by Efron *et al.*[29] Other intrinsic substances, such as neutrophil chemotactic factor, are released in traumatized tissue and help establish an inflammatory reaction.

Observation and Grading

The extent of conjunctival redness can be graded using the grading scales provided in Appendix A. Although illustrative grading scales are not as accurate as objective computer-based image analysis systems, grading scales do offer sufficient sensitivity for general clinical use if clinicians are willing to estimate the grade of redness to the nearest 0.1 grade unit.

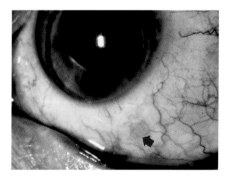

Figure 9.7
Moderate chronic conjunctival hyperemia caused by a fragment of a rigid lens that became embedded in the conjunctiva (arrow) after traumatic injury

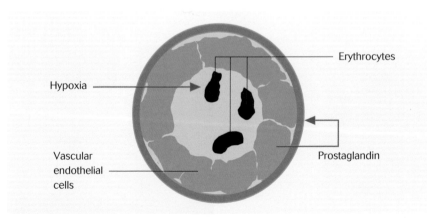

Figure 9.8
Possible mechanism of prostaglandin-mediated vasodilation caused by lens-induced hypoxia

Conjunctival redness typically displays regional variations, so it is important to indicate on the record card the area of conjunctiva being graded. This can be achieved by designating the general zone, such as superior, inferior, temporal or nasal, or a more specific region, by specifying the 'time' with reference to the cornea being the 'clock face' (e.g., 8 o'clock in *Figure 9.9*). It may also be worth noting the time of day that the observation is made, in view of the normal diurnal variation in conjunctival redness.[16]

Management

As described above, numerous factors may result in a red eye and the key factor in a given patient is rarely obvious. In some cases, a variety of actions may need to be taken, either sequentially or simultaneously.

Eye redness may be acute or chronic. Most acute reactions, including the CLARE syndrome,[24] are transient and self-limiting, and in many cases the eye redness resolves before the patient decides to seek the advice of a practitioner. Thus, eye redness as a key presenting complaint from a contact lens patient often suggests a chronic problem that requires active intervention.

Treatment options fall into four broad categories:
- Alterations to the type, design and modality of lens wear;
- Alterations to care systems;
- Improvement of ocular hygiene;
- Prescription of pharmaceutical agents.
Each of these is considered in turn.

Alteration to the lens

All soft lenses – including daily disposable lenses – develop deposits over time. Most of these deposits can be removed by daily surfactant cleaning, but some deposits, such as protein, gradually build up regardless.[30] Protein removal systems may slow the rate of protein build-up, but they do not prevent it. Furthermore, it is the *quality* of protein deposition, rather than the *quantity*, that governs biocompatibility.[31] For example, with type IV (ionic high water) lenses the physiologic compatibility of the protein is preserved, whereas type I (non-ionic low water) lenses attract protein that readily denatures and is therefore more likely to be antigenic to the eye.

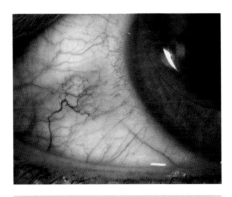

Figure 9.9
Increased eye redness, which is particularly intense at the 8 o'clock location

If it is true that bacteria adherent to protein deposits are the trigger for eye redness, the quantity of protein may be more important – less protein should mean less bacterial attachment.

Assuming protein accumulation to be one cause of red eye in soft lens patients, effective lens-related strategies include changing to a:
- Lens material that deposits a protein film physiologically compatible with the eye;
- Lens material that deposits less protein;
- Rigid lens material;
- Greater lens replacement frequency, with daily disposability being the ultimate modality in this regard.

Alterations to soft lens design may alleviate eye redness if this minimizes the mechanical impact of the lens on the eye. Thus, the fitting of good-quality thin lenses with restricted movement may be beneficial. Rigid lenses with thin interpalpebral designs, smooth edges and restricted movement are most likely to alleviate bulbar conjunctival redness because the lens does not usually come into physical contact with the bulbar conjunctiva.

Covey *et al.*[11] reported that silicone hydrogel lenses, which are highly permeable to oxygen, cause virtually no limbal redness, which indicates that such lenses exert a minimal inflammatory or irritative effect upon the eye.

Alteration to care systems

In the first instance, it is necessary to establish that the patient is fully compliant with the prescribed care regimes, which for soft lenses includes surfactant cleaning, rinsing, disinfection and periodic protein-removal treatment. Any deficiencies in this regard need to be rectified.

A rigorous approach to protein removal may alleviate chronic eye redness. The introduction of protein-removal systems into the regimen of those patients who do not use them, or an increase in frequency of usage (e.g., from weekly to every 3–4 days, or even daily) may be beneficial. This applies to both soft and rigid lens wearers.

If preservatives in contact lens solutions are thought to be of etiologic significance in a particular patient, the employment of preservative-free systems may alleviate the condition (some hydrogen peroxide solutions fall into this category).

Improving ocular hygiene

Improvements to ocular hygiene begin with improvements to personal hygiene. Thus, routine and thorough hand washing prior to lens handling and regular face washing have an impact in reducing eye redness. Some authors[32] have recommended the additional step of conjunctival irrigation with sterile unpreserved saline before and after lens insertion, and periodically during the day, as a way to dilute or remove antigens and generally enhance patient comfort. Although this procedure was advocated to alleviate papillary conjunctivitis induced by contact lenses, the principle can also be applied to the management of chronic red eye.

Attention to lid hygiene could also be of benefit. Encouraging the patient to employ strategies such as lid scrubbing, warm compresses and expression could alleviate eye redness if lid involvement is suspected as being wholly or partially responsible for eye redness.

Pharmaceutical agents

In certain cases, consideration can be given to prescribing ocular decongestants.[33] These drugs all contain vasoconstrictor agents that serve the dual purpose of reducing eye redness and alleviating symptoms. Of course, ocular disease and all other possible lens-related causes of eye redness must be ruled out before decongestants are prescribed, because they could exacerbate the problem by masking and prolonging the real cause of eye redness.

'Over the counter' ocular decongestants include:

- Phenylephrine 0.12% (e.g., P Isopto Frin);
- Naphazoline 0.01% combined with witch hazel 12% (e.g., P Eye Dew);
- Naphazoline 0.01–0.1% combined with antazoline (e.g., P Murine);
- Xylometazoline 0.05% combined with antazoline (e.g., P Otrivine-Antistin);
- Levocabastine 0.05% (e.g., P Livostin Direct).[33]

Phenylephrine in concentrations of 0.12% is insufficient to cause pupil dilation. However, the side effects of phenylephrine include reactive hyperemia (an uncomfortable red eye that can occur after prolonged use), allergic reactions and soft lens discoloration.

Naphazoline is more stable and longer acting, and is less likely to cause an allergic reaction or rebound congestion compared with phenylephrine. However, some patients – especially children – apparently have experienced a sedation effect after prolonged use.

In conclusion, ocular decongestants should generally be avoided and maximum effort be directed toward identifying and rectifying the primary cause of the problem. When all possible causes of eye redness have been ruled out, then decongestants can be prescribed for intermittent use with the primary cosmetic objective of alleviating an unsightly red eye appearance. Patients who use decongestants should be monitored more frequently than normal (say, every 3 months).

Prognosis

Recovery from acute lens-induced conjunctival redness is extremely rapid. In his early writings, Fick[1] recognized this and noted, "The injection of the eyeball disappears with extraordinary rapidity after removal of the [haptic lens]", and "... any possible injection of the conjunctiva will disappear within half an hour." Contemporary research has confirmed the observations of Fick that acute redness dissipates rapidly. For example, Paugh et al.[20] demonstrated that, after the instillation of 800 ppm hydrogen peroxide into the eye, it only took 5 minutes to recover from an eye redness grading of 2.7 down to a normal grading of 0.4.

In general, removal of any acute noxious stimulus, including a contact lens, leads to a very rapid recovery of eye redness to normal levels.

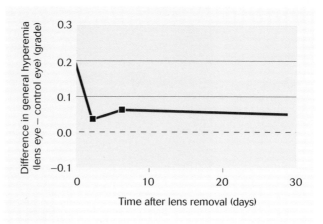

Figure 9.10

Time course of resolution of general conjunctival redness after 5 years extended wear of a hydrogel lens of high-water content in one eye only, relative to control eye not wearing a lens (after Holden et al.[14])

The prognosis for recovery from chronic red eye induced by contact lenses after removal of the lenses and cessation of wear is also reasonably rapid. Holden et al.[17] found that, after approximately 5 years of hydrogel extended lens wear, general conjunctival redness resolved within 2 days of ceasing lens wear (Figure 9.10).

Differential Diagnosis

When a patient wearing contact lenses presents with a red eye as a primary complaint, the initial diagnostic step is to determine whether or not the problem is related to lens wear. This can often be solved simply by removing the lens, whereby eye redness should dissipate rapidly if the problem is purely lens related. However, the possibility that the lens is somehow exacerbating a complication unrelated to lens wear itself should not be discounted.

Another differential diagnosis that may be necessary when presented with an extremely red eye is to determine the extent to which the redness is caused by conjunctival injection or ciliary flush. Two simple tests can be used. A sterile cotton bud can be applied to the bulbar conjunctiva in the region of redness and gently moved from side to side. The conjunctival vessels move, but the ciliary vessels remain in a fixed position. It can therefore be determined whether the redness relates primarily to the 'moving' vessels (indicating conjunctival involvement) or the 'static' vessels (indicating ciliary involvement).

An alternative test is to instil a decongestant into the eye.[34] The effect of a decongestant is limited to the superficial conjunctival vessels; these drugs have no effect on the deeper ciliary vessels. Thus, if the instillation of a decongestant alleviates eye redness, the condition is primarily conjunctival. If the decongestant has no impact on eye redness, the redness can be attributed to excessive ciliary flush.

A sub-conjunctival hemorrhage can be easily differentiated from conjunctival and/or ciliary redness because of the stark appearance of an intensely 'blood red' eye (Figure 9.11). Repeated clumsy insertion and removal of contact lenses by a patient new to contact lens wear – in particular rigid lens wear – can lead to the formation of a sub-conjunctival hemorrhage. Although this condition is benign and self-limiting, its appearance is startling to an unsuspecting lens wearer and may undermine the confidence that such a patient has in contact lens wear, despite assurances to the contrary. Small hemorrhages of individual conjunctival vessels can cause a localized increase in conjunctival redness (Figure

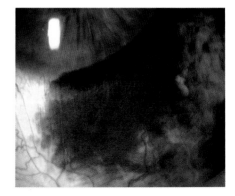

Figure 9.11

Sub-conjunctival ecchymosis

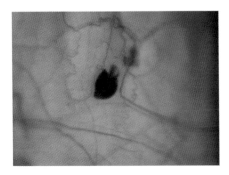

Figure 9.12
Localized conjunctival hemorrhages in a soft lens wearer

9.12), but again these are self-evident and differential diagnosis from vascular engorgement is clear.

Assuming that a given case of eye redness is lens related, it is necessary to determine whether the source of problem is the cornea or conjunctiva. Conjunctival redness associated with a quiet limbus and absence of pain indicates a primary conjunctival problem. Conjunctival redness associated with an injected limbus and corneal pain indicates corneal involvement or, indeed, a problem related *exclusively* to the cornea. Careful slit-lamp examination of the anterior ocular structures, and inspection of the lens at high magnification, generally reveals the cause of the problem. It may also be necessary to prescribe different care systems and differentially diagnose the effects of various solutions over time.

If the red eye is deemed to be unrelated to lens wear, all other possible causes of red eye must be investigated. This may involve a full ocular examination that requires the use of direct and indirect ophthalmoscopy, tonometry, etc. A full account of the differential diagnosis of the red eye in a general ophthalmic context is beyond the scope of this book.

REFERENCES

1 Efron N and Pearson RM (1988). Centenary celebration of Fick's Eine Contactbrille. *Arch Ophthalmol.* **106**, 1370–1377.
2 Pearson RM and Efron N (1989). Hundredth anniversary of August Müller's inaugural dissertation on contact lenses. *Surv Ophthalmol.* **34**, 133–141.
3 Anderson DM (2003). *Dorland's Illustrated Medical Dictionary*, 30th Edition. (Philadelphia: Saunders).
4 Pearsall J (2001). *The Concise Oxford Dictionary*, 10th Edition (Oxford: Oxford University Press).
5 Stapleton F, Dart J and Minassian D (1992). Nonulcerative complications of contact lens wear. Relative risks for different lens types. *Arch Ophthalmol.* **110**, 1601–1606.
6 Papas EB (2000). Key factors in the subjective and objective assessment of conjunctival erythema. *Invest Ophthalmol Vis Sci.* **41**, 687–691.
7 McMonnies CW and Chapman-Davies A (1987). Assessment of conjunctival hyperemia in contact lens wearers. Part I. *Am J Optom Physiol Opt.* **64**, 246–250.
8 McMonnies CW and Chapman-Davies A (1987). Assessment of conjunctival hyperemia in contact lens wearers. Part II. *Am J Optom Physiol Opt.* **64**, 251–255.
9 Fonn D, MacDonald KE, Richter D and Pritchard N (2002). The ocular response to extended wear of a high *Dk* silicone hydrogel contact lens. *Clin Exp Optom.* **85**, 176–182.
10 Morgan PB and Efron N (2002). Comparative clinical performance of two silicone hydrogel contact lenses for continuous wear. *Clin Exp Optom.* **85**, 183–192.
11 Covey M, Sweeney DF, Terry R, *et al.* (2001). Hypoxic effects on the anterior eye of high-*Dk* soft contact lens wearers are negligible. *Optom Vis Sci.* **78**, 95–99.
12 Soni PS, Horner DG and Ross J (1996). Ocular response to lens care systems in adolescent soft contact lens wearers. *Optom Vis Sci.* **73**, 70–85.
13 Villumsen J, Ringquist J and Alm A (1991). Image analysis of conjunctival hyperemia. A personal computer based system. *Acta Ophthalmol (Copenh.)* **69**, 536–539.
14 Willingham FF, Cohen KL, Coggins JM, *et al.* (1995). Automatic quantitative measurement of ocular hyperemia. *Curr Eye Res.* **14**, 1101–1108.
15 Owen CG, Fitzke FW and Woodward EG (1996). A new computer assisted objective method for quantifying vascular changes of the bulbar conjunctivae. *Ophthalmic Physiol Opt.* **16**, 430–437.
16 Guillon M and Shah D (1996). Objective measurement of contact lens-induced conjunctival redness. *Optom Vis Sci.* **73**, 595–605.
17 Holden BA, Sweeney DF, Swarbrick HA, *et al.* (1986). The vascular response to long-term extended contact lens wear. *Clin Exp Optom.* **69**, 112–119.
18 Sherwood L (1989). *Human Physiology – from Cells to Systems*. (New York: West Publishing Company).
19 Mondino BJ, Salamon SM and Zaidman GW (1982). Allergic and toxic reactions of soft contact lens wearers. *Surv Ophthalmol.* **26**, 337–344.
20 Paugh JR, Brennan NA and Efron N (1988). Ocular response to hydrogen peroxide. *Am J Optom Physiol Opt.* **65**, 91–98.
21 Efron N, Brennan NA, Hore J and Rieper K (1988). Temperature of the hyperemic bulbar conjunctiva. *Curr Eye Res.* **7**, 615–618.
22 Efron N, Young G and Brennan NA (1989). Ocular surface temperature. *Curr Eye Res.* **8**, 901–906.
23 Morgan PB, Soh MP, Efron N and Tullo AB (1993). Potential applications of ocular thermography. *Optom Vis Sci.* **70**, 568–576.
24 Binder PS (1980). The physiologic effects of extended wear soft contact lenses. *Ophthalmology* **87**, 745–749.
25 Holden BA, La Hood D, Grant T, *et al.* (1996). Gram-negative bacteria can induce contact lens related acute red eye (CLARE) responses. *CLAO J.* **22**, 47–52.
26 Estrellas PS Jr, Alionte LG and Hobden JA (2000). A *Pseudomonas aeruginosa* strain isolated from a contact lens-induced acute red eye (CLARE) is protease-deficient. *Curr Eye Res.* **20**, 157–165.
27 Efron N and Veys J (1992). Defects in disposable contact lenses can compromise ocular integrity. *Int Contact Lens Clin.* **19**, 8–18.
28 Young G and Coleman S (2001). Poorly fitting soft lenses affect ocular integrity. *CLAO J.* **27**, 68–74.
29 Efron N, Holden BA and Vannas A (1984). Prostaglandin-inhibitor naproxen does not affect contact lens-induced changes in the human corneal endothelium. *Am J Optom Physiol Opt.* **61**, 741–744.
30 Jones L, Senchyna M, Glasier MA, *et al.* (2003). Lysozyme and lipid deposition on silicone hydrogel contact lens materials. *Eye Contact Lens* **29S**, 75–79.
31 Sack RA, Jones B, Antignani A, *et al.* (1987). Specificity and biological activity of the protein deposited on the hydrogel surface. Relationship of polymer structure to biofilm formation. *Invest Ophthalmol Vis Sci.* **28**, 842–849.
32 Farkas P, Kasalow TW and Farkas B (1986). Clinical management and control of giant papillary conjunctivitis secondary to contact lens wear. *J Am Optom Assoc.* **57**, 197–202.
33 Doughty MJ (2001). *Ocular Pharmacology and Therapeutics. A Primary Care Guide*. (Oxford: Butterworth–Heinemann).
34 Jose JG, Polse KA and Holden EK (1984). *Optometric Pharmacology*. (Orlando: Grune and Stratton).

PAPILLARY CONJUNCTIVITIS

Australian ophthalmologist Tom Spring is widely credited as being the first to observe an allergic-like reaction of the upper tarsal conjunctiva, which was later to become known as 'giant papillary conjunctivitis'. In his 1974 letter to the editor of the *Medical Journal of Australia*, Spring noted the presence of large tarsal papillae, accompanied by discomfort and excessive mucus production, in 43% of patients who wore soft lenses.[1]

The term 'giant papillary conjunctivitis' was coined by Allansmith *et al.*[2] to describe papillary changes on the tarsal conjunctiva that were likened to a cobblestone formation (*Figure 10.1*). However, this condition can take on a variety of different appearances, depending on the level of severity and whether it relates to soft or rigid lens wear. In its mild form, this condition has been termed 'lid roughness' and 'papillary hypertrophy'. Even in advances stages the papillary formations may be extensive, but not necessarily 'giant'. Thus, a more appropriate term that encompasses all of the possible manifestations of the same condition is 'contact lens induced papillary conjunctivitis' (CLPC).

Prevalence

In soft lens wearers, CLPC may develop as soon as 3 weeks, or take as long as 4 years, to manifest. In rigid lens wearers, CLPC typically appears after about14 months.

It is difficult to characterize the prevalence of a condition that:
- Has a variable time of onset;
- Varies in severity throughout the seasons of the year (because of its allergic nature);
- Varies over the years as different lens care regimens and lens wear modalities come in and out of vogue.

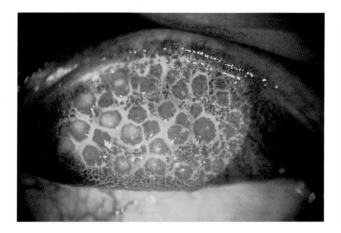

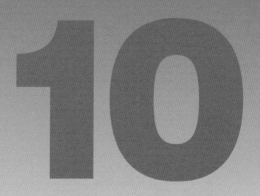

Figure 10.1
'Giant' papillae in a patient wearing soft lenses on a daily wear basis, observed with fluorescein under white light

It is also apparent that the definition of CLPC has changed over time, with the earlier literature (say, pre-1985) focusing on the appearance of very large papillae (consistent with the notion of 'giant' papillae) and the subsequent literature paying more attention to CLPC in its more subtle variants.

The prevalence of overt CLPC in wearers of conventional soft lenses (non-planned replacement) on a daily wear basis (CSDW lenses) has been reported by various authors to be 1.8%,[3] 12%[4] and 15%.[5] The reason for these figures being much lower than that reported by Spring[1] (43%) is probably a reflection of changing times – most of Spring's patients were likely to have been using thermally disinfected hydroxyethyl methacrylate (HEMA) lenses, whereas the patients surveyed in more recent studies[3–5] were using modern lens-care regimens (such as hydrogen peroxide and multipurpose disinfection systems).

Grant[6] reported a prevalence for CLPC of 19% in patients using conventional soft (non-planned replacement) extended wear (CSEW) lenses, versus 3% with disposable soft extended wear (DSEW) lenses. However, Poggio and Abelson[3] found no difference in CLPC between patients who wore CSEW lenses (1.9%) and those who wore DSEW lenses (2.0%) when using disposable lenses. Other authors have reported somewhat higher incidence figures of 6.4%,[7] 6.7%[8] and 6–12%[9] for disposable extended wear lenses.

Alemany and Redal[5] found a lower incidence of overt CLPC in patients wearing daily wear rigid lenses compared with conventional daily wear soft lenses. Grant *et al.*[9] reported that the incidence of CLPC in patients wearing rigid lenses on an extended wear basis was 2%, versus 6–12% for soft disposable extended wear. Fonn *et al.*[10] reported the results of a 4 month clinical trial in which six out of 18 patients (33%) wearing silicone hydrogel lenses on an extended wear basis developed CLPC; two of these patients were discontinued from the study because of the severity of the condition.

Normal Tarsal Conjunctiva

In normals, the tarsal conjunctiva can take on a variety of forms, which may be categorized in different ways. Allansmith[11] described three forms of normal tarsal conjunctival appearance:

- Satin or smooth (14%);
- Small, uniformly sized 'micropapillae', which are less than 0.3 mm in diameter (85%);
- Non-uniform papillae (<1%), in which some papillae can be as large as 0.5 mm in diameter.

An alternative model for classifying the normal tarsal conjunctiva has been proposed by Potvin *et al.*,[12] who conducted a computer-assisted morphometric examination of photographic images of the fluorescein-stained tarsal conjunctiva of eight asymptomatic non-lens wearers. The eight subjects were classified into two distinct groups – those who displayed 'small feature' tarsal plates (with a modal feature area of 25,000–35,000 μm^2 and a restricted range of areas), and those who displayed 'large feature' tarsal plates (with a modal feature area of 50,000–70,000 μm^2 and a wide range of areas). The cells generally appear to be pentagonal and hexagonal in shape.

Allansmith's three-category model[11] is of more relevance to clinicians because it is based upon the appearance of the tarsal conjunctiva under low magnification using the slit-lamp biomicroscope.

Signs and Symptoms

It is important that an assessment be made of the central region of the tarsal plate only, for the following reasons:

- There is often increased 'roughness' of the conjunctiva at the lateral extremities of the everted lid, which is unrelated to lens-induced pathology;
- The process of lid eversion causes the conjunctiva to appear artificially distorted and irregular along the margin of the lid eversion fold (i.e., anatomically superior to the tarsal plate, but paradoxically 'inferior' as the everted lid is viewed);
- The conjunctiva just inside the lid margin (i.e., anatomically inferior to the tarsal plate) is rarely affected by lens wear.

Allansmith[11] noted that the appearance of CLPC was different in soft versus rigid lens wearers. In soft lens wearers, papillae are more numerous; they are located more toward the upper tarsal plate (i.e., closer to the fold of the everted lid), and apexes of the papillae take on a rounded flatter form (*Figure 10.1*). In rigid lens wearers, papillae take on a crater-like form and are located more toward the lash

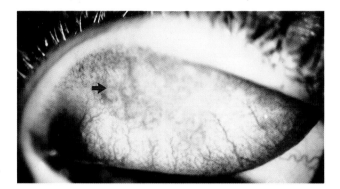

Figure 10.2
CLPC in a rigid lens wearer, with more papillae observed (arrow) toward the lash margin

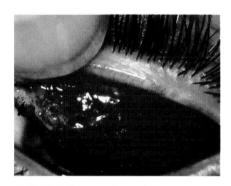

Figure 10.3
Gross redness of tarsal conjunctiva with mucus formation (arrow) in CLPC

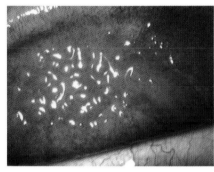

Figure 10.4
Irregular light reflexes in CLPC

margin, with few papillae being present on the upper tarsal plate (*Figure 10.2*). Skotnitsky *et al.*[13] suggest that patients wearing silicone hydrogel lenses for extended wear are more predisposed to develop localized CLPC as a result of the stiffer modulus of these lenses interacting with the superior palpebral conjunctiva.

In the early stages of development, the tarsal conjunctiva in patients who suffer from CLPC may be indistinguishable from the normal tarsal conjunctiva. An important early distinguishing feature is increased redness of the tarsal conjunctiva (*Figure 10.3*). This change can be detected with reference to the

lower palpebral conjunctiva, which is usually unaffected and can therefore act as a 'baseline' against which any change is measured.

In advanced cases, papillae can exceed 1 mm in diameter and often take on a bright red–orange hue. Evidence of papillae often appears in the form of irregular light reflexes (*Figure 10.4*). The hexagonal–pentagonal shape may be lost in favor of a more rounded appearance. The pattern of distribution of papillae may reflect the underlying anatomy of the tarsus; for example, *Figure 10.5* shows a non-uniform CLPC that developed in a soft lens wearer. Three-dimensionally,

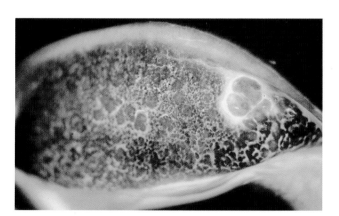

Figure 10.5
Non-uniform CLPC in a soft lens wearer, observed with fluorescein under cobalt blue light

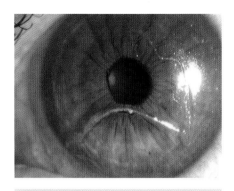

Figure 10.6

Strand of mucus on the surface of a soft lens in a patient with CLPC

giant papillae can be said to take on a 'mushroom' form, with a flattened or even slightly depressed apex or tip.

The conjunctiva is thickened, edematous and often hyperemic, so fine vessels that can normally be observed to traverse the conjunctival surface are obscured, although deep vessels remain visible over the tarsal plate. A tuft of convoluted capillary vessels is often observed at the apexes of papillae; this vascular tuft generally stains with fluorescein.

Other signs that can be observed in severe manifestations of CLPC include conjunctival edema and excessive mucus (*Figure 10.3*), which usually forms into strands that lie in the valleys between papillae. Excess mucus also accumulates at the inner and outer canthus at night and can sometimes be observed as clumps or strands floating across the cornea or on the lens surface (*Figure 10.6*). Prolonged edema may result in a mild ptosis, which is often asymmetric.

Giant papillae can display infiltrates, and if the condition persists for some time, the conjunctival surface at the apexes of the papillae can become scarred and appear a cream–white color (*Figure 10.7*). The cornea may also be compromised and display superficial punctate staining and infiltrates superiorly. Redness of the superior limbus may also be apparent.

There is general concordance between the severity of signs and symptoms. In the early stages of CLPC, patients may complain of discomfort toward the end of the wearing period and of slight itching. Patients may report an increase in mucus production upon awakening. Intermittent blurring is sometimes noted; this results from mucus being periodically smeared across the lens surface. A slight, but non-variable, vision loss is attributable to more tenacious lens deposits, such as protein, which is of etiologic significance in this condition (see later).

In more severe cases, the itching and discomfort can become so marked that the patient is forced to remove the lens. Excessive lens movement and decentration can result from a combination of the large papillae creating greater contact and friction with the coated lens surface, and excess mucus acting as an 'adhesive' between the tarsal conjunctival and lens surfaces.

The signs and symptoms of CLPC, as they manifest with different grades of severity, are summarized in *Table 10.1*.

Pathology

It has been possible to thoroughly document pathologic changes that take place in patients with CLPC because it is a relatively simple matter to biopsy tissue from the tarsal conjunctiva. By the same token, corneal pathology induced by contact lenses is often poorly understood because researchers rarely biopsy tissue specimens from the living human cornea.

The conjunctiva becomes thicker in CLPC (0.2 mm in CLPC versus 0.05 mm in normals). Greiner *et al.*[14] observed dramatic ultrastructural changes in the conjunctival surface in patients with CLPC. Conjunctival surface area is increased by two-fold and epithelial cells are enlarged and distorted, becoming elongated in shape. The microvilli are reduced in number and become distorted, forming aggregated tufts on the surface of papillae. Normally present Crypts of Henle are not observed. The number of mucus-secreting non-goblet cells is increased. More dark cells are observed at the apexes of the papillae.

CLPC is associated with a dramatic redistribution of inflammatory cells between the epithelium and stroma of the conjunctiva. Mast cells, eosinophils and basophils are found in the epithelium (they do not normally reside there) and the number of neutrophils and lymphocytes in the epithelium increased. Eosinophils and basophils are found in the stroma, with an increase in the number of mast cells, plasma cells and neutrophils.

Figure 10.8 illustrates the tissue and cellular pathologic changes that characterize a papilla.

Etiology

A number of factors have been suggested as playing a role in the etiology of CLPC, and it is unlikely that any one causative factor can account for all cases. These factors, summarized below, are:

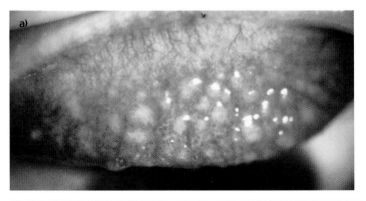

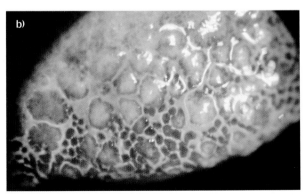

Figure 10.7

Scarring at the apexes of papillae, seen here (a) in white light and (b) in cobalt blue light

- Mechanical trauma;
- Immediate hypersensitivity;
- Delayed hypersensitivity;
- Individual susceptibility;
- Meibomian gland dysfunction (MGD).

Mechanical trauma

Papillary conjunctivitis of an apparently identical form to that induced by contact lenses has been observed in patients who do not wear contact lenses, but whose tarsal conjunctivae have been exposed to various types of mechanical trauma, such as:

- Plastic ocular prostheses;[15]
- Extruded scleral buckle;[16]
- Excessive cyanoacrylate glue used to close a perforated cornea;[17]
- Protruding nylon sutures;[18]
- Rigid contact lens imbedded in the upper fornix;[19]
- Elevated corneal deposits;[20]
- Epithelialized corneal foreign body.[21]

In many of these cases, the papillary conjunctivitis resolved and patient symptoms were alleviated upon removal of the trauma. The reports of Dunn et al.[20] and Greiner[21] are particularly noteworthy because, unlike the other cases that involve trauma induced by synthetic materials, the papillary conjunctivitis was induced by trauma from inert epithelial irregularities.

Trauma is known to cause mast cell degranulation, so the presence of large numbers of degranulated mast cells in the conjunctival epithelium and stroma of patients with CLPC[22] is consistent with trauma being a factor of etiologic significance in this condition. The conjunctivae of patients with CLPC have significantly higher levels of neutrophil chemotactic factor,[23] a substance generally released in traumatized tissue. The decay-accelerating factor (DAF), a membrane-associated complement regulatory protein that inhibits the central C3 amplification convertases of the cascade, is present on both the ocular surface and in tears. Szczotka et al.[24] reported that DAF concentrations were significantly reduced in patients with CLPC compared with normal controls not wearing contact lenses. This reduction may be associated with enhanced complement activation, which contributes to the pathogenesis of CLPC.

Immediate hypersensitivity

Immediate hypersensitivity is an anaphylactic reaction mediated by immunoglobulin type E (IgE) antibodies, which

Table 10.1
Signs and symptoms of papillary conjunctivitis

Grade	Signs	Symptoms
0	Normal tarsal conjunctiva: (a) smooth (b) uniform micropapillae (c) non-uniform micropapillae	None
1	Slight redness of upper tarsus	Occasional itching
2	Slight papillary roughness Slight redness of upper tarsus Slight increase in lens movement	Mild itching Mild lens awareness
3	Moderate papillary roughness Small papillae along lid fold Moderate redness of upper tarsus Infiltrates in vascular tuft Moderate lens movement Moderate lens decentration Fine mucus strands on tarsus Some mucus in tears Slight coating apparent Vision variable	Moderate itching Moderate lens awareness Wearing time reduced Some mucus noted Aware of moderate lens movement Aware of moderate lens decentration Slight intermittent blur with lens
4	Severe papillary roughness Large papillae extending over tarsus Severe redness of upper tarsus Infiltrates may mask vascular tuft Central scarring of papillae Excessive lens movement Excessive lens decentration Mucus pooling between papillae Mucus strands on cornea Mucus strands and clumps in tears Heavy lens coating Vision variable Vision slightly reduced Superficial limbal redness Superficial corneal staining Superficial corneal infiltrates	Severe itching Severe lens awareness Wearing time minimal Excess mucus noted Aware of excessive lens movement Aware of excessive lens decentration Frequent intermittent blur with lens Slight vision loss with lens

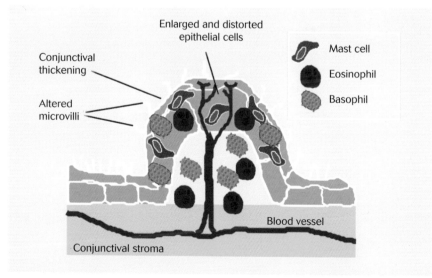

Figure 10.8
Pathologic changes that characterize a papilla

proliferate when the conjunctiva is exposed to certain antigens. The IgE antibodies set off a chain reaction that leads to mast cell degranulation and the release of inflammatory mediators and other substances that can affect tissue damage and repair. Patients with CLPC exhibit large numbers of degranulated mast cells in the conjunctival epithelium,[25] and elevated levels of IgE in tears.[26]

Protein deposition on the lens has been implicated as the antigenic stimulant to IgE production. More specifically, deposits that form on the anterior lens surface are likely to be more significant in that this surface lies in direct apposition with the tarsal conjunctiva. In support of this lens deposition theory, Ballow *et al.*[27] demonstrated that when contact lenses from patients who suffer from CLPC were placed in the eyes of monkeys, a frank papillary conjunctivitis ensued, with elevated IgE levels. These changes did not occur in monkeys that wore new lenses or lenses from patients who did not suffer from CLPC.

A critical issue in formulating strategies to treat or prevent CLPC is to determine the specific causative antigens. Protein deposition on the lens surface is the most popular candidate; however, protein on lenses of patients with CLPC is indistinguishable from that on lenses of patients without CLPC. The antigenic stimulus could also be one of a number of other potential lens contaminants, such as lipids, calcium, mucus and albumin[28]. Microorganisms, such as bacteria (and bacterial endotoxins), may also trigger CLPC.

The type of plastic used to fabricate the contact lens could theoretically have an antigenic role. However, this is difficult to prove.[29] The success or otherwise of various polymers in alleviating or preventing CLPC probably relates more to the propensity of different materials to become deposited and/or the frequency of lens replacement, rather than to any real differences in their intrinsic antigenic potency.

Early generation preservatives, such as thimerosal and benzalkonium chloride, are known to have a causative role in the development of CLPC.[30] Certainly, treatment is more likely to succeed if care systems are free of such preservatives.[31]

Delayed hypersensitivity

In their initial writings, Allansmith *et al.*[2] likened CLPC to vernal conjunctivitis in view of the similar inflammatory cell pro-

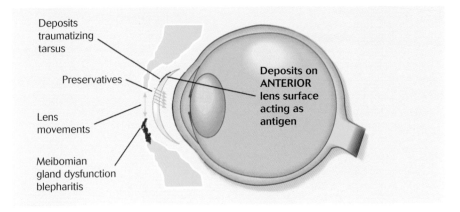

Figure 10.9
Factors of etiologic significance in CLPC

files of the two conditions, a view that still holds today.[32] The unusual presence of large numbers of basophils led Allansmith *et al.*[2] to suggest that these diseases were of the cutaneous basophilic type. This is classically a skin reaction that has a delayed time course and is mediated by sensitized T lymphocytes and antibodies. In support of this proposed etiology, Hann *et al.*[33] induced a CLPC-type reaction in guinea pigs after injection of various antigens into the tarsal plate.

Despite the evidence cited above, the proportion of basophils to the total pool of inflammatory cells in CLPC is significantly less than that observed in a typical cutaneous basophilic hypersensitivity reaction. In view of this, Begley[34] suggests that CLPC may better reflect the classic tuberculin type of delayed hypersensitivity reaction in which variable numbers of basophils can be present.

The antigens discussed in the previous section on the immediate hypersensitivity reaction are likely to be the same as those that mediate the delayed hypersensitivity reaction.

Individual susceptibility

There is disagreement in the literature as to whether atopic individuals are more susceptible to developing CLPC. Some authors have found no connection between atopy and CLPC,[2,25] whereas others have reported an increased prevalence of allergies in patients who exhibit CLPC.[35] Buckley[36] found elevated serum IgE levels in patients who suffered from CLPC, which suggests the presence of an IgE-mediated atopy in these patients.

Indirect evidence of the association of atopy with CLPC comes from the work

of Begley *et al.*,[37] who reported that the onset of this condition was seasonal in a population of 68 patients. The condition peaked during the 'allergy seasons' in mid-western USA, where the study was conducted. These patients reported significantly more overall allergies, in addition to CLPC, than did a control group.

Meibomian gland dysfunction

Some researchers have suggested an association between CLPC and meibomian gland dysfunction (MGD).[38,39] Martin *et al.*[38] found that 42 patients who presented consecutively also suffered from MGD blepharitis, and that the severity of the conditions correlated positively. After treating the MGD blepharitis and refitting new lenses to 32 patients, 28 were judged to be successful 21 months later.

Figure 10.9 illustrates the various factors thought to be of etiologic significance in CLPC.

Observation and Grading

As CLPC manifests in the superior palpebral conjunctiva, it is necessary to evert the lid to detect this condition. This is best performed with the patient positioned in the head-and-brow rest of a slit-lamp biomicroscope, so that the everted lid can be observed readily at low magnification (×10–15) and high illumination. The extent of tarsal redness and edema, and the general position and distribution of papillae, is noted. High magnification can then be employed to examine the conjunctival surface, with particular attention to the distribution of vessels over the surface of the papillae.

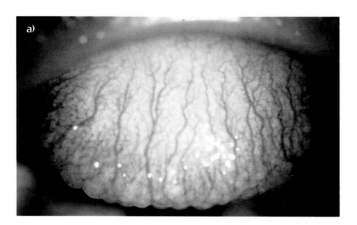
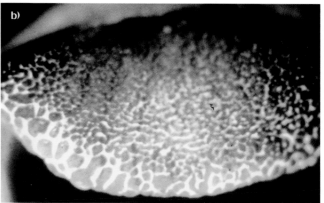

Figure 10.10

CLPC observed under (a) white light and (b) cobalt blue light. Observation with cobalt blue reveals a more extensive pattern of papillae

After observing the tarsal conjunctiva in white light, the lid should be reverted back to its normal form and fluorescein instilled. After a few blinks, the lid should be everted once again and observed under white light and then cobalt blue light (*Figure 10.10*). Fluorescein pools at the base of the papillae, which resolves individual papillae and so the overall pattern of papillary formation is appreciated more readily. Viewing the fluorescein-stained conjunctiva in both white light and blue light is recommended because the 'white light with fluorescein' view represents an intermediate step or 'link' that allows reconciliation of the 'white light without fluorescein' and 'blue light with fluorescein' views. The severity of CLPC can be assessed with reference to the grading scales presented in Appendix A.

The lower lid should be everted by simply pulling downward on the skin just beneath the lashes on the lower eyelid. The exposed lower palpebral conjunctiva will generally be clear and forms a useful baseline reference for assessing the level of tarsal redness and edema of the superior palpebral conjunctiva. However, a mild CLPC will very occasionally be observed in the lower lid (*Figure 10.11*). It is also important to examine the superior cornea carefully, as CLPC can be associated with superior limbal redness, corneal staining, corneal infiltrates and excess tear mucus.

Management

Many possible factors are involved in the etiology of CLPC (and the key factor in a given patient is rarely obvious), so a variety of management options may need to be employed, either sequentially or simultaneously. As a general rule, the earlier the condition is detected and treated, the better is the prognosis for an effective and speedy cure.

In many respects, CLPC is a condition best managed with reference to patient symptoms rather than signs. Many patients are motivated to continue lens wear even in the presence of low-grade CLPC (grades 1 and 2), and they should be allowed to do so. Subtle non-intrusive strategies should be introduced in an attempt to alleviate the condition, while at the same time maintaining patient motivation. The tarsal plate of patients who are largely asymptomatic should be monitored carefully to detect the development of chronic tissue compromise.

Treatment options fall into four broad categories:
- Alterations to the type, design and modality of lens wear;
- Alterations to care systems;
- Improvement of ocular hygiene;
- Pharmaceutical agents.

Each of these is considered in turn.

Alteration to the lens

All soft lenses develop deposits over time. Most of these deposits can be removed by daily surfactant cleaning, but some (such as protein) gradually build up regardless. Protein-removal systems may slow the rate of protein build-up, but they do not prevent it. Furthermore, it is the *quality* of protein deposition, rather than the *quantity*, that governs biocompatibility. For example, Sack *et al.*[40] demonstrated that, although type IV (ionic high water) lenses attract significant amounts of protein, the conformational integrity (i.e., physiologic compatibility) of the protein is preserved. Type I lenses (non-ionic low water) lenses attract much less protein, but the protein is denatured and therefore more likely to be antigenic to the eye.

If it is true that bacteria adherent to protein deposits are the trigger for CLPC, the quantity of protein may be

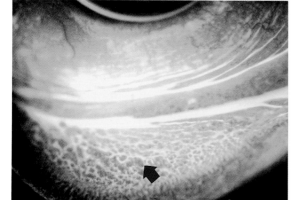

Figure 10.11

An unusual case of CLPC of the lower palpebral conjunctiva (arrow) in response to rigid lens wear, observed with fluorescein under cobalt blue light

more important – less protein should mean less bacterial attachment.

Assuming protein accumulation to be one cause of CLPC in soft lens patients, effective lens-related strategies would include:

- Changing to a lens material that deposits a protein film physiologically compatible with the eye;
- Changing to a lens material that deposits less protein;
- Changing to a rigid lens material;
- Replacing lenses more frequently.

Alterations to soft lens design may alleviate CLPC if the mechanical impact of the lens is minimized. Thus, the fitting of good-quality thin soft lenses with restricted movement may be beneficial.

The ophthalmic literature is devoid of descriptions of properly controlled studies that prove the efficacy of the various treatments described above. Even the ultimate form of regular lens replacement – daily disposable lenses – does not necessarily solve the problem. For example, daily disposable lenses made from type IV materials deposit significant levels of protein within 15 minutes of insertion.[41] The success or otherwise of such lenses in the prevention or cure of CLPC depends on the physiologic compatibility of the protein that rapidly accumulates and/or the rate of attachment of bacteria to the protein.

Cessation of lens wear certainly results in a complete cure, but such an option is generally met with little enthusiasm by patients. In severe cases (grade 3 or 4), ceasing lens wear for a brief period of, say, 2–4 weeks enhances the prospect of success of subsequent treatment strategies. Similarly, a reduction in wearing time in the early phase of treatment optimizes the prospect for recovery.

Certain rigid lenses may attract deposits in a manner less antigenic to the patient (e.g., a lesser amount of protein and/or more physiologically compatible protein). However, rigid lenses potentially have a greater physical impact on the eye, which could exacerbate CLPC. Woods and Efron[42] were unable to demonstrate a difference in the tarsal response in a group of rigid lens wearers who replaced their lenses frequently versus a matched group of rigid lens wearers who did not frequently replace their lenses. This suggests that the mechanical effects of the rigid lenses are the primary determinant of tarsal changes in rigid lens wearers. Lenses with thin interpalpebral designs, smooth edges and restricted movement are most likely to yield a successful outcome. Douglas *et al.*[43] reported that the onset of CLPC could be delayed or prevented by fitting lenses of higher oxygen transmissibility, although the success of this strategy may relate more to the surface effects of the lens materials than to the enhanced oxygen performance of these lenses.

Alteration to care systems

In the first instance, it is necessary to establish that the patient is fully compliant with the prescribed care regime, which for soft lenses includes surfactant cleaning, rinsing, disinfection and periodic protein-removal treatment. Any deficiencies in this regard need to be rectified.

A rigorous approach to protein removal may alleviate CLPC. The introduction of protein-removal systems into the regimes of those patients who do not use them, or an increase in frequency of usage (e.g., from weekly to every 3–4 days or even daily) may be beneficial. This applies to both soft and rigid lens wearers.

If preservatives in contact lens solutions are thought to be of etiologic significance in a particular patient, the employment of preservative-free systems (some hydrogen peroxide solutions fall into this category) may alleviate the condition.

Improvement of ocular hygiene

Improvements to ocular hygiene begin with improvements to personal hygiene. Thus, routine and thorough hand washing prior to lens handling and regular face washing should mitigate against developing CLPC. Some authors[31,44] have recommended the additional step of conjunctival irrigation with sterile unpreserved saline before and after lens insertion, and periodically during the day, as a way to dilute or remove anti-

gens to CLPC and generally enhance patient comfort.

If one accepts the association between CLPC and MGD described earlier,[38,39] attention to lid hygiene should be of benefit. Encouraging the patient to employ strategies such as lid scrubbing, warm compresses and expression will alleviate MGD and presumably have some positive outcome with respect to the CLPC.

Pharmaceutical agents

A variety of medications have been advocated to treat CLPC and provide symptomatic relief. The agent that has received most attention is ocular cromolyn sodium (sodium cromoglycate), which stabilizes mast cell membranes and thus prevents the release of inflammatory mediators, such as histamine. Prescription of this drug is generally used to supplement alternative strategies, such as those described above. An initial dosage of 2% or 4% cromolyn sodium four times a day, tapering off to once a day as the condition improves, has been advocated by various authors.[45,46] The preservative-free form of this drug should be used if there is a poor initial response.

Figure 10.12 shows the tarsal conjunctiva of an atopic individual who presented requesting contact lenses, but who had not worn lenses previously. She had been using cromolyn sodium daily for over 10 years. The scarring and abnormal vascular changes present may reflect a combination of long-term ocular compromise and drug-induced alterations to the normal inflammatory and tissue-repair processes.

Suprofen is another non-steroid anti-inflammatory agent that has been used to treat CLPC. This drug, which inhibits prostaglandin synthesis, was found by Wood *et al.*[47] to have a significant effect on the signs and symptoms of CLPC

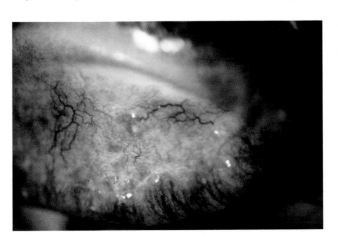

Figure 10.12

Deformities in the tarsal plate of an atopic individual who had not worn contact lenses and had used cromolyn sodium for over 10 years

after 2–3 weeks. Patients instilled two drops of 1% suprofen solution four times daily.

Steroidal agents are sometimes used for short duration in severe cases of CLPC (grade 4); however, in view of the risks of cataract formation, increased intraocular pressure and corneal infection, their use is generally avoided.

A 'soft steroid' known as loteprednol etabonate (a chemical analog of prednisolone) has been found to be as effective in treating CLPC as conventional steroids, but without the untoward side effects. Specifically, Asbell and Howes[48] found that this drug resulted in a significant reduction in both the size of papillae and the extent of itching and lens intolerance in patients with CLPC.

Vaahtoranta-Lehtonen et al.[49] studied the potential effect of ethyl-6-O-decanoylglucoside (EDG), administered as part of the formulation of a contact lens care solution, on papillary hypertrophy in 19 long-term contact lens wearers. The contact lens care solutions were 0.00025% chlorhexidine acetate (CHX) with or without 0.005% EDG. They found that although EDG prevented the development of CLPC, it did not reverse established signs of papillary hypertrophy.

Bailey and Buckley[50] studied 45 patients with CLPC for 6 weeks in a double-mask group comparative study of unpreserved 2% nedocromil sodium eye drops and placebo. There was significantly less itching in the nedocromil sodium group compared with the placebo group during weeks 1–3 of the study, but not during weeks 4–6. Biomicroscopic assessment showed a significant difference in mucus found on the upper tarsal surface in favor of nedocromil sodium by the end of the study. However, 21 patients experienced adverse events during the study, such as an unpleasant taste and/or stinging on insertion of the drops.

Butts and Rengstorff[51] claimed an aqueous preparation that contained the antioxidant 'polysorbate 80' and vitamin A alleviated CLPC in a population of 19 patients; however, the experiment was not masked and lacked controls, and the results were not subjected to statistical analysis. Thus, the efficacy of this therapy is not proved.

Prognosis

The prognosis for recovery from CLPC after removal of lenses and cessation of wear is good. Even in the most severe conditions (grade 4), symptoms disappear within 5 days to 2 weeks of lens removal[2,47] and tarsal redness and excess mucus resolve over a similar period. Resolution of papillae takes place over a much longer time course – typically many weeks and possibly as long as 6 months. The more severe the condition, the longer the recovery period.

In the longer term, however, the prognosis is less good. The condition can recur, especially in atopic patients who appear to have a propensity to develop the condition. Fortunately, such patients have a lower threshold for noticing the early 'warning signs', and typically seek prompt attention, which in turn enhances the probability of successful treatment.

Differential Diagnosis

A key issue in the accurate diagnosis of CLPC is the capacity to differentiate between papillae and follicles (*Figure 10.13*). Papillae are observed in allergic diseases, such as CLPC and vernal conjunctivitis, whereas follicles are indicative of viral or chlamydial conjunctival infections. There is generally little to distinguish between the two conditions, but careful history taking provides the most important diagnostic clues.

The appearance of papillae is described in detail above. According to Allansmith et al.,[31] the side walls of papillae may be perpendicular to the plane of the tarsal plate and not pyramidal as in follicles (*Figure 10.14*).

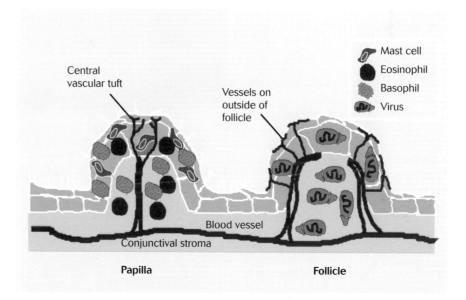

Figure 10.13

Pathologic changes that characterize a papilla (left) and follicle (right)

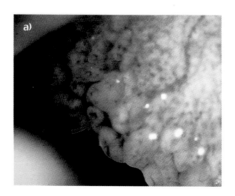 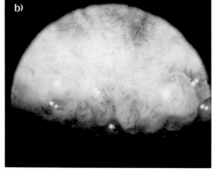

Figure 10.14

Magnified view of (a) papillae and (b) follicles. Note the presence of vascular tufts (arrow) at the apexes of papillae

Other key distinguishing features are:

- Some deep vessels can be observed to traverse the surface of papillae, whereas vessels may be more obvious on the surface of follicles;
- Papillae often display a rich plexus of convoluted vessels (vascular tuft) at the apex, whereas follicles generally do not display this feature.
- Follicles tend to be more pale in color.

In advanced stages, the apexes of the papillae may fill with infiltrates, which thus mask the vascular tuft and give a whitish center. Subsequent scarring also tends to be whitish in appearance; this makes it easy to distinguish papillae from follicles, which usually do not display scar-like areas.

In vernal conjunctivitis unrelated to lens wear, the papillae can be truly gigantic (*Figure 10.15*) and thus differentiated from CLPC. Other distinguishing features of vernal conjunctivitis are the characteristic thick yellow discharge, which consists of mucus, epithelial cells, neutrophils and eosinophils. The condition is usually bilateral and a bilateral ptosis may be present. Long-standing vernal conjunctivitis may result in distorted papillae and disorganized scarring (*Figure 10.16*).

Other pathologies of the tarsal conjunctiva present from time to time, but these are easily distinguishable from the classic cobblestone appearance of multiple papillae formations in CLPC.

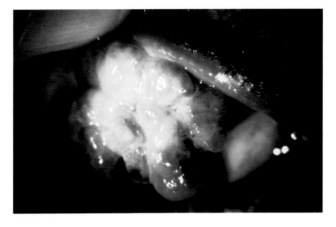

Figure 10.15
Advanced vernal conjunctivitis with characteristic thick yellow discharge

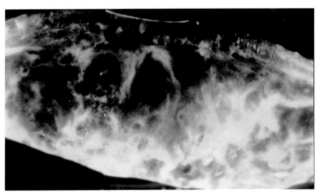

Figure 10.16
Long-standing vernal conjunctivitis with distorted papillae and disorganized scarring, observed with fluorescein under cobalt blue light

REFERENCES

1 Spring TF (1974). Reaction to hydrophilic lenses. *Med J Aust.* **1**, 449–450.
2 Allansmith MR, Korb DR, Greiner JV, *et al.* (1977). Giant papillary conjunctivitis in contact lens wearers. *Am J Ophthalmol.* **83**, 697–708.
3 Poggio EC and Abelson M (1993). Complications and symptoms in disposable extended wear lenses compared with conventional soft daily wear and soft extended wear lenses. *CLAO J.* **19**, 31–39.
4 Nason RJ, Boshnick EL and Cannon WM (1994). Multisite comparison of contact lens modalities. Daily disposable wear vs. conventional daily wear in successful contact lens wearers. *J Am Optom Assoc.* **65**, 774–778.
5 Alemany AL and Redal AP (1991). Giant papillary conjunctivitis in soft and rigid lens wear. *Contactologia* **13**, 14–20.
6 Grant T (1991). Clinical aspects of planned replacement and disposable lenses. In: *The Contact Lens Yearbook 1991*, p. 7–11, Ed. Kerr C. (Saltwood: Medical and Scientific Publishing Ltd).

7 Sankaridurg PR, Sweeney DF, Sharma S, *et al.* (1999). Adverse events with extended wear of disposable hydrogels: Results for the first 13 months of lens wear. *Ophthalmology* **106**, 1671–1680.
8 Rao GN, Naduvilath TJ and Sankaridurg PR (1996). Contact lens related papillary conjunctivitis in a prospective randomised clinical trial using disposable hydrogels. *Invest Ophthalmol Vis Sci.* **37S**, 1129.
9 Grant T, Holden BA, Rechberger J and Chong MS (1989). Contact lens related papillary conjunctivitis (CLPC): Influence of protein accumulation and replacement frequency. *Invest Ophthalmol Vis Sci.* **30S**, 166.
10 Fonn D, MacDonald KE, Richter D and Pritchard N (2002). The ocular response to extended wear of a high *Dk* silicone hydrogel contact lens. *Clin Exp Optom.* **85**, 176–182.
11 Allansmith MR (1987). Pathology and treatment of giant papillary conjunctivitis. The US perspective. *Clin Ther.* **9**, 443–444.
12 Potvin RJ, Doughty MJ and Fonn D (1994). Tarsal conjunctival morphometry of asymptomatic soft contact lens wearers and non-lens wearers. *Int Contact Lens Clin.* **21**, 225–231.
13 Skotnitsky C, Sankaridurg PR, Sweeney DF and Holden BA (2002). General and local contact lens induced papillary conjunctivitis (CLPC). *Clin Exp Optom.* **85**, 193–197.
14 Greiner JV, Covington HI and Allansmith MR (1978). Surface morphology of giant papillary conjunctivitis in contact lens wearers. *Am J Ophthalmol.* **85**, 242–252.

15 Srinivasan BD, Jakobiec FA, Iwamoto T and DeVoe AG (1979). Giant papillary conjunctivitis with ocular prostheses. *Arch Ophthalmol.* **97**, 892–895.
16 Robin JB, Regis-Pacheco LF, May WN, *et al.* (1987). Giant papillary conjunctivitis associated with an extruded scleral buckle. Case report. *Arch Ophthalmol.* **105**, 619.
17 Carlson AN and Wilhelmus KR (1987). Giant papillary conjunctivitis associated with cyanoacrylate glue. *Am J Ophthalmol.* **104**, 437–438.
18 Reynolds RMP (1978). Giant papillary conjunctivitis: A mechanical aetiology. *Aust J Optom.* **61**, 320–323.
19 Stenson S (1982). Focal giant papillary conjunctivitis from retained contact lenses. *Ann Ophthalmol.* **14**, 881–885.
20 Dunn JP Jr, Weissman BA, Mondino BJ and Arnold AC (1990). Giant papillary conjunctivitis associated with elevated corneal deposits. *Cornea* **9**, 357–358.
21 Greiner JV (1988). Papillary conjunctivitis induced by an epithelialized corneal foreign body. *Ophthalmologica* **196**, 82–86.
22 Greiner JV, Peace DG and Baird RS (1985). Effect of eye rubbing on the conjunctiva as a model of ocular inflammation. *Am J Ophthalmol.* **100**, 45–49.
23 Ehlers WH, Fishman JB, Donshik PC, *et al.* (1991). Neutrophil chemotactic factors derived from conjunctival epithelial cells: Preliminary biochemical characterization. *CLAO J.* **17**, 65–68.
24 Szczotka LB, Cocuzzi E and Medof ME (2000). Decay-accelerating factor in tears of contact lens wearers and patients with

contact lens-associated complications. *Optom Vis Sci.* **77**, 586–591.

25 Henriquez AS, Kenyon KR and Allansmith MR (1981). Mast cell ultrastructure. Comparison in contact lens-associated giant papillary conjunctivitis and vernal conjunctivitis. *Arch Ophthalmol.* **99**, 1266–1272.

26 Donshik PC and Ballow M (1983). Tear immunoglobulins in giant papillary conjunctivitis induced by contact lenses. *Am J Ophthalmol.* **96**, 460–466.

27 Ballow M, Donshik PC, Rapacz P, *et al.* (1989). Immune responses in monkeys to lenses from patients with contact lens induced giant papillary conjunctivitis. *CLAO J.* **15**, 64–70.

28 Tan ME, Demirci G, Pearce D, *et al.* (2002). Contact lens-induced papillary conjunctivitis is associated with increased albumin deposits on extended wear hydrogel lenses. *Adv Exp Med Biol.* **506**, 951–955.

29 Donshik PC (2003). Contact lens chemistry and giant papillary conjunctivitis. *Eye Contact Lens* **29S**, 37–39.

30 Roth HW (1991). Studies on the etiology and treatment of giant papillary conjunctivitis in contact lens wearers. *Contactologia* **13**, 55.

31 Allansmith MR, Ross RN and Greiner JV (1985). Giant papillary conjunctivitis: Diagnosis and treatment. In: *Contact Lenses*, p. 43.1–43.17, Ed. Dabezies OH (Boston: Little, Brown and Company).

32 Trocme SD and Sra KK (2002). Spectrum of ocular allergy. *Curr Opin Allergy Clin Immunol.* **2**, 423–427.

33 Hann LE, Cornell-Bell AH, Marten-Ellis C and Allansmith MR (1986). Conjunctival basophil hypersensitivity lesions in guinea pigs. Analysis of upper tarsal epithelium. *Invest Ophthalmol Vis Sci.* **27**, 1255–1260.

34 Begley CG (1992). Giant papillary conjunctivitis. In: *Complications of Contact Lens Wear*, p. 237–252, Ed. Tomlinson A (St Louis: Mosby).

35 Barishak Y, Zavaro A, Samra Z and Sompolinsky D (1984). An immunological study of papillary conjunctivitis due to contact lenses. *Curr Eye Res.* **3**, 1161–1168.

36 Buckley RJ (1987). Pathology and treatment of giant papillary conjunctivitis: II The British perspective. *Clin Ther.* **9**, 451–452.

37 Begley CG, Riggle A and Tuel JA (1990). Association of giant papillary conjunctivitis with seasonal allergies. *Optom Vis Sci.* **67**, 192–195.

38 Martin NF, Rubinfeld RS, Malley JD and Manzitti V (1992). Giant papillary conjunctivitis and meibomian gland dysfunction blepharitis. *CLAO J.* **18**, 165–169.

39 Mathers WD and Billborough M (1992). Meibomian gland function and giant papillary conjunctivitis. *Am J Ophthalmol.* **114**, 188–192.

40 Sack RA, Jones B, Antignani A, *et al.* (1987). Specificity and biological activity of the protein deposited on the hydrogel surface. Relationship of polymer structure to biofilm formation. *Invest Ophthalmol Vis Sci.* **28**, 842–849.

41 Leahy CD, Mandell RB and Lin ST (1990). Initial *in vivo* tear protein deposition on individual hydrogel contact lenses. *Optom Vis Sci.* **67**, 504–511.

42 Woods CA and Efron N (1996). Regular replacement of extended wear rigid gas permeable contact lenses. *CLAO J.* **22**, 172–178.

43 Douglas JP, Lowder CY, Lazorik R and Meisler DM (1988). Giant papillary conjunctivitis associated with rigid gas permeable contact lenses. *CLAO J.* **14**, 143–147.

44 Farkas P, Kasalow TW and Farkas B (1986). Clinical management and control of giant papillary conjunctivitis secondary to contact lens wear. *J Am Optom Assoc.* **57**, 197–202.

45 Donshik PC, Ballow M, Luistro A and Samartino L (1984). Treatment of contact lens-induced giant papillary conjunctivitis. *CLAO J.* **10**, 346–350.

46 Meisler DM, Berzins UJ, Krachmer JH and Stock EL (1982). Cromolyn treatment of giant papillary conjunctivitis. *Arch Ophthalmol.* **100**, 1608–1610.

47 Wood TS, Stewart RH and Bowman RW (1988). Suprofen treatment of contact lens-associated giant papillary conjunctivitis. *Arch Ophthalmol.* **95**, 822–826.

48 Asbell P and Howes J (1997). A double-masked, placebo-controlled evaluation of the efficacy and safety of loteprednol etabonate in the treatment of giant papillary conjunctivitis. *CLAO J.* **23**, 31–36.

49 Vaahtoranta-Lehtonen HH, Lehtonen OP, Harvima I, *et al.* (1999). Papillary hypertrophy of the upper tarsal conjunctiva during contact lens wear: A 4-month study with ethyl-6-*O*-decanoyl-glucoside. *CLAO J.* **25**, 105–108.

50 Bailey CS and Buckley RJ (1993). Nedocromil sodium in contact-lens-associated papillary conjunctivitis. *Eye* **7S**, 29–33.

51 Butts BL and Rengstorff RH (1990). Antioxidant and vitamin A drops for giant papillary conjunctivitis. *Contact Lens J.* **18**, 40–45.

PART V LIMBUS

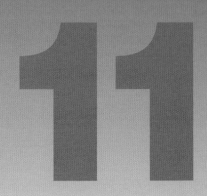

LIMBAL REDNESS

'Limbus' is the Latin word for 'border'. When the eye is viewed macroscopically from a social viewing distance of, say, 50 cm, the limbus appears as a reasonably clear circle that forms the outer limit (or 'border') of the visible iris. However, defining the exact position of the limbus is more problematic, from both a clinical and histologic perspective. When the limbus is viewed under magnification with a slit-lamp biomicroscope, the transition zone between the cornea and conjunctiva is gradual and occurs over a span of about 0.2–0.4 mm, and is generally slightly greater in the vertical meridian.[1]

From a histologic perspective, to define the location of the limbus is even more problematic, but it is defined formally as being about 1.5 mm wide.[2] This is because various histologic features that define the limbal region start and finish at different locations, and some changes are abrupt and some are gradual; a 1.5 mm zone encompasses all these features. Specifically, changes that take place in the transition from the cornea to the conjunctiva and sclera include the following:

- Abrupt termination of Bowman's layer;
- Gradual thickening of the epithelium;
- Introduction of loose connective tissue that underlies the conjunctival epithelium;
- Increasing irregularity of anterior stromal lamellae;
- Appearance of blood vessels in the stroma[1] (*Figure 11.1*).

The last of these features is the topic of this chapter, and for the purposes of a discussion of the limbal redness response to contact lens wear it is convenient to regard the limbus as the region within which the vascular network of the conjunctiva gives way to the avascularity of the cornea.[3]

Signs and Symptoms

Anatomical considerations

That the limbus displays a distinct response to contact lens wear was first recognized by Müller over a century ago.[4] Careful inspection of the superficial blood vessels at the limbus reveals the presence of 'anterior limbal loops' (*Figure 11.2*). In some patients a series of two or three layers of anterior limbal loops can be observed to build on top of each other as the limbal vascular plexus extends toward the cornea, with the vessels that constitute each successive inwardly progressing loop becoming finer and finer. The innermost series of loops are termed 'terminal arcades'.

When the limbus has been physically and/or physiologically stressed (e.g., by some types of contact lens) the limbal vessels dilate and two types of vascular features connected to the terminal arcades can be readily visualized – 'recurrent limbal vessels' and 'spike vessels'. On casual inspection with the slit-lamp biomicroscope, a recurrent limbal vessel may appear as a single vessel, with an accompanying shadow, that connects tangentially from a terminal arcade. On closer inspection, however, it can be seen that two vessels of different caliber are

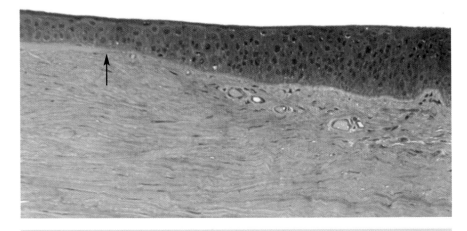

Figure 11.1
Light micrograph of a radial section through the corneoscleral transition in the vertical meridian. The cornea is to the left. The arrow marks the termination of Bowman's layer (it is visible to the left of the arrow)

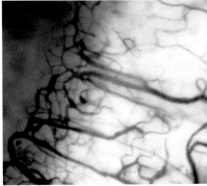

Figure 11.2
Engorged conjunctival and limbal vessels and possible slight neovascularization. The anterior limbal loops are clearly visible at the termination of the vessels in the peripheral cornea

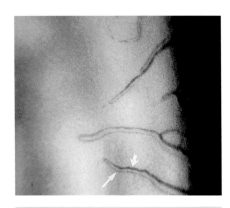

Figure 11.3

High magnification view (×100) of a thick arteriolar component (thick arrow) and thin venular component (thin arrow) of a recurrent limbal vessel

present – a thicker arteriole and a much thinner venule (the 'shadow'; *Figure 11.3*).

Vessel spikes look similar to recurrent limbal vessels, the distinction being that the vessel spike is a single arteriole that does not have a returning venule. The lumen of vessel spikes and recurrent limbal vessels can become so narrow that only clear serum (not red blood corpuscles) can pass through. This raises the question as to whether a vessel spike really represents only the visible arteriolar component of a recurrent limbal vessel, with the venular component being too narrow to allow red blood cells to pass through (and thus it remains invisible). However, electron microscopic evidence (*Figure 11.4*) has confirmed the structure of vessel spikes as single arterioles.[1]

Clinical observations

Holden *et al.*[5] measured the extent of bulbar conjunctival and limbal redness in a group of patients who had worn a conventional (low *Dk*) soft lens with high water content on an extended wear basis in one eye only (the other eye being emmetropic or amblyopic) for an average of 5 years. Bulbar conjunctival redness was graded as 0.9 (vs. 0.7 in non-lens wearing control eyes) and limbal redness was graded as 1.1 (vs. 0.3 in the non-lens wearing control eyes). From this data it can be inferred that extended wear of conventional soft lenses has a much greater impact on limbal redness than on bulbar conjunctival redness.

The time course of development of limbal redness in response to conventional hydrogel lenses and silicone hydrogel (high *Dk*) lenses during open and closed eye wear was investigated by Papas *et al.*[6] Subjects were first monitored without lenses. They then wore a conventional hydrogel lens in one eye and a silicone hydrogel lens in the other eye and were observed after 4 and 16 hours. When not wearing lenses, limbal redness changes averaged 0.2 ± 0.2 and 0.4 ± 0.2 grades at 4 and 16 hours, respectively (inferior quadrant). The corresponding values for conventional hydrogel lens wear were 1.0 ± 0.6 and 1.1 ± 0.6, while for silicone hydrogel lens wear they were 0.2 ± 0.4 and 0.5 ± 0.5 (*Figure 11.5*). Both for the eyes not wearing lenses and those wearing silicone hydrogel lenses, increases in limbal redness were significant only during eye closure. During conventional hydrogel lens wear, significant and larger limbal redness increases were seen after 4 hours of open eye wear, with only relatively small further changes being observed over the next 12 hours. Papas *et al.*[6] concluded that:

• Conventional hydrogel lens wear induces a marked increase in limbal redness during open-eye wear, which is not seen either in the no lens situation or when silicone hydrogel lenses are worn;

• The pattern of limbal redness for both the open and closed eyes during silicone hydrogel lens wear is very similar to that for the no lens situation.

A similar study to that of Papas *et al.*[6] was conducted by Dumbleton *et al.*,[7] whereby the subjects were monitored over a 9 month period rather than a few hours. On a 0 to 100 scale, extended wear of conventional hydrogel lenses resulted in a 16-point increase in limbal redness; no significant change occurred with the silicone hydrogel lenses (*Figure 11.6*). Interestingly, the difference was greatest for subjects wearing conventional hydrogel lenses who initially presented with lower levels of redness. There was a slight resolution of redness in participants who presented initially with higher levels of redness after wearing the silicone hydrogel lenses.

Covey *et al.*[8] were unable to detect any difference in the grade of limbal redness between patients wearing silicone hydrogel lenses (2.6 ± 0.3) on an extended wear basis versus patients who wore no lenses (2.4 ± 0.4) over a 9 month period.

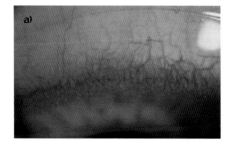

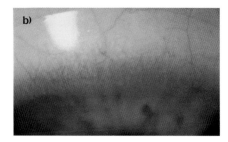

Figure 11.5

Demonstration of the effect of hypoxia on limbal redness. (a) Grade 2.2 limbal redness is evident in this patient wearing a conventional hydrogel lens [38% water content hydroxyethyl methacrylate (HEMA)] contact lens in one eye. (b) The same patient is wearing a silicone hydrogel contact lens in the other eye; the extent of limbal redness (grade 1.0) is much less than that in the eye wearing the HEMA lens

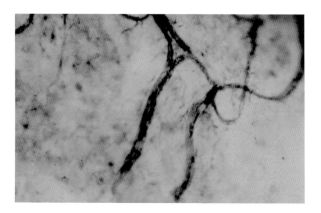

Figure 11.4

Whole-mount gold chloride preparation of anterior limbal vessels that shows two vessel spike formations

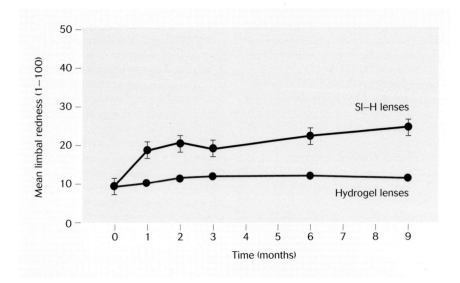

Figure 11.6
Mean change in limbal redness grade over time for silicone hydrogel (Si–H) lenses (blue line) and conventional hydrogel lenses (red line). (Approximate scale: 0, trace redness; 100, extreme redness; after Dumbleton et al.[7])

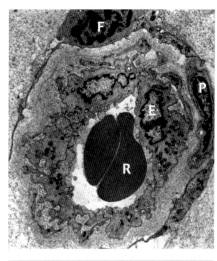

Figure 11.7
Electron micrograph of a non-fenestrated capillary from the limbal conjunctiva, close to the termination of Bowman's membrane (R, red blood cells; E, vascular endothelium; F, fibroblast; P, pericyte)

The development of limbal redness is not thought to be associated with any subjective symptoms, although patients with severe complications induced by contact lenses may coincidentally have limbal redness and suffer from discomfort or pain. None of the short-term or long-term studies referred to above[5–7] reported any symptoms relating to limbal redness during uncomplicated lens wear.

Pathology

Throughout the vascular system, blood flow is adjusted constantly to meet the needs of the local tissue. This is achieved via four basic regulatory mechanisms:
- Neural control – the caliber of vessels is controlled by balancing the input of parasympathetic and sympathetic innervation to vascular smooth muscle in the vessel wall.
- Myogenic control – vessel diameter is altered in response to changes in blood pressure within the vessel. Thus, distension of the vessel wall with increased pressure causes smooth muscle contraction. In the limbus, this mechanism dampens the tendency for increased fluid filtration to cause interstitial edema during periods of raised blood pressure.

- Metabolic control – the accumulation of waste products, such as carbon dioxide and lactic acid, surrounding the vessels causes these to dilate, which increases blood flow and removes the metabolic waste. Local hypoxia has a similar effect.
- Humoral control – agents that circulate in the blood, such as epinephrine, norepinephrine, histamine, serotonin, angiotensin, bradykinin and vasopressin.

However, because microcirculatory fields such as the limbus are devoid of direct neural control and lack smooth muscle in the vessel walls, alternative mechanisms must come into play to control blood flow. Two mechanisms are thought to be involved. First, it is believed that a system of pre-capillary sphincters – defined as the last (most peripheral) smooth muscle cell along any branch of a terminal arteriole – control blood flow into the limbal plexus in a coordinated manner. This implies that capillary flow is not continuous, but will start and stop according to local needs and conditions. Second, small cells that surround capillary vessels, known as pericytes, and vascular endothelial cells appear to have contractile properties that allow them to alter the caliber of limbal vessels.[3]

When fine terminal vessels – comprising either vessel spikes or recurrent limbal vessels – are viewed with the

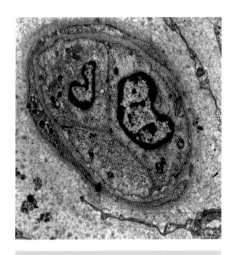

Figure 11.8
Electron micrograph of a limbal conjunctival capillary displaying a closed lumen

electron microscope, they are found to display the usual features of normal limbal capillaries.[1] They are non-fenestrated, with thick endothelial walls surrounded by pericytes (and their processes) and connective tissue cells. Although many vessels possess an open lumen able to allow the passage of formed elements of blood (*Figure 11.7*), many others are observed in which the caliber is reduced so as to prevent the passage of these elements, and in extreme cases the lumen is closed completely (*Figure 11.8*).[1] These observations highlight the dynamic growth patterns with respect to capillary opening and closure.

Etiology

A number of factors may be of etiological significance in the development of limbal redness in contact lens wear:

Hypoxia

Convincing evidence of the role of hypoxia in causing limbal redness has been provided by Papas,[9] who demonstrated a strong inverse relationship between the oxygen transmissibility of contact lenses in the region of the limbus (i.e., the lens periphery) and limbal redness; that is, the lower the local lens oxygen transmissibility, the greater the limbal redness. Since other properties of the lens may have contributed to the limbal redness response, such as lens-induced hypercapnia (carbon dioxide build-up) and lens stiffness, Papas[10] conducted a supplementary experiment in which the eyes of subjects were exposed to atmospheric anoxia in a gas goggle (i.e., no lens wear). These eyes displayed significantly greater levels of limbal redness, which provides evidence that reducing the oxygen concentration at the ocular surface induces more blood flow in limbal vessels.

The precise mechanism by which hypoxia causes increased redness is still unclear; however, Papas[10] has proposed the following sequence of events. Hypoxia may exert an effect on the vascular endothelium that causes the release of nitrous oxide or prostacyclin. These local mediators diffuse toward the smooth muscle cells that comprise the adjacent pre-capillary sphincters, which are induced to relax, resulting in increased blood flow to the hypoxic region. Direct influence of hypoxia on the vascular pericytes, as described above, is another possibility.

Infection

Infection of the cornea leads to a cascade of inflammatory events that induces limbal redness. Increased perfusion of the capillary vessels in the limbus is mediated by the release of vasodilating agents, such as nitrous oxide, histamine and various prostaglandins. This increased blood flow allows immune system cells, such as polymorphonuclear leukocytes (PMNs), to rapidly approach the site of the infection. Chemical mediators, such as cytokines, are involved in the mediation of this process; the cytokines stimulate the release of adhesion molecules, which act to hold the PMNs at the site of the injury for maximum effect. Extravasation occurs, whereby the distended limbal vessel walls increase in permeability and cells and fluid pass out of the vessel into the surrounding tissue. This can sometimes be observed clinically as a milky haze that surrounds engorged limbal vessels[10] (*Figure 11.9*).

Inflammation

An increase in the inflammatory cell population in the conjunctival sac occurs overnight,[11] which may explain why our eyes sometimes appear a little red upon awakening. It is also recognized that contact lenses can alter the concentrations of inflammatory mediators in the tear film.[12] These mild inflammatory effects, taken together, may explain why patients who wear contact lenses on an extended wear basis are more prone to conditions such as contact lens acute red eye (CLARE). That is, the mild inflammatory situation present with closed eye lens wear may predispose the eye to develop more overt inflammatory episodes.

Trauma

Soft contact lenses rest in direct apposition to the limbus. This constant physical presence may cause the direct release of inflammatory mediators and result in increased limbal redness. Clinical observations of local limbal redness in the proximity of a traumatic source, such as a damaged lens edge, supports the notion of direct trauma being of etiological sig-

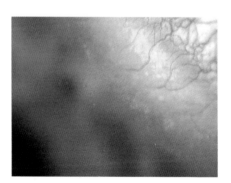

Figure 11.9
Recurrent limbal vessel surrounded by extravascular fluid, seen here as a mottled milky haze

nificance in limbal redness (see *Figure 13.7*). However, the possibility of more subtle physical influences on limbal redness, such as variations in soft lens modulus (stiffness), has been discounted by Dumbleton et al.[7]. As discussed previously, these authors observed that silicone hydrogel lenses cause less limbal redness than conventional soft lenses do, the latter having much lower oxygen transmissibility (which should reduce redness) and lower modulus (which should theoretically tend to increase redness). They concluded that the effects of lens oxygen performance far outweigh the effects of lens modulus on limbal redness.[7]

Solution toxicity or hypersensitivity

The preservatives present in various contact lens care solutions may affect limbal redness. The more noxious forms of preservatives used in early generation systems, such as thimerosal and chlorhexidine, were clearly associated with increased levels of eye redness.[13] However, Soni et al.[14] reported different levels of limbal redness in response to three different 'new generation' lens care systems over an 18 month period; this was likely to be more of a delayed hypersensitivity type of response. The preservatives may act directly as a stimulus on either the pre-capillary sphincters or the vessel walls, causing vessel distension (and limbal redness) to facilitate either an immediate toxic or immediate hypersensitivity reaction, or a more long-term immune response.

Management

As ought to be clear from the above list, the management strategy for the removal or alleviation of limbal redness involves the elimination or modification of the causative agent. This raises two questions:
- What is the acceptable threshold level of limbal redness?
- What is the causative agent in a given patient?

Increased limbal redness in itself is harmless in the immediate sense and does not cause any discomfort for the lens wearer; however, it is an important sign of ocular distress and an indicator that action needs to be taken. The severity of limbal redness can be determined with reference to the grading scales for this tissue change provided in Appendix A.

A level of limbal redness greater than about grade 1.5 should arouse suspicion, although limbal redness up to grade 2.5 may be acceptable in a patient wearing moderate-to-high minus powered hydrogel lenses, as long as the patient is monitored carefully. Fonn et al.[15] plotted the frequency of eyes wearing silicone hydrogel lenses with limbal redness greater than grade 2, which implies that they considered this to be the approximate threshold for clinical significance. It is likely that increased limbal redness, if allowed to persist, is a precursor for corneal neovascularization.

A useful framework for the adoption of possible management strategies to eliminate or alleviate limbal redness is to consider whether the case is (a) acute or chronic, and (b) local or circumlimbal. An example of a possible cause and management strategy with respect to these various scenarios is:

- Acute local limbal redness – keratitis in a region of the cornea near to the local redness. Aggressive anti-infectious and anti-inflammatory treatment may be indicated (management of such conditions is dealt with in Chapter 14).
- Chronic local limbal redness – defect in the edge of a rigid lens designed for constant orientation (e.g., truncated design). Replace the damaged lens.
- Acute circumlimbal redness – contact lens solution immediate hypersensitivity or toxicity reaction. Change lens solutions and change contact lens. A daily disposable lens solves this problem.
- Chronic circumlimbal redness – the result of hypoxia induced by a contact lens. For example, *Figure 11.10* shows grade 4 circumlimbal redness caused by long-term use of a low permeability soft lens used on an extended wear basis.

Prognosis

The prognosis for recovery from chronic limbal redness induced by contact lenses after removal of the lenses and cessation of wear is good. Holden et al.[16] found that, after approximately 5 years of extended lens wear, general conjunctival redness resolved within 2 days and limbal redness had a slightly longer time course, taking about 7 days to resolve fully (*Figure 11.11*).

du Toit et al.[17] measured the limbal vascular response after 8 hours of eye closure while wearing silicone hydrogel and conventional hydrogel lenses compared to control eyes without lenses. They found that, on waking and after lens removal, there were no differences in hyperemia between the eyes wearing silicone hydrogel and conventional hydrogel lenses. However, the reduction in redness over time of the eyes wearing silicone hydrogel lenses was more rapid compared with that for the eyes wearing the conventional hydrogel lens. du Toit et al.[17] suggested that the faster recovery from redness in the eyes wearing the silicone hydrogel lenses may result from the increased oxygen transmissibility of these lenses.

Differential Diagnosis

A primary consideration in differential diagnosis of limbal redness is to determine whether simple increased vascular engorgement or neovascularization is being observed. In the case of increased limbal redness, more blood is flowing through vessels that have become thicker, but the limbal vascular plexus has not become more extensive and/or the vessels have not become longer. Neovascularization implies vessel growth into the normal avascular cornea (see Chapter 21). Although the level of vascular encroachment into a normal cornea is about 0.2 mm in a non-lens wearer, uncomplicated contact lens wear can induce low levels of vascular encroachment that may still be considered 'normal' within certain limits. The only real way to determine if active neovascularization is beginning to occur is to monitor the limbal vasculature carefully over time and measure the degree of vessel penetration into the cornea.

An early sign of contact lens-induced superior limbal keratoconjunctivitis (CL-SLK) or Theodore's SLK (the latter being a condition unrelated to contact lens wear; see Chapter 13 for a discussion of both these conditions) is increased redness of the superior limbus. Thus, detection of increased limbal redness superiorly should raise suspicion that the patient could be suffering from one of these conditions. The observation of associated signs and symptoms of irritation suggest early CL-SLK or Theodore's SLK.

Some patients display prominent palisades of Vogt, which on first inspection give the appearance of a prominent plexus of limbal vessels. Palisades of Vogt consist of an array of connective tissue ridges that commence in the peripheral corneal epithelium and extend into the limbus as spoke-like radiations arranged at right angles to the peripheral cornea[2] (*Figure 11.12*). They measure about 0.5 mm wide and vary in length between individuals, ranging from 2 to 4 mm. Palisades of Vogt are more prominent at the inferior limbus

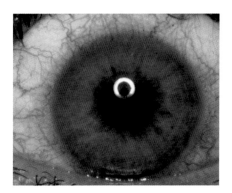

Figure 11.10
Severe circumlimbal redness (grade 4)

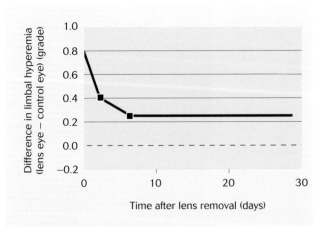

Figure 11.11
Time course of resolution of limbal redness after 5 years extended wear of a hydrogel lens with high water content in one eye only, relative to a control eye not wearing a lens (after Holden et al.[16])

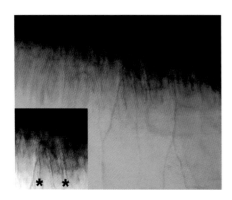

Figure 11.12

High-power slit-lamp view of the palisades of Vogt at the lower limbus. Inset: asterisks highlight two palisades

and in darker races they are more heavily pigmented and thus easier to see. Limbal vessels have a similar appearance, and typically run in parallel to the palisades of Vogt. On careful slit-lamp examination, differential diagnosis between the dark brown palisades of Vogt and red limbal vessels should be clear.

REFERENCES

1 Lawrenson JG, Doshi S and Ruskell GL (1991). Slit-lamp and histological observations of the normal limbal vasculature and their significance for contact lens wear. *J Br Contact Lens Assoc.* **14**, 169–172.

2 Hogan MJ, Alvarado JA and Weddell JE (1971). The limbus. In: *Histology of the Human Eye*, p. 112–182. (Philadelphia: WB Saunders).

3 Papas EB (2003). The limbal vasculature. *Contact Lens Anterior Eye* **26**, 71–76.

4 Pearson RM and Efron N (1989). Hundredth anniversary of August Müller's inaugural dissertation on contact lenses. *Surv Ophthalmol.* **34**, 133–141.

5 Holden BA, Sweeney DF, Vannas A, *et al.* (1985). Effects of long-term extended contact lens wear on the human cornea. *Invest Ophthalmol Vis Sci.* **26**, 1489–1501.

6 Papas EB, Vajdic CM, Austen R and Holden BA (1997). High-oxygen-transmissibility soft contact lenses do not induce limbal hyperaemia. *Curr Eye Res.* **16**, 942–948.

7 Dumbleton KA, Chalmers RL, Richter DB and Fonn D (2001). Vascular response to extended wear of hydrogel lenses with high and low oxygen permeability. *Optom Vis Sci.* **78**, 147–151.

8 Covey M, Sweeney DF, Terry R, *et al.* (2001). Hypoxic effects on the anterior eye of high-*Dk* soft contact lens wearers are negligible. *Optom Vis Sci.* **78**, 95–99.

9 Papas E (1998). On the relationship between soft contact lens oxygen transmissibility and induced limbal hyperaemia. *Exp Eye Res.* **67**, 125–131.

10 Papas EB (2003). The role of hypoxia in the limbal vascular response to soft contact lens wear. *Eye Contact Lens* **29S**, 72–74.

11 Sack RA, Beaton A, Sathe S, *et al.* (2000). Towards a closed eye model of the pre-ocular tear layer. *Prog Retin Eye Res.* **19**, 649–668.

12 Thakur A and Willcox MD (2000). Contact lens wear alters the production of certain inflammatory mediators in tears. *Exp Eye Res.* **70**, 255–259.

13 McMonnies CW and Chapman-Davies A (1987). Assessment of conjunctival hyperemia in contact lens wearers. Part II. *Am J Optom Physiol Opt.* **64**, 251–255.

14 Soni PS, Horner DG and Ross J (1996). Ocular response to lens care systems in adolescent soft contact lens wearers. *Optom Vis Sci.* **73**, 70–85.

15 Fonn D, MacDonald KE, Richter D and Pritchard N (2002). The ocular response to extended wear of a high *Dk* silicone hydrogel contact lens. *Clin Exp Optom.* **85**, 176–182.

16 Holden BA, Sweeney DF, Swarbrick HA, *et al.* (1986). The vascular response to long-term extended contact lens wear. *Clin Exp Optom.* **69**, 112–119.

17 du Toit R, Simpson TL, Fonn D and Chalmers RL (2001). Recovery from hyperemia after overnight wear of low and high transmissibility hydrogel lenses. *Curr Eye Res.* **22**, 68–73.

VASCULARIZED LIMBAL KERATITIS

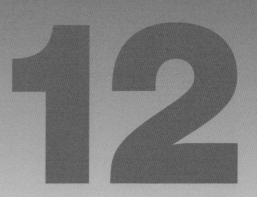

The limbus is prone to pathologic changes for a variety of reasons. Embedded in the limbus is a rich capillary plexus, vessels that may become engorged (see Chapter 11) or could constitute the platform from which vessels may penetrate into the cornea (see Chapter 21). The limbus is the site of the corneal stem cells, which are the primary source for the differentiation and proliferation of the corneal epithelium. A deficiency in limbal stem cells may lead to a plethora of corneal complications.[1] A sharp transition in the topography of the anterior eye occurs at the limbus, whereby there is a pronounced flattening from the corneal surface to the conjunctival surface, to form a physical 'ridge'.[2] These three limbal features – the capillary plexus, stem cells and the limbal ridge – render the limbus susceptible to metabolic, immunologic, toxic and physical insult, and all of these challenges may be induced or exacerbated by contact lenses.

It has long been recognized that the integrity of the limbus is more likely to be compromised by soft lenses because they rest in physical proximity to that tissue.[3] The limbus is less likely to be insulted by rigid lenses, which are invariably smaller than the corneal diameter and only intermittently impinge upon the limbus. Vascularized limbal keratitis (VLK) is an unusual complication of rigid contact lens wear that, as the name suggests, is characterized in its most severe manifestation as an inflammation of the limbus in association with a process of vascularization.[4]

The condition is usually associated with extended rigid lens wear, and has been demonstrated to occur with both low oxygen-permeable lenses[4] and super-permeable rigid lenses[5] – in the latter case with an incidence of only 0.8% of patients per year. VLK has also been observed in patients wearing rigid lenses on a daily wear basis. It is always observed at the 3 and 9 o'clock corneal locations.

Signs and Symptoms

According to Grohe and Lebow,[4] VLK can be characterized as a condition that develops in four grades, which represent stages of increasing severity; these grades are outlined below. This condition typically develops over a period of up to 6 months, but the time course can be more protracted, taking up to 24 months for the condition to become severe.

Grade 1

The patient is asymptomatic. The epithelium adjacent to the limbus appears disrupted, as evidenced by superficial punctate staining. An apparent 'heaping' or accumulation of hyperplastic corneal and/or limbal epithelial tissue can be observed. This appears as an elevated, opaque or whitish elevated mass at the 3 and 9 o'clock corneal location, with a diffuse, ill-defined border. The mass typically appears to bridge from the conjunctiva over the limbus and on to the cornea, although it can form almost exclusively on the cornea or the conjunctiva, but always immediately adjacent to the limbus. The tear film meniscus at the edge of the rigid lens is absent or disrupted (*Figure 12.1*).

Grade 2

The patient typically complains of mild ocular discomfort and increased lens awareness, and may be aware that his or her eyes are red. Corneal infiltrates may be present, as well as mild overlying staining (grade 2) and mild conjunctival redness (grade 2; *Figure 12.2*).

Grade 3

The patient complains of mild-to-moderate discomfort, and may report reduced lens-wearing time. Moderate conjunctival redness (grade 3), more extensive corneal epithelial staining and mild limbal and conjunctival staining are observed. There may also be a greater

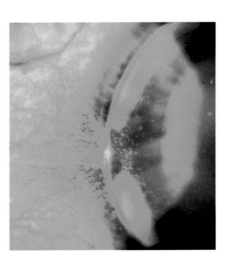

Figure 12.1
Grade 1 VLK viewed in cobalt blue light with fluorescein instilled

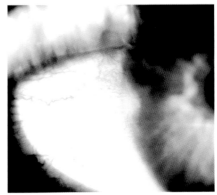

Figure 12.2
Grade 2 VLK

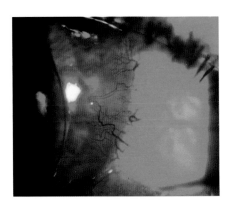

Figure 12.3
Grade 3 VLK viewed in red-free (green) light

infiltrative response. The conjunctiva and limbus may appear to be slightly edematous. A vascular leash, which emanates from the conjunctiva and travels across the limbus, encroaches upon the hyperplastic epithelial mass (*Figure 12.3*).

Grade 4

Patients report considerable discomfort and photophobia. Pain is experienced when the lens edge impinges upon the affected region, and so makes lens wear almost intolerable. Significant conjunctival redness and staining are apparent, often associated with an erosion of the elevated hyperplastic epithelial mass. Superficial and deep vascularization may be present. The patient is aware of the hyperplastic epithelial mass and may refer to this as a 'lump' on the eye (*Figure 12.4*).

Pathology

The precise pathologic changes that are occurring at a cellular level are unknown because studies to this effect have not been reported in the literature. However, it can be deduced from the clinical observations outlined above that there is a syndrome of concurrent tissue pathologies, including epithelial cell hyperplasia (*Figure 12.5*), vessel engorgement and progression, tissue erosion, tissue edema and corneal infiltrates.

Etiology

The etiology of VLK is unknown, but Grohe and Lebow[4] hypothesize that this condition is caused by an interruption to the normal tear-film dynamics at the limbus induced by rigid lenses of inappropriate design. Specifically, they propose that design faults, such as a low lens-edge lift, create abnormal fluid dynamics at the edge of the lens. This could, in turn, compromise the normally full tear meniscus at the lens edge, to produce a desiccation effect and consequent interruption to surface wetting in the region of the limbus. Constant ongoing physical irritation of the poorly lubricated ocular surface by a combination of the eyelids and lens induces a low-grade inflammatory reaction which, if left unchecked, progresses through the various grades of VLK as described above. In a case report, Miller[6] found that VLK was caused by surface crazing on a rigid lens

The theory of the cause of VLK outlined above, and the clinical description

of this condition, strongly suggests that VLK represents a severe clinical sequel of 3 and 9 o'clock staining, albeit uncommon. Indeed, Grohe and Lebow[4] admit that five of the eight VLK patients they described had previously been fitted because of unacceptable peripheral 3 and 9 o'clock corneal staining with rigid lenses, and the patient described by Miller[6] also had a previous case history of 3 and 9 o'clock corneal staining. If this is the case, considerable clinical significance ought to be attached to the early detection and management of 3 and 9 o'clock staining in wearers of rigid contact lenses.

Management

Management of VLK can be outlined with respect to the four grades of severity of the condition.[4]

Grade 1

Instruct the patient to change from extended wear to daily lens wear. If already in daily wear, wearing time should be reduced from all-day wear to 6–8 hours per day. The lens should be redesigned such that the peripheral curve configuration is flattened to create more edge lift and improve the fluid dynamics at the lens edge. Lubricating drops used throughout the day may provide symptomatic relief and help to improve the lens dynamics.

Grade 2

Lens wear should be discontinued for 5 days, and ocular decongestants may be prescribed to alleviate eye redness. The lens should be redesigned as per grade 1, as well as possibly reducing the lens diameter and/or flattening the lens base curve. Efforts should be made to eliminate mechanical bearing at the peripheral cornea. Daily lens wear can be recommended initially, and if the eye remains quiet after a time, extended wear may be resumed.

Grade 3

Lens wear should be discontinued for 5 days, and tissue scrapings should be taken and sent for analysis to differentiate from possible infectious causes (see Differential Diagnosis). Topical corticosteroids may be required if the infiltrative response is severe. The lens should be redesigned utilizing the principles outlined as per grade 2 above. Daily lens

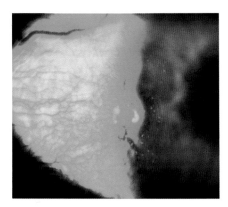

Figure 12.4
Grade 4 VLK viewed in cobalt blue light with fluorescein instilled

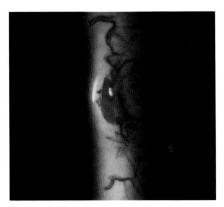

Figure 12.5
Vascularized epithelial mass in VLK

wear can be recommenced initially, but extended wear should only be resumed if there has been a full recovery and there is a pressing need.

Grade 4

Lens wear should be discontinued for 3 weeks. Tissue scrapings should be taken and the eye should be treated with an antibiotic–corticosteroid combination. Topical corticosteroids may be required if the infiltrative response is severe. The lens should be redesigned utilizing the principles outlined as per grade 2 above. Daily lens wear can be recommended initially, but future extended wear is generally contraindicated.

Miller[6] was able to manage a case of VLK by prescribing a new set of lenses of a different material to replace lenses that had suffered surface crazing. The parameters of the replaced lenses were not altered. Thus, changing lens material is a possible alternative strategy to altering the lens parameters in the management of VLK.

Prognosis

If a patient recommences lens wear prematurely after it had been suspended because of VLK, a 'rebound' phenomenon may occur whereby the condition flares up once again and rapidly progresses to the equivalent level of severity at the time of cessation. This situation typically occurs when the patient recommences wearing the original offending lens (i.e., the lens design has remained unaltered). This phenomenon strongly suggests a lens design etiology.

The prognosis for recovery from VLK is generally very good; even severe cases can recover within days[4] or a few weeks.[6] As an illustration of the rapid time course for resolution of this condition, consider the following case. A patient presented 3 months after being fitted with 9.2 mm diameter fluorosilicone acrylate rigid lenses for extended wear; these lenses were worn continuously for up to 7 days at a time. She was assessed as having grade 3 VLK. Objective findings included a raised limbal epithelial mass with fluorescein staining and a prominent vascular leash. The lens edge can be seen impinging against the raised mass in *Figure 12.6*. With the aid of fluorescein, the tear film meniscus at the lens edge can be seen to thin out and vir-

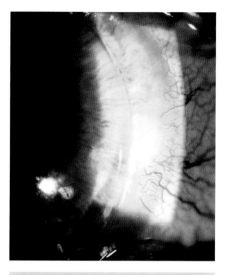

Figure 12.6
Grade 3 VLK in a patient wearing a 9.2 mm diameter rigid lens

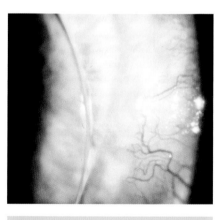

Figure 12.8
Same eye as in *Figure 12.6*, but the patient has been refitted with an 8.0 mm diameter rigid lens, which is no longer impinging upon the raised epithelial mass

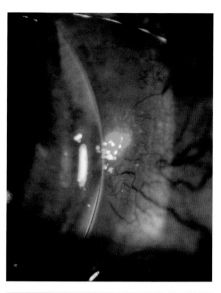

Figure 12.7
Same eye as in *Figure 12.6* after instillation of fluorescein and viewed with a cobalt blue light. The tear film meniscus at the lens edge is virtually absent at the point of contact between the raised epithelial mass and the lens

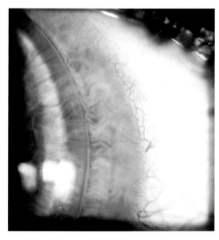

Figure 12.9
Same eye as in *Figure 12.6*, but the wearing schedule was restricted to a maximum of 3 days of extended wear at a time, followed by a cessation of lens wear for 5 days. The raised mass has almost completely resolved

tually disappear in the proximity of the raised mass (*Figure 12.7*).

The lens diameter was subsequently reduced to 8.0 mm; as can be seen in *Figure 12.8*, the lens no longer impinges on the epithelial mass. Comparing *Figure 12.8* with *Figure 12.6*, it can be seen that this strategy resulted in a slight reduction in the size of the epithelial mass, and the vascularization subsided. In a further attempt to resolve the condition, the wearing schedule was restricted to a maximum of 3 days of extended wear at a time; this resulted in a further resolution, but not elimination, of the raised mass and vascular leash. Lens

wear was then ceased for 5 days, which almost completely resolved the raised mass (*Figure 12.9*) and vascular leash (*Figure 12.10*). The patient was subsequently able to resume extended wear for 2 days at a time, and the VLK did not recur.

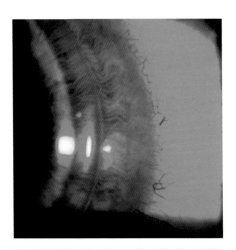

Figure 12.10
Same eye and lens as in *Figure 12.6* viewed with a red-free (green) light, which confirms the absence of vascular leashing

Differential Diagnosis

The key conditions that need to be differentially diagnosed from VLK are phlyctenulosis, peripheral corneal ulceration, pterygium, pseudopterygium and pinguecula.

Phlyctenulosis is an inflammatory disorder that involves the conjunctiva, limbus and/or cornea.[7] It is usually bilateral and primarily affects young children and young adults. Phlyctenules are pinkish white nodules that vary in size from pinpoint to several millimeters. They may be solitary or multiple. The limbus is generally affected first, but there may be isolated involvement of the bulbar conjunctiva or cornea. The condition is generally self-limiting, whereby the phlyctenule progressively becomes grayish, ulcerates and heals completely within 10–15 days to leave residual scarring and vascularization. Symptoms include a foreign body sensation and the reporting of eye redness. The patient reports severe photophobia if the cornea is affected. The pathogenesis of this condition is believed to be a local immunologic reaction of the ocular surface to bacteria-elaborated antigens; the most commonly associated microbial agent is *Staphylococcus aureus*. The condition may be associated with blepharitis. Differential diagnosis between VLK and phlyctenulosis is effected by culturing the eyelid margins and conjunctiva; a positive culture for *Staphylococcus*, and the presence of residual pathology after the active phase of the condition has

resolved, should heighten suspicion of phlyctenulosis. Also, phlyctenules can present at any location around the limbus, whereas VLK only presents at the 3 and 9 o'clock positions.

Peripheral corneal ulcers are considered in detail in Chapters 22 and 23. A microbial peripheral ulcer is extremely painful, and a sterile peripheral ulcer is asymptomatic; the discomfort that results from VLK probably falls equally between the two. The term 'ulcer' implies an erosion of tissue, which is the opposite of the raised tissue mass seen in VLK. However, in the active stages of a microbial peripheral ulcer, the edges of the ulcer may be uneven and slightly raised at certain points, which makes differential diagnosis difficult. As is the case with phlyctenulosis, peripheral corneal ulcers can present at any location around the limbus, whereas VLK only presents at the 3 and 9 o'clock positions. Vascularization of peripheral ulcers usually occurs only when the condition is advanced.

A pterygium is a triangular growth of fibrovascular tissue into the cornea (*Figure 12.11*). It can be differentiated from VLK because of its chronic time course (thought to result from chronic exposure to ultraviolet light), classic triangular shape and extensive corneal encroachment in its late stage. Also, pterygium is asymptomatic. A pseudopterygium is a conjunctival adherence to the cornea caused by limbal or corneal inflammation or trauma. It may have an atypical shape or position that gives a similar appearance to VLK. Differential diagnosis between pseudopterygium and VLK can be effected by determining whether a probe can be passed behind the lesion; this is likely to occur in the case of pseudopterygium because of its lack of adherence to the limbus.[7]

Pinguecula is a horizontal, triangular or oval, elevated milky yellow area of bulbar conjunctival thickening in the palpebral fissure adjacent to the limbus.[7] It may encroach the limbus, but when the cornea is involved it becomes a pterygium. The etiology of pinguecula is uncertain, but may be the same as that for pterygium. A pinguecula that lies close to the limbus can give the appearance of VLK, but these conditions can be differentiated because the raised tissue mass of the pinguecula, by definition, does not fully encroach onto the limbus. The difficulty in differentially diagnosing pinguecula from VLK is illustrated by comparing the pinguec-

ula in *Figure 12.12* with the VLK in *Figure 12.13*. Certain features, such as the yellow color and extensive vascularity of the tissue mass, are almost identical. However, differential diagnosis can be made by noting that the base of the pinguecula is separated by about 1 mm from the limbus, whereas the raised mass in the VLK – although located primarily on the conjunctiva – clearly impinges upon the limbus.

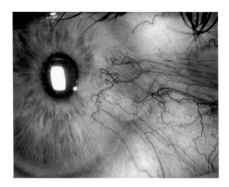

Figure 12.11
Pterygium

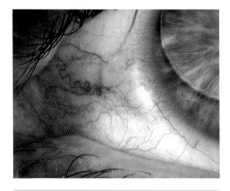

Figure 12.12
Pinguecula, with the raised epithelial mass separated from the limbus by about 1 mm

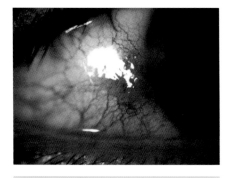

Figure 12.13
VLK, with the raised epithelial mass impinging upon the limbus

REFERENCES

1 Dua HS, Saini JS, Azuara-Blanco A and Gupta P (2000). Limbal stem cell deficiency: Concept, aetiology, clinical presentation, diagnosis and management. *Indian J Ophthalmol.* **48**, 83–92.

2 Wichterle K, Vodnansky J and Wichterle O (1991). Shape of the cornea and conjunctiva. *Optom Vis Sci.* **68**, 232–235.

3 Harrer S and Rubey F (1982). Limbal and perilimbal changes in wearers of HEMA lenses. *Klin Monatsbl Augenheilkd.* **181**, 341–343.

4 Grohe RM and Lebow KA (1989). Vascularized limbal keratitis. *Int Contact Lens Clin.* **16**, 197–209.

5 Gleason W, Tanaka H, Albright RA and Cavanagh HD (2003). A 1-year prospective clinical trial of menicon Z (tisilfocon A) rigid gas-permeable contact lenses worn on a 30-day continuous wear schedule. *Eye Contact Lens* **29**, 2–9.

6 Miller WL (1995). Rigid gas permeable surface defects associated with an isolated case of vascularized limbal keratitis. *Int Contact Lens Clin.* **22**, 209–212.

7 Kaufman HE, Barron BA and McDonald MB (1998). *The Cornea*, Second Edition. (Boston: Butterworth–Heinemann).

SUPERIOR LIMBIC KERATO-CONJUNCTIVITIS

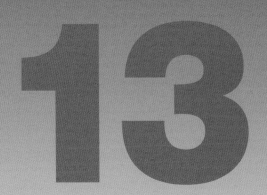

Contact lens induced superior limbic keratoconjunctivitis (CLSLK) is a syndrome that comprises a combination of tissue pathologies. Tissues affected include the corneal epithelium and stroma, the limbus and the bulbar and tarsal conjunctiva. Although this condition was first described fully in the literature in the early 1980s,[1–11] a similar syndrome unrelated to contact lens wear, known as Theodore's superior limbic keratoconjunctivitis (or 'Theodore's SLK'), had been described about 20 years prior to this.[12]

The strong association between the development of CLSLK and the use of contact lens care solutions that contain thimerosal means this condition has also been called 'thimerosal keratoconjunctivitis'[1] or 'thimerosal keratopathy'.[13]

In its mild form, CLSLK is easy to overlook (*Figure 13.1*). The condition is confined to the superior limbal area and as such is hidden by the upper lid in primary gaze. The correct procedure to observe this condition is to lift the upper lid while the patient gazes down. Such an examination technique should be part of the routine procedure during every contact lens aftercare examination.

Prevalence

Although the prevalence of CLSLK in the general population is not known, the prevalence of this condition among symptomatic contact lens wearers has been investigated. Wilson-Holt and Dart[1] reported the results of a retrospective evaluation of the record cards of 312 patients with complications related to contact lenses who presented consecutively to an eye clinic. They found that 42 patients (13.5%) presented with a typical CLSLK and 13 (4.1%) presented with an atypical CLSLK. Thus, a total of 55 patients (17.6%) were afflicted with this condition.

Stapleton *et al.*[14] found that, of 1104 patients with disorders related to contact lenses who presented to an eye clinic, only five (0.5%) displayed a classic CLSLK; however, 67 patients (6%) displayed what was described as 'thimerosal keratopathy/conjunctivitis'. The description given by these authors[14] of the pathologic changes at the superior limbus that characterized this latter condition indicated that they were observing an atypical form of CLSLK. Thus, combining these figures gives a prevalence of CLSLK-associated disease among symptomatic contact lens wearers of about 6.5%.

Thimerosal was commonly used as a preservative in contact lens solutions up until the mid-1980s; its use declined thereafter as a result of practitioners and industry taking note of the increasing number of reports that linked thimerosal to CLSLK. This may explain why the prevalence of this condition declined from 17.6%[1] to 6.5%[14] between 1989 and 1992. It is likely that the prevalence of CLSLK in the UK has reduced even further, since the introduction in 1994 of solutions that do not contain preservatives that could be toxic or allergenic to the cornea, such as thimerosal. Instead, these solutions contain safe chlorhexidine-based preservatives, such as Dymed and Polyquad; such products, together with disinfecting systems based on hydrogen peroxide, now dominate the market.[15] It appears that all contact lens manufacturers in the UK have ceased using noxious preservatives, such as thimerosal, in contact lens care products.[16] The prevalence of CLSLK in patients using modern disinfection systems devoid of thimerosal is thought to be very low.

Signs and Symptoms

Symptoms of CLSLK include increased lens awareness, lens intolerance, foreign body sensation, burning, itching, photophobia, redness and increased lacrimation. Although an occasional slight mucus secretion might be observed, there is no heavy discharge such as that seen in bacterial conjunctivitis. Some loss of vision (by three or more lines of Snellen acuity[1,3]) has been reported in advanced cases, such as with extensive pannus formation.

A myriad of signs is observed in patients with CLSLK, which include:

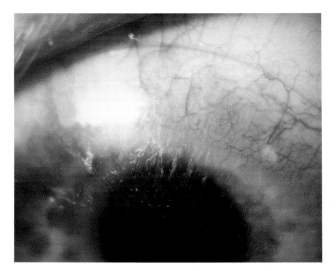

Figure 13.1
CLSLK in a patient wearing soft lenses (grade 2)

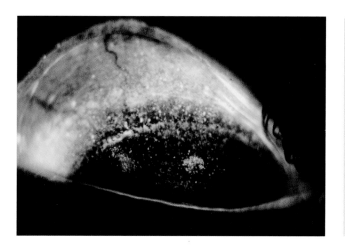

Figure 13.2
Corneal, limbal and conjunctival fluorescein staining in CLSLK in a patient wearing hydrogel bifocal contact lenses (grade 3)

- Punctate epithelial fluorescein staining (*Figure 13.2*) – typically in the upper third to half of the cornea, which can be coarse in some patients, and sometimes is in a swirled pattern;[2]
- Epithelial rose bengal staining of the superior cornea;
- Intraepithelial opacities;
- Subepithelial haze in the superior cornea – extending in a V-shaped pattern toward the pupil;
- Epithelial dulling of the superior cornea;
- Epithelial microcysts of the superior cornea;
- Epithelial infiltrates in the superior cornea (*Figure 13.3*);
- Epithelial irregularity of the superior cornea;
- Stromal opacification;

- Fibrovascular micropannus – a plexus of vessels that advance from the superior cornea in the form of a V-shape, with the apex toward the pupil and an even, linear leading edge parallel with the upper lid margin (see *Figures 13.1* and *13.4*);
- Fine subepithelial linear opacities at the periphery of the superior cornea – aligned with the general direction of blood vessels in the pannus;
- Superior limbal edema;
- Superior limbal hypertrophy;
- Superior limbal fluorescein staining;
- Superior limbal vascular injection;
- Poor wetting of the superior bulbar conjunctiva;
- Superior bulbar conjunctival punctate staining;
- Superior bulbar conjunctival redness;
- Superior bulbar conjunctival chemosis – described as a 'boggy apron' of bulbar conjunctiva that forms redundant folds over the superior limbus;[3]

- Irregular thickening of the superior bulbar conjunctiva;
- Papillary hypertrophy of the upper tarsal conjunctiva – in 25% of cases;[3]
- Follicular hypertrophy of the upper tarsal conjunctiva;
- Redness of the upper tarsal conjunctiva;
- Scattered petechiae on the upper tarsal conjunctiva;
- Corneal filaments – said to be present in 13% of patients who suffer from CLSLK;[3]
- Corneal warpage;
- Corneal astigmatism;
- Pseudodendrites – bilateral dendritic corneal lesions that lack the terminal bulbs characteristic of herpetic disease.

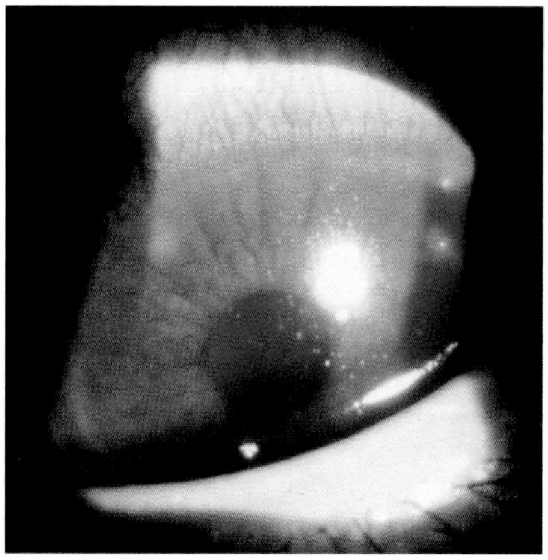

CLSLK is almost always bilateral and the specific signs often display symmetry between the eyes. There is considerable variability in the time course of onset of the condition; signs usually become manifest between 2 months and 2 years of commencement of lens wear.[3,5] The approximate sequence of manifestation of signs of increasing severity is shown in the grading scales in Appendix A.

It is interesting to compare the clinical presentation of CLSLK with that of Theodore's SLK, which also occurs in eyes not wearing contact lenses. *Table 13.1* summarizes the similarities and differences between the two conditions.

There have been a few reports of CLSLK in patients wearing rigid contact lenses. Wilson-Holt and Dart[1] reported two cases in which the patients were using a wetting solution containing thimerosal. One patient had previously worn soft lenses. Both patients suffered from lens intolerance and red eyes, although the overall signs and symptoms were less severe compared with those observed in patients wearing soft lenses.

Pathology

Sendele *et al.*[3] used light microscopy to examine biopsy material from the superior bulbar conjunctiva of five patients who suffered from CLSLK and five normal control subjects. The following observations were made of the affected specimens:
- Epithelial keratinization (two patients);
- Intracellular epithelial edema (three patients);
- Acanthosis (three patients);
- Pseudo-epitheliomatous hyperplasia (three patients);

Figure 13.3
CLSLK in a soft lens patient who displays superior limbal redness, focal infiltrates and increased lacrimation. The hazy corneal reflex indicates an uneven epithelium (grade 1.5)

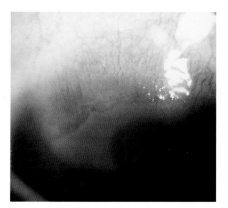

Figure 13.4
Fibrovascular pannus in CLSLK stained with rose bengal (grade 1.5)

- Acute inflammatory cells in the epithelium (three patients);
- Acute inflammatory cells in the stroma (three patients);
- Plasma cells in stroma, which indicates chronic inflammation (five patients);
- Mononuclear cells in stroma, which indicates chronic inflammation (five patients);

- Absence of goblet cells (four patients). Transmission electron microscopy of the same tissue samples confirmed light microscopic observations and revealed the following additional pathologic changes:
- Flattening of surface microvilli;
- Accumulation of intracytoplasmic keratin filaments;
- Condensed cytoplasm;

- Fibrillogranular inclusions (probably lipoproteinaceous);
- Epithelial infiltration of polymorphonuclear leukocytes

Sendele *et al.*[3] pointed out that, although their findings provided evidence of acute and chronic inflammation typical of Theodore's SLK, they did not observe marked epithelial keratinization, nuclear degeneration or glycogen accumulation – which have been reported by other researchers to be representative of Theodore's SLK. However, Stenson[5] observed pre-keratinized epithelial cells as well as a neutrophilic response in conjunctival and corneal scrapings of CLSLK patients.

Figure 13.5 highlights the differences between the normal bulbar conjunctiva and the bulbar conjunctiva of a patient who suffers from CLSLK.

Etiology

The primary etiological factor in the development of CLSLK is thimerosal hypersensitivity. Provocative tests in thimerosal-sensitized patients result in general conjunctival redness[1,3] (not confined to the superior limbus only), which means that contact lens wear has impacted the clinical presentation. Therefore, other factors perhaps play a minor role by initiating, modulating or exacerbating this condition. Evidence that relates to the significance of these etiological factors is considered in turn.

Thimerosal hypersensitivity

Thimerosal is an organic mercury compound that interacts with living tissue (such as bacteria or corneal epithelial cells) by binding to sulfhydryl groups of enzymes and other proteins. Compared with other traditional preservatives, such as chlorhexidine, thimerosal has relatively inferior antibacterial potency, but superior anti-fungal potency.[17]

There is some confusion in the literature concerning the use of the word 'thimerosal', which sometimes appears as 'thiomersal'. These are different solutions – thimerosal being the American formulation, and thiomersal (or thiomersolate) being the British formulation.[18] As the American formulation is used almost universally in solutions, 'thimerosal' is the preferred spelling (and is thus used throughout this book).

The key evidence that links thimerosal to CLSLK comes from clinical stud-

Table 13.1
Comparison of Theodore's SLK and CLSLK

Feature	Theodore's SLK	CLSLK
Age	Usually middle-aged (over 40 years)	Younger (under 40 years)
Sex	More common in females	Equal male:female distribution
Associated factors	Linked to thyroid disease	Usually soft contact lens wear Increased lens movement Soiled lenses Thimerosal in lens solutions
Symptoms	Mild-to-severe irritation without lenses Vision rarely affected	Mild-to-severe irritation with lenses Vision can be reduced
Signs	Mild superior corneal staining Superior bulbar conjunctival redness Superior bulbar conjunctival chemosis Limbal redness Grade 3 papillary hypertrophy Corneal filaments frequently observed	Severe superior corneal staining Superior bulbar conjunctival redness Superior bulbar conjunctival chemosis Limbal redness Grade 1 papillary hypertrophy Corneal filaments rarely observed
Staining	Superior corneal fluorescein staining	Superior corneal rose bengal staining
Pathology	Epithelial keratinization Nuclear degeneration	Epithelial keratinization Neutrophilic response Reduced number of goblet cells
Management	Lubricants Silver nitrate application Bandage lens therapy Pressure patching Conjunctival resection Conjunctival cauterization	Temporary cessation of lens wear Interim corticosteroids Interim lubricants Interim prostaglandin inhibitors Change lens design Use non-thimerosal regimen Regular lens replacement Daily disposable lenses

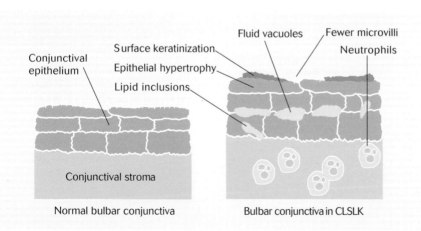

Figure 13.5

Normal bulbar conjunctiva and bulbar conjunctiva in CLSLK

ies that have sought to identify a common causative factor in patients who present with this condition. Wright and Mackie[6] observed that all 61 patients who suffered from CLSLK in their sample were using solutions that contained thimerosal. All of 10 patients subjected to a provocative test [a challenge dose of 0.005% thimerosal (in normal saline) applied topically] showed a rapid adverse response. Sendele et al.,[3] reported 40 cases of CLSLK; in every case, patients were using thimerosal-preserved care solutions. In all 40 CLSLK patients of Sendele et al.,[3] all six CLSLK patients of Miller et al.,[7] all 15 CLSLK patients of Fuerst et al.[8] and all 31 CLSLK patients of Wilson et al.,[9] thimerosal was a component of care solutions being used.

Further evidence that implicates thimerosal in the etiology of CLSLK includes:

- The condition is always bilateral;
- Signs and symptoms resolve when the patient ceases using thimerosal-preserved solutions;[1,3]
- The syndrome recurs if thimerosal is reintroduced into the care regimen;
- The syndrome does not recur if thimerosal-free solutions are used.

The results of 'patch testing' have confounded the thimerosal argument. For example, Sendele et al.[3] applied the following three challenge tests to patients who suffer from CLSLK:

- Two drops of 0.001% and 0.01% thimerosal (the latter being 10 times the concentration normally used in contact lens solution formulations), balanced in saline, instilled into the eyes of 15 patients every hour during waking hours;
- An occlusive skin patch test soaked in 0.001% thimerosal applied to the forearm;
- 0.1 ml of 0.001% thimerosal injected into the forearm.

Only five of the 15 patients tested (and none of the control subjects) developed a reaction to the thimerosal within 72 hours. Similarly, Miller et al.[7] noted a positive skin-test reaction to thimerosal in only one of six patients examined.

Wilson-Holt and Dart[1] adopted a different approach to provocative testing. They instilled one drop of a saline solution that contained 0.005% thimerosal into the eye, four times each day. Conjunctival redness was observed in all patients – usually within 12 hours, but sometimes taking up to 72 hours to develop. The inconclusive nature of patch testing results may be because the thimerosal molecule is too small for skin testing of an antibody-medicated response.[2]

There have been reports of patients who have recovered from CLSLK, but have suffered a recurrence when lens wear has been resumed in the *absence* of thimerosal.[8] Such reports are inconclusive because in many cases the same lens was reused. Despite thorough cleaning, not all of the offending antigen may have been purged completely from the lens.

Of the four patients in the study of Stenson,[5] three experienced a resolution of signs of CLSLK after lens removal and were able to resume a limited wearing schedule with thinner lenses, presumably while still using thimerosal-preserved solutions. However, that it was necessary to restrict wearing time suggests that the condition was not resolved fully. A shorter wearing schedule would have minimized the time of contact of thimerosal with the ocular surface, and thus reduced the severity of the condition. Any additional strategy to minimize the overall physiologic challenge of lens wear, such as the use of thinner lenses (of necessarily superior oxygen performance), would be expected to have a general beneficial effect on ocular signs and symptoms (such as eye redness), independently of any direct effect in curing CLSLK.

Thimerosal has long been known to cause an intense delayed hypersensitivity reaction. The mechanism of a delayed hypersensitivity reaction requires that affected patients be previously sensitized to an offending antigen and then be re-exposed to that antigen for a prolonged period before the condition flares up. Likely mechanisms for pre-sensitization that involve thimerosal include previous vaccine injections (such as those for diphtheria and tetanus), topical antiseptics and ophthalmic preparations.

Once a patient has been sensitized to thimerosal, a re-exposure of minute concentrations later in life results in the onset of symptoms and signs over a period of weeks or months. This is typical of a hypersensitivity reaction, as distinct from a toxicity reaction, which is dose dependent and immediate. Furthermore, Langerhans' cells are present in the limbus and adjacent tissues; such cells are known to mediate cutaneous hypersensitivity reactions to a variety of chemicals.[13] Patch-testing studies have revealed that the incidence of skin hypersensitivity to thimerosal is about 7% in the USA[19] and 25% in Sweden.[20]

Mackie[13] argues that CLSLK can present as a Type I (immediate) or Type IV (delayed) hypersensitivity reaction, primarily based upon clinical evidence that some patients display an immediate reaction and some display a delayed response.

The precise mechanism by which thimerosal induces a hypersensitivity reaction in CLSLK is not known, but Wilson-Holt and Dart[1] advanced the following theory: hydrogel lenses absorb thimerosal (which is highly water soluble) during the disinfection procedure, and the thimerosal is slowly re-released back into the eye during lens wear. This prolonged ocular contact with thimerosal induces a local delayed hypersensitivity reaction initiated by sensitized T lymphocytes.

Thimerosal toxicity

Thimerosal is only mildly cytotoxic, but to a degree that is much less than other preservative systems.[21] A true toxicity reaction would affect all of the ocular surface and would not be restricted to the superior cornea and conjunctiva, as occurs in CLSLK. It is for these reasons that CLSLK is not considered to be a toxic reaction.

Mechanical effects

Evidence for a significant mechanical component in the etiology of CLSLK is weak and largely anecdotal. Stenson[5] noted that some of her CLSLK patients displayed excessive lens movement. Abel et al.[10] noted excess lens movement in the majority of their patients, which indicates a poor fit and may be associated with increased mechanical influences.

Stenson[5] also reported that refitting with thinner lenses resulted in some alleviation of CLSLK; however, as explained earlier, the reason for this improvement may be more physiologic (increased oxygen) than physical (mechanical).

Abel et al.[10] reported one case in which a patient had apparently been successfully wearing spin-cast lenses cared for with thimerosal-based preservatives. CLSLK developed after switching to a lathe-cut design. These authors surmised that the new lens may have created a mechanical heaping of the superior bulbar conjunctiva, which resulted in poor wetting of the superior cornea and eventual epithelial pathology.

That CLSLK occurs at the site of the superior limbus lends some support to the theory of a mechanical etiology because of the physical bearing of the upper lid against the lens, which would exacerbate any ocular irritation caused by, for example, lens surface deposits. Certainly, blink-induced 'microtrauma' is thought to be a cause of superior limbic keratoconjunctivitis in the absence of contact lens wear.[22]

Ocular lubricants provide some symptomatic relief,[10] which suggests that mechanical irritation is a component of the CLSLK syndrome.

Lens deposits

Lens deposits, such as protein, are of potential significance in the etiology of adverse ocular reactions to lens wear because these deposits can:

• Act as a mechanical abrasive;
• Support bacterial colonization;
• Absorb or attract extraneous contaminants, such as metal ions, preservatives and other components of care systems.

It is thought that the latter mechanism in particular may be relevant to CLSLK because of the possible absorption of the mercuric component of thimerosal into lens surface deposits and its subsequent release onto the ocular surface during wear.

To examine the role of lens deposition in CLSLK, Barr et al.[23] conducted a thorough protein and elemental analysis of contact lenses worn by 12 patients who suffered from this condition. Apart from one case in which high levels of mercury were found in a lens, no clear association between deposit type and the genesis of CLSLK could be demonstrated. Thus, the role of lens spoilation in the etiology of CLSLK remains unclear.

Hypoxia beneath upper lid

That the ocular response in CLSLK is confined to the region of the superior limbus suggests that hypoxia induced by the upper lid may be a contributing factor to the etiology of this condition.[24] The upper lid normally covers the superior third of the cornea. The oxygen supply to the superior limbus during normal open-eye lens wear comes from the capillary plexus of the superior palpebral conjunctiva. The partial pressure of oxygen at the lens surface beneath the upper eyelid is 55 mmHg,[25] versus 155 mmHg in the absence of the eyelid.

Of course, lid-induced hypoxia cannot be the sole or primary cause of CLSLK,

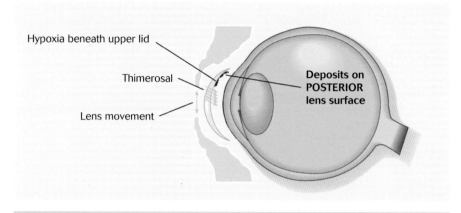

Figure 13.6
Factors of etiological significance in CLSLK

otherwise all contact lens wearers would be affected. Nevertheless, partial oxygen deprivation may be an exacerbating factor that compromises the physiologic status of the superior cornea and limbus so that this region is more prone to immunologic challenge. Holden et al.[26] provided evidence for this by demonstrating that lens-induced hypoxia inhibits respiration and growth of the corneal epithelium and stroma.

Figure 13.6 illustrates the various etiological factors thought to lead to the development of CLSLK.

Management

The accumulated clinical evidence that implicates thimerosal as the prime cause of CLSLK provides an excellent focus for managing this condition.

Suspension of lens wear

After the suspension of lens wear, the signs and symptoms of CLSLK immediately begin to resolve because the ocular surface is no longer in contact with thimerosal. The recommended period of cessation of lens wear is related to the severity of the condition. Patients who suffer from CLSLK may be advised to cease lens wear for 2–4 weeks in mild cases and up to 3 months in severe cases. The time course of resolution is discussed under 'Prognosis'.

As criteria for the resumption of lens wear, Boruchoff and Bajart[27] suggested there must no longer be any epithelial haze, surface irregularity or peripheral revascularization. These criteria may be a little too stringent. Certainly, it would

be prudent to wait until corneal haze has largely resolved and the corneal surface is smooth; however, a vascular pannus may be permanent. Lens wear can be resumed in the presence of a vascular pannus as long as the patient is monitored closely to check for the absence of further vascular encroachment.

Elimination of thimerosal

In the unlikely event that a patient is using a contact lens care product that contains thimerosal (this preservative is no longer used in contact lens care systems), the total elimination of thimerosal will almost certainly cure CLSLK, and the patient should be cautioned against the future use of any form of contact lens care solution that contains thimerosal. The patient should also be interrogated carefully as to whether he or she uses any other topical ocular medications – even those not related to contact lens wear. If thimerosal is an ingredient of any product being used, the patient should be advised to cease using them. In cases where the patient is using a prescription product that contains thimerosal, the prescribing practitioner should be notified and advised to alter the medication. Patients should be warned specifically of their allergy to thimerosal and should be told to in future always check that thimerosal is not an ingredient of any product to be applied to the eye.

Alteration to the lens

Any lens that has been worn by a patient who suffers from CLSLK – soft or rigid – should be discarded and a new lens prescribed, because no matter how thoroughly such a lens is cleaned, it requires only a trace amount of residual thimerosal to induce a reaction.

Assuming that subsequent lens wear is prescribed in the absence of thimerosal-preserved solutions, there are no constraints on the design of the replacement lenses or the modality of lens wear. However, for patients who have not recovered completely from CLSLK and who are commencing lens wear again, it is advisable to prescribe a lens of minimum thickness profile, so as to reduce the potential for mechanical irritation. Silicone hydrogel lenses should be prescribed if hypoxia is thought to be related to the development of the condition. More frequent lens replacement, including the use of daily disposable lenses, may be beneficial if protein or elemental deposition is thought to be related to the problem. Changing to rigid lenses is unlikely to be of any additional benefit, as CLSLK is known to occur in patients who wear rigid lenses.[9]

Pharmaceutical agents

As there is no infectious component to CLSLK, there is no point in prescribing antibiotics or antiviral agents during the active phase of the condition. Opinion is divided as to the value of prescribing corticosteroids to dampen the immunologic response. Abel et al.[10] found that corticosteroids helped in severe cases, whereas other authors[3,9,13] found that such drugs had no beneficial effect. Wilson-Holt and Dart[1] did not attempt to use any other therapeutic agents in the management of their CLSLK cases.

For patients whose eyes are particularly red and uncomfortable, Mackie[13] recommended the prescription of oxytetracycline 250 mg twice daily or oral doxycycline 100 mg on alternate days for their anti-inflammatory effect on the conjunctiva. In severe cases, the cornea can be treated with silver nitrate to remove the affected cells and promote regrowth of a new healthy epithelium.

Ocular lubricants in the form of drops or ointments may provide symptomatic relief during the recovery phase,[10] further to a positive placebo effect in a naturally anxious patient.

Bandage lenses and pressure patching

Paradoxically, bandage lenses have been advocated for patients who suffer from Theodore's SLK.[28,29] Adapting this approach to CLSLK would mean a rapid resumption of lens wear in the absence of thimerosal-preserved care systems. The main beneficiary of such an approach is a patient who suffers from a concurrent tarsal hypertrophy whose limbus would be protected from mechanical insult caused by the roughened tarsus. Similarly, pressure patches provide symptomatic relief by limiting eye movement and consequent mechanical irritation.[28]

Surgery

Sendele et al.[3] removed the involved superior corneal epithelium in two CLSLK patients with incapacitating reduction of vision attributed to corneal epithelial irregularity. This was achieved by mechanical scraping with a scalpel blade. They reported that, although this procedure may have hastened visual recovery, it did not seem to otherwise affect the clinical course.

Kenyon and Tseng[30] described three severe cases of CLSLK in which two free grafts of limbal tissue were transplanted from the most affected to the least affected eye, the latter having been prepared by limited conjunctival resection and superficial dissection of the fibrovascular pannus. Subsequent impression cytology confirmed restoration of the corneal epithelium. It is curious that this procedure is possible in view of the perfect symmetry that is encountered in virtually all cases of CLSLK.[13] With the absence of thimerosal in contact lens care solutions and the virtual elimination of severe cases of CLSLK, such radical surgical procedures are less likely to be necessary in the future.

Prognosis

In the 42 patients who suffered from CLSLK and were examined by Wilson-Holt and Dart,[1] the time for resolution of clinical signs after cessation of lens wear was from 3 weeks to 9 months, with a mean of 4.2 months. Sendele et al.[3] reported a similar time course of resolution, as did Abel et al.,[10] who noted that recovery took from 5 days to 10 months in the eight patients they followed. In these patients, edema and redness subsided first, followed by clearing of the epitheliopathy. Papillary changes took the longest to resolve, and persisted for months in several cases. Sendele et al.[3] reported that one patient took 2 years to recover in the absence of lens wear; fortunately, such a prolonged period of recovery is rare.

Recovery of visual acuity after severe cases of CLSLK was reported by Sendele et al.[3] to be 'gradual'. These authors inferred that visual acuity had only recovered to 6/9 in some subjects, even after several months.

Differential Diagnosis

In the early stages, CLSLK may be mistaken for increased redness of the superior conjunctiva or limbus, or neovascularization of the superior cornea – conditions that could be caused by a variety of insults. For example, *Figure 13.7* depicts superior limbal redness in a 24-year old asymptomatic man wearing rigid lenses. The edge of the lens was chipped, which led to irritation of the superior limbus between the 8 and 12 o'clock positions. A case of conjunctivitis that affects the superior globe is

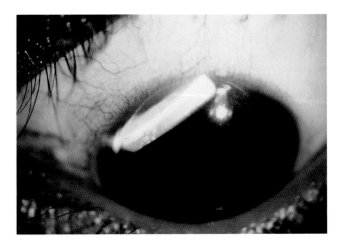

Figure 13.7

Increased redness of the superior limbus caused by irritation from the edge of a chipped rigid lens, which has a similar appearance to that of CLSLK shown in *Figure 13.8*. Neovascularization of the superior cornea induced by a soft lens is shown in *Figure 13.9*. All of these conditions display pathology in common with certain features of CLSLK.

Wilson-Holt and Dart[1] reported that they had misdiagnosed two CLSLK patients as having bacterial conjunctivitis; these patients were unfortunately treated with thimerosal-preserved topical antibiotics, which of course exacerbated the condition.

CLSLK can also be mistaken for infiltrative keratitis. A culture-positive scraping provides verification of an infectious keratitis. True CLSLK should be suspected if thimerosal-preserved care solutions were being used.

The key difference between CLSLK and Theodore's SLK is that the latter generally occurs in the absence of lens wear. Theoretically, a contact lens wearer can coincidentally develop Theodore's SLK in the presence or absence of thimerosal-preserved care systems. The distinguishing features between these two conditions are outlined in *Table 13.1*.

In general, the clinical presentation of a severe case of CLSLK is unambiguous, with a host of corneal, limbal and conjunctival pathologies confined to the region of the superior limbus.

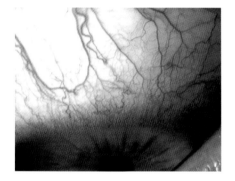

Figure 13.8
Conjunctivitis affecting the superior globe, with a similar appearance to that of CLSLK

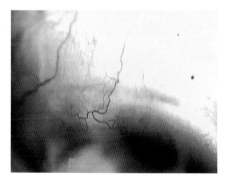

Figure 13.9
Neovascularization of the superior cornea induced by a soft lens, which has a similar appearance to that of CLSLK

REFERENCES

1 Wilson-Holt N and Dart JK (1989). Thiomersal keratoconjunctivitis, frequency, clinical spectrum and diagnosis. *Eye* **3**, 581–587.
2 Wallace W (1985). Soft contact lens associated superior limbic keratoconjunctivitis. *Int Eyecare* **1**, 302–303.
3 Sendele DD, Kenyon KR, Mobilia EF, *et al.* (1983). Superior limbic keratoconjunctivitis in contact lens wearers. *Ophthalmology* **90**, 616–622.
4 Bloomfield SE, Jakobiec FA and Theodore FH (1984). Contact lens induced keratopathy: A severe complication extending the spectrum of keratoconjunctivitis in contact lens wearers. *Ophthalmology* **91**, 290–294.
5 Stenson S (1983). Superior limbic keratoconjunctivitis associated with soft contact lens wear. *Arch Ophthalmol.* **101**, 402–404.
6 Wright P and Mackie I (1982). Preservative-related problems in soft contact lens wearers. *Trans Ophthalmol Soc UK* **102**, 3–6.
7 Miller RA, Brightbill FS and Slama SL (1982). Superior limbic keratoconjunctivitis in soft contact lens wearers. *Cornea* **1**, 293–297.
8 Fuerst DJ, Sugar J and Worobec S (1983). Superior limbic keratoconjunctivitis associated with cosmetic soft contact lens wear. *Arch Ophthalmol.* **101**, 1214–1216.
9 Wilson LA, McNatt J and Reitschel R (1981). Delayed hypersensitivity to thimerosal in soft contact lens wearers. *Ophthalmology* **88**, 804–809.
10 Abel R, Shovlin JP and DePaolis MD (1985). A treatise on hydrophilic lens induced superior limbic keratoconjunctivitis. *Int Contact Lens Clin.* **12**, 116–121.
11 Binder PS, Rasmussen DM and Gordon M (1981). Keratoconjunctivitis and soft contact lens solutions. *Arch Ophthalmol.* **99**, 87–90.
12 Theodore FH (1963). Superior limbic keratoconjunctivitis. *Ear Nose Throat J.* **42**, 25–36.
13 Mackie IA (1993). Thiomersal keratopathy. In: *Medical Contact Lens Practice. A Systematic Approach*, p. 128–132 (Oxford: Butterworth–Heinemann).
14 Stapleton F, Dart J and Minassian D (1992). Nonulcerative complications of contact lens wear. Relative risks for different lens types. *Arch Ophthalmol.* **110**, 1601–1606.
15 Morgan PB and Efron N (2003). Trends in UK contact lens prescribing 2003. *Optician* **225**(5904), 34–35.
16 Kerr C and Meyler J (2003). *The ACLM Contact Lens Yearbook 2003*. (London: Association of Contact Lens Manufacturers).
17 Tragakis MP, Brown SI and Pearce DB (1973). Bacteriologic studies of contamination associated with soft contact lenses. *Am J Ophthalmol.* **75**, 496–499.
18 Stapleton FS, Phillips AJ and Hopkins GA (1997). Drugs and solutions in contact lens practice and related microbiology. In: *Contact Lenses*, Fourth Edition, p. 93–153, Ed. Phillips AJ and Speedwell L (Oxford: Butterworth–Heinemann).
19 Rudner EJ, Clendenning WE and Epstein E (1973). Epidemiology of contact dermatitis in North America. *Arch Dermatol.* **108**, 537–542.
20 Hansson H and Moller H (1970). Patch test reactions to merthiolate in healthy young subjects. *Br J Dermatol.* **83**, 349–356.
21 Gasset AR, Ishii Y, Kaufman HE and Miller T (1974). Cytotoxicity of ophthalmic preservatives. *Am J Ophthalmol.* **78**, 98–105.
22 Cher I (2003). Blink-related microtrauma: When the ocular surface harms itself. *Clin Exp Ophthalmol.* **31**, 183–190.
23 Barr JT, Dugan PR, Reindel WR and Tuovinen OH (1989). Protein and elemental analysis of contact lenses of patients with superior limbic keratoconjunctivitis or giant papillary conjunctivitis. *Optom Vis Sci.* **66**, 133–140.
24 Baum JL (1997). The Castroviejo Lecture. Prolonged eyelid closure is a risk to the cornea. *Cornea* **16**, 602–611.
25 Efron N and Carney LG (1979). Oxygen levels beneath the closed eyelid. *Invest Ophthalmol Vis Sci.* **18**, 93–95.
26 Holden BA, Sweeney DF, Vannas A, *et al.* (1985). Effects of long-term extended contact lens wear on the human cornea. *Invest Ophthalmol Vis Sci.* **26**, 1489–1501.
27 Boruchoff SA and Bajart AM (1989). The superior limbic manifestations of contact lens intolerance. In: *Contact Lenses. The CLAO Guide to Basic Science and Clinical Practice*, Vol. 2, p. 44.1–44.3, Ed. Dabezier Jr OH. (Boston: Little, Brown & Co).
28 Mondino BJ, Zaidman GW and Salamon SW (1982). Use of pressure patching and soft contact lenses in superior limbic keratoconjunctivitis. *Arch Ophthalmol.* **100**, 1932–1934.
29 Watson S, Tullo AB and Carley F (2002). Treatment of superior limbic keratoconjunctivitis with a unilateral bandage contact lens. *Br J Ophthalmol.* **86**, 485–486.
30 Kenyon KR and Tseng SCG (1989). Limbal autograft transplantation for ocular surface disorders. *Ophthalmology* **96**, 709–713.

PART IV

CORNEAL EPITHELIUM

CORNEAL STAINING

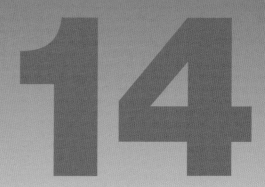

The use of fluorescein in the examination of corneal integrity was introduced by Pflüger[1] in 1882, just 6 years before the first fitting of contact lenses to humans was reported by Fick.[2] However, it is only in the past 35 years that fluorescein has been used routinely by clinicians for this purpose.[3]

Corneal staining is probably the most familiar of all potential contact lens complications, since its clinical importance is well established and it is easily observed. Strictly speaking, epithelial staining is not a condition in itself – rather, it is a general term that refers to the appearance of tissue disruption and other pathophysiologic changes in the anterior eye as revealed with the aid of one or more of a number of dyes, such as fluorescein, rose bengal or lissamine green. These dyes are sometimes referred to as 'vital stains', which suggests that they stain living things; however, this is a misleading term because such stains can be taken up by dead cells and even by inorganic material.[4]

It has become a convention among clinicians to use the term 'corneal staining' to describe the appearance of bright areas of fluorescence in the epithelium after instillation of the dye fluorescein and illumination with cobalt blue light (*Figure 14.1*). Throughout this chapter,

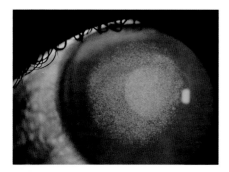

Figure 14.1
Punctate staining of the central cornea

corneal staining refers to staining with *fluorescein*, unless otherwise stated.

Prevalence

Non-lens wearers
Before considering the extent of corneal staining in contact lens wearers, the extent of staining in the normal population must be recognized. Schwallie *et al.*[5] evaluated corneal fluorescein staining in 16 normal subjects not wearing lenses over a 2-week period. The average duration for an episode of staining above the group median (grade 0.5) was found to be 1.2 ± 0.4 days. For both eyes, the most prevalent location of staining was the inferior region (50%), followed by the nasal region (20%). Overall, a mean staining grade of 0.5–0.6 was found. In a similar study, Dundas *et al.*[6] found some degree of corneal staining on 79% of the corneas of 102 normal subjects they examined.

Lens wearers
The prevalence of corneal staining of any degree of severity in a population of contact lens wearers is thought to be as high as 60%,[7] but often staining is of a low level and generally clinically insignificant. Indeed, corneal staining is frequently observed in non-lens wearers.[7,8]

Begley *et al.*[9] found that the average overall staining grade for both eyes of 98 asymptomatic soft contact lens wearers was 0.5. Corneal staining between the two eyes was positively and significantly correlated. One-third of the subjects who participated in the study had notable corneal staining. Jalbert *et al.*[10] measured levels of corneal staining over a 2 year period in response to successful daily wear and extended wear of disposable hydrogel contact lenses. Their results were similar to those of Begley *et al.*;[9] overall levels of corneal staining

were low with median values below or equal to grade 0.5 in all groups. There was no difference in the extent, depth or geographic distribution of corneal staining between the daily wear and extended wear groups. Staining was recorded more frequently in the superior and inferior areas of the cornea than in the central, nasal or temporal regions.

In perhaps the largest survey ever undertaken of the ocular response to contact lens wear (66,218 patients), Hamano *et al.*[11] determined the prevalence of clinically significant staining [corneal erosion or superficial punctate keratitis (SPK) greater than grade 2; see below] to be 0.9% in soft lens wearers, 0.5% in rigid lens wearers and 1.3% in polymethyl methacrylate (PMMA) lens wearers.

Signs and Symptoms

Vital stains
A variety of vital stains can be used to highlight various aspects of surface-tissue pathology, and the types of stains and their applications for staining the conjunctival surface are discussed in detail in Chapter 8. Below is given a brief overview of the use of the three main stains used in contact lens practice to investigate various abnormalities and the pathology of the corneal surface.

Fluorescein
Fluorescein is combined with sodium salt to make it more soluble in water.[12] Although it is available as a 2% solution, fluorescein is rarely used in this form because it supports the growth of bacteria that are potentially pathogenic to the eye, such as *Pseudomonas aeruginosa*.[13] Therefore, paper strips impregnated with fluorescein are preferred; these strips have an orange–yellow color. Fluorescein can be instilled by wetting the strip with two drops of

sterile unpreserved saline, having the patient look up and briefly and gently touching the strip on the inferior bulbar conjunctiva.

When examining a fluorescein-stained eye, it is important to prompt the patient to blink frequently. If the patient blinks infrequently, the tear film breaks up to leave large dark areas of non-fluorescence, which could either mask true staining or be misinterpreted as non-staining background fluorescence. Fluorescein break-up in the absence of blinking is the basis of an important test of tear film stability.[14]

Fluorescein has a molecular weight of 376, so it is smaller than the pore size of many hydrogels and can be absorbed into the lens, which results in a yellow stain. Therefore, as a precaution, the eye should be irrigated with sterile saline prior to inserting a soft lens after examination of the eye with fluorescein. If a lens does become stained with fluorescein, it usually washes out following the next disinfection cycle.

Fluorescein of high molecular weight, known as Fluorexon[15] (molecular weight 710) is available, but it is not used widely because it has relatively low fluorescent properties and causes discomfort and stinging in some patients.[16]

Sequential fluorescein staining

Sequential staining refers to the repeated application of fluorescein over a period of minutes, followed by observation with the slit-lamp biomicroscope in the usual way.[17] This has been suggested as a more sensitive technique that is predictive of the epithelial complications of contact lens wear, although this link has not been proved. It is likely that sequential staining merely results in

high concentrations of fluorescein in the eye that cause a toxic epithelial response. The value of this technique is therefore questionable.

Rose bengal

Rose bengal is a mildly toxic, bright red stain that is adsorbed to and absorbed by compromised epithelial cells, mucus and fibrous tissue (*Figure 14.2*).[4] It is available as a 1% solution or as impregnated filter strips. Davis and Lebow[16] suggest that much better results are obtained if the solution form is used. Following instillation, the eye is observed in white light.

In the absence of a complete tear film – and especially in the case of mucus deficiency – rose bengal is taken up by healthy epithelial cells.[4] Accordingly, this stain is especially useful for investigating dry eye conditions; that is, a dry eye may display extensive staining with rose bengal, especially if there is a mucus deficiency.

Lissamine green

An alternative stain with similar properties to rose bengal is lissamine green; both of these agents stain degenerated and dead epithelial cells and mucus.[18] The stained regions appear as a vivid green color (*Figure 14.3*). Lissamine green is better tolerated by patients than is rose bengal, but is equally as effective as rose bengal in evaluating the surface of the eye. However, Emran and Sommer[19] believe that lissamine green is an inadequately sensitive test for practical use.

Slit-lamp biomicroscope appearance

Corneal staining after instillation of fluorescein is observed as a bright green

fluorescence and may present in an infinite combination of shapes, locations, depths and intensities. The position is generally noted as superior, inferior, temporal, nasal or central, and the depth of staining is noted as deep or superficial. A large number of terms have been used to describe the various forms of appearance of the staining. Some of these have assumed the status of 'syndromes' based on frequently observed characteristic patterns of tissue damage. These are considered briefly below.

Punctate staining

Perhaps the form of disturbance noted most often is punctate staining, whereby small superficial discrete dots are observed on the corneal surface (see *Figure 14.1*). This is also referred to as micropunctate staining, superficial punctate erosion (SPE) or SPK. Intense punctate staining is sometimes called 'stipple staining'.

Diffuse staining

A vast array of closely separated punctate spots gives rise to a 'diffuse' appearance. The terms SPE and SPK are also used to describe this appearance (*Figure 14.4*).

Coalescent staining

The overall pattern of fluorescence may be so diffuse as to obscure the constituent elements of staining, which produces an appearance described as confluent or coalescent staining (*Figure 14.5*).

3 and 9 o'clock staining

The classic form of staining in rigid lens wearers is known as 3 and 9 o'clock staining, which refers to a triangular area

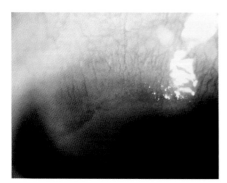

Figure 14.2
Rose bengal staining the leading edge of a fibrovascular pannus

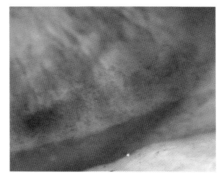

Figure 14.3
Diffuse lissamine green staining of the inferior cornea

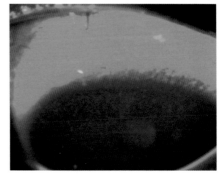

Figure 14.4
Diffuse staining of the superior cornea

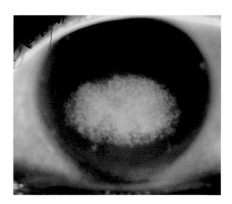

Figure 14.5
Coalescent superficial corneal staining

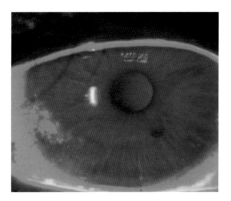

Figure 14.6
3 and 9 o'clock corneal staining caused by rigid lens wear

of staining (apex away from the central cornea) at the nasal and temporal cornea outside the lens periphery (*Figure 14.6*).[20] Although this condition may result in part from incomplete or infrequent blinking, it occurs primarily as a result of corneal non-wetting caused by the lids being bridged away from the cornea by the lens edge.[21]

Dimple-veil 'staining'

Dimple-veil 'staining' is not true staining, in that fluorescein is not taken up by the corneal tissue; instead, fluorescein pools in indentations in the epithelial surface. This condition is caused by air bubbles that become trapped between the back surface of the lens and the corneal epithelium (*Figure 14.7*) and is caused by a poor lens–cornea fitting relationship. Dimple-veil 'staining' is usually observed centrally in steep-fitting rigid lenses or peripherally in high-riding lenses in cases of high with-the-rule astigmatism. Patients are asymptomatic and the indentations in the corneal epithelium are similar in appearance to the stippled surface of a golf ball. Improving the fitting relationship immediately eliminates the signs.[22]

Inferior epithelial arcuate lesion ('smile stain')

In 1975, Kline and DeLuca[23] reported a study in which 46% of 72 eyes fitted with soft lenses displayed superficial epithelial arcuate staining located in an area between 4 and 8 o'clock locations on the cornea. This pattern of staining has come to be known as an 'inferior epithelial arcuate lesion', or 'smile stain'.[24] Zadnik and Mutti[24] described this condition as an arcuate band of coarse, white, punctate epithelial disruption (*Figure 14.8*). Many authors[24–26] have subsequently reported this finding in soft lens wearers, and all believe the condition has a metabolic and/or desiccation etiology that relates to a combination of factors, such as an insufficient post-lens tear film, lens adherence and/or lens dehydration. Watanabe and Hamano[26] suggested that inferior epithelial arcuate lesions are found in 3.3% of disposable lens wearers.

Superior epithelial arcuate lesion

Superior epithelial arcuate lesions (SEALs) are an infrequent and often asymptomatic complication of conventional soft contact lens wear.[27,28] The characteristic arcuate pattern of the full-thickness corneal epithelial lesion usually occurs in the area covered by the upper eyelid, within 2–3 mm of the superior limbus in the 10 and 2 o'clock region[28] (*Figure 14.9*). The reported low incidence of SEALs is partly because this condition, which has also been referred to as 'epithelial splitting',[29,30] is not usually symptomatic.

The etiology of SEALs is multifactorial.[31] It is thought that SEALs are produced by mechanical chaffing at the peripheral cornea. This chaffing occurs as a result of inward pressure of the upper lid, in an area in which the peripheral corneal topography and lens design, rigidity and surface characteristics combine to create excessive 'frictional' pressure and abrasive shear force on the epithelial surface.[31] Patient characteristics, such as gender, age and specific corneal and lid topographies, also appear to influence the occurrence of SEALs.[28] Silicone hydrogel lenses are made from higher modulus materials with surfaces that seem to differ subtly in wettability in some patients; these factors are thought to contribute to the increased prevalence of SEALs with these lenses.[30,32]

Epithelial plug

Perhaps the most devastating form of staining that can be observed is the 'epithelial plug', which is a large discrete area (typically round in shape) of full-thickness epithelial loss (*Figure 14.10*). This rare condition is observed in some patients who have suffered severe

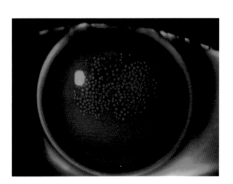

Figure 14.7
Dimple-veil 'staining' caused by rigid lens wear

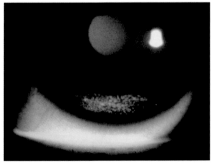

Figure 14.8
Inferior epithelial arcuate lesion, or 'smile stain'

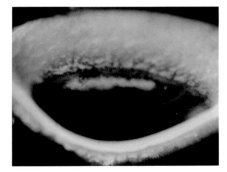

Figure 14.9
Superior epithelial arcuate lesion (SEAL), otherwise known as 'epithelial splitting'

corneal metabolic compromise, presumably because of prolonged lens-induced hypoxia.

Madigan and Holden[33] investigated the basis for this condition in a feline model. The corneas of both eyes of cats that had worn low-oxygen transmissibility thick parallel-design hydrogel contact lenses only in one eye for 8–121 days were examined using both light and transmission electron microscopy. A circular trephined section of the epithelium could be lifted away effortlessly from the stromal bed of all corneas that wore lenses (*Figure 14.11*). Contact lens wear induces many changes in the epithelium, including a decrease in the number of cell layers and appearance of cuboidal rather than columnar basal cell shapes. In addition, electron microscopy revealed that the number of hemidesmosomes per micrometer of basement membrane was reduced significantly after contact lens wear. Anchoring fibrils in lens-wearing corneas appeared normal, and the reduction in epithelial adhesion occurred without obvious epithelial edema. Madigan and Holden[33] concluded that decreased epithelial adhesion after contact lens wear, which is presumably the cause of epithelial plug formation, appears to be related directly to the reduced numbers of hemidesmosomes.

Other forms of staining

Other terms used to describe staining include linear abrasions, dimple stains and exposure keratitis. Severe staining (grades 3 and 4) may be accompanied by bulbar conjunctival redness and chemosis, limbal redness, excessive lacrimation and, in some cases, stromal infiltrates, depending on the cause of the problem.

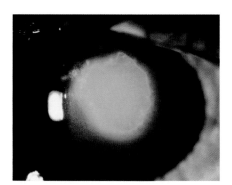

Figure 14.10
Focal area of full thickness epithelial loss, known as an 'epithelial plug'

Vision

Visual acuity is generally unaffected by corneal staining, although a slight loss might be expected in extreme cases (such as grade 4 staining, as depicted in *Figure 14.10*). As is described below, epithelial recovery is generally rapid so any vision loss is also restored quickly.

Comfort

A paradox of the corneal staining response is that there is no clear relationship between the severity of staining and the degree of ocular discomfort. For example, an exposure keratitis in the form of an extensive inferior arcuate diffuse staining pattern can be virtually asymptomatic, whereas a small tracking stain caused by a foreign body trapped beneath a rigid lens can be excruciatingly painful. Photophobia may be present in the case of an infection.

Pathology

Fluorescence observed in the cornea after the instillation of fluorescein indicates one of three phenomena:

- Fluorescein has entered damaged cells;
- Fluorescein has entered intercellular spaces;
- Fluorescein has filled gaps in the epithelial surface, created when epithelial cells are displaced.

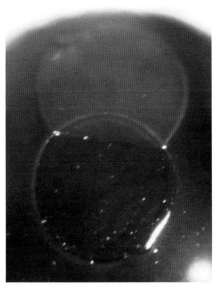

Figure 14.11
Epithelial layer lifted away from the stromal bed (cat model)

To determine precisely what it is that fluorescein stains, Wilson *et al.*[34] examined rabbit corneas stained with fluorescein with the biomicroscope and later with a higher magnification epifluorescent microscope following incision. They determined that fluorescein primarily reveals cells that have taken up fluorescein optimally. Typically, this means degenerated or devitalized cells; however, this is not always the case. The bright fluorescent appearance is concentration dependent, whereby concentrations greater or lesser than an optimum level produce a lower level of fluorescence. Thus, cells with a dull fluorescence could actually contain a higher *or* lower concentration of fluorescein than cells that display bright fluorescence.

In many of their preparations, Wilson *et al.*[34] observed a dull background fluorescence, which indicates that fluorescein enters intercellular spaces, presumably in low concentrations, and on occasions enters the anterior stroma. This background fluorescence can result in a 'salt and pepper' appearance, whereby the 'salt' indicates cells that have filled with an optimum concentration of fluorescein, and the 'pepper' indicates cells that are filled with a higher or lower fluorescein concentration that 'blend in' with the background fluorescence.

More controversially, Wilson *et al.*[34] suggested that bright fluorescence is unlikely to represent pooling of fluorescein as a result of missing cells, because repeated irrigation did not change the bright fluorescent appearance (which indicates that such fluorescence must come from within the cell). Certainly, in cases of gross epithelial detachment, such as occurs with an epithelial plug (*Figure 14.10*), fluorescein clearly fills the void.

Figure 14.12 illustrates the way in which the corneal epithelium is stained by fluorescein and rose bengal.

Etiology

Numerous causes of epithelial staining related to contact lenses can be classified broadly into six etiologic categories: mechanical, exposure, metabolic, toxic, allergic and infectious. In many cases the pattern of staining can provide a clue to the cause. Each of these etiologic factors is considered below.

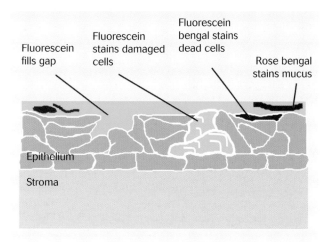

Fluorescein fills gap

Fluorescein stains damaged cells

Fluorescein bengal stains dead cells

Rose bengal stains mucus

Epithelium

Stroma

Figure 14.12
Mechanism of fluorescein and rose bengal staining of corneal epithelium

Mechanical

Sources of mechanical staining include lens defects, poor lens finish (e.g., rough edge),[35] lens binding (e.g., as can occur with overnight rigid lens extended wear lenses),[36] excessive lens bearing (e.g., tight rigid lens fit, bearing of a poorly blended optic zone junction, or decentered lens, as depicted in *Figure 14.13*), foreign bodies beneath the lens, deposits on the posterior lens surface or abrasion that occurs during lens insertion or removal.

Staining induced by lens defects or posterior lens deposits usually takes the form of discrete areas of fluorescence that correspond to the location of the defect or deposit.[35] The staining may be arcuate as a result of natural lens rotation during wear. Staining caused by lens binding appears as an arc that corresponds to the lens edge, whereas excessive lens bearing can result in a more diffuse form of staining.

A foreign body often leaves a zig-zag track, which indicates the path it has taken across the corneal surface as a result of blinking (*Figure 14.14*). This phenomenon is rarely observed in soft lens wearers.

Staining incurred during lens insertion or removal is often of a linear form. Since such staining is characteristically a 'chance occurrence', it is typically unilateral.

Exposure

In soft lens wearers, exposure keratitis manifests typically as a band of inferior arcuate staining. This is caused by epithelial disruption as a result of drying of the corneal surface.[37] Such staining patterns are observed when soft lenses decenter superiorly, to leave an inferior band of exposed cornea that is not properly wetted because of less frequent blinking.

Desiccation staining with soft lenses can be categorized as a form of exposure keratitis.[38] This condition appears as a central stipple stain. It occurs when lenses of high water content are made too thin, which causes water to be drawn out of the cornea when the lens dehydrates during wear.[39] All forms of exposure keratitis are typically bilateral.

The classic pattern of 3 and 9 o'clock staining in rigid lens wearers is also primarily thought to represent a form of exposure keratitis, whereby the eyelids are bridged away from the corneal surface at the lens edge at the 3 and 9 o'clock corneal locations (see *Figure 14.6*).[21]

Metabolic

All contact lenses are known to induce various levels of epithelial hypoxia (oxygen deprivation) and hypercapnia (excessive carbon dioxide),[40] which results in the production of metabolites (e.g., lactic acid) that can adversely affect epithelial structure and function, and lead to tissue acidosis.

For lenses of low oxygen transmissibility and/or lens overwear, such changes can be exacerbated, and the epithelial decompensation is observed as a generalized, diffuse staining that encompasses most of the cornea; it is typically bilateral. The spontaneous focal loss of epithelium depicted in *Figure 14.10* was attributed to the effects of severe hypoxia in a soft lens patient wearing −9.00D soft lenses of low water content (38%).

Fine punctate staining can be observed when epithelial microcysts break through the anterior epithelial surface (see Chapter 15).

Toxic

Preservatives used in contact lens disinfection systems are generally formulated in low concentrations so that direct application to the eye is non-toxic. Single-bottle multiple-purpose solutions contain surfactant cleaning elements that are below the threshold for ocular toxicity. However, some preservatives, such as chlorhexidine, can bind strongly and reversibly to many hydrogel polymers or to protein deposits on the lens surface, especially in lenses that are disposed of infrequently.[41] This can eventually lead to a toxic reaction, which in severe cases can present as diffuse staining across the whole cornea (*Figure 14.15*). Hydrogen peroxide, when introduced directly into the eye, can result in a severe and painful toxic reaction.[42]

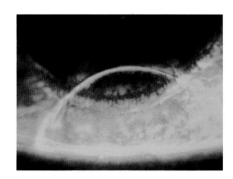

Figure 14.13
Corneal and conjunctival imprint of edge of decentered rigid lens as revealed by fluorescein

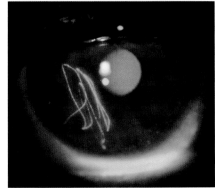

Figure 14.14
Foreign body track in rigid lens wearer

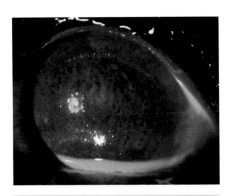

Figure 14.15
Severe toxicity staining in a patient who
inadvertently used a contact lens cleaner as
a wetting solution

Allergic

An allergic reaction can take the form
of a delayed or immediate hypersensitivity response. This is an acquired cell-
mediated (antibody) immunologic
reaction that generally requires previous
exposure and sensitization to the offending antigen. In the immediate form, it
may resemble a toxic response. Delayed
hypersensitivity can manifest months or
years after continued use of an apparently harmless product.

Thimerosal, benzalkonium chloride
and chlorhexidine have all been implicated in the etiology of allergic reactions
to contact lens solutions. Fortunately,
these substances are now virtually obso-
lete, and sophisticated preservatives
that are essentially non-toxic and non-
allergenic, such as polyaminopropyl
biguanide (Dymed), now dominate the
market.[43] Chlorine-based disinfection
systems are also largely non-toxic and
non-allergenic, although concerns have
been expressed about the disinfection
capacity of some formulations of these
solutions.[44]

Infectious

Infection by a variety of pathogens can
result in corneal staining. Indeed, an
infectious corneal ulcer is only defined as
such if the affected region of stromal
degradation is accompanied by an overlying epithelial defect and the ulcer is
culture positive. In such cases, staining
is usually confined to the region of ulceration, which, in the early stages, can be
quite small (*Figure 14.16*). Fluorescein
may also diffuse into the stroma, which
results in a dull background fluorescence.

Observation and Grading

In many cases, epithelial defects can be
observed using the slit-lamp biomicroscope under white light without the aid
of fluorescein. As a general rule, observation in white light should always precede observation after instillation of
fluorescein. Once the fluorescein is
instilled, the cornea should be examined
with a broad beam at low magnification
(×10, to give a full view of cornea)
under cobalt blue light to determine the
overall level of staining. This is the preferred technique, for example, to assess
pan-corneal conditions such as 3 and 9
o'clock staining or desiccation staining.
Closer examination using a 1 mm beam
at higher magnification (×40) is required
to detect more subtle forms of staining
(such as fine foreign-body tracks) as well
as the depth of staining.

Fluorescein has a maximum absorption spectrum at 460–490 nm, with a
maximum emission spectrum at 520
nm.[12] Based on this knowledge, filters
can be interposed in the observation and
illumination system of a slit-lamp biomicroscope to enhance conditions for
viewing corneal staining.[45] Specifically,
a Wratten #47B excitation filter should
be placed in the illumination system;
this has a peak transmission between
400 and 500 nm. A Wratten #12 filter
(which absorbs all wavelengths below
500 nm and provides maximum transmission at 530 nm and beyond) placed
in the observation system further
enhances the observed fluorescence.

A grading scale to assess the severity of corneal staining is provided in
Appendix A. Although this scale depicts

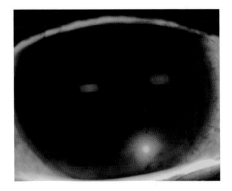

Figure 14.16
Staining of a sterile peripheral ulcer that
reveals involvement of epithelium (central
intense fluorescence) and stroma (diffuse
background glow)

fluorescein staining, the images can be
applied to any stain, as only the color of
the dye is different.

Management

Unlike various other forms of ocular compromise with contact lens wear, it is often
possible to identify the cause of corneal
staining from the patient history, knowledge of the lenses worn and maintenance
system used, inspection of the lens and
analysis of the form of staining. Clinical
intervention is generally not required if
the level of staining is less than grade 2.

Minor staining is observed commonly in contact lens wearers; it is typically
transient and in a daily lens wearer will
disappear by the following morning.
However, persistent minor staining that
forms a characteristic pattern, as well as
staining greater than grade 2, may
require intervention.

It is, of course, not possible to detail
all of the possible strategies to alleviate
corneal staining deemed to be clinically
excessive, but the general principles outlined below according to probable etiology should provide some guidance.
Whatever strategy is adopted, lens wear
need only be ceased for 1 or 2 days for
low-level staining (less than grade 2), and
perhaps 4 or 5 days for more intense
staining (greater than grade 2).

Mechanical

Strategies to resolve staining of a mechanical etiology are generally self-evident. In
the case of disposable lenses with persistent edge defects or poor surface finish, an alternative lens type should be
tried. If the mechanical problem relates
to posterior lens deposits, the lenses
should be replaced more frequently.
With rigid lenses, light polishing may
solve the problem, but lens replacement
is generally the best option.

Numerous and often conflicting strategies have been advocated to alleviate
rigid lens binding after overnight wear.
Woods and Efron[46] demonstrated that
regular rigid lens replacement (say, every
6 months) significantly reduces the incidence of binding. Excessive rigid lens
bearing is alleviated by modifying the
lens fit. Foreign bodies are dealt with by
rinsing the lens and sometimes also the
eye. Abrasion that occurs during lens
insertion or removal may necessitate re-
education of the patient with respect to
lens insertion and removal techniques.

Exposure

Exposure keratitis in soft lens wearers is usually caused by a lens that decenters superiorly. This is managed by fitting a larger diameter lens or perhaps a lens of different design that centers better.

In rigid lens wearers, the general principle to be followed in attempting to alleviate 3 and 9 o'clock staining is to ensure that the stained region is wetted properly. Numerous strategies have been advocated to alleviate this condition,[21] include adopting a lens design that allows for greater movement (typically, a smaller, looser lens fit), blinking instructions, use of in-eye lubricants[47] or changing to soft lenses.

Desiccation staining, which is generally observed in association with the wearing of thin soft lenses of high water content, is prevented by designing lenses with greater average thickness according to the guidelines provided by McNally *et al.*,[48] and/or using a material of lower water content.

Metabolic

Corneal staining attributed to epithelial hypoxia and hypercapnia is alleviated by following the general guidelines to alleviate metabolic stress, as described in Chapter 18. In general, treatment options include refitting a lens of higher gas transmissibility (such as a silicone hydrogel lens), reducing wearing time or changing from extended wear to daily wear.

Toxic

The obvious strategy to treat corneal staining caused by solution toxicity is to change to a solution that is non-toxic for that patient. Corneal burns from the instillation of hydrogen peroxide may require patient re-education in the use of peroxide systems or the prescription of a different system. Associated strategies include more frequent lens replacement to avoid a build-up of deposits that can absorb and concentrate preservatives, and the use of a lens made from a different polymer that is less likely to absorb and concentrate the offending preservatives.

Allergic

Similar strategies to those described above to treat toxicity staining are applied to the treatment of corneal staining caused by solution allergy; that is, change to a solution that is non-allergenic for that patient, replace lenses more frequently and prescribe lenses made from a different polymer. Atopic patients who are prone to suffer a reaction to a variety of preservatives are best fitted with daily disposable lenses so as to avoid contact with solutions all together.

Infectious

It is essential that the offending agent involved in an infectious episode of corneal pathology be killed as quickly as possible to avoid widespread corneal damage. Resolution of the infection generally results in the re-establishment of a normal epithelium. The issue of corneal infection related to contact lenses and ulceration is dealt with in detail in Chapter 23.

Prognosis

Recovery from corneal staining is generally quite rapid after removal of the causative agent. Light staining (less than grade 2) can recover within a few hours, and certainly overnight, assuming that lens wear has ceased. The foreign body track depicted in *Figure 14.14* completely resolved in 24 hours. More severe cases of corneal staining (greater than grade 2) may take up to 4 or 5 days to disappear.

Resolution of epithelial staining is slower if lenses are worn during the recovery period because the lenses inevitably induce a certain measure of anterior corneal hypoxia and mechanical insult, which gives a sub-optimal environment for epithelial growth and repair.

Differential Diagnosis

There are two main issues concerning the differential diagnosis of corneal staining, both of which relate to determining the etiology of various forms of staining (rather than to differentiating corneal staining from other phenomena that could theoretically take on a similar appearance). The first issue is the clinical interpretation of *different* patterns of staining – a topic that has already been dealt with in some detail in this chapter. The distribution, depth and intensity of staining, whether the staining is unilateral or bilateral, and the associated history can provide strong clues as to the cause of the condition.

Secondly, differentiation of the etiology of corneal staining can be aided by the application of other vital stains – the most common being rose bengal. Dead cells, fibrotic tissue and excess mucus stain heavily with rose bengal, which makes this stain especially useful for identifying degenerative conditions and dry eye.

REFERENCES

1 Pflüger F (1882). Zur ernährung der cornea. *Klin Monatsbl Augenheilkd.* **20**, 69–73.
2 Efron N and Pearson RM (1988). Centenary celebration of Fick's Eine Contactbrille. *Arch Ophthalmol.* **106**, 1370–1377.
3 Korb DR and Korb JME (1970). Corneal staining prior to contact lens wearing. *J Am Optom Assoc.* **41**, 228–233.
4 Feenstra RP and Tseng SC (1992). Comparison of fluorescein and rose bengal staining. *Ophthalmology* **99**, 605–617.
5 Schwallie JD, McKenney CD, Long WD Jr and McNeil A (1997). Corneal staining patterns in normal non-contact lens wearers. *Optom Vis Sci.* **74**, 92–98.
6 Dundas M, Walker A and Woods RL (2001). Clinical grading of corneal staining of non-contact lens wearers. *Ophthalmic Physiol Opt.* **21**, 30–35.
7 Guillon JP, Guillon M and Malgouyres S (1990). Corneal desiccation staining with hydrogel lenses: Tear film and contact lens factors. *Ophthalmic Physiol Opt.* **10**, 343–348.
8 Norn MS (1970). Micropunctate fluorescein vital staining of the cornea. *Acta Ophthalmol (Copenh.)* **48**, 108–118.
9 Begley CG, Barr JT, Edrington TB, *et al.* (1996). Characteristics of corneal staining in hydrogel contact lens wearers. *Optom Vis Sci.* **73**, 193–200.
10 Jalbert I, Sweeney DF and Holden BA (1999). The characteristics of corneal staining in successful daily and extended disposable contact lens wearers. *Clin Exp Optom.* **82**, 4–10.
11 Hamano H, Kitano J, Mitsunaga K, *et al.* (1985). Adverse effects of contact lens wear in a large Japanese population. *CLAO J.* **11**, 141–146.
12 Romanchuk KG (1982). Fluorescein. Physicochemical factors affecting its fluorescence. *Surv Ophthalmol.* **26**, 269–276.
13 Vaughan DG (1955). The contamination of fluorescein solutions – with special reference to *Pseudomonas aeruginosa*. *Am J Ophthalmol.* **39**, 55–60.
14 Lemp MA and Hamill JR Jr (1973). Factors affecting tear film breakup in normal eyes. *Arch Ophthalmol.* **89**, 103–105.
15 Refojo MF, Korb DR and Silverman HI (1972). Clinical evaluation of a new fluorescent dye for hydrogel lenses. *J Am Optom Assoc.* **43**, 321–326.
16 Davis LJ and Lebow KA (2000). Noninfectious corneal staining. In: *Anterior Segment Complications of Contact Lens Wear*, p. 67–94, Ed. Silbert JA. (Boston: Butterworth–Heinemann).
17 Korb DR and Herman JP (1979). Corneal staining subsequent to sequential fluorescein instillations. *J Am Optom Assoc.* **50**, 316–322.

18 Manning FJ, Wehrly SR and Foulks GN (1995). Patient tolerance and ocular surface staining characteristics of lissamine green versus rose bengal. *Ophthalmology* **102**, 1953–1957.

19 Emran N and Sommer A (1979). Lissamine green staining in the clinical diagnosis of xerophthalmia. *Arch Ophthalmol.* **97**, 2333–2335.

20 Korb DR and Korb JME (1970) A study of three and nine o'clock staining after unilateral lens removal. *J Am Optom Assoc.* **41**, 7–14.

21 van der Worp E, De Brabander J, Swarbrick H, *et al.* (2003). Corneal desiccation in rigid contact lens wear: 3- and 9-o'clock staining. *Optom Vis Sci.* **80**, 280–290.

22 Jones LW and Jones DA (2001). Slit lamp biomicroscopy. In: *The Cornea. Its Examination in Contact Lens Practice*, p. 1–49, Ed. Efron N. (Oxford: Butterworth–Heinemann).

23 Kline LN and DeLuca TJ (1975). An analysis of arcuate staining with B&L Soflens. Part II. *J Am Optom Assoc.* **46**, 1129–1132.

24 Zadnik K and Mutti DO (1985). Inferior arcuate staining in soft contact lens wearers. *Int Contact Lens Clin.* **12**, 110–113.

25 Little SA and Bruce AS (1995). Role of the post-lens tear film in the mechanism of inferior arcuate staining with ultrathin hydrogel lenses. *CLAO J.* **21**, 175–181.

26 Watanabe K and Hamano H (1997). The typical pattern of superficial punctate keratopathy in wearers of extended wear disposable contact lenses. *CLAO J.* **23**, 134–137.

27 Sankaridurg PR, Sweeney DF, Sharma S, *et al.* (1999). Adverse events with extended wear of disposable hydrogels: Results for the first 13 months of lens wear. *Ophthalmology* **106**, 1671–1680.

28 Holden BA, Stephenson A, Stretton S, *et al.* (2001). Superior epithelial arcuate lesions with soft contact lens wear. *Optom Vis Sci.* **78**, 9–12.

29 Malinovsky V, Pole JJ, Pence NA and Howard D (1989). Epithelial splits of the superior cornea in hydrogel contact lens patients. *Int Contact Lens Clin.* **16**, 252–256.

30 Jalbert I, Sweeney DF and Holden BA (2001). Epithelial split associated with wear of a silicone hydrogel contact lens. *CLAO J.* **27**, 231–233.

31 O'Hare N, Stapleton F, Naduvilath T, *et al.* (2002). Interaction between the contact lens and the ocular surface in the etiology of superior epithelial arcuate lesions. *Adv Exp Med Biol.* **506**, 973–980.

32 Dumbleton K (2003). Noninflammatory silicone hydrogel contact lens complications. *Eye Contact Lens* **29S**, 186–189.

33 Madigan MC and Holden BA (1992). Reduced epithelial adhesion after extended contact lens wear correlates with reduced hemidesmosome density in cat cornea. *Invest Ophthalmol Vis Sci.* **33**, 314–323.

34 Wilson G, Ren H, Laurent J (1995) Corneal epithelial fluorescein staining. *J Am Optom Assoc.* **66**, 435–439.

35 Efron N and Veys J (1992). Defects in disposable contact lenses can compromise ocular integrity. *Int Contact Lens Clin.* **19**, 8–18.

36 Swarbrick HA and Holden BA (1987). Rigid gas permeable lens binding: Significance and contributing factors. *Am J Optom Physiol Opt.* **64**, 815–823.

37 Barr JT (1985), Peripheral corneal desiccation staining – lens materials and designs. *Int Contact Lens Clin.* **12**, 139–142.

38 Holden BA, Sweeney DF and Seger RG (1986). Epithelial erosions caused by thin high water contact lenses. *Clin Exp Optom.* **69**, 103–106.

39 Mirejovsky D, Patel AS and Young G (1993). Water properties of hydrogel contact lens materials: A possible predictive model for corneal desiccation staining. *Biomaterials* **14**, 1080–1088.

40 Ang JH and Efron N (1990). Corneal hypoxia and hypercapnia during contact lens wear. *Optom Vis Sci.* **67**, 512–521.

41 Refojo MF (1976). Reversible binding of chlorhexidine gluconate to hydrogel contact lenses. *Contact Intraocul Lens Med J.* **2**, 47–50.

42 Paugh JR, Brennan NA and Efron N (1988). Ocular response to hydrogen peroxide. *Am J Optom Physiol Opt.* **65**, 91–98.

43 Morgan PB and Efron N (2003). Trends in UK contact lens prescribing 2003. *Optician* **225**(5404), 34–35.

44 Lowe R, Vallas V and Brennan NA (1992). Comparative efficacy of contact lens disinfection solutions. *CLAO J.* **18**, 34–40.

45 Courtney RC and Lee JM (1982). Predicting ocular intolerance of a contact lens solution by use of a filter system enhancing fluorescein staining detection. *Int Contact Lens Clin.* **9**, 302–307.

46 Woods CA and Efron N (1996). Regular replacement of rigid contact lenses alleviates binding to the cornea. *Int Contact Lens Clin.* **23**, 13–18.

47 Itoi M, Kim O, Kimura T, *et al.* (1995). Effect of sodium hyaluronate ophthalmic solution on peripheral staining of rigid contact lens wearers. *CLAO J.* **21**, 261–264.

48 McNally JJ, Chalmers R and Payor R (1987). Corneal desiccation staining with thin high water contact lenses. *Clin Exp Optom.* **70**, 106–111.

EPITHELIAL MICROCYSTS

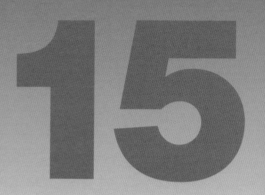

The first report of the appearance of corneal epithelial microcysts in association with contact lens wear was published in 1976 in the *British Journal of Ophthalmology* by Ruben *et al.*[1] As is outlined in this chapter, these authors were correct in surmising that "Corneal microcysts are evidence of chronic changes in the ... epithelium ...". This observation was confirmed in 1978 by Zantos and Holden[2] (who used the term 'microvesicles') in a report of a clinical trial, and in 1979 by Josephson[3] in a published case report. Numerous scientific papers since then have carefully documented, and in many cases quantified, the appearance of microcysts in patients wearing different types of contact lenses.

Epithelial microcysts can be observed readily with the slit-lamp biomicroscope (*Figure 15.1*). This sign is considered to be an important indicator of chronic metabolic stress in the corneal epithelium in response to contact lens wear.

Prevalence

As many as 10 microcysts[4–6] can be observed in the corneal epithelium of about 50% of non-wearers of contact lenses.[7] Thus, the appearance of a small number of microcysts in a contact lens wearer should be considered a normal occurrence.

A number of authors have published estimates, summarized in *Table 15.1*, of the prevalence of a significant microcyst response in association with various types and modalities of lens wear;[1,4,8–17]. Bearing in mind the different methodologies, lens types and study durations employed by the various authors, the concordance of estimates of prevalence is good. In general, a lower prevalence of microcysts is associated with daily wear of contact lenses, compared with hydrogel extended lens wear. The prevalence of microcysts associated with both hydrogel lens extended wear and low-*Dk* rigid lens extended wear approaches 100%, and is zero with silicone hydrogel lenses.

Signs and Symptoms

Slit-lamp biomicroscope appearance

Microcysts can be seen in the central and paracentral cornea at low magnification (×15). They appear as minute scattered gray opaque dots with focal illumination and as transparent refractile inclusions with indirect retroillumination (*Figure 15.2*). Microcysts are often said to be irregular in shape, but all of the photomicrographs of microcysts examined by this author suggest that they are generally of a uniform spherical or ovoid shape. Zantos[18] suggested that they can vary in size from 15 to 50 μm[3]; however, microcysts as large as the full thickness of the epithelium (50–75 μm) have not been reported, so it is likely that microcysts are in the order of 5–30 μm in diameter.

Careful observation at high magnification (×40) is required to differentiate epithelial microcysts from other epithe-

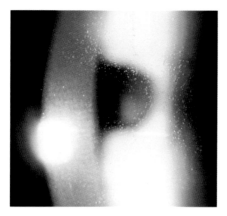

Figure 15.1

Extensive formation of epithelial microcysts, which can be clearly seen against the background of the pupil margin.

Table 15.1
Prevalence of contact lens-induced epithelial microcysts*

Lens type	Mode of lens wear	Lens Dk	Prevalence of microcysts (%)
No lens wear	–	–	26[4]
PMMA	DW	Zero	29[4]
Rigid	DW	'Low'	29[8]
	DW	'High'	0.7[17]
	EW	'Very low'	97[4]
	EW	'Low'	23,[9] 93,[10] 100[4]
	EW	'Low'	84[4]
	EW	'Medium'	29[4]
	EW	'High'	1.6[17]
Hydrogel	DW	'Very low'	0.9,[17] 26,[1] 34[4]
	EW	'Low'	7,[17] 43–77,[11] 71,[10] 86,[4] 97,[4] 100[8,12,13]
	CW	'Low'	41[4]
Silicone hydrogel	CW	'High'	0[14–16]

*PMMA, polymethyl methacrylate; DW, daily wear; EW, extended wear; CW, continuous wear

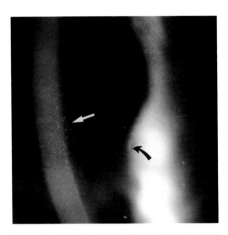

Figure 15.2
Epithelial microcysts appear as gray dots in focal illumination (white arrow) and refractile inclusions in retroillumination (black arrow)

lial inclusions, such as vacuoles or bullae, which superficially take on a similar appearance. The preferred observation technique is marginal retroillumination. The observation and illumination arms should be set at least 45° apart. A 2 mm wide beam should be directed to one of the lateral margins of the pupil so that, when focused on the cornea, the background is split evenly between the illuminated iris and the black pupil. Microcysts are then observed readily in the region of the epithelium that lies in front of the border of the iris and pupil. By slowly scanning laterally from side to side, an overall estimate of the number of microcysts can be derived.

The greater the number of microcysts, the greater is the probability of detecting slight superficial punctate staining, which represents a breaking open of the anterior epithelial surface as microcysts emerge from the deeper layers and are expunged from the cornea.

Once it has been established under high magnification (×40) that the inclusions being observed are indeed microcysts (see Differential diagnosis below), the severity of the overall response can be quantified by once again observing the cornea at a low enough magnification for it to fill the field of view (perhaps ×10 magnification). By scanning back and forth with a 1 mm vertical beam, it is possible to view the microcysts in direct focal illumination. Holden *et al.*[4] advocate quantifying the severity of a microcyst response by counting the number of microcysts, which at this low level of magnification

appear as minute gray dots. An alternative strategy is to grade the response using a grading scale for epithelial microcysts, such as that provided in Appendix A.

Optical effects

Epithelial microcysts display a characteristic optical phenomenon known as 'reversed illumination' when viewed using the above observation technique; that is, the distribution of light within the microcyst is opposite to the light distribution of the background[18] (*Figure 15.3*). It must be emphasized that the illuminated optic section of the cornea adjacent to the area of interest must be ignored; that is, concentrate only on the microcyst with respect to the brightness and darkness of background features (the pupil and iris). Other inclusions (such as vacuoles and bullae) or mechanical epithelial defects (such as dimple veiling, which creates fluid-filled epithelial pits) display 'unreversed illumination' (*Figure 15.3*).

Simple optical principles can be used to demonstrate the significance of the optical appearance of microcysts and other epithelial inclusions (*Figure 15.4*). The 'reversed illumination' appearance indicates that the inclusion acts as a converging refractor; therefore, it must consist of material that is of a higher refractive index than the surrounding epithelium.[19] Conversely, the 'unreversed illumination' appearance indicates that the inclusion acts as a diverging refractor; therefore, it must consist of material that is of a lower refractive index than the surrounding epithelium.

The inclusions observed predominantly in association with all forms of contact

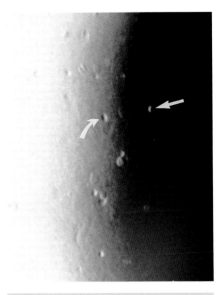

Figure 15.3
High magnification slit-lamp photomicrograph showing microcysts (displaying reversed illumination; curved arrow) and vacuoles (displaying unreversed illumination; straight arrow)

lens wear and that display characteristic patterns in terms of the time course of onset and resolution are those that display reversed illumination. These observations and features, together with our current understanding of the pathology and etiology of the microcyst response, allow inclusions that display reversed illumination to be defined as 'microcysts'.

Vision

Visual acuity is generally unaffected by microcysts, although in extreme cases (the number of microcysts approaches

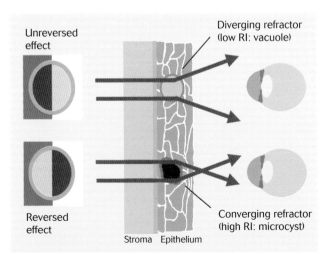

Unreversed effect

Reversed effect

Diverging refractor (low RI: vacuole)

Converging refractor (high RI: microcyst)

Stroma   Epithelium

Figure 15.4
Optical theory illustrating how (top) vacuoles act as diverging refractors and display unreversed illumination, and (bottom) microcysts act as converging refractors and display reversed illumination (after Zantos[18]). RI, refractive index

200) there might be a slight loss of vision. Zantos and Holden[2] reported a case in which vision decreased by one line of acuity.

Comfort

Microcysts are asymptomatic: patients are unaware that they have a microcyst response. Patients who display an extensive microcystic response may experience some ocular discomfort and lens intolerance; however, this is likely to be the result of concurrent pathology. For example, a patient with a severe microcyst response may also have a mild anterior uveal reaction as part of an overall hypoxia-driven syndrome, which could cause ocular pain.

Time course of onset

Microcysts can be detected as early as 1 week after commencing extended lens wear;[20] however, the rate of onset is generally slow and microcysts do not begin to appear in significant numbers until lenses have been worn for about 2 months. The number of microcysts then increases at a more rapid rate over the next 2–4 months[5,16] (*Figure 15.5*). Fonn and Holden[10] reported that the prevalence of microcysts in new patients fitted with extended wear hydrogel lenses was 5% after 5 weeks, 33% after 8 weeks and 71% after 13 weeks.

The number of microcysts eventually reach a steady-state level, although cyclic patterns of microcysts have been reported in some patients.[5]

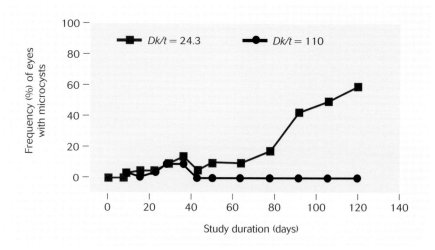

Figure 15.5

Percentage of eyes that develop epithelial microcysts over 140 days while wearing low *Dk/t* (red) and high *Dk/t* (blue) lenses (after Fonn et al.[16])

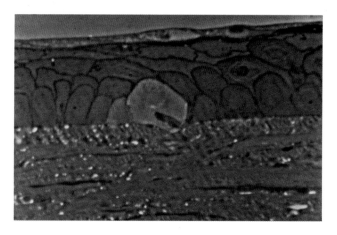

Figure 15.6

Epithelial microcyst forming in the basal epithelium (rabbit model)

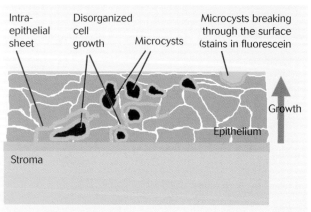

Intra-epithelial sheet | Disorganized cell growth | Microcysts | Microcysts breaking through the surface (stains in fluorescein | Growth | Epithelium | Stroma

Figure 15.7

Pathogenesis of epithelial microcysts, which are formed in the basal epithelium and transported anteriorly as the epithelium grows in that direction

Pathology

The optical phenomenon of reversed illumination, which microcysts display, suggests that they contain material of a higher refractive index than the surrounding tissue.[19,21] Bergmanson[22] postulated that microcysts represent an extracellular accumulation of broken down cellular material trapped in the basal epithelial layers. In a process similar to that which occurs in Cogan's microcystic dystrophy,[23] the epithelial basement membrane reduplicates and folds to form intraepithelial sheets that eventually detach from the basement membrane and encapsulate the cellular debris.

Based on her findings of the effects of 15 months of soft lens extended wear in cats, Madigan[24] suggested that microcysts are not an accumulation of extracellular debris, but rather represent apoptotic (dead) cells which either become phagocytosed (ingested) by living neighboring cells, or remain involuted in the intercellular spaces (*Figure 15.6*).

Figure 15.7 illustrates the likely pathologic process by which microcysts are produced. Microcysts are thought to originate in the deepest layers of the epithelium, where they are difficult to observe because they are only partially formed. They are then carried to the surface of the epithelium, which is constantly growing in the anterior direction. Microcysts that approach the corneal surface are observed more easily because they are now fully formed. They eventually break through the epithelial surface, to leave a minute pit that stains with fluorescein.

Etiology

An abundance of evidence now exists to suggest that microcysts primarily represent visible evidence of chronic metabolic tissue stress and altered cellular growth patterns caused by the direct and/or indirect (acidosis) effects of hypoxia and/or hypercapnia.[25] The primary evidence to support this theory is that the prevalence of microcysts, as well as the number of microcysts present, correlates with the modality of lens wear (more microcysts occur with extended versus daily wear),[4] length of lens wear (the number of microcysts increases with length of wear)[1,10] and the gas transmissibility (Dk/t) of the lens (lenses of lower Dk/t induce more microcysts).[4,26]

Holden *et al.*[12] demonstrated that, after 5 years of soft lens extended wear, the epithelium suffers a 15% reduction in oxygen uptake and a 6% reduction in thickness (*Figure 15.8*). These findings concur with the observation of Hamano *et al.*[27] that hydrogel lenses cause a 94% suppression of mitosis after only 48 hours in rabbit cornea. Therefore, microcysts indicate that the corneal epithelium is not respiring or growing normally.

Other factors have been suggested as playing a role in the etiology of microcysts. Efron and Veys[20] provided evidence that lens-induced mechanical trauma can produce microcysts. Also,

Rah *et al.*[28] reported a significant microcyst response after 3 months of reverse geometry rigid lens wear in an orthokeratology study. Reverse geometry lenses exert forces on the cornea to change the corneal shape via a combination of direct mechanical effects and indirect fluid forces. Dart[29] suggested that microcysts are a toxic response to preservatives or other foreign substances in contact lens care solutions; however, this is unlikely because microcysts have been observed in patients who use disposable lenses for which no preservatives are used.

Management

While the actual presence of microcysts is not thought to be dangerous, their existence in large numbers is worrying as this represents epithelial metabolic distress. Based on the working hypothesis that the severity of the microcyst response is related to the level of hypoxia and/or hypercapnia induced by lens wear, a variety of strategies can be employed in an attempt to minimize the number of microcysts:

- Increase Dk/t – the number of microcysts diminishes if lenses of higher Dk/t are fitted.[4,26]
- Decrease the frequency of overnight wear – the number of microcysts diminishes if lenses are worn only one or two nights per week, instead of every night.[30]
- Increase the frequency of lens replacement – this strategy is controversial. Pritchard *et al.*[31] fitted 119 non-wearers of contact lens with 0.04 mm thick

hydroxyethyl methacrylate (HEMA; water content, 38%) lenses and randomly assigned them to 1 or 3 month replacement schedules or a non-replacement (control) group. The lenses were worn on a daily wear basis only and a single multipurpose solution was prescribed for cleaning and disinfection. Over a 2 year period, significantly fewer subjects in the groups with more regular replacement exhibited microcysts. In contrast to this finding, Grant *et al.*[30] reported that the frequency of lens disposal had no effect on the cumulative hypoxic microcyst response of the cornea.

- Change from extended wear to daily wear – the number of microcysts diminishes if lenses are not worn overnight.[4]
- Change from hydrogel to rigid lenses – rigid lenses induce fewer microcysts than hydrogel lenses of the same Dk/t because, first, corneal oxygenation beneath rigid lenses is enhanced by the blink-activated tear pump that does not function with soft lenses and, second, rigid lenses leave a significant area of the cornea exposed directly to the atmosphere.[4,10]
- Change to silicone hydrogel lenses – these lenses have such a high Dk/t that hypoxia is obviated and there is no microcyst response.[14–16]
- Change to hyperpermeable rigid lenses – these lenses also have a very high Dk/t and negligible microcyst response.[17]
- Avoid defective lenses – since lens defects are known to induce epithelial microcysts, the fitting of lenses that can induce mechanical trauma to the cornea should be avoided.[20]
- Avoid reverse geometry lens fits – reverse geometry rigid lenses induce a microcyst response after 3 months;[28] this adverse response can be avoided, if significant, by fitting conventional lenses instead.

It is perhaps also worth noting strategies that are unlikely to be successful at alleviating the microcyst response. Kenyon *et al.*[8] demonstrated that the number of microcysts was unaffected by the wearing schedule (lens removal every 4, 7, 14 or 28 days); thus, altering the extended wear overnight removal schedule is of no benefit. The number of microcysts is unaffected by the solutions used in conjunction with lens wear, so changing the lens maintenance system similarly fails to alleviate the microcyst response.

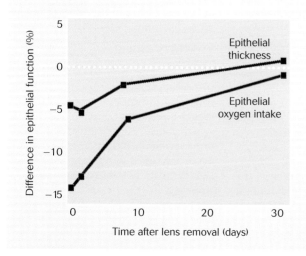

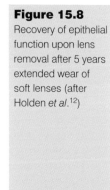

Figure 15.8

Recovery of epithelial function upon lens removal after 5 years extended wear of soft lenses (after Holden *et al.*[12])

Prognosis

Ceasing hydrogel extended lens wear

The prognosis for eliminating micro-cysts is good, although the immediate response after ceasing lens wear may alarm the unwary clinician. Holden *et al.*[12] observed an average of 17 micro-cysts in the corneal epithelium of 27 patients who had worn hydrogel lenses of high water content on an extended wear basis for 5 years. On lens removal, the number of microcysts at first *increased* to a peak of 34 after 7 days; the number of microcysts then decreased gradually toward total recovery within 3 months[3] (*Figure 15.9*). This phenomenon – of an initial increase followed by a decrease in the microcyst response – was noted earlier by Zantos.[18]

The initial increase and subsequent decrease in the number of microcysts after cessation of lens wear is thought to result from the following mechanism. When the lens is removed, epithelial metabolism begins to return to normal, as evidenced by the recovery of epithelial oxygen consumption and thickness (refer again to *Figure 15.8*). Regular cell mitosis resumes. This resurgence in epithelial metabolism and growth results in an accelerated removal of cellular debris (formation of microcysts) and a rapid movement of microcysts toward the surface. As microcysts are more visible in the superficial epithelium (as a consequence of being fully formed), more microcysts are observed a few days after lens removal.

As the epithelium continues to function normally, the remaining microcysts are brought to the surface. In the absence of further microcystic development, the number of microcysts gradually decreases until they are eliminated completely from the cornea.

Microcyst 'rebound'

A phenomenon known as 'microcyst rebound' has been observed in about 33% of patients who are re-fitted from low *Dk/t* lenses to silicone hydrogel lenses or hyperpermeable rigid lenses. The patients develop large numbers of microcysts within the first few weeks of being refitted; the number of microcysts then decreases to normal levels over the following month.[6]

The mechanism for this reaction is the same as that which underpins the normal process of recovery after ceasing

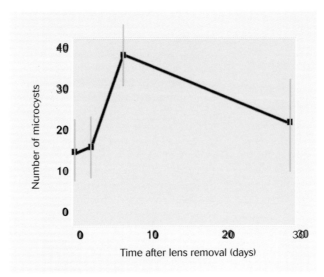

Figure 15.9
Pattern of recovery of epithelial microcysts upon lens removal after 5 years extended wear of soft lenses (after Holden *et al.*[12])

wear of low *Dk/t* lenses, as described above. That is, silicone hydrogel lenses or hyperpermeable rigid lenses have such high *Dk/t* values that it is as though lenses are not being worn. In the absence of ongoing hypoxic stress while wearing silicone hydrogel lenses or hyperpermeable rigid lenses, the number of microcysts at first increases and then decreases, in a similar time course to that shown in *Figure 15.9*. It is therefore not necessary to discontinue lens wear with patients who transfer from low to high *Dk/t* lenses because the increase in microcysts is transitory.[6]

Differential Diagnosis

On casual observation, it is easy to overlook epithelial microcysts, which can take on the appearance of tear film debris. A differential diagnosis can be made after a blink; debris is washed across the corneal surface, whereas microcysts remain in a fixed position.

Once it is established that *fixed* entities in the epithelium are being observed, differential diagnosis is more problematic. Microcysts need to be differentiated from vacuoles, bullae, dimple veiling, mucin balls and fluid-filled pits (left behind when mucin balls dislodge). Differential diagnosis can be effected by considering the size, shape, color, distribution and optical configuration of the entity being observed, whether or not it stains with fluorescein, and the types of lenses that induce the response. A scheme for applying these considerations to differentiate the above features

is outlined in Chapter 7 and summarized in *Table 7.1*.

Deposits on the endothelium, such as endothelial bedewing, also take on the 'reversed illumination' appearance when viewed using retroillumination; however, these *endothelial* deposits can be differentiated from *epithelial* microcysts by determining, using an optic section, whether they are at the posterior (endothelial) or anterior (epithelial) surface of the cornea.

Microcysts can also be observed in certain dystrophies. For example, Lisch *et al.*[32] described five family members and three unrelated patients (four women, four men, 23–71 years of age) who had a dystrophy of the corneal epithelium. Direct slit-lamp examination showed bilateral or unilateral, gray, band-shaped and feathery opacities that sometimes appeared in whorled patterns. Retroillumination showed intraepithelial, densely crowded, clear microcysts. Light and electron microscopy disclosed diffuse vacuolization of the cytoplasm of epithelial cells in the affected area. Visual acuity was so reduced in three patients that abrasion of the corneal epithelium was performed. The corneal abnormalities recurred within months, with the same reduction in visual acuity as before. The authors found no other ophthalmic irregularities or associated systemic abnormalities and no indication of drug-induced keratopathy.

Interestingly, Lisch *et al.*[32] found that the microcyst response *diminished* noticeably in one patient after he began wearing rigid lenses. Bourne[33] reported a similar phenomenon whereby soft contact lens wear decreased the number of epithelial microcysts in a patient with Meesmann's corneal dystrophy. The reason for this apparent therapeutic effect of contact lenses on microcysts in patients with corneal epithelial dystrophies is unclear.

REFERENCES

1 Ruben M, Brown N, Lobascher D, *et al.* (1976). Clinical manifestations secondary to soft contact lens wear. *Br J Ophthalmol.* **60**, 529–531.

2 Zantos SG and Holden BA (1978). Ocular changes associated with continuous wear of contact lenses. *Aust J Optom.* **61**, 418–426.

3 Josephson JE (1979). Coalescing microcysts after long-term use of extended-wear lenses. *Int Contact Lens Clin.* **6**, 24–28.

4 Holden BA, Grant T, Kotow M, *et al.* (1987). Epithelial microcysts with daily and extended wear of hydrogel and rigid gas permeable contact lenses. *Invest Ophthalmol Vis Sci.* **28S**, 372.

5 Holden BA and Sweeney DF (1991). The significance of the microcyst response: A review. *Optom Vis Sci.* **68**, 703–707.

6 Keay L, Sweeney DF, Jalbert I, *et al.* (2000). Microcyst response to high *Dk/t* silicone hydrogel contact lenses. *Optom Vis Sci.* **77**, 582–585.

7 Hickson S and Papas E (1997). Prevalence of idiopathic corneal anomalies in a non-contact lens-wearing population. *Optom Vis Sci.* **74**, 293–297.

8 Kenyon E, Polse KA and Seger RG (1986). Influence of wearing schedule on extended-wear complications. *Ophthalmology* **93**, 231–236.

9 Polse KA, Rivera RK and Bonanno J (1988). Ocular effects of hard gas-permeable-lens extended wear. *Am J Optom Physiol Opt.* **65**, 358–364.

10 Fonn D and Holden BA (1988). Rigid gas-permeable vs. hydrogel contact lenses for extended wear. *Am J Optom Physiol Opt.* **65**, 536–542.

11 Fonn D, Gauthier C and Sorbara L (1990). Adverse response rates in concurrent short-term extended wear and daily wear clinical trials of hydrogel lenses. *Int Contact Lens Clin.* **17**, 217–223.

12 Holden BA, Sweeney DF, Vannas A, *et al.* (1985). Effects of long-term extended contact lens wear on the human cornea. *Invest Ophthalmol Vis Sci.* **26**, 1489–1501.

13 Humphreys JA, Larke JR and Parrish ST (1980). Microepithelial cysts observed in extended contact-lens wearing subjects. *Br J Ophthalmol.* **64**, 888–889.

14 Sweeney DF (2003). Clinical signs of hypoxia with high-*Dk* soft lens extended wear: Is the cornea convinced? *Eye Contact Lens* **29S**, 22–25.

15 Morgan PB and Efron N (2002). Comparative clinical performance of two silicone hydrogel contact lenses for continuous wear. *Clin Exp Optom.* **85**, 183–192.

16 Fonn D, MacDonald KE, Richter D and Pritchard N (2002). The ocular response to extended wear of a high *Dk* silicone hydrogel contact lens. *Clin Exp Optom.* **85**, 176–182.

17 Gleason W, Tanaka H, Albright RA and Cavanagh HD (2003). A 1-year prospective clinical trial of menicon Z (tisilfocon A) rigid gas-permeable contact lenses worn on a 30-day continuous wear schedule. *Eye Contact Lens* **29**, 2–9.

18 Zantos SG (1983). Cystic formations in the corneal epithelium during extended wear of contact lenses. *Int Contact Lens Clin.* **10**, 128–134.

19 Bron AJ and Tripathi RC (1973). Cystic disorders of the corneal epithelium. I. Clinical aspects. *Br J Ophthalmol.* **57**, 361–375.

20 Efron N and Veys J (1992). Defects in disposable contact lenses can compromise ocular integrity. *Int Contact Lens Clin.* **19**, 8–18.

21 Tripathi RC and Bron AJ (1973). Cystic disorders of the corneal epithelium. II. Pathogenesis. *Br J Ophthalmol.* **57**, 376–390.

22 Bergmanson JP (1987). Histopathological analysis of the corneal epithelium after contact lens wear. *J Am Optom Assoc.* **58**, 812–818.

23 Cogan DG, Kuwabara T, Donaldson DD and Collins E (1974). Microcystic dystrophy of the cornea. A partial explanation for its pathogenesis. *Arch Ophthalmol.* **92**, 470–474.

24 Madigan M (1989). *Cat and Monkey as Models for Extended Hydrogel Contact Lens Wear in Humans*. PhD Thesis (Sydney: University of New South Wales).

25 Covey M, Sweeney DF, Terry R, *et al.* (2001). Hypoxic effects on the anterior eye of high-*Dk* soft contact lens wearers are negligible. *Optom Vis Sci.* **78**, 95–99.

26 Rivera RK and Polse KA (1991). Corneal response to different oxygen levels during extended wear. *CLAO J.* **17**, 96–101.

27 Hamano H, Hori M, Hamano T, *et al.* (1983). Effects of contact lens wear on mitosis of corneal epithelium and lactate content in aqueous humor of rabbit. *Jpn J Ophthalmol.* **27**, 451–458.

28 Rah MJ, Jackson JM, Jones LA, *et al.* (2002). Overnight orthokeratology: Preliminary results of the Lenses and Overnight Orthokeratology (LOOK) study. *Optom Vis Sci.* **79**, 598–605.

29 Dart J (1986). Complications of extended wear hydrogel contact lenses. *Contax* March/April, 11–16.

30 Grant T, Chong MS and Holden BA (1988). Which is best for the eye: Daily wear, 2 nights or 6 nights? *Am J Optom Physiol Opt.* **65S**, 40.

31 Pritchard N, Fonn D and Weed K (1996). Ocular and subjective responses to frequent replacement of daily wear soft contact lenses. *CLAO J.* **22**, 53–59.

32 Lisch W, Steuhl KP, Lisch C, *et al.* (1992). A new, band-shaped and whorled microcystic dystrophy of the corneal epithelium. *Am J Ophthalmol.* **114**, 35–44.

33 Bourne WM (1986). Soft contact lens wear decreases epithelial microcysts in Meesmann's corneal dystrophy. *Trans Am Ophthalmol Soc.* **84**, 170–182.

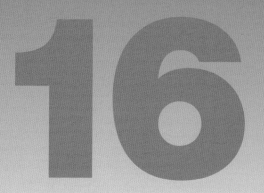

A small number of vacuoles and/or bullae can sometimes be observed in the corneas of contact lens wearers. Although they appear to be clinically innocuous, vacuoles and bullae can be confused with other small epithelial inclusions that have potentially more serious clinical ramifications, and it is for this reason that their clinical presentation is given due consideration in this book.

One of the earliest recorded visual disturbances of contact lens wear was the appearance of haloes. Research conducted periodically throughout the past 50 years has concluded that the source of these haloes is a pathologic disturbance to the corneal epithelium, in the form of edema.[1-7] Epithelial vacuoles and/or bullae may represent an exaggerated clinical manifestations of the tissue abnormalities that cause epithelial edema.

Signs and Symptoms

Gleason et al.[8] monitored the level of epithelial edema in patients who wore various lens types over a 12 month period (Figure 16.1). Epithelial edema was found to occur at an incidence

(expressed as the percentage of eyes per year) of 0.3% for daily wear of superpermeable rigid lenses, 1.1% for extended wear of superpermeable rigid lenses, 1.0% for daily wear low Dk (58% water content) hydrogel lenses and 3.6% for extended wear low Dk (58% water content) hydrogel lenses.

Vacuoles

According to Hickson and Papas,[9] epithelial vacuoles can be observed in 10% of the normal (not wearing lenses) population. Zantos[10] reported that the prevalence of vacuoles in patients wearing low Dk/t extended wear hydrogel lenses is about 32%. He also suggested that this value may be higher in aphakic patients.

When viewed under high magnification with the slit-lamp biomicroscope, vacuoles appear to be spherical bodies located within the corneal epithelium, about the same size as epithelial microcysts (5–30 µm in diameter). They are almost perfectly round in shape and have distinct edges.[10] When viewed using indirect illumination against the background of a dark pupil and illuminated iris, vacuoles display 'unreversed illumination'; that is, the distribution of light within the vacuole is the same as that of the background (Figure 16.2).

Zantos[10] noted that fewer than 10 vacuoles were observed in a given eye of a patient wearing hydrogel lenses on an extended wear basis. He noted that they may occur concurrently with – but apparently unrelated to – microcysts in the same eye (see Figure 15.3).

Vacuoles are usually observed toward the mid-periphery of the cornea. They occur as discrete units in most cases, but occasionally are observed in clusters of two or four vacuoles. Apart from this, there is no particular pattern or distribution. Single epithelial vacuoles are sometimes observed in non-lens wearers, but almost invariably these are

located at the corneal periphery.[10] A curious feature of vacuoles is that they tend to occur in areas that directly overlie corneal opacities in aphakic patients.[10]

Bullae

Zantos[10] described a form of epithelial inclusion that is similar to vacuoles, known as epithelial 'bullae'. The prevalence of bullae in contact lens wearers is very low.[10] On close inspection these are differentiated from vacuoles by their irregular shape (roughly oval) and less distinct edges. They appear as flattened, pebble-like formations in the epithelium. Bullae can present as single entities (Figure 16.3) or they can coalesce into clusters that contain many distinct elements. They can be widespread, or confined to a small area, typically near the centre of the cornea.

The severity of vacuole or bullae formation can be graded using the grading scale for microcysts in Appendix A. Although individual vacuoles and bullae have a different appearance to that

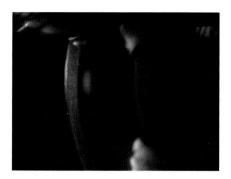

Figure 16.1
Haziness of the epithelium may indicate epithelial edema

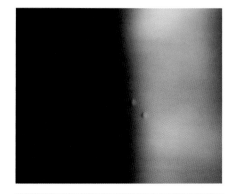

Figure 16.2
Two vacuoles viewed under high magnification (×40) with the slit-lamp biomicroscope. The dark background to the left is the pupil, and the brighter background to the right is the illuminated iris. The vacuoles display unreversed illumination

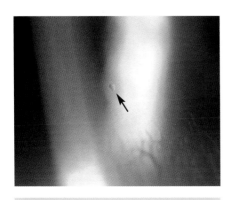

Figure 16.3
A single bulla in a non-lens wearer (arrow)

of microcysts, the progressive increase in the number of microcysts, as depicted in the grading scale, can be considered to have universal application for all forms of epithelial inclusions.

Vision

Vacuoles and bullae as such do not cause vision loss. However, epithelial edema – which may represent a sub-clinical manifestation of vacuoles and bullae – has been demonstrated to reduce contrast sensitivity. Specifically, Cox and Holden[6] demonstrated that osmotically induced epithelial edema produced halo formation, which was associated with a loss of contrast sensitivity (*Figure 16.4*). Furthermore, they demonstrated that the source of the visual disturbance was likely to be edema of the basal cells of the corneal epithelium, which act as a diffraction grating.

Pathology

Inferences from clinical observations

As is the case with microcysts, the pathology of vacuoles and bullae can be inferred only from their optical configuration and clinical appearance. As they display unreversed illumination, their contents must be of a lower refractive index than that of the surrounding epithelium, which is primarily water. Thus, they must be gaseous or liquid in nature. Zantos10 believes that vacuoles are more likely to be gaseous, since the distinct edges of the vacuoles indicate that the refractive index difference between them and the surrounding tissue is greater than would be expected if the vacuoles had a fluid composition.

Zantos[10] has applied the same logic to infer the likely composition of bullae. Since bullae also display unreversed illumination, they also must be of a lower refractive index than that of the surrounding epithelium. However, unlike vacuoles, bullae have indistinct edges, which indicates that the refractive index difference between them and the surrounding medium is not great. Therefore, bullae are more likely to be composed of fluid than gas.

Electron microscopic studies

Bergmanson[11] has demonstrated the co-existence of epithelial edema and thinning after periods of rigid lens wear (*Figure 16.5*). Extracellular edema is evident around the apex of the basal cells. This appearance can be compared with that of the normal cornea (not wearing lenses; *Figure 16.6*). This evidence is consistent with the notion that vision loss and haloes induced by rigid lens wear are caused by lens-induced edema of the basal cells of the corneal epithelium.[7]

Etiology

The etiology of vacuoles and bullae is not known. Zantos[10] suggests that vacuoles may be associated with depressions in the epithelium, as occurs with dimple veiling (*Figure 16.7*); he based this assumption on his observation that dimple veiling has been observed to precede the occurrence of vacuoles. Bullae seem to occur in cases in which there is excessive or persistent edema during contact lens wear, and as such may serve as an indicator of edematous stress induced by contact lenses.[10]

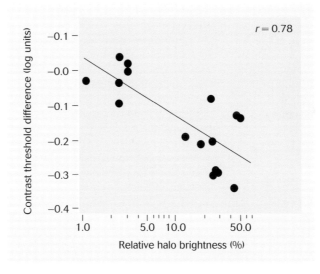

Figure 16.4
Relationship between contrast sensitivity and relative halo brightness (after Cox and Holden[6])

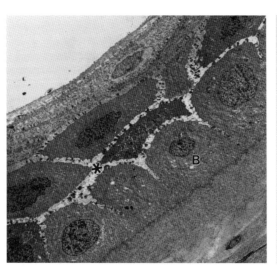

Figure 16.5
Transmission electron micrograph of the epithelium after 24 hours of wear of a polymethyl methacrylate (PMMA) contact lens in a rhesus monkey. This transverse section illustrates epithelial thinning and edema. Epithelial thinning is largely caused by partial collapse of cellular shape; the tall columnar basal cells (B) have become almost cuboidal in shape. The epithelial edema (asterisk) is intercellular with little or no fluid within the cells. Magnification ×5000

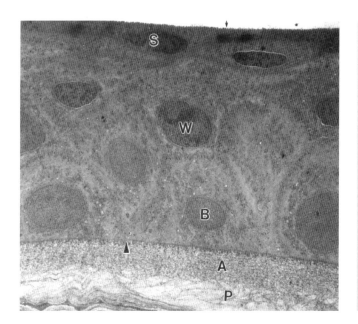

Figure 16.6
Transverse section through a normal epithelium (no lens wear). The epithelial surface is anteriorly lined by microvilli (arrow) and posteriorly by a basement membrane (triangle). The cells that form the epithelium are classified according to their shape and location as basal (B), wing (W) and squamous (S) cells; here the letters 'B', 'W' and 'S' are overlaid on the cell nuclei. Internally, the basement membrane faces the anterior limiting lamina (A), which itself internally merges into the stroma (P). Primate. electron micrograph, magnification ×5100

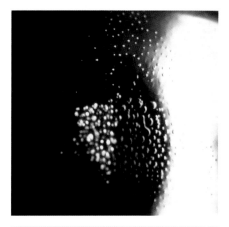

Figure 16.7
Dimple veiling that results from bubbles previously trapped beneath a rigid lens

The etiology of epithelial edema is two-fold. First, epithelial edema follows the traumatic loss of surface epithelial cells. The fluid barrier (zonula occludens) is found between surface epithelial cells and, thus, when it is removed fluid may enter deeper corneal layers. Since the cells fit tightly and attach snugly together, the edema may neither occur instantly nor be widespread. Second, epithelial edema follows hypotonic ocular exposure, which has an inhibiting effect on the fluid barrier. Reflex tears, which are of low tonicity, may disrupt the fluid barrier and provoke epithelial edema, for instance during adaptation to rigid lenses.[11] Note that epithelial edema does not occur in response to lens-induced hypoxia.[12]

Management

Epithelial vacuoles appear to be innocuous and are not apparently associated with any adverse symptoms.[10] It is always prudent, however, to note their appearance on the patient's record card and to monitor the patient carefully to confirm that they eventually disappear.

Although far less common, bullae are potentially more problematic because they may indicate the presence of chronic epithelial edema. This being the case, other tests of epithelial edema should be conducted. This could involve the measurement of corneal sensitivity, which is expected to be reduced.[6] Also, the patient can simply be directed to look at a bright point source of light (e.g., a penlight held at distance of 3 m) in a darkened room, and to report what he or she sees. If the patient reports seeing haloes, the tentative diagnosis of epithelial edema is confirmed. The brighter the haloes, the more extensive the edema.

Hypotonic stress rather than hypoxia is more likely to be the cause of epithelial edema,[6] and the most likely cause of tear hypotonicity is excess lacrimation. Although there are many causes of excess lacrimation (being in a windy environment, emotional tearing, noxious smells, etc.) the most likely cause in a contact lens wearer is lens discomfort. Increased lacrimation during adaptation to rigid contact lenses is an obvious candidate. Should adaptation be especially difficult or prolonged for a patient, reverting to soft lenses is likely to alleviate the problem.

Prognosis

The corneal epithelium has a rapid turnover rate, and cells are constantly moving in the anterior direction, differentiating and eventually sloughing off the corneal surface. By virtue of this process, any inclusion within the epithelium is removed within a few days. Thus, the prognosis for the recovery of vacuoles is good, assuming they occur as the result of an *ad hoc* disturbance to the epithelium.

The prognosis for the recovery from epithelial bullae is also good, assuming that the cause can be identified and removed. Failing that, the presence of chronic edema results in a continual turnover of bullae, which may persist but appear to change location as they are reformed in various regions of affected epithelium.

In severe cases, vacuoles and bullae may break through the epithelial surface *en masse*. *Figure 16.8* is the cornea of a 42-year-old male Caucasian, and highlights the eruption of vacuoles through the anterior layers of the epithelium. The patient had been wearing low-*Dk* hydrogel lenses on an extended wear basis for 3 years. He awoke with a stinging sensation and blurred vision. The epithelial disturbance was characterized by localized edema, staining and poor wetting.

Differential Diagnosis

Vacuoles and bullae need to be differentiated from other inclusions that can

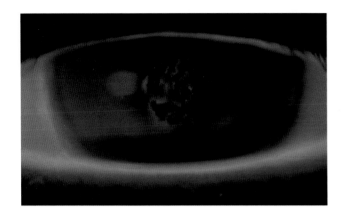

Figure 16.8
Heavy central corneal staining because of vacuoles and bullae breaking through the epithelial surface

be observed in the epithelium of contact lens wearers, such as microcysts, dimple veiling, mucin balls and fluid-filled pits (left behind when mucin balls dislodge). Differential diagnosis can be effected by considering the size, shape, color, distribution and optical configuration of the entity being observed, whether or not it stains with fluorescein, and the types of lenses that induce the response. A scheme to apply these considerations in differentiating the above features is outlined in Chapter 7 and summarized in *Table 7.1*.

REFERENCES

1 Finkelstein IS (1952). The biophysics of corneal scatter and diffraction of light induced by contact lenses. Part I. *Trans Opt Soc (London)* **29**, 185–208.
2 Finkelstein IS (1952). The biophysics of corneal scatter and diffraction of light induced by contact lenses. Part II. *Trans Opt Soc (London)* **29**, 231–259.
3 Smelser GK and Ozanics V (1952). Importance of atmospheric oxygen for maintenance of the optical properties of the human cornea. *Science* **115**, 140.
4 Lambert SR and Klyce SD (1981). The origins of Sattler's veil. *Am J Ophthalmol.* **91**, 51–56.
5 Wilson G and Stevenson R (1981). Corneal recovery from osmotic and anoxic stress. *Am J Optom Physiol Opt.* **58**, 797–802.
6 Cox IG and Holden BA (1990). Can vision loss be used as a quantitative assessment of corneal edema? *Int Contact Lens Clin.* **17**, 176–179.
7 Caldicott A and Charman WN (2002). Diffraction haloes resulting from corneal oedema and epithelial cell size. *Ophthalmic Physiol Opt.* **22**, 209–213.
8 Gleason W, Tanaka H, Albright RA and Cavanagh HD (2003). A 1-year prospective clinical trial of menicon Z (tisilfocon A) rigid gas-permeable contact lenses worn on a 30-day continuous wear schedule. *Eye Contact Lens* **29**, 2–9.
9 Hickson S and Papas E (1997). Prevalence of idiopathic corneal anomalies in a non contact lens-wearing population. *Optom Vis Sci.* **74**, 293–297.
10 Zantos SG (1983). Cystic formations in the corneal epithelium during extended wear of contact lenses. *Int Contact Lens Clin.* **10**, 128–134.
11 Bergmanson JPG (2001). Light and electron microscopy. In: *The Cornea. Its Examination in Contact Lens Practice*, p. 136–177, Ed. Efron N. (Oxford: Butterworth–Heinemann).
12 Wang J, Fonn D, Simpson TL and Jones L (2002). The measurement of corneal epithelial thickness in response to hypoxia using optical coherence tomography. *Am J Ophthalmol.* **133**, 315–319.

Epithelial wrinkling is a severe ocular complication of contact lens wear, and is characterized by the appearance of a series of deep parallel grooves in the corneal surface that give the impression of a 'wrinkled' effect (*Figure 17.1*). This condition was originally described as 'epithelial folds' by Quinn,[1] and was later more fully described by Lowe and Brennan,[2] who coined the term 'corneal wrinkling'. Epstein[3] refers to this condition as 'epithelial wrinkling'.

As is discussed under 'Pathology' below, there is a difference of opinion in the literature as to the depth of the wrinkles in the cornea. Specifically, it is unclear whether the phenomenon occurs purely at the level of the epithelium, or whether there is also some stromal involvement. Since two of the above-mentioned authors[1,3] have adopted a name for this condition that implies primarily epithelial involvement, and two authors have adopted the word 'wrinkling',[2,3] the term 'epithelial wrinkling' is used in this book. It follows, therefore, that this condition is discussed in this section on 'Corneal epithelium'.

Prevalence

Epstein[3] deems epithelial wrinkling to be 'a very rare complication of soft lens wear'. However, in a prospective clinical trial of 330 subjects wearing disposable hydrogel lenses on a six-night extended wear and replacement schedule, Sankaridurg *et al.*[4] found a prevalence of 1.7 events of 'corneal wrinkling' per year of lens wear, which eventually resolved without sequelae. It is unclear whether Sankaridurg *et al.*[4] were observing true epithelial wrinkling as characterized in this chapter, or an unrelated form of pathology, such as edematous folds in the deeper corneal layers.

Signs

The case described by Lowe and Brennan[2] took the form of two linear wave patterns of fluorescein that pooled across the central cornea and intersected at an angle of 70° (*Figure 17.2*). Several discrete spots were observed at the points of intersection of the two wave patterns. The intensity of fluores-

cein within the troughs of the wrinkles was observed to increase with time following the blink. The patient was wearing a very thin (0.036 mm center thickness) mid-water content (52.5% water) custom-designed hydrogel lens in one eye. The lens was said to be made of a highly elastic material ('Snoflex 50', Smith & Nephew, Australia), with a power of –0.50D and a back optic zone radius (BOZR) of 8.20 mm. The patient had a keratometer reading of 8.00/7.92 mm; thus, the lens was fitted very steep in relation to the cornea.

Lowe and Brennan[2] assessed the extent of corneal distortion by observing the reflected mires of an optical keratoscope. The formation of ridges and troughs can be seen to mimic clearly the observed fluorescein pattern (*Figure 17.3*).

Burnett-Hodd[5] reported the case of a patient wearing a very thin, custom-designed hydrogel toric lens. The lenses had a BOZR of 7.40 mm and the patient had a mean keratometer reading of 7.80 mm. The reason for fitting this lens very steep in relation to the cornea was to stop the rotation of the lens that had occurred with flatter designs. These

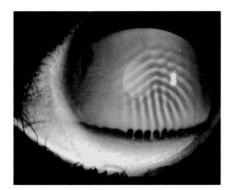

Figure 17.1
Epithelial wrinkling with two sets of furrows arranged orthogonally

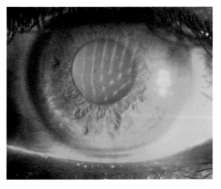

Figure 17.2
Epithelial wrinkling that displays a remarkably similar pattern to that shown in *Figure 17.1*

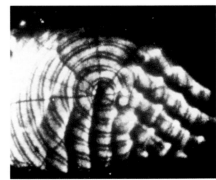

Figure 17.3
Photokeratogram of a cornea that displays epithelial wrinkling

lenses displayed profound wrinkling during wear, an effect that is shown for one eye in *Figure 17.4*. When this lens was removed and fluorescein instilled, a series of linear wrinkles could be observed both in white light (*Figure 17.5*) and cobalt blue light (*Figure 17.6*), which corresponding to the previously observed wrinkling of the lens.

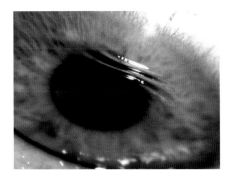

Figure 17.4
Wrinkling of a contact lens

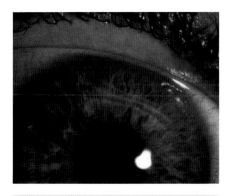

Figure 17.5
Epithelial wrinkling highlighted with fluorescein and observed in white light (same case as shown in *Figure 17.4*)

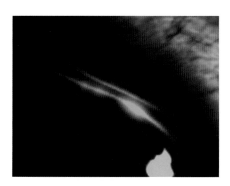

Figure 17.6
Epithelial wrinkling highlighted with fluorescein and observed in cobalt blue light (same case as shown in *Figure 17.4*)

Wrinkles can occur in any orientation, or indeed in multiple orientations in the one eye. In the case reported by Burnett-Hodd[5] (*Figure 17.6*), the wrinkles were at an angle of about 160° (ophthalmic lens axis notation). In another case shown in *Figure 17.7*, the wrinkles are at an angle of about 80°. The wrinkles run in different directions in the same eye in the case depicted in *Figures 17.1* and *17.2*.

Giese[6] described a 17-year-old patient with Marfan's syndrome who developed central epithelial wrinkling in his right eye while he was wearing hydrogel lenses of low water content. No visual discomfort or distortions were noted. The patient was refitted with a non-hydroxyethyl methacrylate (HEMA) hydrogel contact lens, with no further episodes of wrinkling observed during subsequent care of the patient. Although Giese[6] expressed the view that the wrinkling was unrelated to Marfan's syndrome, there may be a link because Marfan's syndrome is primarily a heritable connective tissue disorder. Bowman's layer, which is composed almost entirely of collagen (a connective tissue), is implicated in the appearance of wave-like patterns that mimic epithelial wrinkling induced by contact lenses[7] (see 'Differential diagnosis'). Therefore, the corneas of patients with Marfan's syndrome may well be prone to displaying wrinkle-like patterns when the cornea is subjected to the physical stresses of contact lens wear.

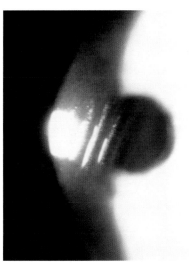

Figure 17.7
Epithelial wrinkling of the central cornea after removal of a 42.5% water-content lens of 0.035 mm center thickness

Symptoms

As one would expect with such a dramatic distortion of the cornea, vision loss in patients who exhibit epithelial wrinkling can be dramatic. It appears that the extent of vision loss is proportional to the degree of epithelial distortion. Lowe and Brennan[2] reported that vision dropped to less than 6/60 within 5 minutes of lens insertion. Burnett-Hodd[5] noted that vision was poor 10 minutes after lens insertion. In the case reported by Quinn,[1] the 15-year-old male reported a gradual reduction in vision over a number of months.

Epithelial wrinkling is also extremely painful, with the time course of discomfort and vision loss occurring in parallel.

Pathology

Lowe and Brennan[2] argue that wrinkling involves the epithelium and anterior stroma. This view is based upon their observations of the extreme variance in intensity of fluorescence across the ridges of a wrinkled cornea (*Figure 17.2*), which implies deep troughs, and the extreme distortion of photokeratometric mires reflected off a wrinkled cornea (*Figure 17.3*). The intensity of the wrinkling pattern increases with time after a blink, which indicates fluorescein pooling within the deep troughs.

With the lens removed from the eye, vision improves momentarily after each blink, and declines rapidly to a steady-state level thereafter.[2] This phenomenon is consistent with the apparent smoothing of the anterior refracting surface immediately after a blink, whereby fresh tears are swiped across the cornea and fill the troughs of the wrinkled epithelium. As the eye is held open, the tears drain from the troughs, to leave an uneven corneal surface that degrades vision.

Epstein[3] draws a distinction between epithelial wrinkling and full-thickness corneal folds. It appears from his analysis that Epstein[3] may be describing different severities of the same condition. A case of severe epithelial wrinkling (and what Epstein[3] might refer to as 'full-thickness epithelial folds') is shown in *Figure 17.8*. When viewed in white light, the vertical furrows are so deep as to give the impression that the whole cornea is involved. The depth of the furrows is confirmed with the aid of fluorescein

(*Figure 17.9*). The extreme distortion of the surface of the contact lens is evident from the photokeratogram shown in *Figure 17.10*. Considerable distortion of the corneal surface can be observed in the keratoscope mires after removal of the lens (*Figure 17.11*).

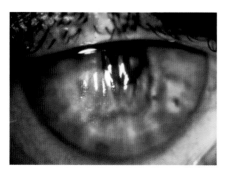

Figure 17.8
Severe epithelial wrinkling observed in white light

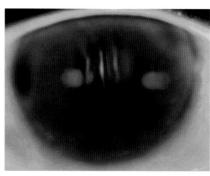

Figure 17.9
Severe epithelial wrinkling highlighted with fluorescein and observed in cobalt blue light (same case as shown in *Figure 17.8*)

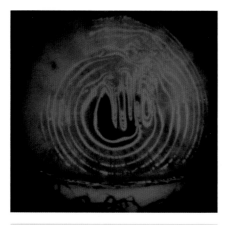

Figure 17.10
Photokeratogram of lens surface that displays a heavy wrinkled pattern (same case as shown in *Figure 17.8*)

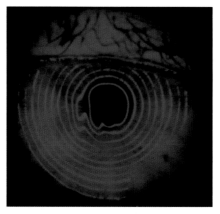

Figure 17.11
Photokeratogram of cornea that displays a severe epithelial wrinkling after lens removal (same case as shown in *Figure 17.8*)

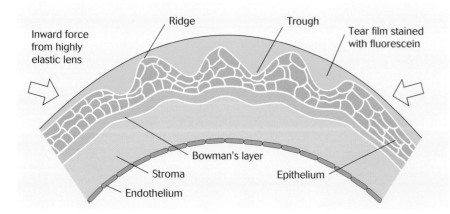

Figure 17.12
The forces that act to cause the corneal tissue to collapse in a concertina-like action. The epithelium and Bowman's layer, and to a lesser extent the anterior stroma, become wrinkled. The posterior stroma is largely unaffected. (Not to scale)

Etiology

It is interesting to observe that in all reported cases of epithelial wrinkling in which the details of the lenses worn are known,[1,2,5] the features of the type of lens that caused the problem were remarkably similar. Specifically, the offending lenses typically exhibited these properties:
- Highly elastic hydrogel material;
- Custom design;
- Extremely thin;
- Mid-water content (50–55% water);
- Steep fitting.

Lowe and Brennan[2] propose that excessive elastic forces draw corneal tissue inward from the limbus, which causes the superficial corneal tissue to collapse in a concertina-like action and so creates a wrinkled appearance (*Figure 17.12*). They suggest that the force is derived from an intrinsic elastic force created when a relatively steep lens is compressed against the eye; in an attempt to return to its original shape, an inward force is created.

If the lens also displays a high propensity for dehydration, lens dehydration (and associated base-curve steepening) and lens-diameter reduction provide an additional inward force. However, in the case reported by Lowe and Brennan,[2] the lens was made of a vinyl pyrrolidone–methyl methacrylate (VP-MMA) copolymer and thus would be categorized using the FDA system as Group II (high water content, non-ionic). Such lenses are characteristically dehydration resistant.[8]

Epithelial wrinkling is observed in patients who wear highly elastic, ultra-thin mid-water content lenses. In the three reported cases discussed in this chapter,[1,2,5] the lenses that induced epithelial wrinkling were either specifically designed by the practitioner or were experimental; that is, they were apparently not standard commercially available products.

Bruce and Brennan[9] suggested that epithelial wrinkling may also have an osmotic etiology in view of the observation of Dixon[10] that complete evaporation of the tear film in normal humans can cause an almost identical epithelial wrinkling and vision loss to that observed in cases of lens-induced epithelial wrinkling.

Lowe and Brennan[2] noted that no wrinkling was observed in subjects who wore the offending lenses overnight; the

Figure 17.12 labels: Ridge, Trough, Tear film stained with fluorescein, Inward force from highly elastic lens, Bowman's layer, Stroma, Epithelium, Endothelium

effect was only observed in subjects who wore the lenses during the day. This observation led Lowe and Brennan[2] to propose that lid movement, and the specific lens–cornea bearing relationship, are integral to the cause of this effect.

Epstein[3] proposes an alternative theory to explain the appearance of epithelial wrinkling. He suggests that epithelial edema is the cause, whereby epithelial swelling pushes the cornea up against the lens such that it folds back on itself. According to Epstein,[3] full-thickness corneal folds are likely to be a combination of mechanical and osmotic pressures that combine to produce both suction and molding forces.

Management

The management protocol for a patient who experiences epithelial wrinkling is to cease lens wear immediately. Patients who suffer from this condition may be alarmed at the extreme discomfort and loss of vision; it is therefore important to reassure patients that this is only a transient problem and that vision and comfort will be restored within 24 hours.

Although the appearance of wrinkling will indeed disappear within 24 hours, the patient should not wear lenses for 1 week as a precaution to allow possible sub-clinical compromise to resolve. The patient should then be refitted with a soft lens that is devoid of inherently high elastic forces. Specifically, lenses should not be designed and fitted in accordance with the combination of parameters listed in 'Etiology' above. True epithelial wrinkling does not occur with rigid lenses, although the pressure induced by rigid lenses can cause a transient pattern of linear formations (see 'Differential diagnosis' below).

Prognosis

The prognosis for recovery of the cornea after an episode of epithelial wrinkling is good. The time course of recovery from epithelial wrinkling has been shown to be related directly to the period of lens wear that induced the changes. Lowe and Brennan[2] noted that epithelial wrinkling took 3, 90 and 240 minutes to recover after 5, 90 and 300 minutes of lens wear, respectively. In the two cases of full-thickness epithelial folds

reported by Epstein,[3] the cornea recovered to normal within about 60 minutes. Epithelial folds took about a week to resolve in the case reported by Quinn.[1]

Differential Diagnosis

A clinical phenomenon that appears remarkably similar to epithelial wrinkling is the Fischer–Schweitzer polygonal mosaic, which can sometimes be observed after rigid lens extended wear, thick hydrogel lens wear or aggressive rubbing of the eyes through the closed eyelid (*Figure 17.13*).[11] This pattern, which may be localized or cover the whole corneal surface, appears as minute branching lines or furrows in the epithelial surface that are revealed with fluorescein. It is thought to result from epithelial groove formation caused by wrinkling of Bowman's membrane during physical deformation of the cornea. The Fischer–Schweitzer mosaic disappears within 10 minutes of removing the initiating corneal stress. The appearance of this mosaic in rigid lens wearers may indicate that the lens exerts undue pressure on the cornea, and an alternative fit might need to be sought. The Fischer–Schweitzer polygonal mosaic is asymptomatic, and in that way can be differentiated from epithelial wrinkling, which is extremely painful.

Tripathi and Bron[7] described the clinicopathologic features and pathogenesis of a chronic secondary mosaic degeneration of the cornea known as the anterior crocodile shagreen of Vogt. According to these authors,[7] the structural basis for a normal anterior corneal mosaic pattern is attributed to the particular arrangement of many prominent collagen lamellae of the anterior stroma. These lamellae take an oblique course to gain insertion into Bowman's layer. Since, at normal intraocular pressure, Bowman's layer is under tension, when viewed from the anterior surface the cornea appears smooth. By releasing the tension, however, a reproducible polygonal ridge pattern becomes manifest. It is suggested that a prolonged phthisical state of the eye is one condition wherein the mosaic pattern may become permanent. As a secondary event, this is followed by irregular calcification of Bowman's layer, which particularly involves the ridges that project into the epithelium. Biomicroscopically, these ridges corresponded to the branching reticular arrangement of the mosaic opacities.[7] This phenomenon is therefore only seen in severely and chronically diseased eyes and is unlikely to be seen in contact lens wearers.

A single large wrinkle, presumed to be in Bowman's membrane, is shown in *Figure 17.14*. This event occurred in a 47-year-old female Caucasian patient, and was seen after 1 month of daily rigid lens wear. The patient suffered no discomfort, but experienced a slight reduction in low contrast visual acuity. It took 2 weeks for the condition to resolve.

REFERENCES

1 Quinn TG (1982). Epithelial folds. *Int Contact Lens Clin.* **9**, 365.
2 Lowe R and Brennan NA (1987). Corneal wrinkling caused by a thin medium water content lens. *Int Contact Lens Clin.* **10**, 403–406.

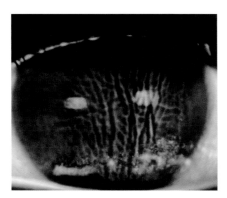

Figure 17.13
Fischer–Schweitzer polygonal mosaic after removal of a thick hydrogel lens

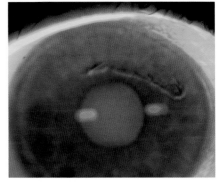

Figure 17.14
A single large horizontal wrinkle in a patient wearing a rigid lens

3 Epstein AB (1996). Contact lens complications (Appendix 4). In: *Specialty Contact Lenses: A Fitter's Guide*, p. 292–293, Ed. Schwartz CA. (Philadelphia: WB Saunders).

4 Sankaridurg PR, Sweeney DF, Sharma S, *et al.* (1999). Adverse events with extended wear of disposable hydrogels: Results for the first 13 months of lens wear. *Ophthalmology* **106**, 1671–1680.

5 Burnett-Hodd (2003). Making the specialist practice special. CIBA Vision Specialist Club Meeting, March 11, 2003. (Coventry: CIBA Vision Specialist Club).

6 Giese MJ (1997). Corneal wrinkling in a hydrogel contact lens wearer with Marfan syndrome. *J Am Optom Assoc.* **68**, 50–54.

7 Tripathi RC and Bron AJ (1975). Secondary anterior crocodile shagreen of Vogt. *Br J Ophthalmol.* **59**, 59–63.

8 Efron N and Morgan PB (1999). Hydrogel contact lens dehydration and oxygen transmissibility. *CLAO J.* **25**, 148–151.

9 Bruce AS and Brennan NA (1990). Corneal pathophysiology with contact lens wear. *Surv Ophthalmol.* **35**, 25–58.

10 Dixon J (1964). Ocular changes due to contact lenses. *Am J Ophthalmol.* **58**, 424–433.

11 Bron AJ and Tripathi RC (1969). Anterior corneal mosaic. Further observations. *Br J Ophthalmol.* **53**, 760–764.

PART VII CORNEAL STROMA

STROMAL EDEMA

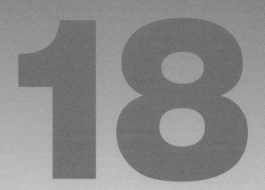

Corneal edema induced by contact lenses was recognized in the first two written accounts of the clinical application of contact lenses over a century ago. In his original treatise on contact lenses, published in 1888, Adolf Fick noted that the cornea became cloudy within hours of insertion of a glass haptic shell.[1] Although Fick would not have been aware of the exact cause of this disturbing pathologic change, it is clear that he was observing corneal edema induced by contact lenses. Even more remarkably, Fick observed that the onset of corneal clouding could be delayed by trapping an air bubble between the lens and cornea.[1]

In his inaugural dissertation to the University of Kiel in Germany in 1889, August Müller provided a graphic subjective description of what was undoubtedly a marked corneal edema induced by contact lenses.[2] Müller correctly identified inadequate tear exchange beneath the lens as the cause of this problem, but was unable to find a solution.

These pioneering works signaled the beginning of the battle against corneal edema – yet, despite numerous significant advances in lens materials, designs, fitting techniques and possible modalities of wear, we are still unable to claim an absolute victory over lens-induced edema.

Definition

Edema refers to an increase in the fluid content of tissue. Since the cornea is only able to swell in the anterior–posterior direction as a result of the collagen fiber network in the stroma, the physical dimensions of the cornea can only increase in that dimension – that is, in thickness. Corneal edema is usually expressed as the percentage increase in corneal thickness. Thus, for example, a cornea that swells from a thickness of 550 µm before lens wear to become 605 µm thick after lens wear has swollen 55 µm, or has experienced 10 per cent edema. As discussed in this chapter, it is typically the corneal stroma that swells. The corneal epithelium can also become edematous, but it usually swells in response to osmotic stress (see Chapter 16), whereas the stroma swells in response to hypoxic stress. As a result of this analysis, it can be seen that in a cornea that suffers from stromal edema only, the percentage increase in total corneal thickness slightly underestimates the percentage increase in stromal thickness.

Laboratory scientists have developed techniques for the precise measurement of corneal thickness and have noted that edema is a reliable and repeatable index of the physiologic integrity of the cornea. Indeed, corneal edema has become established as *the* reference against which other measures of corneal integrity are gauged.

Central Corneal Clouding

Early textbook accounts that described the detection of corneal edema associated with the wearing of contact lenses made from polymethyl methacrylate (PMMA) cited central corneal clouding (CCC) as the key diagnostic criterion to indicate corneal compromise.[3] This condition occurred in patients wearing tightly fitted PMMA lenses that restricted tear exchange beneath the lens and hence created hypoxic edema. A discrete, round area of clouding could be observed clearly in the central cornea (*Figure 18.1*).

CCC indicates a gross level of edema rarely observed in modern contact lens practice. Careful observation of the cornea using a slit-lamp biomicroscope reveals the existence of more subtle signs that can be used to predict the level of edema in response to lens wear. In this chapter, the edema response to contact lens wear is reviewed, techniques available to the clinician to evaluate the extent of edema are described and management alternatives to minimize the edema response are provided.

Prevalence

Every human experiences corneal edema during sleep. Upon awakening in the morning, the cornea immediately begins to reduce in thickness ('deswell'). A new steady-state thickness – representing a thinning of about 3 per cent – is reached after about 4 hours, which indicates that the cornea swells about 3 per cent overnight.[4]

The prevalence of edema induced by contact lenses is essentially 100 per cent, since *all* contact lenses induce some level of edema, including silicone elastomer lenses.[5] The amount of edema is related primarily to the extent of corneal hypoxia induced by the lens (see later). With low *Dk* hydrogel and rigid lenses, daytime central corneal edema typical-

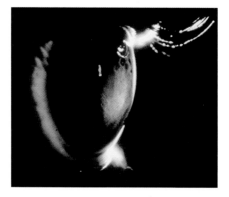

Figure 18.1
Profile view of a cornea, illuminated using sclerotic scatter technique, that displays marked CCC

ly varies between 1 and 6 per cent, and the level of overnight central edema measured upon awakening generally falls in the range 10–15 per cent.[6] Silicone hydrogel lenses induce less than 3 per cent overnight central corneal edema,[7] similar to the level of overnight edema without lenses.

Although central corneal swelling data are usually quoted in the literature, the edema response across the cornea is not uniform,[8] because of:

- Variation in thickness across powered contact lenses, whereby blink-induced tear mixing does *not* act to equalize the distribution of oxygenated tears beneath the lens;[9]
- Resistance of the peripheral cornea to swell as a result of 'limbal clamping'.[10]

Topographic corneal swelling plots for a silicone hydrogel lens and a conventional mid-water hydrogel lens are shown in *Figures 18.2* and *18.3*, respectively. The apparently greater swelling of the temporal and nasal mid-peripheral cornea compared with the central cornea may be an artifact of the experimental methodology; nevertheless, the difference in overall swelling induced by these lenses is substantial.

Signs and Symptoms

A variety of sophisticated clinical and laboratory techniques can be employed to measure precisely the extent of lens-induced corneal edema, the most popular being optical pachometry and ultrasonic recording.[11] Specular microscopy, confocal microscopy, optical coherence tomography,[8] femtosecond laser ranging and interferometry can also be used to measure corneal thickness. It is often necessary to use these more sophisticated techniques in clinical trials and laboratory research on contact lenses, or to provide baseline information prior to corneal surgery, but their clinical application is limited by the cost and inconvenience of the procedures.

Clinicians can estimate the magnitude of corneal edema via careful observation with the slit-lamp biomicroscope, as a number of structural changes can be identified that correlate with various levels of edema. These structural changes – striae, folds and haze – act as useful reference points or 'yardsticks' to form the basis of clinical decision making.

Striae

When viewed using direct focal illumination, striae appear as fine, wispy, white, vertically oriented lines (*Figure 18.4*), and are always located in the posterior stroma.[12] They can also appear as dark lines against the orange fundus pupillary reflex when observed using retro-illumination. Striae are observed only when the level of edema reaches about 5 per

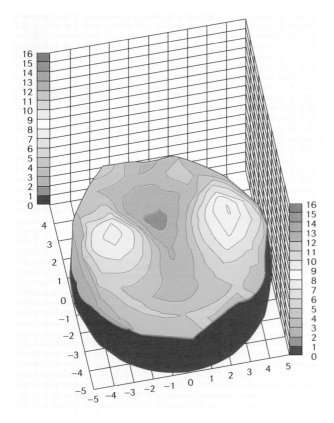

Figure 18.2

Three-dimensional representation of the topographic corneal edema response to the wear of silicone hydrogel lenses under closed eye conditions. To the right is the nasal direction, and the closer region is the inferior cornea. The vertical scale is the percentage increase in corneal thickness over baseline

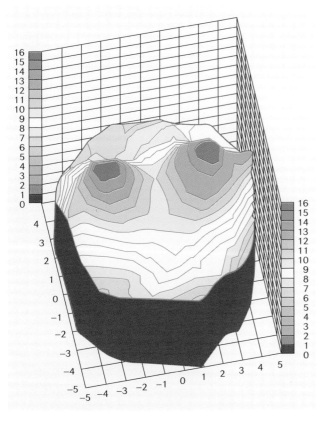

Figure 18.3

Three-dimensional representation of the topographic corneal edema response to the wear of conventional mid-water hydrogel lenses under closed eye conditions. To the right is the nasal direction, and the closer region is the inferior cornea. The vertical scale is the percentage increase in corneal thickness over baseline

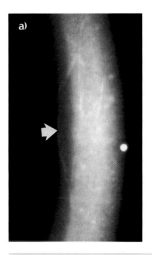 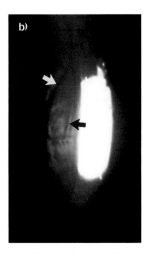 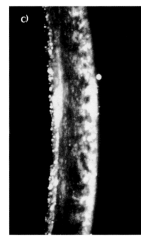

Figure 18.4

Slit-lamp photographs that depict corneal signs of increasing edema from left to right. (a) Striae – a vertical striate line (arrow) observed in the posterior stroma in direct focal illumination. (b) Folds – a depressed groove (white arrow) and raised ridge (black arrow) observed in specular reflection. (c) Haze – the stroma takes on a granular appearance at high levels of edema, as viewed in direct focal illumination

cent. As the level of edema increases, striae become grayer and thicker, and they increase in number.[13] Striae do not cause vision loss.

Folds

Folds can be observed in the endothelial mosaic as a combination of depressed grooves or raised ridges, or as a general area of apparent buckling, when the level of edema reaches about 8 per cent (*Figure 18.4*). They also increase in number as the level of edema increases.[13] Folds are best observed using specular reflection. Vision is thought to be unaffected by folds.

Haze

The stroma takes on a hazy, milky or granular appearance when the level of edema reaches about 15 per cent (*Figure 18.4*). In essence, the stroma has suffered a loss of transparency. This can be viewed using a variety of observation techniques. The milky appearance is evident when the cornea is viewed against the pupil using indirect illumination. Instead of the normal dark appearance, a fine gray haze is detected and fine iris detail is partially obscured. Sclerotic scatter technique enhances this clinical picture. Stromal haze induced by contact lenses can cause a slight degradation of vision when the level of edema exceeds 20 per cent.

In a clinical setting, stromal haze indicates gross edema and is often associated with other signs and symptoms of ocular distress. It would perhaps be more appropriate to consider edema of this level as a frank bullous keratopathy. Contact lens wear is more likely to be an exacerbating factor than the primary cause of the development of stromal haze, so other possible causes of this complication ought to be investigated.

Pathology

The cornea is a sophisticated five-layered tissue of which 78 per cent is water. The stroma, which constitutes 90 per cent of the thickness of the cornea, has a con-

stant tendency to imbibe water and swell. This tendency is counteracted by a fluid control mechanism (described as the 'pump–leak' model[14]) located in the endothelium, which acts to move water out of the stroma and back into the aqueous via a bicarbonate ion pump. If this mechanism is disrupted, or other physiologic challenge is offered to the cornea, the demand on the endothelial pump to maintain deturgescence may become too great. Water then enters the stroma, and the cornea increases in thickness.[15]

Striae

Striae are thought to be represent fluid separation of the predominantly vertically arranged collagen fibrils in the posterior stroma (*Figure 18.5*). This creates a local refractile optical effect whereby stromal transparency is reduced in the immediate vicinity of the separated fibrils. It was postulated originally that the vertical orientation of striae is an artifact of the vertical orientation of the slit beam of the biomicroscope and/or the horizontal binocular displacement of the eyepieces of the objective; however, rotating the beam to a horizontal orientation does not alter this appearance (i.e., horizontally oriented striae do not suddenly appear).

Folds

It is thought that folds indicate a physical buckling of the posterior stromal layers in response to high levels of edema (*Figure 18.5*). The inherent transparency of the stroma means it is not possible to observe folding of stromal tissue directly. Instead, folding can be seen as

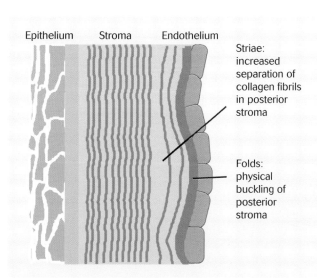

Epithelium   Stroma   Endothelium

Striae: increased separation of collagen fibrils in posterior stroma

Folds: physical buckling of posterior stroma

Figure 18.5

Striae and folds

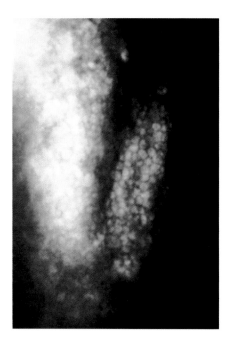

Figure 18.6
High-magnification slit-lamp photomicrograph of deep folds in the endothelial mosaic, which indicates buckling of the posterior stroma through excessive edema

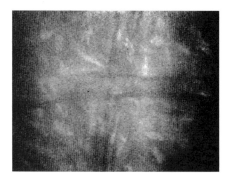

Figure 18.7
Confocal micrograph of vertical and horizontal folds in an eye that had worn a hydrogel contact lens overnight (the image was captured within 30 minutes of awakening)

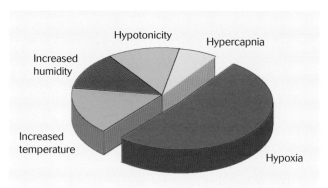

Figure 18.8
Factors that contribute to corneal edema after sleep; hypoxia is the major cause

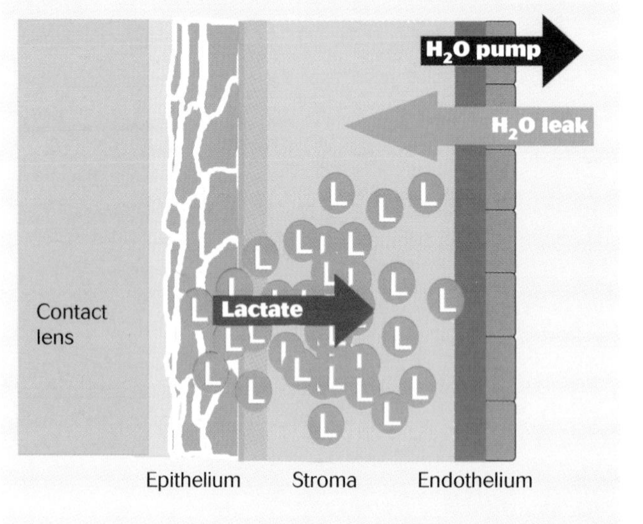

Figure 18.9
Etiology of edema induced by a contact lens. Excess lactate in the stroma that results from anaerobic respiration of the epithelium draws water osmotically into the stroma

an alteration to the topography of the endothelial layer observed in specular reflection (*Figure 18.6*). Efron *et al.*[16] confirmed the appearance of edematous formations using the confocal microscope (*Figure 18.7*). These appeared as long, straight, dark, orthogonal lines in the posterior stroma of the eyes of patients who had worn hydrogel lenses overnight. That both vertical and horizontal lines were observed supports the notion that the appearance of only ver-

tically oriented striae and folds with the slit-lamp biomicroscope is an artifact of the configuration of the slit-lamp biomicroscope, as suggested above.

Haze
Haze is essentially a more advanced form of striae, whereby a gross separation of collagen fibers occurs throughout the full thickness of the stroma, which disrupts the regular geometry and orderly arrangement of the stromal lamellae. This causes a failure of the optical coherence of the stromal collagen layers, and transparency is reduced.[14] The greater the edema, the greater this disruption and the greater is the extent of haze.

Etiology

A number of possible mechanisms have been suggested as playing a role in lens-induced corneal edema. These include hypoxia,[15,17,18] retardation of carbon dioxide efflux (which leads to tissue acidosis),[17] mechanical effects,[19] tempera-

ture changes,[20] hypotonicity,[21] inflammation[22] and increased humidity. The extent to which these factors contribute to overnight corneal edema[23] is indicated in *Figure 18.8*. While the factors that contribute to corneal edema induced by *contact lenses* have not been investigated in this manner, it seems reasonable to explain lens-induced edema primarily in terms of the effects of epithelial hypoxia.

Contact lenses restrict corneal oxygen availability, and so create a hypoxic environment at the anterior corneal surface. To conserve energy, the corneal epithelium begins to respire anaerobically. Lactate, a by-product of the anaerobic metabolism, increases in concentration and moves posteriorly into the corneal stroma. This creates an osmotic load that is balanced by an increased movement of water into the stroma. The sudden influx of water cannot be matched by the removal of water from the stroma by the endothelial pump, which results in corneal edema[24,25] (*Figure 18.9*).

Nguyen *et al.*[26] showed that the variability in corneal swelling induced by contact lenses is associated with both corneal metabolic activity and endothelial function (percentage of recovery per hour). This suggests that individuals with larger levels of corneal metabolic activity produce more lactic acid (i.e., more swelling), whereas stronger endothelial function resists swelling.

Observation and Grading

The level of corneal edema in a contact lens wearer can be assessed using the grading scale for corneal edema shown in Appendix A. An analysis of the clinical changes depicted in each level of grading is given below.

Grade 0
Grade 0 is the normal non-lens wearing situation of 0 per cent edema during the day.

Grade 1
Grade 1 denotes slight changes, up to 4 per cent edema, which could include the normal 3 per cent edema experienced by all humans overnight. Pachometric techniques must generally be employed to detect grade 1 edema; however, trace levels of striae formation may be present.

Grade 2
Observation of between one and three striae in the posterior stroma is designated to represent grade 2 edema, which represents 5–7 percent swelling. In the clinic, grade 2 edema is observed only in patients who:
• Wear contact lenses of extremely low oxygen transmissibility;
• Have slept in low *Dk* lenses.
Examples of the former case include low *Dk* lenses used to correct high hyperopic (over +8.00D) or high myopic (over –12.00D) prescriptions. In the case of patients with hydrogel lenses for extended wear, striae are observed typically within 4 hours only of awakening, because the cornea deswells back to steady-state thickness within this time frame.[27] It is advisable to schedule patients who sleep in lenses to present for early morning appointments so that the full impact of overnight lens wear on the cornea can be assessed.

Grade 3
If between one and 10 folds are detected, the edema is classified as grade 3. A significant number of striae (between

five and 14) should also be observed. Some folds may be present as well, which indicates edema levels of 8 per cent or greater. Since the cornea deswells at such a rapid rate upon eye opening, folds are observed within only 1 hour of awakening in patients who have slept in low *Dk* lenses. Lenses worn in daytime only are unlikely to induce edema levels as high as 8 per cent, even for the correction of high myopia.

Grade 4
Corneal swelling of 15 per cent or greater is typically associated with the presence of at least 15 striae and 11 folds (*Figure 18.10*). The stroma takes on a hazy appearance, the degree of which increases with increasing edema. The epithelium may appear cloudy, with possible bullous formations. The severe CCC (viewed by the sclerotic scatter technique) depicted in *Figure 18.11* is classified as grade 4.

Management

Since oxygen starvation is the primary cause of edema induced by contact lenses, strategies to reduce the edema response are generally directed toward mechanisms that increase corneal oxygen availability during lens wear. There are some important differences between rigid and soft lenses in the way oxygen reaches the cornea; thus, it is necessary to consider alternative edema-reducing strategies for rigid and soft lenses separately, along with general strategies that apply equally to both types of lenses.

Alleviating rigid lens edema
Material Dk
Materials of higher oxygen permeability (*Dk*) allow greater levels of oxygen to reach the cornea. However, increasing the *Dk* of rigid lenses can have drawbacks, such as increased lens flexibility (which reduces lens stability), increased susceptibility to scratching,[28] reduced wettability and lower deposit resistance.

Lens thickness
A thinner lens has a higher oxygen transmissibility (*Dk/t*) than a thicker lens made of the same material.[29] Again, there are some drawbacks to reducing lens thickness; a thinner lens is more flexible (tending to reduce lens stability), masks less astigmatism and offers less resistance to breakage.

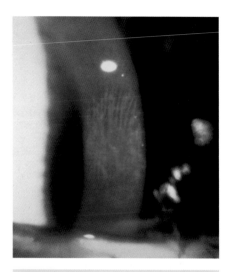

Figure 18.10
Grade 4 edema, showing extensive formation of striae and folds

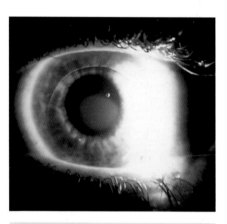

Figure 18.11
Frontal view of severe CCC viewed by sclerotic scatter technique

Base curve
A flatter base curve allows the lens to move more freely, which results in a greater tear exchange and increased corneal oxygenation.[30]

Edge lift
Increasing the edge lift may enhance tear exchange by affording a larger reservoir of oxygenated tears at the lens periphery.[31] However, increasing edge lift may also increase lens awareness.

Lens diameter
A smaller lens, as well as covering a smaller area of the cornea, allows greater lens movement and therefore enhances tear exchange and oxygenation.[32]

Fenestrations

It was originally thought that fenestrations in rigid lenses reduce edema by providing additional avenues for oxygen passage to the cornea.[33] However, this does not seem to be the case. Fenestrations are now thought to act by altering the fluid forces between the lens and cornea; this serves to enhance lens movement, which in turn leads to an increased tear exchange and greater corneal oxygenation.

Alleviating soft lens edema
Material Dk

With hydrogels, increasing the material Dk essentially means increasing the lens water content.[29] The potential drawbacks of hydrogel lenses with higher water content is that they are more fragile and therefore need to be thicker, which can reduce comfort slightly. Silicone hydrogel lenses have such high Dk levels[34] that corneal oxygen availability is almost unimpeded.

Lens thickness

Reducing lens thickness increases Dk/t.[29] However, thinner lenses are more fragile and can lead to unacceptable corneal staining, particularly with materials of higher water content.

Base curve

There has been some debate as to whether flattening the base curve of hydrogel lenses results in an increased tear exchange, despite the observation that flatter lenses move more freely over the cornea.[35] Florkey *et al.*[36] showed that blink-induced tear exchange enhances corneal oxygenation beneath silicone hydrogel lenses, which generally have a higher modulus than hydrogel lenses. Flatter lenses allow tear film debris and desquamated epithelial cells to be flushed out more readily from beneath the lens, and thus minimize metabolic disturbance to the cornea and reduce the potential to induce edema.

Lens diameter

A smaller lens moves more freely over the cornea, which may allow more oxygen to reach the cornea via an increased tear pump.

Microfenestrations

Conventional fenestrations (0.2–1.0 mm in diameter) in hydrogel lenses can increase corneal oxygenation[37] and reduce edema,[38,39] but fenestrated lens-

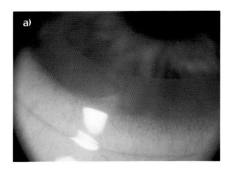 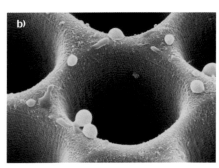

Figure 18.12

(a) An array of thousands of microfenestrations in the mid-periphery of a soft lens.
(b) Microfenestrations (40 µm diameter) viewed under the electron microscope reveal smooth, rounded edges

es are very uncomfortable.[40] A strategically positioned array of microfenestrations can significantly reduce the corneal edema induced by lenses.[40] In particular, microfenestrations positioned toward the lens edge may be useful in reducing peripheral corneal edema when medium-to-high minus hydrogel lenses (say, over –3.00D) are worn. Microfenestration arrays have also been shown to improve tear mixing in silicone hydrogel lenses,[41] although the benefit being sought in these studies related more to revealing strategies to remove debris and waste products from beneath the lens, rather than to enhance corneal oxygenation[42] (*Figure 18.12*). The clinical viability of microfenestrations has yet to be established fully.

General strategies to reduce edema
Change from extended to daily wear

Overnight wear of hydrogel lenses is generally associated with increased levels of edema, because corneal oxygen availability is reduced significantly when the eyelid is closed. Thus, converting a patient from extended wear to daily wear reduces the overall edema response.

Change from soft to rigid lenses

For soft and rigid lenses of the same Dk/t, rigid lenses generally deliver more oxygen to the cornea during open-eye wear because of the lid-activated tear pump.[43] For the extended wear patient, converting from a soft lens to a rigid lens of the same Dk/t alleviates the physiologic impact of lens wear as it allows a more rapid edema reduction after awakening.

Reduce wearing time

After lens insertion, edema initially increases rapidly and then more gradually over the first 6–8 hours of lens wear. Limiting the time that lenses may be worn each day therefore reduces both the magnitude and the duration of corneal edema.

Anti-inflammatory drugs

A possible strategy to reduce lens-induced edema is the use of non-steroid anti-inflammatory drugs. While it is not feasible to use such drugs on a routine basis, they may prove useful for the treatment of acute episodes of severe (grade 4) edema. At this time, there is no conclusive evidence to indicate that edema induced by contact lenses can be modified by drug therapy.[22]

Postpone lens wear

It may be prudent to cease lens wear temporarily after an acute edema episode, especially if associated with other pathologic changes, such as limbal redness, infiltrates or corneal staining. Lens wear should be ceased until all pathologic signs and associated symptoms have resolved.

Abandon lens wear

Clearly a last resort, abandonment of lens wear must be considered if chronic edema persists after all other possible treatment alternatives have failed.

General considerations

The various strategies described above for reducing lens-induced edema should be employed in a systematic manner, with respect to (a) the severity of edema as gauged biomicroscopically (based on the appearance of striae, folds and haze) and

(b) the modality of lens wear (rigid vs. soft; daily wear vs. extended wear). Consideration should also be given to the time of day – morning or afternoon – that the observations of edema are made.

Holden and Mertz[44] provided criteria for the minimum contact lens *Dk/t* required to avoid excessive levels of edema – these are 24×10^{-9} (cm × mlO$_2$)/(s × ml × mmHg) for daily lens wear and 87×10^{-9} (cm × mlO$_2$)/(s × ml × mmHg) for extended lens wear (*Figure 18.13*). Harvitt and Bonanno[45] found that, to prevent anoxia throughout the entire corneal thickness, the *Dk/t* requirements are 35×10^{-9} (cm × mlO$_2$)/(s × ml × mmHg) for the open eye and 125×10^{-9} (cm × mlO$_2$)/(s × ml × mmHg) for the closed eye. Only silicone hydrogel soft lenses and hyperpermeable rigid lenses meet the Holden–Mertz criterion for extended wear.

Prognosis

In general, the prognosis for recovery of the cornea from lens-induced edema is excellent. In laboratory experiments, it can be demonstrated that the edema induced when a patient wears a contact lens for the first time resolves within 4 hours when the lens is removed.[27] Conversely, it was demonstrated by

Holden *et al.*[46] that edema took 7 days to resolve after lens removal from patients who had worn extended wear lenses for 5 years.

The cases cited above are likely to represent the two extremes (4 hours versus 7 days) of rate of recovery from lens-induced edema. It may be that, within this range, the rate of recovery of edema after lens wear is related to the total accumulated lens wear experience.[47,48] There do not appear be any reports of the failure of edema induced by contact lenses to resolve.

The rate at which the cornea recovers from lens-induced edema has been suggested as a test of the health of the cornea. It is known, for example, that the corneas of patients who suffer from Fuchs' endothelial dystrophy[49] and of diabetic patients[50,51] have an impaired capacity to eliminate excess edema. Specifically, the corneal deswelling rate is thought to reflect the integrity of the endothelium, which is responsible for corneal hydration control.

Differential Diagnosis

Striae can take on a similar appearance to ghost vessels and nerve fibers. The characteristics that allow these entities to be differentiated are discussed fully in Chapter 21. Fonn and Gauthier[52]

described the presence of fibrillary lines in both lens wearers and non-lens wearers; these seem to be very similar to edema-related striae, but are thought to be neural in origin and are apparently permanent.

Folds can occur naturally in a small proportion of normal patients and are often observed in diabetic patients.[53] Folds observed in diabetic daily lens wearers do not alter their appearance over a number of months.[54] Again, the capacity of lens-induced folds to resolve rapidly after lens removal is a key diagnostic criterion.

Various corneal dystrophies and diseases of the cornea and associated ocular structures, as well as iatrogenic interventions (such as ophthalmic surgery or drug therapy) can result in stromal edema. While it is beyond the scope of this chapter to review all these possible causes of edema, in most instances there are associated signs and symptoms that cannot be reconciled with edema induced by contact lenses. For example, in addition to stromal edema, Fuchs' endothelial dystrophy is characterized by permanent and pronounced endothelial guttata, bullous keratopathy (large fluid vacuoles in the stroma), loss of vision and pain.

A condition known as acute hydrops can occur in severe keratoconus, whereby there is an acute influx of aqueous into the cornea as a result of a rupture in Descemet's membrane. This causes a sudden drop of visual acuity and is associated with discomfort and watering. This condition is treated initially with hypertonic saline and either patching or a bandage contact lens. Acute hydrops usually clears within 6 weeks, although a variable amount of stromal scarring may remain.[55]

The key feature that distinguishes the signs of corneal edema induced by contact lenses – striae, folds and haze – from other clinical entities that take on a similar appearance is that lens-induced edema resolves soon after lens removal.

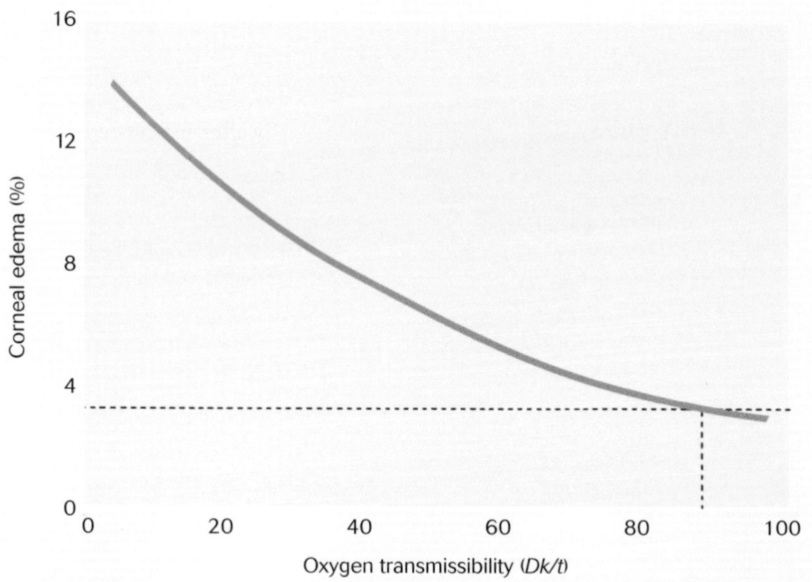

Figure 18.13
Relationship between *Dk/t* versus edema for daily and extended wear (adapted from Holden and Mertz[44])

REFERENCES

1 Efron N and Pearson RM (1988). Centenary celebration of Fick's Eine Contactbrille. *Arch Ophthalmol.* **106**, 1370–1377.
2 Pearson RM and Efron N (1989). Hundredth anniversary of August Müller's inaugural dissertation on contact lenses. *Surv Ophthalmol.* **34**, 133–141.

3 Goldberg JB (1970). *Biomicroscopy for Contact Lens Practice: Clinical Procedures*. (Chicago: Professional Press).

4 Mandell RB and Fatt I (1965). Thinning of the human cornea on awakening. *Nature* **208**, 292–293.

5 LaHood D, Sweeney DF and Holden BA (1988). Overnight corneal edema with hydrogel, rigid gas-permeable and silicone-elastomer contact lenses. *Int Contact Lens Clin.* **15**, 149–153.

6 Holden BA, Mertz GW and McNally JJ (1983). Corneal swelling response to contact lenses worn under extended wear conditions. *Invest Ophthalmol Vis Sci.* **24**, 218–226.

7 Fonn D, du Toit R, Simpson TL, *et al.* (1999). Sympathetic swelling response of the control eye to soft lenses in the other eye. *Invest Ophthalmol Vis Sci.* **40**, 3116–3121.

8 Wang J, Fonn D and Simpson TL (2003). Topographical thickness of the epithelium and total cornea after hydrogel and PMMA contact lens wear with eye closure. *Invest Ophthalmol Vis Sci.* **44**, 1070–1074.

9 Efron N and Fitzgerald JP (1996). Distribution of oxygen across the surface of the human cornea during soft contact lens wear. *Optom Vis Sci.* **73**, 659–665.

10 Bonanno JA and Polse KA (1985). Central and peripheral corneal swelling accompanying soft lens extended wear. *Am J Optom Physiol Opt.* **62**, 74–81.

11 Chan-Ling T and Pye DC (1994). Pachometry: Clinical and scientific applications. In: *Contact Lens Practice*, p. 407–435, Eds Ruben M and Guillon M. (London: Chapman and Hall Medical).

12 Sarver MD (1971). Striate corneal lines among patients wearing hydrophilic contact lenses. *Am J Optom Arch Am Acad Optom.* **48**, 762–763.

13 LaHood D and Grant T (1990). Striae and folds as indicators of corneal oedema. *Optom Vis Sci.* **67S**, 196.

14 Fatt I and Weissman BA (1992). *Physiology of the Eye. An Introduction to the Vegetative Functions*. (Boston: Butterworth–Heinemann).

15 Bonanno JA (2001). Effects of contact lens-induced hypoxia on the physiology of the corneal endothelium. *Optom Vis Sci.* **78**, 783–790.

16 Efron N, Mutalib HA, Perez-Gomez I and Koh HH (2002). Confocal microscopic observations of the human cornea following overnight contact lens wear. *Clin Exp Optom.* **85**, 149–155.

17 Ang JH and Efron N (1990). Corneal hypoxia and hypercapnia during contact lens wear. *Optom Vis Sci.* **67**, 512–521.

18 Stickel TE and Bonanno JA (2002). The relationship between corneal oxygen tension and hypoxic corneal edema. *Optometry* **73**, 598–604.

19 Thoft RA and Friend J (1975). Biochemical aspects of contact lens wear. *Am J Ophthalmol.* **80**, 139–145.

20 Martin DK and Fatt I (1986). The presence of a contact lens induces a very small increase in the anterior corneal surface temperature. *Acta Ophthalmol (Copenh.)* **64**, 512–518.

21 Hill RM (1975). Osmotic edema associated with contact lens adaptation. *J Am Optom Assoc.* **46**, 897–899.

22 Efron N, Holden BA and Vannas A (1984). Prostaglandin-inhibitor naproxen does not affect contact lens-induced changes in the human corneal endothelium. *Am J Optom Physiol Opt.* **61**, 741–744.

23 Sweeney DF and Holden BA (1991). The relative contributions of hypoxia, osmolality, temperature and humidity to corneal oedema with eye closure. *Invest Ophthalmol Vis Sci.* **32S**, 739.

24 Klyce SD (1981). Stromal lactate accumulation can account for corneal oedema osmotically following epithelial hypoxia in the rabbit. *J Physiol.* **321**, 49–64.

25 Iskeleli G, Karakoc Y, Akdeniz-Kayhan B, *et al.* (1999). Comparison of tear lactate dehydrogenase activities of different types of contact lens wearers and normal control group. *CLAO J.* **25**, 101–104.

26 Nguyen T, Soni PS, Brizendine E and Bonanno JA (2003). Variability in hypoxia-induced corneal swelling is associated with variability in corneal metabolism and endothelial function. *Eye Contact Lens* **29**, 117–125.

27 O'Neal MR and Polse KA (1985). *In vivo* assessment of mechanisms controlling corneal hydration. *Invest Ophthalmol Vis Sci.* **26**, 849–856.

28 Tranoudis I and Efron N (1996). Scratch resistance of rigid contact lens materials. *Ophthalmic Physiol Opt.* **16**, 303–309.

29 Efron N (1991). Understanding oxygen: *Dk/L*, EOP, oedema. *Trans Br Contact Lens Assoc.* **14**, 65–69.

30 Fink BA, Hill RM and Carney LG (1992). Influence of rigid contact lens base curve radius on tear pump efficiency. *Optom Vis Sci.* **69**, 60–65.

31 Fink BA, Hill RM and Carney LG (1991). Effects of rigid contact lens edge lift changes on tear pump efficiency. *Optom Vis Sci.* **68**, 409–413.

32 Fink BA, Carney LG and Hill RM (1991). Rigid contact lens design: Effects of overall diameter changes on tear pump efficiency. *Optom Vis Sci.* **68**, 198–203.

33 Stewart CR (1976). Effect of corneal lens fenestration on edema and spectacle blur. *J Am Optom Assoc.* **47**, 952–957.

34 Alvord L, Court J, Davis T, *et al.* (1998). Oxygen permeability of a new type of high *Dk* soft contact lens material. *Optom Vis Sci.* **75**, 30–36.

35 Paugh JR, Stapleton F, Keay L and Ho A (2001). Tear exchange under hydrogel contact lenses: Methodological considerations. *Invest Ophthalmol Vis Sci.* **42**, 2813–2820.

36 Florkey L, Fink BA, Mitchell GL and Hill RM (2003). Tear exchange and oxygen reservoir effects in silicone hydrogel systems. *Eye Contact Lens* **29S**, 90–92.

37 Efron N and Carney LG (1983). The effect of fenestrating soft contact lenses on corneal oxygen availability. *Am J Optom Physiol Opt.* **60**, 503–508.

38 Brennan NA, Efron N and Carney LG (1986). The effects of fenestrating soft contact lenses on corneal swelling: A re-examination. *Clin Exp Optom.* **69**, 120–123.

39 Litoff D, Pristaw AI, Smith RS and Gold RM (1992). Argon laser fenestration of a Softperm contact lens. *CLAO J.* **18**, 95–96.

40 Ang JHB and Efron N (1987). Comfort of fenestrated hydrogel lenses. *Clin Exp Optom.* **70**, 117–120.

41 Miller KL, Polse KA and Radke CJ (2003), Fenestrations enhance tear mixing under silicone-hydrogel contact lenses. *Invest Ophthalmol Vis Sci.* **44**, 60–67.

42 Efron N (1992). Microfenestration of soft contact lenses. *Optician* **204**(5371), 27–30.

43 O'Neal MR, Polse KA and Sarver MD (1984). Corneal response to rigid and hydrogel lenses during eye closure. *Invest Ophthalmol Vis Sci.* **25**, 837–842.

44 Holden BA and Mertz GW (1984). Critical oxygen levels to avoid corneal edema for daily and extended wear contact lenses. *Invest Ophthalmol Vis Sci.* **25**, 1161–1167.

45 Harvitt DM and Bonanno JA (1999). Re-evaluation of the oxygen diffusion model for predicting minimum contact lens *Dk/t* values needed to avoid corneal anoxia. *Optom Vis Sci.* **76**, 712–719.

46 Holden BA, Sweeney DF, Vannas A, *et al.* (1985). Effects of long-term extended contact lens wear on the human cornea. *Invest Ophthalmol Vis Sci.* **26**, 1489–1501.

47 McMahon TT, Polse KA, McNamara N and Viana MA (1996). Recovery from induced corneal edema and endothelial morphology after long-term PMMA contact lens wear. *Optom Vis Sci.* **73**, 184–188.

48 Nieuwendaal CP, Odenthal MT, Kok JH, *et al.* (1994). Morphology and function of the corneal endothelium after long-term contact lens wear. *Invest Ophthalmol Vis Sci.* **35**, 3071–3077.

49 Mandell RB, Polse KA, Brand RJ, *et al.* (1989). Corneal hydration control in Fuchs' dystrophy. *Invest Ophthalmol Vis Sci.* **30**, 845–852.

50 Weston BC, Bourne WM, Polse KA and Hodge DO (1995). Corneal hydration control in diabetes mellitus. *Invest Ophthalmol Vis Sci.* **36**, 586–595.

51 Ziadi M, Moiroux P, d'Athis P, *et al.* (2002). Assessment of induced corneal hypoxia in diabetic patients. *Cornea* **21**, 453–457.

52 Fonn D and Gauthier C (1991). Prevalence of superficial fibrillary lines of the cornea in contact lens wearers and nonwearers. *Cornea* **10**, 507–510.

53 Henkind P and Wise GN (1961). Descemet's wrinkles in diabetes. *Am J Ophthalmol.* **52**, 371–372.

54 O'Donnell C and Efron N (1995). Corneal endothelial folds in diabetes. *Optom Vis Sci.* **72S**, 57.

55 Kanski JJ (2003). *Clinical Ophthalmology*. Fifth Edition. (Oxford: Butterworth–Heinemann).

STROMAL THINNING

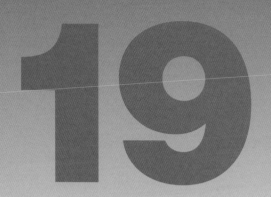

As discussed in Chapter 18, corneal edema is a reliable indicator of the level of hypoxic stress induced by contact lens wear. It is an acute response, in that the edema increases to a steady state within a few hours when the cornea is subjected to hypoxic stress, and returns to baseline within a few hours of the hypoxic stress being removed. Of course, edema can be considered to be chronic if a patient wears edema-inducing lenses over long periods, but even in these circumstances the edema still resolves when the cornea is no longer subjected to hypoxia.

Stromal thinning is an insidious chronic change often masked by acute lens-induced edema. Indeed, the only way that stromal thinning can be assessed properly is to measure stromal thickness after a long period of cessation of lens wear (at least 1 week). This chapter examines the phenomenon of stromal thinning induced by contact lenses and considers its clinical implications.

Signs

Longitudinal lens wearing trials

Stromal thinning was defined formally for the first time in 1995 by Holden *et al.*,[1] although this phenomenon had been observed anecdotally by previous workers. For example, Millodot[2] noted that the corneas of patients who had worn polymethyl methacrylate (PMMA) contact lenses on a daily wear basis for 10–21 years became thinner, after ceasing lens wear, than the corneas of a matched control group of non-lens wearers. Lebow and Plishka[3] reported apparent corneal thinning in an 11 month longitudinal extended wear study of 22 myopic patients who wore low *Dk* hydrogel contact lenses (Hydrocurve II, CIBA Vision; *Figure 19.1*). These authors were unsure of the cause of the progressive decrease in

corneal thickness over the course of their study. It was thought at the time that these changes may have represented either some form of physiologic adaptation or a methodological artifact related to the progressive drop-out of subjects who exhibited adverse responses that were partially or wholly characterized by excessive corneal edema.

Schoessler and Barr[4] monitored corneal thickness changes in eight myopic patients who wore low *Dk* hydrogel contact lenses (Permalens, CooperVision) continuously for 18 months. The averaged results showed maximum corneal swelling after 1 week of wear, with the cornea gradually returning to near pre-fitting thickness levels. These authors noted that "some patients [showed] chronic corneal thickening and some [showed] corneal thinning after the 18-month wearing period."

Holden's group[1] detected stromal thinning by measuring the presenting stromal thickness of patients who had been wearing a lens in one eye only on an extended wear basis for an average of 5.2 ± 2.4 years. A lens was worn in one eye only in these patients because they were suffering from either unilateral myopia, or amblyopia in the contralateral eye. Upon ceasing lens wear after having worn lenses for 5.2 years, it was noted that the stroma in the lens-wearing eye decreased in thickness to a steady-state level *thinner* than that of the fellow non-wearing eye (*Figure 19.2*).

Theoretical analysis

Presuming that the stromal thicknesses of both eyes were the same prior to lens wear (this was validated in a control group of unilateral myopes and amblyopes not wearing lenses), the only conclusion that can be drawn is that contact lenses induce stromal thinning. It can be seen from *Figure 19.2* that the stroma had thinned an average of 11 μm in 5.2

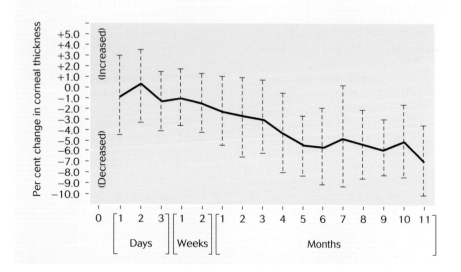

Figure 19.1

Change in corneal thickness over time in patients wearing low *Dk* hydrogel extended wear lenses (after Lebow and Plishka[3])

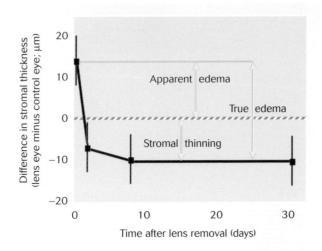

years of lens wear, which represents an average of 2.1 μm thinning per year of lens wear. The revelation of stromal thinning by Holden *et al.*[1] has facilitated interpretation of data from earlier longitudinal lens-wearing studies that failed to take this phenomenon into account. The following equation, derived from *Figure 19.2*, can be applied to establish to the actual extent of lens-induced edema and thinning of the stroma:

True edema = Apparent edema +
Stromal thinning

It is important for clinicians to recognize that the phenomenon of stromal thinning induced by contact lenses does *not* confound or invalidate the interpretation of clinical signs of acute edema discussed in Chapter 18. The signs of striae, folds and haze represent a given level of acute edema, irrespective of whether or not the stroma has thinned; that is, these signs still indicate the level of true edema.

Cross-sectional studies

Liu and Pflugfelder[5] evaluated the effect of long-term contact lens wear on corneal thickness in 35 subjects who had been wearing contact lenses for 13.5 ± 6 years; these data were compared with 40 control eyes. They observed that the mean corneal thickness in the center and in eight peripheral areas measured in subjects wearing contact lens was reduced significantly, by about 30–50 μm, compared with normal subjects, and that these changes were unrelated to the degree of myopia. Liu and Pflugfelder[5] concluded, as did Holden *et al.*[1], that long-term contact lens wear appears to cause a decrease in corneal thickness.

Myrowitz *et al.*[6] measured corneal thickness in 124 consecutive patients (248 eyes) who underwent comprehensive evaluations in consideration of refractive surgery. They observed that 39 patients (78 eyes) who had previously worn soft contact lenses for an average of 16 years had a mean corneal thickness of 543.2 ± 3.8 μm (standard error), 23 patients (46 eyes) who had worn rigid contact lenses for an average of 19 years had a mean corneal thickness of 509.4 ± 6.9 μm and 62 patients (124 eyes) who had not previously worn contact lenses had a mean corneal thickness of 546.4 ± 3.5 μm. These authors[6] concluded that long-term rigid contact lens wear is associated with a decrease in the average central corneal thickness of 37 μm compared with no contact lens wear. They were unable to confirm the earlier findings of Holden *et al.*[1] and Liu and Pflugfelder[5] of such an effect among soft lens wearers.

Methodological considerations

An important methodological issue needs to be taken into account when considering the reported data of lens-induced corneal thinning. Whereas Holden *et al.*[1] specifically measured *stromal* thickness, all of the other researchers referred to above[2–6] measured total *corneal* thickness; that is, the combined thickness of the stroma (typically 550 μm thick) and the epithelium (typically 50 μm thick). Long-term contact lens wear is also known to induce epithelial thinning, which is estimated to be 5.6 per cent by Holden *et al.*[1] and between 8.7 and 18.4 per cent by Perez *et al.*[7] Therefore, some published estimates of stromal thinning may be confounded by

the effects of lens wear on the epithelial thickness.

Consider the results of Liu and Pflugfelder,[5] who observed 40 μm of corneal thinning (taking the mid-point of their reported range of 30–50 μm thinning). Their subjects may also have suffered about 10 per cent of epithelial thinning, or about 5 μm assuming a 50 μm thick epithelium. This would leave about 35 μm of *stromal* thinning, which represents about 2.6 μm/year of stromal thinning over the 13.5 years of lens wear in the subject cohort of Liu and Pflugfelder.[5] The same analysis can be applied to the data of Myrowitz *et al.*,[6] whose 37 μm of corneal thinning in rigid lens wearers may equate to 32 μm of stromal thinning. The calculated rate of stromal thinning over the 19 years of lens wear is therefore 1.7 μm per year. The calculated stromal thinning rates of 2.1, 2.6 and 1.7 μm per year based on the data of Holden *et al.*,[1] Liu and Pflugfelder[5] and Myrowitz *et al.*,[6] respectively, are remarkably similar.

Symptoms

None of the studies that reported stromal thinning have noted any symptomatic associations. However, should the stroma become so thin that corneal warpage takes place, some loss of visual function might be expected (see Chapter 24).

Pathology

Of course, recognition that the stroma has become thinner is in itself a statement of pathologic change, but further to this, subtle ultrastructural changes that result from contact lens wear have been observed in the cornea. These changes may offer valuable insights into the process of stromal thinning.

A good starting point from which to consider lens-induced structural changes that may be of relevance to stromal thinning is to note the critical role of stromal keratocytes in the synthesis and maintenance of the collagen and extracellular matrix that comprise the bulk of the stroma.[8] Any disruption to the ability of keratocytes to function normally might be expected to compromise the structural integrity of the cornea. Specifically, if keratocytes do not lay down and maintain the collagen and extracellular matrix, there will be a gradual reduction in tissue mass, which may manifest as stromal thinning.

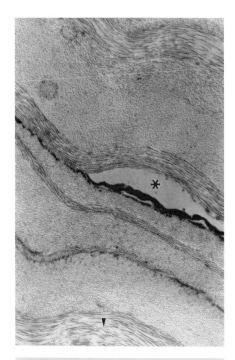

Figure 19.3
After PMMA lens wear, stromal edema is most conspicuous around keratocytes and between lamellae, where pooling of extracellular fluid (asterisk) may be present. Intralamellar swelling (triangle) is also evident in places. Primate, electron micrograph, magnification ×8500

Electron microscopy
In a primate model, Bergmanson and Chu[9] found that PMMA lens wear induces changes in stromal keratocytes, including the formation of clear zones around the keratocytes along with spaces filled with granular tissue (*Figure 19.3*). The theoretical background outlined above, coupled with the experimental observations of Bergmanson and Chu,[9] highlighted the need to focus attention on the effect of contact lens wear on stromal keratocytes in human subjects; however, keratocytes are beyond the resolution of the slit-lamp biomicroscope, which precludes clinical studies using this instrument. It was only through the development of the corneal confocal microscope in the 1990s that the monitoring of keratocytes in the corneas of human subjects became possible.

Confocal microscopy
Studies of keratocyte populations in humans using the confocal microscope revealed a loss of keratocytes through contact lens wear (*Figure 19.4*). Bansal *et al.*[10]

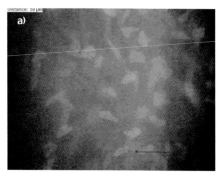
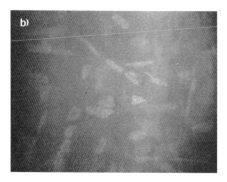

Figure 19.4
Confocal microscope images of the posterior corneal stroma. The white shapes are keratocytes. (a) Control eye (not wearing a lens) and (b) lens-wearing eye

reported that the anterior stromal keratocyte density (KD, 757 ± 243 cells/mm^2) in patients who wore contact lenses for daily wear was significantly less than that in non-lens wearers (925 ± 276 cells/mm^2). Jalbert and Stapleton[11] used the confocal microscope to measure stromal KD in nine subjects wearing extended wear hydrogel lenses and nine age- and sex-matched control subjects not wearing lenses. They reported that stromal KD was lower in the lens-wearing group in both the anterior stroma (544 ± 206 cells/mm^2, versus 804 ± 145 cells/mm^2 in the group not wearing lenses) and posterior stroma (514 ± 111 cells/mm^2, versus 628 ± 101 cells/mm^2 in the group not wearing lenses). They also described haziness around some keratocytes in the lens-wearing group, which may denote areas of edema. Jalbert and Stapleton[11] concluded that extended wear of hydrogel lenses reduces stromal KD.

Edema artifact
A potential error in the studies of Bansal *et al.*[10] and Jalbert and Stapleton[11] is the failure when using the confocal microscope to account for a methodological problem that relates to the confounding influence of edema on estimates of KD.[12] Simply put, the confocal microscope samples the keratocyte population by capturing an image within a fixed depth of field (10 µm). If the stroma swells and the keratocytes redistribute evenly with the swelling, fewer keratocytes will be counted within the fixed depth of field, assuming that the total number of keratocytes has remained constant. Thus, the presence of edema leads to an underestimation of KD unless measures are taken to account for this effect (*Figure 19.5*). A binomial expansion model applied to this problem suggests that the magnitude of the apparent loss of keratocytes should be roughly

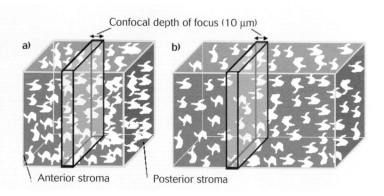

Figure 19.5
(a) Stromal keratocytes (white) can be seen in the 10 µm thick section (yellow) of stromal tissue (blue) with the confocal microscope. (b) The stromal tissue has become swollen and expanded in one dimension (along the anterior–posterior axis). Assuming that the number of keratocytes has remained constant, fewer keratocytes will be seen in the 10 µm thick swollen section with the confocal microscope, which gives rise to the illusion of a reduction in the number of keratocytes

equivalent to the level of edema;[12] thus, for example, 10 per cent corneal swelling would lead to an apparent loss of 10 per cent of keratocytes.

Efron *et al.*[13] followed 23 neophyte myopic subjects who wore a high *Dk/t* lens (PureVision) in one eye and a low *Dk/t* lens (Acuvue 2) in the other eye on an extended wear basis for 6 months. Confocal microscopy and ultrasonic pachometry were performed on both eyes at baseline (before lens wear), after 3 and 6 months of lens wear and 1 week after cessation of lens wear (the 'post-cessation' visit). No differences were established between the two lenses or between the three study visits for anterior stromal KD. Posterior stromal KD was similar for the two lenses throughout the study. However, there was an overall drop in posterior KD of 14 per cent in both eyes at the 6 month visit, compared with the initial visit (*Figure 19.6*). Posterior KD at the 6 month visit was no different from that at the post-cessation visit. Corneal thickness was similar for the two lenses at the initial and post-cessation visits, but was 3 per cent greater for the eye wearing the Acuvue 2 lens at the 6 month visit. Efron *et al.*[13] concluded that extended contact lens wear causes a loss of kera-tocytes, and they pointed out that their finding could not be attributed to hypoxia and/or edema induced by contact lenses, or to the artifact of confocal microscopy related to the presence of edema discussed above.

Conflicting findings

Patel *et al.*[14] examined the corneas of 20 daily contact lens wearers (who had worn lenses for more than 10 years) and 20 corneas of 20 age-matched control subjects who had not worn contact lenses. Full-thickness central and temporal KDs in contact lens wearers were $22,122 \pm 2676$ cells/mm^3 and $20,731 \pm 2627$ cells/mm^3, respectively, and were not significantly different from central and temporal KDs in control subjects. These authors[14] concluded that long-term daily contact lens wear has no demonstrable effect on KD. This 'negative' result may relate to the fact that lenses were worn on a daily wear basis, whereas the subjects in the studies of Jalbert and Stapleton[11] and Efron *et al.*[13] wore lenses on an extended wear basis. However, the negative results of Patel *et al.*[14] disagree with the positive findings of keratocyte loss reported by Bansal *et al.*,[10] in that the subjects in both studies were using daily wear lenses.

It is unclear why baseline estimates of anterior KD differ between the studies of Efron *et al.*[13] (1112 ± 96 cells/mm^2), Bansal *et al.*[10] (925 ± 276 cells/mm^2) and Jalbert and Stapleton[11] (804 ± 145 cells/mm^2). These differences may be related to the different methods used for cell counting. Interpretation of the data of Bansal *et al.*[10] and Jalbert and Stapleton[11] has been confounded by the fact that the loss of keratocytes could be attributable, at least in part, to an artifact related to the presence of residual edema in the cornea at the time confocal microscopy was undertaken,[12] as outlined above. Although Bansal *et al.*[10] and Jalbert and Stapleton[11] did remove the contact lenses a few hours prior to performing confocal microscopy, the presence of residual edema cannot be discounted in view of the demonstration by Holden *et al.*[1] that chronic lens-induced edema can take up to 7 days to dissipate.

The study by Efron *et al.*[13] of the effects of extended contact lens wear on stromal keratocyte populations was designed to account for the potential confounding effects of hypoxic edema on the determination of KD.[12] This was achieved by comparing the performance of a hydrogel lens of relatively low oxygen performance [Acuvue 2 (*Dk/t* = 26), a lens expected to render the cornea hypoxic and induce edema] fitted to one eye, with that of a silicone hydrogel lens of relatively high oxygen performance [PureVision (*Dk/t* = 110), a lens not expected to induce significant hypoxia or edema] fitted to the other eye. Indeed, the corneal thickness changes observed at the 6 month visit were entirely consistent with the relative oxygen performances of the two lens types. That is, corneal thickness with the Acuvue 2 lens was overall about 3 per cent greater at the 6 month visit than at the initial visit, whereas there was no change with the PureVision lens.

The 14 per cent reduction in posterior stromal KD with the extended wear of both the Acuvue 2 and PureVision lens reported in the study of Efron *et al.*[13] is in close agreement with the earlier observations of Jalbert and Stapleton,[11] who reported an 18 per cent drop. The results of the study of Efron *et al.*[13] indicated that this decrease is not dependent on the oxygen performance of the lens or on the effects of edema; that is, that hypoxia and/or edema are not of etiologic significance in the lens-induced reduction of poste-

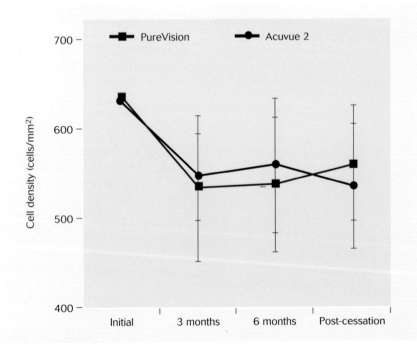

Figure 19.6
Posterior stromal keratocyte density (mean ± standard deviation) at the initial, 3 month and 6 month visits and 1 week post-cessation visit (after Efron *et al.*[13])

rior stromal KD. Furthermore, the reduction in posterior stromal KD cannot be explained by an artifact related to the presence of residual edema,[12] because the decrease noted at 6 months in the edematous cornea of the eye wearing the Acuvue 2 lens was still evident 1 week after ceasing lens wear, at which time the residual edema had resolved. It is unclear why Bansal et al.[10] and Jalbert and Stapleton[11] reported a reduction in anterior stromal KD of 18 per cent and 32 per cent, respectively, whereas no change in anterior stromal KD was found in the study of Efron et al.[13]

Etiology

It was originally presumed that stromal thinning is caused by the effects of chronic edema, and Holden et al.[1] proposed two possible mechanisms. First, stromal keratocytes may lose their ability to synthesize new stromal tissue through the direct effects of lens-induced tissue hypoxia, and/or the indirect effects of chronic lens-induced tissue acidosis caused by an accumulation of lactic acid and carbonic acid. Second, constantly elevated levels of lactic acid associated with chronic lens-induced edema may lead to some dissolution of the mucopolysaccharide ground substance of the stroma.

Mechanical effects of lens wear

The first mechanism referred to above implies that a full appreciation of keratocyte dysfunction induced by contact lenses is fundamental to developing an understanding of lens-induced stromal thinning. As described above, the confocal microscope has allowed attention to be focused on the fate of keratocytes during lens wear. Jalbert and Stapleton[11] attributed keratocyte loss induced by contact lenses to three possible etiologies – hypoxia, cytokine-mediated effects and mechanically induced effects. In view of the results of Efron et al.,[13] hypoxia and edema can be discounted. An obvious common influence of the Acuvue 2 and PureVision lenses on the cornea that could explain the loss of keratocytes in the posterior stroma is that the physical presence of the lenses creates a direct (mechanical) or indirect (cytokine mediated) effect. Certainly, it has been reported that other mechanical effects on the cornea, such as epithelial debridement, are associated with keratocyte loss.[15]

Refractive surgery

Erie et al.[16] noted a reduction in anterior stromal KD of 25–45 per cent during a 36 month period after photorefractive keratectomy (PRK). Mitooka et al.[17] and Perez-Gomez and Efron[18] observed a 22 per cent and 34 per cent drop in anterior stromal keratocytes 6 and 12 months after myopic laser in-situ keratomileusis (LASIK), respectively. Differences in the severity and duration of these two different forms of mechanical and laser interventions – epithelial debridement and photoablation versus lens-induced epithelial microtrauma – could account for the differences in extent of keratocyte loss between contact lens[10,11,13] and refractive surgery studies.[15,16,18] Nevertheless, these findings serve to confirm that a combination of mechanical and photorefractive interventions alter keratocyte populations, perhaps in some ways analogous to the effects induced by contact lenses.

Mechanical scrape wounds

Wilson et al.[19] detected cell shrinkage, blebbing with formation of membrane bound bodies, condensation and fragmentation of the chromatin, and DNA fragmentation in anterior stromal keratocytes after the epithelium had been damaged by creating scrape wounds. The authors concluded that the disappearance of keratocytes from the underlying anterior stroma after epithelial debridement is mediated by apoptosis. Clearly, any mechanical effect induced by contact lens wear will be less severe than the overt epithelial damage induced by the experiment of Wilson et al.;[19] nevertheless, this work establishes the principal of keratocyte apoptosis being governed by changes in the epithelium. In any case, the above analogy may not apply because the reduction in stromal KD induced by contact lenses reported in the study of Efron et al.[13] only occurred in the posterior stroma, and the results of Wilson et al.[19] relate primarily to the anterior stroma.

The loss of posterior keratocytes reported in the 6 month study of Efron et al.[13] was not associated with stromal thinning; this is perhaps because stromal thinning is a long-term change that may not become apparent until lenses have been worn for many years. Long-term studies of stromal thickness changes in patients who wear silicone hydrogel contact lenses (which do not induce corneal

hypoxia) may provide valuable insights into the etiology of stromal thinning; the absence of stromal thinning in such circumstances will point strongly to hypoxia as the cause, whereas the presence of stromal thinning associated with silicone hydrogel lenses will suggest an etiology that relates to the physical presence of the lens.

Management

The standard strategy to alleviate any condition related to contact lenses is to remove the cause. However, the application of this general strategy in the case of stromal thinning is problematic because the cause is presently unknown. Certainly, Holden et al.[20] failed to develop a predictive model for stromal thinning based on their experimental data.[1]

If it is determined in the future that hypoxia is of etiologic significance in stromal thinning, the solution to this problem will be to fit lenses that optimize corneal oxygen availability. If the physical presence of a contact lens is deemed to be a key determinant of stromal thinning, then the design and fit of lenses that minimize physical contact with the eye will provide the solution. Of course, it is difficult to see how a perfect solution to the avoidance of physical contact could be found; the device is, after all, called a contact lens!

Estimating stromal thinning

There are important clinical ramifications of stromal thinning induced by contact lenses, in addition to this being of interest from the standpoint of understanding the fundamental mechanisms of corneal physiology. Stromal thinning may be associated with a structural weakening of the cornea, which leads to a greater susceptibility to corneal warpage induced by contact lenses and to refractive changes (see Chapter 24). Thus, measurement of corneal thickness may, at least, assist practitioners to reconcile clinical phenomena thought to be related to structural weakening of the cornea.

Assuming that the cornea of a contact lens wearer is 550 µm thick before commencing lens wear, the epithelium thins by a total of about 5 µm and the stroma thins by about 2.5 µm per year of lens wear, one might expect the presenting corneal thickness of a lens wearer to be:

Presenting corneal thickness = 545 –
[2.5 × (Years of lens wear)] µm
To take an example, a patient who has
been wearing lenses for 16 years might
be expected to have a corneal thickness
of 505 µm (i.e., 545 – [2.5 × 16]).

Advice regarding refractive surgery

A significant percentage of patients who
contemplate corneal refractive surgery
wear contact lenses. Lens-induced stromal thinning may preclude a myopic
patient from undergoing refractive surgery because there may be insufficient
corneal tissue available for ablation to
create the desired refractive change
safely. Indeed, pachometry is an important pre-screening test for all potential
refractive surgery patients, and Seiler *et
al.*[21] suggest that the minimum residual
corneal thickness after ablation should
be 250 µm to avoid ectasia. Thus, contact lens wearers should be warned at an
early stage that long-term lens wear may
preclude refractive surgery at a later
date because of lens-induced stromal
thinning.

Prognosis

In the study of Holden *et al.*,[1] subjects
discontinued lens wear for 1 month so
that recovery of any lens-induced changes
over this period could be monitored. As
can be seen from *Figure 19.2*, the stromal
thinning that was evident after 7 days
(once the acute lens-induced edema had
subsided) displayed no signs of recovery
over the subsequent 23 days. Five subjects were convinced by Holden *et al.*[22]
to refrain from wearing lenses for a
further 5 months, and it was observed
that stromal thickness appeared to be
gradually returning to normal. These
authors[22] concluded, therefore, that
lens-induced stromal thinning is 'very
long lasting'.

Microdots

In what may be a corollary of stromal
thinning, Bohnke and Masters[23] described
a condition that they termed 'stromal
microdot degeneration' (*Figure 19.7*).
They suggested that numerous small
white dots seen with the confocal
microscope in long-term contact lens
wearers may be a sign of stromal degeneration, and that this "… may be the
early stage of a significant corneal disease, which eventually may affect large

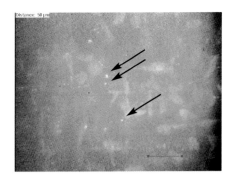

Figure 19.7
Stromal microdot degeneration. Some
microdots are indicated by arrows

numbers of patients after decades of
contact lens wear." This rather bleak
prognosis must be tempered by the fact
that Bohnke and Masters[23] apparently
failed to notice that microdots can also
be observed in normal non-lens wearers,
albeit in lower numbers.[24] Nevertheless,
stromal microdots may represent visible
evidence of accelerated keratocyte apoptosis. If keratocyte apoptosis is associated with stromal thinning, stromal
microdots may be an associated feature
in advanced cases. Further research is
required to validate such an association.

Differential Diagnosis

Stromal thinning induced by contact
lenses needs to be differentiated from
stromal thinning associated with corneal
diseases and dystrophies.

Keratoconus

An obvious candidate for differential
diagnosis is keratoconus, a condition
characterized by apical corneal thinning
(*Figure 19.8*), distortion and steepening,
irregular astigmatism and poor spectacle visual acuity. Pflugfelder[25] demonstrated that two indices generated
from measurements obtained from the
Orbscan Corneal Topography System
(CTS; Orbscan, Inc., Salt Lake City, UT)
can be used to distinguish corneal thinning induced by contact lenses from
keratoconus. These are the 'corneal
thickness index' and a mathematically
derived 'discriminant function'.

Pellucid marginal degeneration

Pellucid marginal degeneration is an
uncommon variant of keratoconus. A

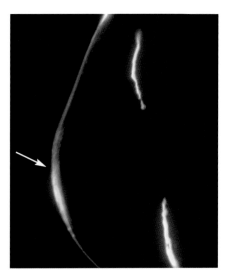

Figure 19.8
Keratoconus displaying stromal thinning
(arrow)

corneal protrusion occurs inferiorly, usually above a narrow band of clear, neovascularized, thinned corneal stroma,
and is concentric with the limbus. The
corneal protrusion is steepest directly
above the band of corneal thinning,
which results in a 'beer belly' appearance, and the thinning can also occur
superiorly. In *Figure 19.9*, the classic inferior 'beer belly' appearance is evident, as
well as superior thinning. The key aspect
of differential diagnosis is that stromal
thinning induced by contact lenses occurs
across the whole cornea, whereas thinning occurs at the corneal margin in pellucid marginal degeneration.

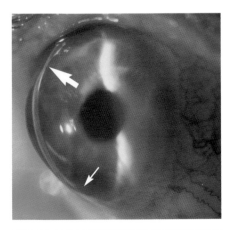

Figure 19.9
Pellucid marginal degeneration, with
thinning of the superior cornea (thick arrow)
and inferior cornea (thin arrow)

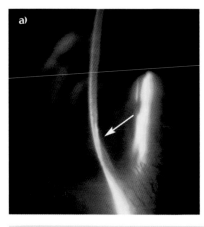
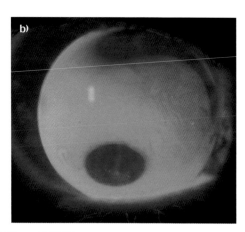

Figure 19.10

Terrien's marginal corneal degeneration. (a) Stromal thinning (arrow) and (b) fluorescein pattern of rigid lens fit on the cornea in (a), showing heavy bearing inferiorly at the region of protrusion

Terrien's marginal corneal degeneration

Peripheral corneal thinning is also a characteristic of Terrien's marginal corneal degeneration. This is a symmetric, ectatic, marginal corneal dystrophy, seen more often in middle-aged men.[8] The degeneration usually occurs in the superior cornea, but may occur anywhere around the limbus. It begins as a fine, punctate stromal opacity similar to corneal arcus. The affected region becomes vascularized and an indentation develops parallel to the limbus, followed by progressive thinning (*Figure 19.10a*). The thinned region may eventually bulge ectatically (*Figure 19.10b*). As in the case of pellucid marginal degeneration, differential diagnosis relates to the identification of pan-corneal versus marginal stromal thinning.

Conclusions

Further studies are required to document more fully lens-induced stromal thinning, to:

- Shed light on the etiology of this phenomenon;
- Determine if this is linked to stromal keratocyte loss;
- Discover if there are any other clinical ramifications.

REFERENCES

1 Holden BA, Sweeney DF, Vannas A, *et al.* (1985). Effects of long-term extended contact lens wear on the human cornea. *Invest Ophthalmol Vis Sci.* **26**, 1489–1501.
2 Millodot M (1978). Long-term wear of hard contact lenses and corneal integrity. *Contacto* **22**, 7–12.
3 Lebow KA and Plishka K (1980). Ocular changes associated with extended wear contact lenses. *Int Contact Lens Clin.* **7**, 49–55.
4 Schoessler JP and Barr JT (1980). Corneal thickness changes with extended contact lens wear. *Am J Optom Physiol Opt.* **57**, 729–733.
5 Liu Z and Pflugfelder SC (2000). The effects of long-term contact lens wear on corneal thickness, curvature, and surface regularity. *Ophthalmology* **107**, 105–111.
6 Myrowitz EH, Melia M and O'Brien TP (2002). The relationship between long-term contact lens wear and corneal thickness. *CLAO J.* **28**, 217–220.
7 Perez JG, Meijome JM, Jalbert I, *et al.* (2003). Corneal epithelial thinning profile induced by long-term wear of hydrogel lenses. *Cornea* **22**, 304–307.
8 Kaufman HE, Barron BA and McDonald MB (1998). *The Cornea*, Second Edition. (Boston: Butterworth–Heinemann).
9 Bergmanson JP and Chu LW (1982). Corneal response to rigid contact lens wear. *Br J Ophthalmol.* **66**, 667–675.
10 Bansal AK, Mustonen RK and McDonald MB (1997). High resolution *in vivo* scanning confocal microscopy of the cornea in long term contact lens wear. *Invest Ophthalmol Vis Sci.* **38S**, 138.
11 Jalbert I and Stapleton F (1999). Effect of lens wear on corneal stroma: Preliminary findings. *Aust NZ J Ophthalmol.* **27**, 211–213.
12 Efron N, Mutalib HA, Perez-Gomez I and Koh HH (2002). Confocal microscopic observations of the human cornea following overnight contact lens wear. *Clin Exp Optom.* **85**, 149–155.
13 Efron N, Perez-Gomez I and Morgan PB (2002). Confocal microscopic observations of stromal keratocytes during extended contact lens wear. *Clin Exp Optom.* **85**, 156–160.
14 Patel SV, McLaren JW, Hodge DO and Bourne WM (2002). Confocal microscopy *in vivo* in corneas of long-term contact lens wearers. *Invest Ophthalmol Vis Sci.* **43**, 995–1003.
15 Campos M, Raman S, Lee M and McDonnell PJ (1994). Keratocyte loss after different methods of de-epithelialization. *Ophthalmology* **101**, 890–894.
16 Erie JC, Patel SV, McLaren JW, *et al.* (2003). Keratocyte density in the human cornea after photorefractive keratectomy. *Arch Ophthalmol.* **121**, 770–776.
17 Mitooka K, Ramirez M, Maguire LJ, *et al.* (2002). Keratocyte density of central human cornea after laser *in situ* keratomileusis. *Am J Ophthalmol.* **133**, 307–314.
18 Perez-Gomez I and Efron N (2003). Change to corneal morphology after refractive surgery (myopic laser *in situ* keratomileusis) as viewed with a confocal microscope. *Optom Vis Sci.* **80**, 690–697.
19 Wilson SE, He YG, Weng J. *et al.* (1996). Epithelial injury induces keratocyte apoptosis: Hypothesized role for the interleukin-1 system in the modulation of corneal tissue organization and wound healing. *Exp Eye Res.* **62**, 325–327.
20 Holden BA, Swarbrick HA, Sweeney DF, *et al.* (1987). Strategies for minimizing the ocular effects of extended contact lens wear – a statistical analysis. *Am J Optom Physiol Opt.* **64**, 781–789.
21 Seiler T, Koufala K and Richter G (1998). Iatrogenic keratectasia after laser *in situ* keratomileusis. *J Refract Surg.* **14**, 312–317.
22 Holden BA, Vannas A, Nilsson K, *et al.* (1985). Epithelial and endothelial effects from the extended wear of contact lenses. *Curr Eye Res.* **4**, 739–742.
23 Bohnke M and Masters BR (1997). Long-term contact lens wear induces a corneal degeneration with microdot deposits in the corneal stroma. *Ophthalmology* **104**, 1887–1896.
24 Efron N, Hollingsworth J, Koh HH, *et al.* (2001). Confocal microscopy. In: *The Cornea: Its Examination in Contact Lens Practice*, p. 86–135, Ed. Efron N. (Oxford: Butterworth–Heinemann).
25 Pflugfelder SC, Liu Z, Feuer W and Verm A (2002). Corneal thickness indices discriminate between keratoconus and contact lens-induced corneal thinning. *Ophthalmology* **109**, 2336–2341.

DEEP STROMAL OPACITIES

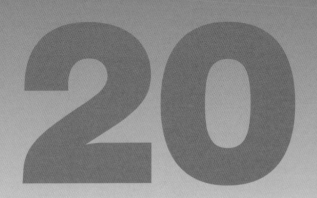

20

A limited number of reports published in the literature detail the appearance of deep stromal opacities in the eyes of contact lens wearers. As discussed in this chapter, the evidence in some of these reports to support the notion that deep stromal opacities are caused by contact lens wear is not entirely convincing. However, the possibility of a causative relationship in some of the reported cases cannot be discounted. In view of the uncertainty that surrounds the cause, this condition is referred to as contact lens *associated* deep stromal opacification (CLADSO).

Signs

Reports of deep stromal opacities can be traced as far back as 1982,[1] but relatively few published reports describe this condition, and descriptions of the clinical presentation vary considerably.

It is therefore not possible to provide a definitive description of CLADSO. In view of this, an account is given below of each of the major reports of this condition in chronologic sequence of their date of publication.

Pinckers *et al.*[2] observed whitish dots in the stroma of the cornea, which resembled a cloudy dystrophy, in four patients wearing hydroxyethyl methacrylate (HEMA) contact lenses. They referred to this condition as 'contact lens induced pseudo-dystrophy of the cornea'. A lattice-like corneal pattern was seen in another patient wearing HEMA contact lenses. Corneal sensitivity was normal or reduced.

In 32 long-term contact lens wearers (up to 19 years), deep whitish opacities directly adjacent to Descemet's membrane were seen by Remeijer *et al.*[3] in the central part of the cornea. These

opacities were seen in HEMA and polymethyl methacrylate (PMMA) contact lens wearers. Endothelial cell density was normal, but there was marked polymegethism of the endothelium, commensurate with the duration of lens wear.

A case of deep stromal opacities is shown in *Figure 20.1*. This 24-year-old female patient had been wearing HEMA lenses for only 4 years. There were no visual complaints or reports of discomfort. Viewed using a thin optic section (*Figure 20.2*), it can be seen that the opacities are confined to the posterior stroma.

In their review of CLADSO, Loveridge and Larke[4] reported the case of a 42-year-old white Caucasian female who displayed deep stromal opacification centrally and slightly inferior to the pupil, and just anterior to Descemet's membrane (*Figure 20.3*). Stellate folds were visible in Descemet's membrane. The patient had a history of 19 years of PMMA lens wear, followed by 6 years of soft HEMA lens wear. There was a degree of polymegethism and pleomor-

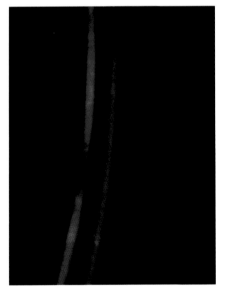

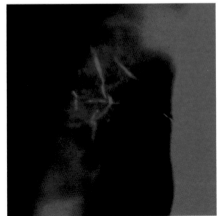

Figure 20.1
Deep stromal opacities observed in a contact lens wearer

Figure 20.2
Optic section of the cornea shown in *Figure 20.1*, demonstrating the posterior location of the opacification

Figure 20.3
Deep stromal opacities observed in a contact lens wearer

phism of the endothelium consistent with the duration of lens wear. Her contact lenses had a prescription of R –3.75D, L –5.00D, and she had worn lenses 13 hours per day without any apparent problems. The patient had been using a care system that contained the preservatives chlorhexidine and thimerosal.

Brooks et al.[5] described two patients with deep corneal stromal opacities that occurred after prolonged contact lens wear. The opacities were associated with folds or striae in Descemet's membrane, which they overlay. Although the corneal endothelial cell counts were within the normal range, the count was reduced in the affected eye in the patient with the unilateral deep stromal opacity and there was mild polymegethism of the endothelial cells.

Hoang-Xuan et al.[6] reported the cases of two patients who had worn soft contact lenses for 5 and 8 years on a daily wear basis. They presented with bilateral central avascular haze immediately anterior to Descemet's membrane, which was associated with mild stromal edema and Descemet's folds. Endothelial polymegethism was observed with the specular microscope.

Holland et al.[7] reported six patients who presented with a mottled cyan opacification at the level of Descemet's membrane. These opacities were located in the peripheral and mid-peripheral cornea. All the patients had bilateral findings, and all the patients had worn soft contact lenses bilaterally for periods that ranged from 7 to 14 years.

Pimenides et al.[8] reported the cases of one male and three female long-term HEMA contact lens wearers (mean age 30.3 years, range 26–33) who demonstrated deep stromal opacities that were predominantly just anterior to Descemet's membrane. None had any history of corneal dystrophy. These opacities were more common centrally, but were also identified in the corneal periphery. Lenses had been worn for a mean of 14.3 years (range 10–17), and for a mean of 14.3 hours per day (range 12–16). Specular microscopy disclosed cell densities within normal limits (mean 3041.5 cells/mm²) and the coefficient of variation of mean cell area was 0.31. Refractive errors ranged from –12.25 D to +6.25 D best-vision sphere.

Symptoms

Comfort

Although Brooks et al.[5] noted that the development of the opacities was associated with ocular discomfort and photophobia, other authors suggest that deep stromal opacities are asymptomatic.[2,7]

Vision

The degree of vision loss is variable. Pinckers et al.[2] reported that visual acuity was normal in the four patients they examined. All four patients in the case series reported by Pimenides et al.[8] attained at least 6/9 Snellen visual acuity. The six patients examined by Holland et al.[7] had visual acuities of 6/6 or better.

Some authors reported reduced vision in cases of deep stromal opacification. Vision loss was severe in the two cases reported by Hoang-Xuan et al.[6], and in the case report of Loveridge and Larke[4] the patient had corrected visual acuity of R6/18+ L6/12. Remeijer et al.[3] noted that deep stromal opacities could reduce visual acuity, and the patients examined by Brooks et al.[5] suffered from reduced vision.

Pathology

Comparison with pre-Descemet's dystrophies

There do not appear to have been any published ultrastructural studies of corneal tissue from patients who suffer from CLADSO. However, an important defining characteristic of this condition is that the region of affected tissue is just anterior to Descemet's membrane and the endothelium (*Figure 20.4*) – a characteristic that also defines a spectrum of sporadically appearing degenerative

changes collectively referred to as pre-Descemet's dystrophies.[9]

The opacities in pre-Descemet's dystrophies usually appear between the fourth and seventh decades of life and may show a variety of morphologies. Familial occurrences have been described, but not in all cases. Histopathologic studies obtained in one case of pre-Descemet's dystrophy showed the pathologic involvement to be limited to the posterior stromal keratocytes, with vacuolization and enlargement of the affected cells and histochemical staining of lipid-like material.[10] Transmission electron microscopy showed cytoplasmic membrane-bound vacuoles that contained a fibrillogranular material and electron-dense lamellar inclusions,[10] which suggests an accumulation of lipofuscin-like material. No extracellular deposition of a similar material was noted.

Endothelial involvement

Brooks et al.[5] advance the interesting hypothesis that that the long-term effects of subtle endothelial cell changes induced by lens wear cause a keratopathy with later scarring and opacification; that is, lens-induced endothelial dysfunction is the *cause* of deep stromal opacities (see Part VIII, Corneal endothelium). An alternative explanation is that long-term contact lens wear induces the formation of deep stromal opacification, which in turn adversely affects the endothelium.

Although it is unclear which of the above hypotheses is true, deep stromal opacities are in such close proximity to the endothelium that the function of this tissue layer may be affected adversely. This possibility was examined by Gobbels et al.,[11] who used a com-

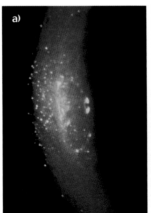
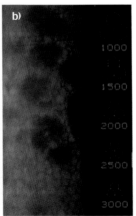

Figure 20.4

(a) Pre-Descemet's dystrophy, appearing on slit-lamp biomicroscopic examination as a localized region of deep stromal opacities just anterior to the endothelium. (b) Pre-Descemet's dystrophy, appearing on specular microscopic examination as a series of dark shadows just anterior to, and obscuring, the endothelium

puterized automated fluorophotometer to measure corneal endothelial permeability in 21 patients who had worn HEMA contact lenses on a daily wear basis for more than 10 years and who displayed deep stromal and pre-endothelial corneal opacities. They made the same measurements on an age-matched group of eight healthy individuals with no ocular disease. These authors[11] found that the corneal endothelial permeability of contact lens wearers with deep stromal opacities was increased significantly when compared with those of contact lens wearers without this condition. Also, contact lens wearers without stromal opacities showed no significant increase in endothelial permeability compared with the control group.[11]

Microdot deposits

Bohnke and Masters[12] used confocal *in vivo* real-time microscopy to study the corneal morphology in long-term contact lens wearers, and observed features (presumed to be of a pathologic nature) that they termed 'microdot deposits' (see *Figure 19.7*). Specifically, this was a cross-sectional study in which the following patient groups were examined:

- 13 patients with a history of up to 26 years of soft contact lens wear;
- 11 patients with a history of up to 25 years of rigid contact lens wear;
- A control group of 29 normal subjects who had not worn contact lenses.

The extent of microdot deposition was quantified using a scoring system ranging from 0 (no microdots) to 4 (heavy deposition). In the control group, 0 of 29 patients had stromal microdot deposits. In the soft contact lens group, 13 of 13 patients had panstromal microdot deposits with a mean score of 3.1 (range 1–4) and in the rigid contact lens group, 11 of 11 had a mean score of 1.9 (range 1–4) for corneal microdot deposits. Since subjects with soft contact lens wear had a more pronounced corneal degeneration than did subjects with rigid lenses, the authors[12] assumed the deposits to be induced by chronic hypoxia.

Bohnke and Masters[12] stated that the condition of stromal microdot degeneration as observed with confocal microscopy may be the early stage of a significant corneal disease. It is possible that stromal microdot degeneration is a precursor to some forms of CLADSO, especially in view of the demonstration by Curran *et al.*[10] that pathologic involvement in this condition is limited to the posterior stromal keratocytes, as discussed above.

Etiology

There does not appear to be any consensus among the authors of case reports of deep stromal opacities as to the cause of this condition. Indeed, a wide variety of etiologic factors has been advanced, including the following:

- Long-term contact lens wear;[3,5,7]
- Exposure to heavy metals;[7]
- Allergic reaction to thimerosal;[3]
- Exposure to chlorhexidine;[3]
- Chronic hypoxia;[3,5,6]
- Chronic hypercapnia;[3,5]
- Endothelial dysfunction;[3–6]
- Suction effects by the lens.[5]

Management

Recommendations offered by the authors of case histories of deep stromal opacification regarding management of this condition generally relate to the perceived etiology. Brooks *et al.*[5] emphasize the importance of early recognition and treatment, particularly with a better fitting lens of high oxygen transmissibility. Avoidance of the use of solution preservatives such as chlorhexidine and thimerosal is no longer an issue because these chemicals are not used in modern contact lens care systems.

In cases where the cornea appears to be severely compromised, lens wear should be ceased for up to 12 months,[4,6] or discontinued permanently. Loveridge and Larke[4] obtained apparent success by refitting a patient who had suffered from deep stromal opacities with rigid lenses, after the patient had ceased lens wear for 12 months. Pinckers *et al.*[2] and Remeijer *et al.*[3] also achieved success after the replacement of HEMA lenses by rigid lenses.

Prognosis

The prognosis for recovery from deep stromal opacities is at best protracted. Pimenides *et al.*[8] reported that the density of the stromal opacities diminished over a period of months following cessation of contact lens wear in two cases. Hoang-Xuan[6] observed that more than 1 year after the removal of contact lenses, only one patient fully recovered her initial visual acuity. Remeijer *et al.*[3] noted that the lesions gradually diminished and resolved completely in most patients. According to Brooks *et al.*,[5] once the opacities develop they regress only slowly and may result in permanent visual impairment. Pinckers *et al.*[2] reported that the pseudo-dystrophies vanished after changing the lens type.

Loveridge and Larke[4] monitored their patient for 12 months after ceasing lens wear because of deep stromal opacities. Although the appearance of folds and corneal distortion slowly resolved and vision improved – factors that would normally discount the possibility of the condition being diagnosed as a dystrophy – this resolution may have related more to the subsidence of lens-induced edema than the regression of stromal opacities.

Differential Diagnosis

Corneal dystrophies

It is highly likely that some of the cases reported as deep stromal opacification in contact lens wearers are, in fact, stromal dystrophies that present coincidentally with, but are unrelated to, contact lens wear. Perhaps it is this uncertainty that led Pinckers *et al.*[2] and Hoang-Xuan *et al.*[6] to refer to this condition as a 'pseudo-dystrophy' of the cornea. Consider, for example, the report of Loveridge and Larke[4] of an apparent case of CLADSO. The photograph of that condition (*Figure 20.3*) is almost identical to Figure 18.34 in Kaufman *et al.*,[13] which depicts lattice dystrophy of the stroma.

The three major stromal dystrophies are described as granular dystrophy (*Figure 20.5*), macular dystrophy and lattice dystrophy. The characteristics of these dys-

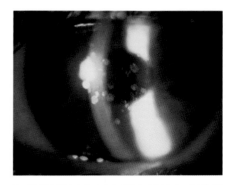

Figure 20.5
Granular dystrophy

Table 20.1
Characteristics of the three major stromal dystrophies (after Kaufman et al.[13])

Feature	Granular dystrophy	Macular dystrophy	Lattice dystrophy
Age of onset of deposits	First decade	First decade	First decade
Age of onset of symptoms	Third decade	First decade	Second decade
Age of onset of vision loss	Fourth decade	First decade	Second decade
Heredity	Autosomal dominant	Autosomal recessive	Autosomal dominant
Erosions	Uncommon	Common	Frequent

Opacities	Discrete with sharp borders
	Intervening stroma clear early, but becoming progressively cloudy
	Not to limbus
		Indistinct margins
		Hazy intervening stroma early
		
		Extends to limbus
		Endothelium affected
		Central lesions more anterior
		Peripheral lesions more posterior
			Early:
			  tiny refractile lines and dots
			  subepithelial spots
			  diffuse central haze
			Late:
			  lattice lines with knobs
			  amorphous various-sized deposits
			  stromal haze
			Limbal zone clear except in extreme cases

Corneal thickness	Normal	Thinned	Normal
Characteristic histochemical stains	Masson's trichrome Luxol fast blue Antibodies to microfibrillar protein	Periodic acid–Schiff Colloidal iron Alcian blue Metachromatic dyes	Periodic acid–Schiff Congo red Thioflavine-T Crystal violet Positive birefringence and dichroism
Material accumulated	Phospholipids Microfibrillar protein	Glycosaminoglycans	Amyloid
Ultrastructure	Electron-dense, rod-shaped structures surrounded by 8–10 nm microfibrils	Intracytoplasmic membrane-limited vacuoles filled with fibrillogranular material or lamellar bodies Similar vacuoles in endothelium	Characteristic 8–10 nm electron-dense, non-branching amyloid fibrils
Distinguishing clinical characteristics	Clear limbal zone	Opacities reach limbus Cornea thinned unless decompensated	Lattice lines

trophies are presented in *Table 20.1*. Comparison of the features observed in a suspected case of CLADSO with the characteristics of stromal dystrophies described in *Table 20.1* facilitates the differentiation of these conditions.

Stromal dystrophies characterized by additional distinct features that have been described in the literature[13] include:
- Central crystalline dystrophy of Schnyder;
- Fleck dystrophy;
- Central cloudy corneal dystrophy of Francois;
- Posterior amorphous corneal dystrophy;
- Congenital hereditary stromal dystrophy;
- Pre-Descemet's dystrophy.

The wide variety of appearances of both CLADSO and stromal dystrophies means it is not possible to define differentiating features of these conditions in terms of appearance, except to state that CLADSO, by definition, is located deep in the stroma. This consideration at least facilitates the differentiation of CLADSO from some dystrophies characteristically located at a more anterior location in the stroma.

Perhaps the key feature that differentiates CLADSO from corneal dystrophies is that dystrophies are invariably irreversible and progressive, whereas CLADSO appears to have the ability to resolve once lens wear has ceased.

Other causes

A variety of other influences can cause stromal opacification, which in turn can manifest in various forms. A number of these are likely to be observed in contact lens practice. For example, stromal scarring is often evident in advanced cases of keratoconus (*Figure 20.6*), and it is like-

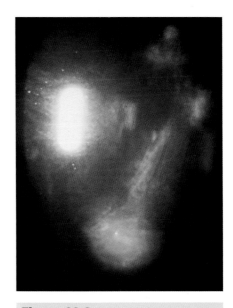

Figure 20.6
Stromal scarring in keratoconus

ly that the extent of opacification is exacerbated by rigid lens wear. Confirmation of other signs of keratoconus facilitates differentiation of this cause of stromal opacification from CLADSO.

Figure 20.7 shows the cornea of an aphakic female patient referred for soft contact lenses because of band calcification of the cornea. The calcification is suspected to have resulted from incomplete lid closure because of a partial upper lid paresis. The patient history and characteristic band appearance of the opacity allows this condition to be differentiated from CLADSO.

A bizarre case of a defined, bilateral and symmetric ring of stromal opacification in the mid-peripheral stroma is shown in *Figure 20.8*. The rings had been present for 8 years and the cause is unknown.

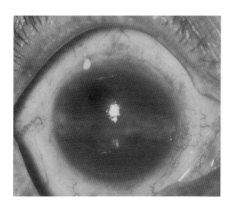

Figure 20.7
Band keratopathy

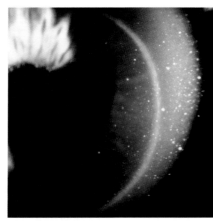

Figure 20.8
Idiopathic ring of stromal opacification in the mid-peripheral stroma

REFERENCES

1 Kilp H, Konen W, Zschausch B and Lemmen K (1982). [Deep corneal stromal opacities after contact lens wear]. *Fortschr Ophthalmol.* **79**, 116–117.
2 Pinckers A, Eggink F, Aandekerk AL and van't Pad Bosch A (1987). Contact lens-induced pseudo-dystrophy of the cornea? *Doc Ophthalmol.* **65**, 433–437.
3 Remeijer L, van Rij G, Beekhuis WH, *et al.* (1990). Deep corneal stromal opacities in long-term contact lens wear. *Ophthalmology* **97**, 281–285.
4 Loveridge R and Larke JR (1992). Deep stromal opacification: A review. *J Br Contact Lens Assoc.* **15**, 109–114.
5 Brooks AM, Grant G, Westmore R and Robertson IF (1986). Deep corneal stromal opacities with contact lenses. *Aust NZ J Ophthalmol.* **14**, 243–249.
6 Hoang-Xuan T, Laroche JM, Robin H, *et al.* (1994). [Corneal pseudo-dystrophic complication caused by contact lenses]. *J Fr Ophthalmol.* **17**, 231–237.
7 Holland EJ, Lee RM, Bucci FA Jr, *et al.* (1995). Mottled cyan opacification of the posterior cornea in contact lens wearers. *Am J Ophthalmol.* **119**, 620–626.
8 Pimenides D, Steele CF, McGhee CN and Bryce IG (1996). Deep corneal stromal opacities associated with long term contact lens wear. *Br J Ophthalmol.* **80**, 21–24.
9 Grayson M and Wilbrandt H (1967). Pre-Descemet dystrophy. *Am J Ophthalmol.* **64**, 276–282.
10 Curran RE, Kenyon KR and Green WR (1974). Pre-Descemet's membrane corneal dystrophy. *Am J Ophthalmol.* **77**, 711–716.
11 Gobbels M, Wahning A and Spitznas M (1989). [Endothelial function in contact lens-induced deep corneal opacities]. *Fortschr Ophthalmol.* **86**, 448–450.
12 Bohnke M and Masters BR (1997). Long-term contact lens wear induces a corneal degeneration with microdot deposits in the corneal stroma. *Ophthalmology* **104**, 1887–1896.
13 Kaufman HE, Barron BA and McDonald MB (1998). *The Cornea*, Second Edition. (Boston: Butterworth–Heinemann).

CORNEAL NEOVASCULAR-IZATION

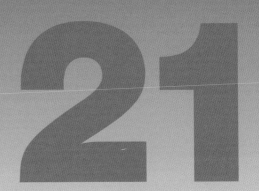

Although reports of corneal neovascularization induced by contact lenses can be traced back as far as 1929,[1] it is only in the past three decades that this problem has attracted the attention of contact lens practitioners at large. A variety of terms can be used to describe the vascular response of the cornea to lens wear. This has, unfortunately, resulted in some ambiguity in the literature, with various authors using different terms to describe the same phenomenon or using the same term to describe different phenomena. Some of the more commonly used terms used to define the presence of blood vessels in the cornea are:

- *Vascularization:* the normal existence of vascular capillaries within the cornea (encroaching no more that 0.2 mm into the cornea from the limbus).
- *Neovascularization:* the formation and extension of vascular capillaries within and into previously unvascularized regions of the cornea.
- *Limbal hyperemia* (also known as limbal redness): increased blood flow results in distension of the limbal blood vessels. Hyperemia may be active, when caused by dilation of blood vessels, or it may be passive, when the drainage is hindered. (It is also termed limbal injection or limbal engorgement.)
- *Vessel penetration:* apparent ingrowth of vessels, typically toward the corneal apex, measured from an arbitrary reference at the corneoscleral junction.
- *Vasoproliferation:* increase in the number of vessels.
- *Vascular pannus:* vascularization and connective-tissue deposition beneath the epithelium, usually in the superior limbal region. Pannus is Latin for 'cloth'; an advancing vessel plexus has the appearance of a cloth draping over the cornea.
- *Vascular response:* a general term that encompasses any alteration to the normal vasculature, including those entities described above.

Prevalence

The original haptic lenses could induce corneal neovascularization, although there is little data on the magnitude of the problem apart from isolated case reports.[1-4] Certainly, the prevalence of corneal neovascularization among wearers of polymethyl methacrylate (PMMA) lenses was very low.[5]

Reports of the prevalence of corneal neovascularization among patients who wear hydrogel lenses on an extended wear basis for cosmetic reasons are inconsistent; retrospective studies indicate substantially fewer cases of abnormal vascularization than do prospective studies. The prevalence of neovascularization during rigid (gas permeable) lens wear appears to be extremely small.

Corneal neovascularization has a greater prevalence in patients who use extended wear hydrogel lenses for aphakic correction[6] than in cosmetic lens wearers. Such a finding is not unexpected in view of the surgical trauma that the cornea has endured, the compromised physiologic status of the cornea as a result of surgery,[7] and the necessarily thick lenses that must be worn to provide the optical correction for an aphakic eye.

The reported prevalence of corneal neovascularization in patients who wear soft lenses for therapeutic reasons varies markedly. The extent of neovascularization in such patients may be related to the underlying corneal pathology being treated, the type of lens fitted and the mode and duration of lens wear.

Published estimates[5,8-21] of the prevalence of lens-induced neovascularization are presented in *Table 21.1*. When considering the data presented in this table, it is important to bear in mind that there are significant differences between studies

Table 21.1
Prevalence of corneal neovascularization induced by contact lenses

Lens type	Mode of lens wear	Lenses replaced regularly?	Patient type	Prevalence of vascularization (%)
PMMA	Daily wear	No	Cosmetic	0.03[5]
Low *Dk* rigid	Daily wear	No	Cosmetic	0.0[9]
	Extended wear	No	Cosmetic	0.0[9,10]
High *Dk* rigid	Daily wear	No	Cosmetic	7.3[19]
	Extended wear	No	Cosmetic	7.4[19]
Hydrogel	Daily wear	No	Cosmetic	0.64,[11] 1.25,[12] 14.2[19]
	Extended wear	Yes	Cosmetic	0.86,[11] 14.5,[19] 65[20]
	Extended wear	No	Cosmetic	0.0,[13] 0.2,[15] 1.75,[11] 7.0,[14] 8.7[8]
	Extended wear	No	Aphakic	14.2[16]
	Extended wear	No	Therapeutic	2.88,[17] 35.0[18]
Silicone hydrogel	Extended wear	Yes	Cosmetic	0[20,21]

with respect to sample sizes, experimental protocols, patient characteristics and criteria chosen to indicate whether a vascular response is normal or abnormal.

Signs and Symptoms

'Normal' vascular response

Using the limit of visible iris as a reference point, McMonnies et al.[22] found the mean linear extent of limbal vessel filling, measured inferiorly, to be 0.13 mm in non-wearers, 0.22 mm in rigid lens wearers and 0.47 mm in hydrogel lens wearers (daily wear). Stark and Martin[8] and Holden et al.[23] reported an increased vascular response of 0.52 mm and 0.50 mm, respectively, associated with hydrogel extended lens wear.

Whether reports of vascular responses represent the filling of capillaries that were empty, the dilation of fine vessels that were barely visible, true penetration of vessels into the stroma or a combination of these is often unclear. Nevertheless, that a number of authors[8,22,23] have established independently that various modes of lens wear can alter the appearance of the limbal vasculature provides support for the concept of a normal (although in many cases undesirable) lens-induced vascular response.

'Abnormal' vascular response

Adjacent to the limbus there exists a vascular plexus at all levels from which ingrowing vessels typically emerge. A variety of neovascularization patterns can occur, which are best considered under the three headings: superficial neovascularization, deep stromal neovascularization and vascular pannus.

Superficial neovascularization

Superficial neovascularization is the most common form of vascular response induced by contact lenses.[24] In the undisturbed eye, episcleral branches of the anterior ciliary artery form a plexus around the limbus, known as the superficial marginal arcade. Minute branches form at right angles to this plexus, and thus encroach the cornea and then loop inward toward the corneal apex (*Figure 21.1*). The resultant vascular loops or arcades are typically semicircular; they tend to anastomose, with each successive arc becoming smaller, and ultimately form a rich vascular plexus around the limbus.[24]

New vessels often leak a creamy, lipid-like fluid, which can be seen around vessels on high magnification (see *Figure 11.5*). The combination of extensive vessel formation surrounded by this extravascular fluid can lead to vision loss; however, vision loss in the case of superficial neovascularization is rare and only occurs if vessels encroach the pupillary axis.

Deep stromal neovascularization

Contact lenses can induce neovascularization at all levels of the stroma, from just beneath the anterior-limiting lamina (Bowman's membrane) down to the posterior-limiting lamina (Descemet's membrane).[24–26] It develops insidiously and may progress in the absence of acute symptoms.[27] The typical appearance is that of a large feeding vessel that emerges sharply from the limbus, usually in the mid-stroma, rapidly develops into finer, wildly tortuous branches and ends in buds with numerous small-vessel anastomoses (*Figure 21.2*). This irregular pattern is thought to result from a breakdown of structure of the stroma.[27]

Rozenman et al.[28] observed five eyes (five patients) with deep stromal neovascularization and scarring in patients wearing soft contact lenses during a 6 month period. There was no evidence suggestive of other causes of interstitial keratitis. Two patients were aphakic and required a penetrating keratoplasty. Weinberg[6] reported the case of a 61-year-old man who developed deep corneal neovascularization, decreased visual acuity and associated corneal opacity at the level of Descemet's membrane after prolonged wear of an aphakic soft contact lens. The vascularization markedly diminished and the vision improved after cessation of soft lens use; however, the associated opacity remained.

Loss of vision can occur when there has been leakage of lipid into the stroma.[29] Donnenfeld et al.[29] documented five cases of hemorrhaging of deep corneal vessels induced by contact lens wear (*Figure 21.3*); in one of these cases, a penetrating keratoplasty was required for visual rehabilitation.

Vascular pannus

A pannus is an extensive ingrowth of tissue from the limbus onto the peripheral cornea. The penetration occurs between the epithelium and anterior-limiting lamina, which results in a separation of these layers, and often leads to

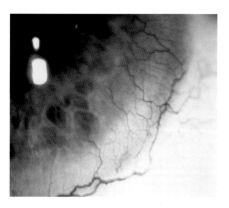

Figure 21.1
Extensive superficial neovascularization that extends approximately 2.5 mm into the cornea

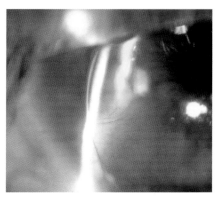

Figure 21.2
Deep stromal neovascularization in a patient who has been refitted with rigid lenses

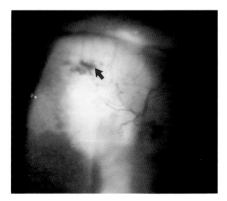

Figure 21.3
Hemorrhaging of a deep stromal vessel

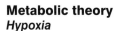

destruction of the anterior-limiting lamina.[30] The term 'micropannus' is used when the extent of invasion is less than 2.0 mm from the limbus[31] (*Figure 21.4*).

There are two forms of pannus – active (inflammatory) and fibrovascular (degenerative); both types may be observed in contact lens wearers.[32] An active pannus is avascular and is composed of subepithelial inflammatory cells. In the later stages it may be associated with secondary scarring of the stroma.

A fibrovascular pannus consists of an ingrowth of collagen and vessels, and often contains fatty plaques.[30] The clinical appearance of a fibrovascular pannus is a congested band of vessels that penetrate in an orderly fashion in the cornea, with the limit of penetration remaining even across its width. The invading end of the pannus often contains a considerable amount of fibrotic tissue, which stains brightly with rose bengal (*Figure 21.5*). This condition is observed in con-

tact lens patients in association with superior limbic keratoconjunctivitis.[33] As this name suggests, the pannus is observed at the superior limbus.

Pathology

The ultrastructural tissue changes observed in corneal neovascularization induced by contact lenses were described by Madigan *et al.*[34] in a primate model. Vessel lumina were approximately 15–80 μm in diameter and contained erythrocytes and sometimes leukocytes. Numerous extravascular leukocytes were observed around blood vessels, and the surrounding stromal lamellae were disorganized and separated with lines of keratocytes lying between them (*Figure 21.6*). The overlying corneal epithelium was often affected, with general edema, cell loss and the presence of large fluid-filled vesicles. The underlying Descemet's layer and endothelium apparently were unaffected.

The likely sequelae of events in the development of a vascular response can be predicted based upon general vascular response studies in lower animals. In particular, detailed investigations of corneal neovascularization in the rat[35] after focal injury caused by chemical cautery have enabled three distinct phases of vessel formation to be defined – the prevascular latent period, neovascularization and vascular regression.

Etiology

Numerous theories have been advanced to explain why corneal neovascularization occurs, all of which are potentially relevant to the vascular response induced by contact lenses. These theories are summarized below.

Metabolic theory
Hypoxia
Lack of oxygen is known to induce neovascularization in other body tissues; it seems obvious that similar mechanisms could also occur in the cornea.[36] Certainly, contact lenses are known to cause corneal hypoxia,[37] and hypoxia has been shown to upregulate the expression of vascular endothelial growth factor in the eye and promote neovascularization.[38]

There is, however, evidence that factors other than hypoxia must be involved in corneal neovascularization. Imre[39] points out that some hypoxic tissues do not vascularize. Michaelson *et al.*[40] found that the development of neovascularization after chemical burns in rabbits was unaffected by the ambient oxygen tension. Josephson and Caffery[41] provided evidence of progressive corneal neovascularization associated with the extended wear of a silicone elastomer contact lenses, which allow full oxygenation of the cornea because of their extremely high oxygen transmissibility.

Lactic acid
Lactic acid could be implicated in lens-induced corneal neovascularization in two ways: first, contact lenses can create hypoxia in the cornea leading to lactic acid production[42] and, second, tightly fitting soft lenses may indent the conjunctiva and restrict venous drainage, which causes lactic acid to accumulate in the peripheral cornea.[43]

Edema
The presence of excess fluid in the cornea (edema) is thought by Cogan[44] to be sufficient to induce neovascularization. This is supported by the finding of Thoft *et al.*[45] that edema facilitates anterior stromal neovascularization in rab-

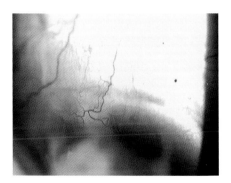

Figure 21.4
Vascular micropannus. Slight loss of tissue transparency between the vessels indicates early fibrovascular degeneration

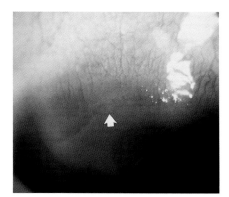

Figure 21.5
Fibrovascular pannus, with an even leading edge of fibrous tissue stained with rose bengal

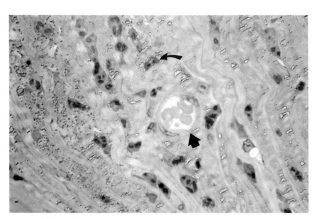

Figure 21.6
Light micrograph of single blood vessel (thick arrow) induced by contact lens wear in primate stroma. Note the erythrocytes within the vessel lumen, the single endothelial cell wall, distorted stromal lamellae and lines of keratocytes (curved arrow)

bits. Clinically, corneal edema is frequently present prior to neovascularization,[46] and some authors are of the opinion that corneal neovascularization does not occur in the absence of swelling.[47] Certainly, contact lenses can induce significant levels of edema, particularly during extended wear.[48] The etiologic role of edema can be challenged on the basis of the absence of neovascularization in conditions in which there is permanent edema (i.e., congenital endothelial dystrophy and long-term extended lens wear). Baum and Martola[49] suggest that stromal edema alone is insufficient stimulus for corneal neovascularization.

Stromal softening
Chronic edema as a result of contact lens wear may cause a breakdown of stromal ground substance or individual collagen fibrils, which results in stromal thinning (see Chapter 19). Edema could also cause the stroma to soften, or lose compactness, and thus reduce the physical barrier to vessel penetration. Sholley et al.[50] suggested that infiltrating neutrophils could release collagenases, proteases and elastases, which degrade the stroma and facilitate the ingrowth of vascular endothelial cells. While this theory could have some relevance to the normal vascular response to contact lens wear described earlier, experimental verification of a physical degradation or softening of stromal tissue in response to contact lens wear has not been produced.

The growth of vessels from the limbus along radial keratotomy scars (Figure 21.7) lends support to the 'stromal softening' theory in that loose and disorganized scar tissue can be considered as

an avenue of weakness through the normally compact stroma, and thus has the same effect as a softened stroma.

Vasogenic homeostasis model
It is now recognized that the normally avascular corneal state represents an exquisite balance between many endogenous positive and negative mediators of neovascularization. This may be referred to as the 'vasogenic homeostasis' model.

Vasogenic stimulation
According to this aspect of the model, corneal neovascularization is produced by locally generated or introduced vasostimulatory factors,[35] and vessels grow in the direction of a concentration gradient of these substances. Neovascularization is usually preceded by inflammation, and so it is likely that infiltrating leukocytes provide these vascular-stimulating factors.[51] An extensive scientific literature describes numerous candidates as vasostimulatory agents, the most important of which are listed in Table 21.2.

Vasogenic suppression
This aspect of the model proposes that the normal cornea contains substances that inhibit neovascularization.[52,53] Some of the key anti-angiogenic factors are identified in Table 21.2. These substances need to be inactivated if neovascularization is to occur. However, this part of the model lacks solid experimental support, and Fromer and

Klintworth[51] argue that positive chemotaxis toward a vasostimulating factor is a more suitable explanation of the observed patterns of corneal neovascularization.

Neural control theory
Cassel and Groden[54] suggest that there may be a neural influence on corneal vascularization. They have provided experimental support for this theory by examining the limbal vascular response to a cautery burn within a central trephined area of the cornea in rabbits. Limbal vessel growth was more advanced in the trephined corneas compared with matched controlled corneas that were not trephined. Since trephination produces denervation within the trephined zone,[55] the impaired limbal vascular response in the trephinated cornea could be attributed to an absence of neural influence. The effects of contact lenses on corneal neurology and sensitivity have been well documented.[56] If one accepts the neural control theory of Cassel and Groden,[54] it could be argued that the vascular response to lens wear is mediated by lens-induced changes to corneal neurology.

Overall model
No single theory can account for corneal neovascularization in response to contact lens wear. Indeed, virtually all of the mechanisms discussed above can be triggered by some aspect of contact lens usage. Many of these theories can be incorporated into a model of lens-induced

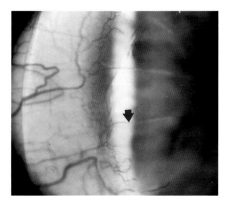

Figure 21.7
Ingrowth of vessels (arrow) from the limbus along radial keratotomy scars

Table 21.2
Factors that promote and inhibit corneal neovascularization (after Weissman[26])

Angiogenic factors	Anti-angiogenic factors
Vascular endothelial growth factor	Angiostatin
Basic fibrovascular growth factor	Endostatin
Acidic fibrovascular growth factor	Thrombospondin
Transforming growth factor alpha	Platelet factor 4
Transforming growth factor beta	Fibronectin
Tumor necrosis factor alpha	Prolactin
Platelet-derived endothelial cell growth factor	Interleukin-12
Angiogenin	Corticosteroids
Interleukin-1	Heparin
Interleukin-8	
Prostaglandin E1	
Biogenic amines	
Bradykinin	
Histamine	
Serotonin	

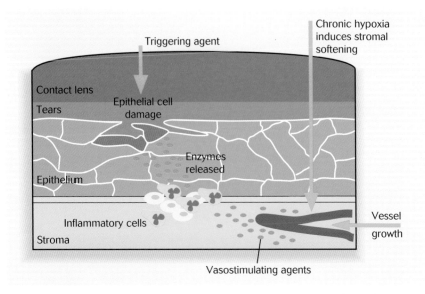

Figure 21.8

Dual etiology model of neovascularization induced by contact lenses, depicting chronic hypoxia that leads to stromal softening as a precursor, and epithelial irritation that acts as a stimulus to vessel growth

neovascularization. Such a model is given in *Figure 21.8*, in which two main etiologic factors are presented. First, the contact lens creates tissue hypoxia, which leads to corneal edema and stromal softening. Second, the contact lens has somehow contributed to a mechanical injury to the epithelium, which results in a release of enzymes. Inflammatory cells migrate to this site and release vasostimulating agents that

cause vessels to grow in that direction. As is obvious from the preceding discussion, this is only one of a number of possible models that could be proposed to explain stromal neovascularization in response to contact lens wear.

Observation and Grading

The distinguishing characteristic of superficial vessels is that they can be seen to be continuous with the superficial marginal arcade. They can be observed using direct focal illumination, but are best observed using either direct or indirect retro-illumination (*Figure 21.9*). High magnification (×40)

is often required to trace the path of the returning venules deeper in the cornea. Individual blood corpuscles can usually be observed at this magnification. Fine vessels can be observed more easily under red-free illumination (i.e., a green filter), because the red vessels appear very dark and are therefore seen in higher contrast[27] (*Figure 21.10*).

The extent of corneal neovascularization can be designated using the grading scales provided in Appendix A. The 'normal' or expected vascular encroachment observed in response to different types and modalities of lens wear discussed above means the grading in an uncomplicated lens wearer is low, but not necessarily zero. A guide to the expected level of vascular encroachment can be derived from published data.[57] Calculation of the mean-plus-one standard deviation gives the range within which approximately 85 per cent of the population falls, which is an acceptable criterion to adopt for 'normality'. Thus, the limits of 'normal' vascular ingrowth, measured from the limit of visible iris, should be (rounded upward) 0.2 mm for no lens wear or silicone hydrogel lens wear, 0.4 mm for daily wear of rigid lenses, 0.6 mm for daily wear of hydrogel lenses and 1.4 mm for extended wear of hydrogel lenses, respectively.

The maximum level of neovascularization induced by contact lenses in a cosmetic lens wearer should not exceed grade 1.5 (see Appendix A). This equates to about 0.7 mm of superficial vessel encroachment. That being the case, the 'normal' level of encroachment observed with hydrogel lenses worn on an extended wear basis is considered to be unacceptable.

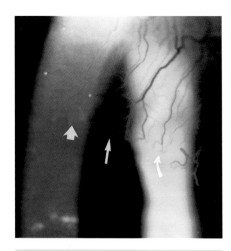

Figure 21.9

Extensive superficial neovascularization at the level of the anterior stroma, viewed by direct focal illumination (thick arrow), direct retro-illumination (curved arrow) and indirect retro-illumination (thin arrow)

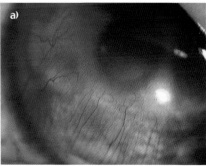
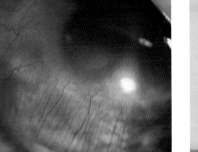
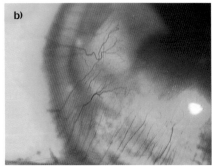

Figure 21.10

Extensive superficial neovascularization induced by contact lenses. (a) Observed in white light, and (b) observed in red-free (green) light

Figure 21.11 shows the various patterns of corneal neovascularization induced by contact lenses. The various levels of 'normal' superficial neovascularization are depicted.

Management

Needless to say, the best form of treatment of corneal neovascularization is prevention. Adherence to this maxim could be achieved by fitting a lens that does not touch the cornea, provides no resistance to the passage of oxygen or carbon dioxide (and therefore creates no edema or tissue acidosis) and does not involve the use of any form of chemical. As such a lens does not exist, practitioners are faced with a compromise.

General principles

If corneal neovascularization is a primary concern, lens design features known to provide minimal interference with corneal physiology are required, namely high oxygen transmissibility (to minimize hypoxic edema and hypercapnic acidosis), minimal mechanical effect (as judged by patient comfort[58]) and good movement (to avoid venous stasis that results from limbal compression in soft lenses[43]). Care systems likely to induce toxic or allergic responses should be avoided, and regular aftercare visits are essential.

If neovascularization of grade 1.5 or more develops, action should be taken to arrest and possibly reverse the vascular ingrowth. Since it is rarely possible to identify the specific cause of the vascular response, a systematic trial and error approach must be adopted. If an epithelial injury and/or localized keratitis is present, lens wear should be ceased until the condition resolves. In the absence of obvious concurrent pathology, the most prudent action is to replace the lens with one likely to provide an optimal physiologic response. For example, a silicone hydrogel lens might be fitted to optimize corneal oxygen availability. If chemical toxicity or allergy is thought to be the cause of a neovascular response, it may be advisable to change to a lens type (e.g., daily disposable lenses) or a care system (e.g., hydrogen peroxide system) that virtually eliminates exposure of the eye to chemicals.

Other options to be considered include changing from extended wear to daily wear, using frequent replacement or dis-posable lenses, reducing wearing time or even ceasing lens wear. In view of the extremely low prevalence of corneal neovascularization in patients who wear rigid contact lenses, a change to rigid lenses should be considered if the problem persists with soft lenses. Certainly, Chan and Weissman[32] demonstrated that conversion from hydrogel contact lenses to daily wear rigid lenses successfully reversed vascular pannus formation (*Figure 21.12*).

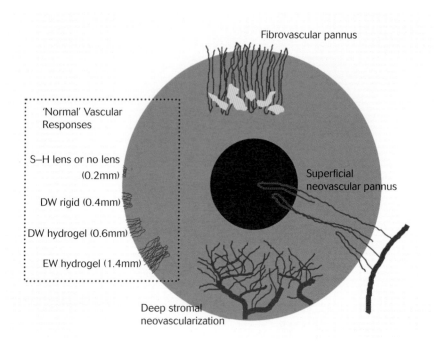

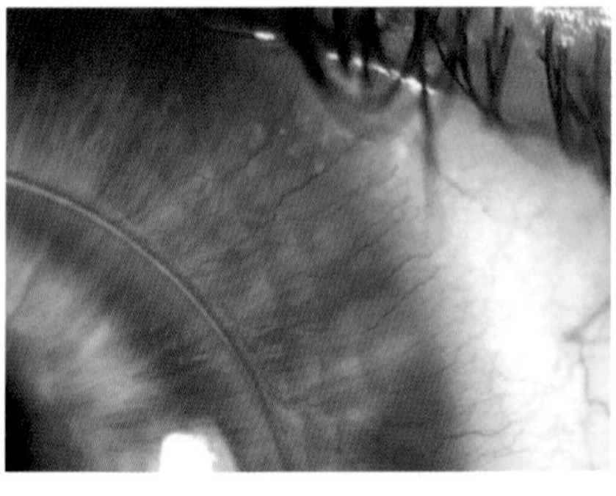

Figure 21.11

Various patterns of contact lens-induced corneal neovascularization. Si–H, silicone hydrogel; DW, daily wear; EW, extended wear

Toric lenses

Toric soft lenses are typically designed with asymmetric thickness profiles because of the cylindrical power requirement and the need to provide thick and thin zones for stabilization purposes. Even with the best lens designs, sections of the lens are relatively thick. In some toric lens designs that employ inferior prism ballast, the thick zone is located inferiorly, which can result in low oxygen transmissibility in these regions, especially if the lens material has a low Dk.[59] Westin *et al.*[60] noted the formation of inferior corneal neovascularization associated with extended wear of prism-ballasted toric hydrogel contact lenses. Changing to a different lens design or a rigid lens should solve such a problem.

Therapeutic agents

It is clear that certain drugs can control or reduce corneal neovascularization. For example, Duffin *et al.*[61] demonstrated that topical administration of a non-corticosteroid anti-inflammatory agent (flurbiprofen, a prostaglandin inhibitor) significantly suppressed corneal neovascularization induced by contact lenses in rabbits wearing rigid lenses. Topical corticosteroids can also prevent vascular ingrowth of the cornea.[62] However, Ruben[24] warns that the use of

Figure 21.12

Extensive superficial neovascularization induced by hydrogel lenses, which was treated by refitting the patient with rigid lenses

such drugs is not without danger; for example, the use of corticosteroids in patients with dry eye syndrome can result in viral and fungal infections.

Hyperbaric treatment

Other radical approaches have been applied to the treatment of neovascularization induced by contact lenses. Nishida *et al.*[63] reported the case of a 39-year-old man who suffered from corneal neovascularization that was thought to have resulted from hypoxia caused by improper use of PMMA lenses. The condition was treated successfully by hyperbaric oxygenation of the corneas under swimming goggles.

Fluorescein angiography

Visualization of the pattern of vascular progression in contact lens wearers can be enhanced with the use of fluorescein angiography.[3] Mackman *et al.*[64] used this technique to study the corneas of two aphakic patients who had undergone penetrating keratoplasty and subsequently wore extended wear hydrogel lenses. The vascularization was demonstrated to be more extensive than apparent by observing the cornea using conventional methods of illumination and observation techniques with a slit-lamp biomicroscope. Further, the ingrowing vessels were shown to be leaky, which was thought to have contributed to graft edema and graft rejection.

Surgical interventions

In extreme cases, surgical intervention may be required, such as diathermy, bipolar galvanic electrolysis or laser or microcautery occlusion of the vessels.[24,65,66] Where vision loss caused by secondary fibrosis has occurred, keratoplasty may be necessary to restore useful vision.[29]

Suspending or abandoning lens wear

Grade 2 or greater neovascularization indicates that there may be a serious threat to vision, and immediate action is required. Lens wear should be ceased for an extended period – at least until the vessels no longer lie in the pupillary area. Patients should be monitored carefully if lens wear is recommenced, as ghost vessels may refill rapidly and the neovascularization process may recur (see below). If vessels remain in the pupillary area, the patient should be counselled as to the possibility of abandoning lens wear permanently.

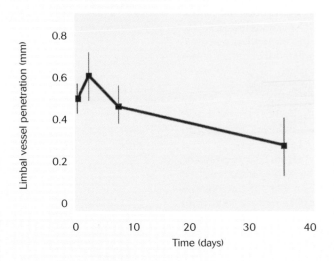

Figure 21.13

Regression of neovascularization after cessation of lens wear for 1 month after 5 years of soft lens extended wear (adapted from Holden *et al.*[67]).

Prognosis

The 'normal' form of peripheral vascular ingrowth may undergo regression when contact lens wear is ceased. Holden *et al.*[67] observed that, 1 month after removal of extended wear hydrogel lenses worn for an average of 5 years, the extent of limbal vessel penetration appeared to decrease. However, Holden's group[67] was unable to provide statistical verification of this observation (*Figure 21.13*).

Klintworth and Burger[35] noted that large vessels which invaded the rat cornea after chemical cautery injury persisted for as long as 2 months. Ausprunk *et al.*[68] observed complete regression of vessels in rabbit corneas 10 weeks after the vascularizing stimulus had been removed. Madigan *et al.*[34] reported a gradual decrease in visibility of vessels after cessation of lens wear in vascularized monkey corneas; larger vessels emptied to leave 'ghost vessels' of reduced diameter (10–25 μm), while the smaller, superficial vessels apparently regressed (*Figure 21.14*). Only a few ghost vessels were observed 14 months after lens removal. McMonnies[27] noted that fully established corneal vessels do not seem to regress in human eyes and can persist indefinitely, remaining as ghost vessels (*Figure 21.15*).

While the rate of vascular regression in humans is still open to debate, practitioners should note that cessation of

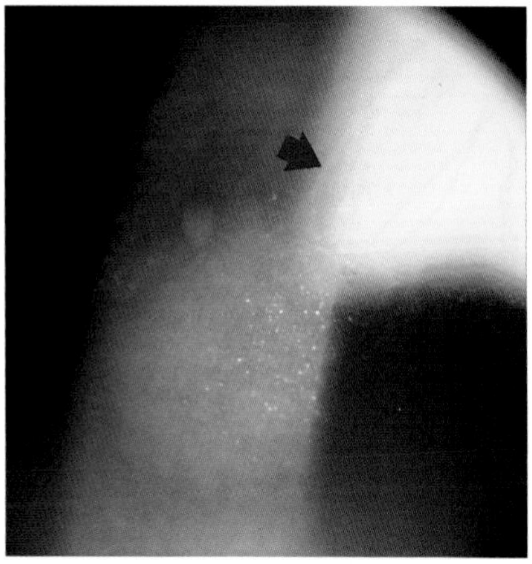

Figure 21.14

Ghost vessels (arrow) in primate cornea 3 months after lens wear was ceased

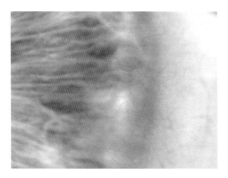

Figure 21.15

Extensive plexus of ghost vessels

lens wear will at least halt the progression of vessel infiltration into the cornea. Madigan et al.[34] reinserted lenses into monkey eyes that had suffered neovascularization induced by contact lenses 9 months previously. Within 36 hours, the existing 'ghost vessels' had refilled and the overall appearance, including associated epithelial edema, was similar to that observed during the original phase of neovascularization.

Resumption of lens wear must be treated with extreme caution and be accompanied by a rigorous and frequent aftercare protocol, since it is evident from the primate model of Madigan et al.[34] that ghost vessels refill rapidly if a stimulus to neovascularization – which may simply be lens wear – is reintroduced.

Differential Diagnosis

Stromal neovascularization has a distinct appearance so it is unlikely that this condition will be confused with other complications of contact lens wear. It is perhaps more important to distinguish between the various forms of vascular response with a view to determining the etiology of the condition. This is not always straightforward; for example, the only difference between neovascularization induced by contact lens wear versus that which may occur coincidentally as part of an unrelated pathologic process may be the extent of the reaction.

Ghost vessels have a similar appearance to nerve fibers, but are less like striae. The distinguishing features of these three structures are compared in *Table 21.3*.

Table 21.3
Differential diagnosis of ghost vessels

	Ghost vessels	Nerve fibers	Striae
Connected to limbus	Yes	Yes	No
Color	Gray/white	Gray/white	Gray/white
Bifurcations	Yes	Yes	No
Stromal depth	Any	Any	Deep
Orientation	Radial	Radial	Vertical
Form	Discrete, abrupt end	Discrete, can be long	'Feathery', faded ends
Diameter	10–25 μm	0.1–0.25 μm	5 μm
Permanence	Resolution in months	Permanent	Resolution in minutes

REFERENCES

1 Lauber H (1929). Praktische durchfurung von myopiekorrektion mit kontaktglasern. *Klin Monatsbl Augenheilkd.* **82**, 535–542.

2 Strebel J (1937). Objektive nachweise der orthopadischen heilwirkung der haftglasser beim hornhautkegel. *Klin Monatsbl Augenheilkd.* **99**, 30–38.

3 Dixon WS and Bron AJ (1973). Fluorescein angiographic demonstration of corneal vascularization in contact lens wearers. *Am J Ophthalmol.* **75**, 1010–1015.

4 Dixon JM and Lawaczek E (1963). Corneal vascularization due to contact lenses. *Arch Ophthalmol.* **69**, 72–79.

5 Dixon JM (1967). Corneal vascularization due to corneal lenses: The clinical picture. *Trans Am Ophthalmol Soc.* **65**, 333–339.

6 Weinberg RJ (1977). Deep corneal vascularization caused by aphakic soft contact lens wear. *Am J Ophthalmol.* **83**, 121–122.

7 Holden BA, Polse KA, Fonn D and Mertz GW (1982). Effects of cataract surgery on corneal function. *Invest Ophthalmol Vis Sci.* **22**, 343–350.

8 Stark WJ and Martin NF (1981). Extended-wear contact lenses for myopic correction. *Arch Ophthalmol.* **99**, 1963–1966.

9 Levy B (1985). Rigid gas-permeable lenses for extended wear – a 1-year clinical evaluation. *Am J Optom Physiol Opt.* **62**, 889–894.

10 Kamiya C (1986). Cosmetic extended wear of oxygen permeable hard contact lenses: One year follow-up. *J Am Optom Assoc.* **57**, 182–184.

11 Poggio EC and Abelson M (1993). Complications and symptoms in disposable extended wear lenses compared with conventional soft daily wear and soft extended wear lenses. *CLAO J.* **19**, 31–39.

12 Roth HW (1978). The etiology of ocular irritation in soft lens wearers: Distribution in a large clinical sample. *Contact Intraocul Lens Med J.* **4**, 38–46.

13 Maguen E, Nesburn AB and Verity SM (1984). Myopic extended wear contact lenses in 100 patients. A retrospective study. *CLAO J.* **10**, 335–342.

14 Binder PS (1983). Myopic extended wear with the Hydrocurve II soft contact lens. *Ophthalmology* **90**, 623–626.

15 Lamer L (1983). Extended wear contact lenses for myopes. A follow-up study of 400 cases. *Ophthalmology* **90**, 156–161.

16 Spoor TC, Hartel WC, Wynn P and Spoor DK (1984). Complications of continuous-wear soft contact lenses in a nonreferral population. *Arch Ophthalmol.* **102**, 1312–1313.

17 Dohlman C, Bouchoff SA and Mobilia EE (1973). Complications in use of soft contact lenses in corneal disease. *Arch Ophthalmol.* **90**, 367–375.

18 Schecter DR, Emery JM and Soper JW (1975). Corneal vascularization in therapeutic soft-lens wear. *Contact Intraocul Lens Med J.* **1**, 141–145.

19 Gleason W, Tanaka H, Albright RA and Cavanagh HD (2003). A 1-year prospective clinical trial of menicon Z (tisilfocon A) rigid gas-permeable contact lenses worn on a 30-day continuous wear schedule. *Eye Contact Lens* **29**, 2–9.

20 Fonn D, MacDonald KE, Richter D and Pritchard N (2002). The ocular response to extended wear of a high *Dk* silicone hydrogel contact lens. *Clin Exp Optom.* **85**, 176–182.

21 Morgan PB and Efron N (2002). Comparative clinical performance of two silicone hydrogel contact lenses for continuous wear. *Clin Exp Optom.* **85**, 183–192.

22 McMonnies CW, Chapman-Davies A and Holden BA (1982). The vascular response to contact lens wear. *Am J Optom Physiol Opt.* **59**, 795–799.

23 Holden BA, Sweeney DF, Swarbrick HA, et al. (1986). The vascular response to long-term extended contact lens wear. *Clin Exp Optom.* **69**, 112–119.

24 Ruben M (1981). Corneal vascularization. In: *Complications of contact lenses*, p. 27–35, Eds Miller D and White PF. (Boston: Little, Brown and Co.)

25 Shah SS, Yeung KK and Weissman BA (1998). Contact lens related deep stromal vascularization. *Int Contact Lens Clin.* **25**, 128–136.

26 Weissman BA (2001). Corneal vascularization: The superficial and the deep. *Contact Lens Ant Eye* **24**, 3–8.

27 McMonnies CW (1983). Contact lens-induced corneal vascularization. *Int Contact Lens Clin.* **10**, 12–21.

28 Rozenman Y, Donnenfeld ED, Cohen EJ, et al. (1989). Contact lens-related deep stromal neovascularization. *Am J Ophthalmol.* **107**, 27–32.

29 Donnenfeld ED, Ingraham H, Perry HD, et al. (1991). Contact lens-related deep stromal intracorneal hemorrhage. *Ophthalmology* **98**, 1793–1796.

30 Apple DJ and Rabb MF (1978). *Clinicopathologic Correlation of Ocular Disease. A Text and Stereoscopic Atlas*, Second Edition. (St Louis: Mosby).

31 Grayson M (1983). *Diseases of the Cornea*, Second Edition. (St Louis: Mosby).

32 Chan WK and Weissman BA (1996). Corneal pannus associated with contact lens wear. *Am J Ophthalmol.* **121**, 540–546.

33 Sendele DD, Kenyon KR, Mobilia EF, et al. (1983). Superior limbic keratoconjunctivitis in contact lens wearers. *Ophthalmology* **90**, 616–622.

34 Madigan MC, Penfold PL, Holden BA and Billson FA (1990). Ultrastructural features of contact lens-induced deep corneal neovascularization and associated stromal leukocytes. *Cornea* **9**, 144–151.

35 Klintworth GK and Burger PC (1983). Neovascularization of the cornea: Current concepts of its pathogenesis. In: *Noninfectious Inflammation of the Anterior Segment*, 27–44, Ed. Foulks GN (Boston: Little, Brown and Co).

36 Ashton N and Cook C (1983). Mechanisms of corneal vascularization. *Br J Ophthalmol.* **37**, 193–205.

37 Efron N and Carney LG (1981). Models of oxygen performance for the static, dynamic and closed lid wear of hydrogel contact lenses. *Aust J Optom.* **64**, 223–230.

38 Shweiki D, Itin A, Soffer D and Keshet E (1992). Vascular endothelial growth factor induced by hypoxia may mediate hypoxia-initiated angiogenesis. *Nature* **359**, 843–845.

39 Imre G (1972). Neovascularization of the eye. In: *Contemporary Ophthalmology*, p. 88–102, Ed. Bellows JG. (Baltimore: Williams & Wilkins).

40 Michaelson IC, Herz N and Kertesz D (1954). Effect of increased oxygen concentration on new vessel growth in the adult cornea. *Br J Ophthalmol.* **38**, 588–594.

41 Josephson JE and Caffery BE (1987). Progressive corneal vascularization associated with extended wear of a silicone elastomer contact lens. *Am J Optom Physiol Opt.* **64**, 958–959.

42 Hamano H, Hori M, Hamano T, *et al.* (1983). Effects of contact lens wear on mitosis of corneal epithelium and lactate content in aqueous humor of rabbit. *Jpn J Ophthalmol.* **27**, 451–458.

43 McMonnies CW (1984). Risk factors in the etiology of contact lens induced corneal vascularization. *Int Contact Lens Clin.* **5**, 286–293.

44 Cogan DG (1949). Vascularization of the cornea. *Arch Ophthalmol.* **41**, 406–416.

45 Thoft RA, Friend J and Murphy HS (1979). Ocular surface epithelium and corneal vascularization in rabbits. I. The role of wounding. *Invest Ophthalmol Vis Sci.* **18**, 85–92.

46 Arentsen JJ (1986). Corneal neovascularization in contact lens wearers. In: *Contact Lenses and External Disease*, p. 15–25, Ed. Cohen EJ. (Boston: Little, Brown and Co).

47 Berggren L and Lempberg R (1973). Neovascularization in the rabbit cornea after intracorneal injections of cartilage extracts. *Exp Eye Res.* **17**, 261–273.

48 Holden BA, Mertz GW and McNally JJ (1983). Corneal swelling response to contact lenses worn under extended wear conditions. *Invest Ophthalmol Vis Sci.* **24**, 218–226.

49 Baum JL and Martola EL (1968). Corneal edema and corneal vascularization. *Am J Ophthalmol.* **65**, 881–884.

50 Sholley MM, Gimbrone MA Jr and Cotran RS (1978). The effects of leukocyte depletion on corneal neovascularization. *Lab Invest.* **38**, 32–40.

51 Fromer CH and Klintworth GK (1976). An evaluation of the role of leukocytes in the pathogenesis of experimentally induced corneal vascularization. III. Studies related to the vasoproliferative capability of polymorphonuclear leukocytes and lymphocytes. *Am J Pathol.* **82**, 157–170.

52 Maurice DM, Zauberman H and Michaelson IC (1966). The stimulus to neovascularization in the cornea. *Exp Eye Res.* **5**, 168–184.

53 Kaminiski M and Kaminska G (1978). Inhibition of lymphocyte-induced angiogenesis by enzymatically isolated rabbit cornea cells. *Arch Immunol Theor Exp.* **26**, 1079–1085.

54 Cassel GH and Groden LR (1984). New thoughts on ocular neovascularization: A neurally controlled regenerative process? *Ann Ophthalmol.* **16**, 138–141.

55 Rozsa AJ, Guss RB and Beuerman RW (1983). Neural remodeling following experimental surgery of the rabbit cornea. *Invest Ophthalmol Vis Sci.* **24**, 1033–1051.

56 Millodot M (1984). A review of research on the sensitivity of the cornea. *Ophthalmic Physiol Opt.* **4**, 305–318.

57 Efron N (1987). Vascular response of the cornea to contact lens wear. *J Am Optom Assoc.* **58**, 836–846.

58 Efron N, Brennan NA, Currie JM, *et al.* (1986). Determinants of the initial comfort of hydrogel contact lenses. *Am J Optom Physiol Opt.* **63**, 819–823.

59 Eghbali F, Hsui EH, Eghbali K and Weissman BA (1996). Oxygen transmissibility at various locations in hydrogel toric prism-ballasted contact lenses. *Optom Vis Sci.* **73**, 164–168.

60 Westin E, McDaid K and Benjamin WJ (1989). Inferior corneal vascularization associated with extended wear of prism ballasted toric hydrogel contact lenses. *Int Contact Lens Clin.* **16**, 20–22.

61 Duffin RM, Weissman B and Ueda J (1982). Complications of extended-wear hard contact lenses on rabbits. *Int Contact Lens Clin.* **9**, 101–105.

62 Olson CL (1966). Subconjunctival steroids and corneal hypersensitivity. *Arch Ophthalmol.* **75**, 651–658.

63 Nishida T, Yasumoto K, Morikawa Y and Otori T (1991). Hard contact lens-induced corneal neovascularization treated by oxygenation. *Cornea* **10**, 358–360.

64 Mackman G, Polack FM and Sidrys L (1985). Fluorescein angiography of soft contact lens induced vascularization in penetrating keratoplasty. *Ophthalmic Surg.* **16**, 157–161.

65 Cherry PM and Garner A (1976). Corneal neovascularization treated with argon laser. *Br J Ophthalmol.* **60**, 464–472.

66 Epstein RJ, Hendricks RL and Harris DM (1991). Photodynamic therapy for corneal neovascularization. *Cornea* **10**, 424–432.

67 Holden BA, Sweeney DF, Vannas A, *et al.* (1985). Effects of long-term extended contact lens wear on the human cornea. *Invest Ophthalmol Vis Sci.* **26**, 1489–1501.

68 Ausprunk DH, Falterman K and Folkman J (1978). The sequence of events in the regression of corneal capillaries. *Lab Invest.* **38**, 284–294.

Few of the ocular complications induced by contact lenses discussed in this book lead to a permanent loss of sight; indeed, many conditions (e.g., corneal staining, epithelial microcysts and stromal edema) resolve if lens wear is ceased. Stromal infiltrates, in the absence of significant epithelial compromise or associated pathology, are usually benign;[1] however, they can also be a key sign of microbial keratitis, which is potentially sight-threatening and often must be dealt with as a medical emergency. This chapter concentrates on sterile keratitis induced by contact lenses; that is, the appearance of stromal infiltrates in the absence of microbial infection.

General Definitions

A variety of terms are used to describe conditions in which corneal infiltrates are observed:

- Infiltrate – material that has passed into tissue spaces or cells, which may include fluids, cells or other substances. The 'other substances' may be natural to the tissue spaces or cell (but in excess) or foreign to the tissue spaces or cell.[2]
- Infiltrative keratitis – an inflammation of corneal tissue characterized in part (or in total) by the presence of infiltrates.
- Ulcerative keratitis – an inflammation of corneal tissue characterized in part (or in total) by extensive epithelial compromise and underlying epithelial and/or stromal infiltrates, and possible stromal melting.
- Microbial keratitis – an inflammation of corneal tissue as a result of the direct involvement of microbial agents, such as a bacteria, virus, fungus or protozoa.
- Infectious keratitis – an inflammation of corneal tissue attributable to the processes of direct microbial infection.

- Sterile keratitis – an inflammation of corneal tissue attributable to processes other than direct microbial infection.
- Culture-positive – microorganisms positively identified from a culture or scraping of the affected tissue.
- Culture-negative – no microorganisms identified from a culture or scraping of the affected tissue.
- Intraepithelial infiltrates – infiltrates (predominantly inflammatory cells) within the epithelium.
- Subepithelial infiltrates – infiltrates (predominantly inflammatory cells) lying between the epithelial basement membrane and Bowman's membrane and/or in the anterior stroma.
- Stromal infiltrates – infiltrates (predominantly inflammatory cells) in any part of the stroma.

Signs and Symptoms

According to Zantos,[3] infiltrates appear as a diffuse band of haziness near the limbus (*Figure 22.1*), as focal spots of haziness in any region of the cornea or

as a combination of the two. In most cases the infiltrates are 'subepithelial'; that is, beneath the epithelium, but almost always in the anterior half of the stroma. Less frequently, intraepithelial infiltrates can be observed. On slit-lamp examination, the areas of infiltration appear as hazy, gray areas that give a dull, grainy appearance (*Figure 22.1*). Infiltrates are best examined initially under diffuse illumination at low magnification, to gain an appreciation of the scope and general distribution of the infiltration. Small faint focal infiltrates can be more difficult to see and are perhaps best observed using indirect illumination. A fine optic section is used at high magnification to determine the depth of the infiltrates (*Figure 22.2*). Infiltrates are often located in the proximity of local bulbar conjunctival and limbal redness. The extent of infiltration can be assessed with reference to the grading scales in Appendix A.

Over the past two decades the literature that describes the different types of infiltrative events that occur during contact lens wear, as either a direct or an indirect result of the involvement of microorganisms, has been confusing. For

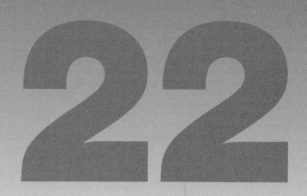

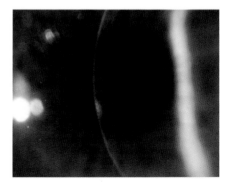

Figure 22.1
Broad band of infiltrates in the mid-peripheral cornea

Figure 22.2
Thin optic section reveals that infiltrates are located in the epithelium and anterior stroma

example, previous classification systems concentrated on whether an infiltrative episode was culture-negative or culture-positive;[4] the problem with this approach is that a culture-negative result does not necessarily imply the absence of infectious organisms (they could have been missed by chance), and a culture-positive result could have been derived from natural biota of the ocular surface unrelated to the problem being investigated. Classification systems based on the presence or absence of a corneal ulcer – or the size of an ulcer if one was present[5–7] – is also problematic because of the difficulty in precisely defining an ulcer (as distinct from an epithelial erosion) and the continuum of severity of epithelial erosions and stromal involvement.[4]

It is only since the beginning of the twenty-first century that some clarity has been given to this difficult area of contact lens management. Sweeney *et al.*[8] reviewed all the cases of corneal infiltrative events in 916 patients who wore low *Dk* soft lenses seen between 1987 and 1997 at major clinical trial sites in Australia and India. A total of 269 corneal infiltrative events were recorded, and a thorough analysis of these cases formed the basis of a classification

scheme for sterile keratitis.[8] This classification scheme, represented in a flow diagram in *Figure 22.3*, is adopted here as the basis for considering infiltrative events related to contact lenses.

Essentially, infiltrative events induced by contact lenses can be divided into microbial keratitis (MK) and sterile keratitis. The two most common forms of MK are bacterial (e.g., *Pseudomonas aeruginosa*) and protozoal (e.g., *Acanthamoeba*); MK is dealt with in Chapter 23. Five forms of sterile keratitis associated with contact lenses have been identified, and these can be classified as being symptomatic (clinically significant) or asymptomatic (clinically insignificant), as follows.

Symptomatic forms of sterile keratitis
Contact lens induced peripheral ulcer

Contact lens induced peripheral ulcer (CLPU) is a unilateral inflammatory reaction of the cornea characterized in the active stage by focal excavation of the epithelium, and by infiltration and necrosis of the anterior stroma. It is only observed in patients who wear lenses on an extended wear basis, often immediately upon waking in the morning. A

small (typically 0.5–1.0 mm diameter), single, circular focal infiltrate with a slight diffuse infiltration surrounding the focal infiltrate is present in the mid-periphery to periphery of the cornea. The region of infiltration may extend from the limbus to beyond the location of the focal infiltrate. Diffuse infiltration usually presents as a triangular pattern and appears to stream from the limbal vessels. The infiltration is limited to the anterior stroma, but there may also be slight anterior chamber involvement.

In most cases an erosion with full loss of epithelium is seen to overlie the focal infiltrate. If fluorescein is instilled into the eye of a patient during the acute, active phase of a CLPU, fluorescein fills the excavated erosion in the epithelium and a bright spot of fluorescence is seen with cobalt blue light. In addition, because of the compromised epithelial cell junction barriers, fluorescein diffuses into the surrounding stroma, to create a fluorescent halo that encircles the focal excavation. The surrounding fluorescent halo is brightest immediately around the excavation, and fades away over a radial distance of about 2 mm (see *Figure 14.16*).

Symptoms include limbal and bulbar redness and tearing. Patients experience

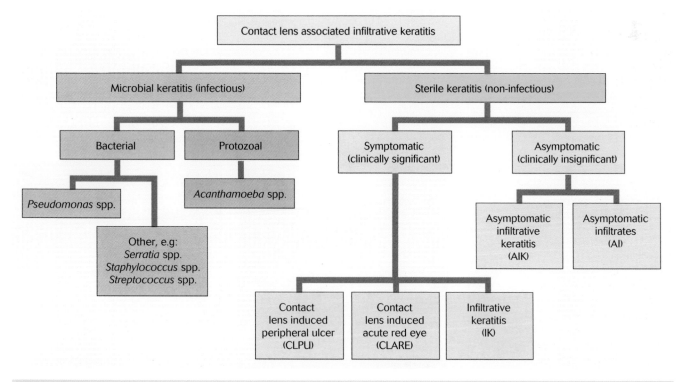

Figure 22.3
Schema for the classification of infiltrative keratitis associated with contact lenses

moderate-to-severe pain, foreign body sensation or irritation, although the condition may be asymptomatic. Some patients may report having observed a 'white spot' on their cornea.

Contact lens induced acute red eye

Contact lens induced acute red eye (CLARE) is an inflammatory reaction of the cornea and the conjunctiva observed immediately after a period of eye closure (typically overnight sleep). A combination of multiple small focal infiltrates (up to 60 may be seen) and diffuse infiltration in the mid-periphery to periphery of the cornea are present, generally without punctate staining overlying the infiltrate. The diffuse infiltration appears to stream from the limbal vessels with no clear space between the infiltrates and the limbus. It appears that the infiltration is restricted to the

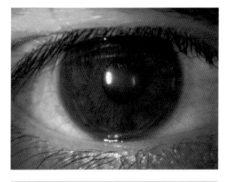

Figure 22.4
Contact lens-induced acute red eye (corneal involvement not visible at this level of magnification).

subepithelium and/or anterior stroma. Staining is not usually observed to overlie the infiltrates, and anterior chamber involvement is rare. Symptoms include moderate-to-severe circumlimbal redness (*Figure 22.4*), irritation or moderate pain, tearing and photophobia. Patients are typically awakened by their symptoms or they are noticed soon after waking. Vision can be affected adversely during the acute phase of the event. Sweeney *et al.*[9] reported that 10 per cent of 49 cases of CLARE were bilateral and the mean time to the first occurrence of CLARE after being fitted with extended wear hydrogel lenses was 8.8 ± 10.3 months.

Infiltrative keratitis

Infiltrative keratitis (IK) is a unilateral inflammatory reaction of the cornea characterized by anterior stromal infiltration, with or without epithelial involvement, in the mid-periphery to periphery of the cornea (*Figure 22.5*). Any epithelial staining that is present is usually punctate, but it may be severe enough to represent an erosion. IK is associated with both daily and extended lens wear, but events occur during the day; it is not associated with sleep and is rarely reported in the morning. Infiltrates are small, possibly multiple, with or without accompanying mild-to-moderate diffuse infiltration and restricted in depth to the subepithelium. There is no anterior chamber involvement. Symptoms include redness and mild-to-moderate irritation, but rarely pain. A watery and sometimes purulent discharge may be present.

Asymptomatic forms of sterile keratitis
Asymptomatic infiltrative keratitis
Asymptomatic infiltrative keratitis (AIK) is an inflammatory event characterized by infiltration of the cornea without patient symptoms. The condition is typically unilateral, but can present in both eyes. It is seen in association with daily and extended lens wear. Signs include small, focal, sometimes multiple, infiltrates (up to 0.4 mm in diameter) with or without mild-to-moderate diffuse infiltration in the periphery of the cornea (*Figure 22.6*). The events may be associated with punctate staining after instillation of fluorescein and sometimes involve mild-to-moderate limbal and bulbar redness. There is no anterior chamber involvement or residual scarring.

Asymptomatic infiltrates
Asymptomatic infiltrates (AI) refer to the appearance of infiltrates in the cornea with no patient signs or symptoms. They can be seen in one or both eyes, and in association with daily or extended lens wear. The event is characterized by a low number (typically two) of very small focal infiltrates (<0.2 mm) and/or mild diffuse infiltration with no staining overlying the infiltrates after instillation of fluorescein (*Figure 22.7*). There may be slight conjunctival redness. As with AIK, there is no anterior chamber involvement or residual scarring. Sweeney *et al.*[8] infer that this is not a true inflammatory event; however, some authorities[2] believe that the very presence of

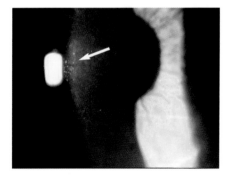

Figure 22.5
Infiltrative keratitis (arrow). Unusually, infiltrates have occurred in the central cornea. The infiltration is diffuse and restricted to the anterior cornea

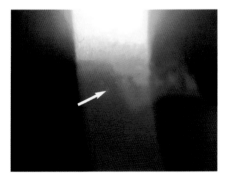

Figure 22.6
Asymptomatic infiltrative keratitis. A group of small, faint focal infiltrates can be seen near the superior limbus, in the center of the slit beam (arrow)

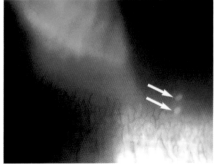

Figure 22.7
Asymptomatic infiltrates. Two small focal infiltrates can be seen near the inferior limbus (arrows), and the surrounding cornea is slightly hazy

infiltrates, by definition, implies that AI is an inflammatory event, albeit extremely mild.

Other forms of sterile keratitis

As is discussed under 'Etiology', all of the forms of sterile keratitis described above are attributed to either the direct or indirect effects of microorganisms. It is important to note, however, that infiltrates can accumulate in the corneal stroma as a result of other stimuli. Infiltrative events in this category include those induced by trauma, solution toxicity, immediate or delayed solution hypersensitivity and allergic reactions to environmental antigens. Autoimmune reactions to intrinsic cellular debris trapped beneath a tight contact lens are another source of stromal infiltrates.

The meaning of 'peripheral' ulcers

There is good reason to believe that CLPUs occur in the cornea periphery, rather than the central cornea, because any immune reaction induced by corneal insult is likely to be mediated by cellular elements derived from the limbal vasculature. The central cornea is too far from the limbus for the timely pathogenesis of a cell-mediated infiltrative event.

Notwithstanding the above argument, it is yet to be proved that CLPU is more likely to occur in the peripheral cornea than in the central cornea, simply because there is much more peripheral cornea than central cornea by way of area. It can be calculated that for a mean human corneal diameter[10] of 12.9 mm and corneal curvature[11] of 7.8 mm – and taking a pupil diameter of 4 mm as representing the 'central region of the cornea' (which might be the yardstick adopted when clinically recording central versus peripheral corneal phenomena) – the peripheral cornea represents approximately 87 per cent of the total surface area of the cornea. Thus, if infiltrative events occur at random locations on the cornea, 87 per cent of these events would be characterized as 'peripheral events'. It is difficult to disassociate this statistical artifact from the collective anecdotal clinical notion, albeit entirely rational, that a physiologic basis for CLPU occurs in the lens periphery.

Relative Frequency and Clinical Severity

An indication of the relative frequency with which the infiltrative events described above are seen in hydrogel lens wearers can be gained by considering the percentage distribution of occurrence of these events in the large sample of Sweeney et al.[8] (*Figure 22.8*). MK is relatively uncommon. Of the sterile forms of keratitis, CLPU is seen least frequently and AI is seen most frequently.

Sweeney et al.[8] asked a panel of ophthalmologists, optometrists and other biological scientists to review all 269 events of sterile keratitis in their series of cases. The majority of panel members reviewed patient records and had access to the attending eye care practitioners for any issues that required clarification. All events were rated by the panel for severity as an eye disease on a decimal scale from 0.0 to 4.0, whereby the 0 and the five integer grades corresponded to the following descriptors:

- 0 – None;
- 1 – Very slight;
- 2 – Slight;
- 3 – Moderate;
- 4 – Serious event (such as central MK).

The results of this analysis are displayed in *Table 22.1*. On average, all cases were considered to be less than moderately severe. Cases of MK, CLPU and CLARE were considered to be between slightly severe and moderately severe, the severity of cases of IK was considered to be very slight and cases of AIK and AK were essentially not considered to be clinically serious events.

Prevalence

In what was one of the first properly controlled studies of continuous wear contact lenses, Zantos[12] reported that 41 per cent of 34 patients wearing low *Dk* hydrogel lenses developed corneal infiltrates over a 2 year period. In a retrospective evaluation of the records of 500 extended wear patients wearing low *Dk* hydrogel lenses examined between 1977 and 1983, 10 per cent of patients were found by Gordon and Kracher[13] to have suffered from an episode of sterile keratitis. Josephson and Caffery[1] reported that 4 per cent of all of their hydrogel lens patients developed sterile keratitis, but they did not report the lens wear modality.

Hamano et al.[14] reported the incidence of sterile keratitis in patients wearing various lens types and modalities to be:

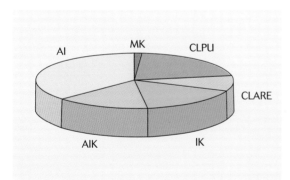

Figure 22.8
Relative frequency of the various forms of infiltrative keratitis. (AI, asymptomatic infiltrates; AIK, asymptomatic infiltrative keratitis; CLARE, contact lens induced acute red eye; CLPU, contact lens induced peripheral ulcer; IK, infiltrative keratitis; MK, microbial keratitis)

Table 22.1
Clinical severity of different forms of sterile keratitis (after Sweeney et al.[8])

Condition	Clinical severity between 0 (none) and 4 (serious event)
Microbial keratitis	2.8 ± 0.3
Contact lens induced peripheral ulcer	2.5 ± 0.4
Contact lens induced acute red eye	2.1 ± 0.7
Infiltrative keratitis	1.2 ± 0.7
Asymptomatic infiltrative keratitis	0.4 ± 0.2
Asymptomatic infiltrates	0.2 ± 0.2

- Polymethyl methacrylate (PMMA), 0.4 per cent;
- Rigid, 0.2 per cent;
- Silicone elastomer lenses, 0.8 per cent;
- Hydroxyethyl methacrylate (HEMA), 0.4 per cent;
- Hydrogel lenses with high water content, <0.1 per cent;
- Weekly disposable hydrogel lenses, 0.1 per cent;
- Daily disposable hydrogel lenses, 0.1 per cent.

Vajdic et al.[15] reported much higher incidence figures: disposable daily wear hydrogel lenses 15 per cent, disposable extended wear soft lenses 7 per cent, daily wear rigid lenses 3 per cent and extended wear rigid lenses 2 per cent. Higher incidence figures are likely to be reported from closely monitored clinical trials, such as that of Vajdic et al.,[15] versus incidence figures derived from retrospective clinical surveys, as in the case of the work of Hamano et al.[14]

In the cases reviewed by Sweeney et al.,[8] the incidence of 'clinically significant' events (CLPU, CLARE and IK), expressed as a percentage of eye years, was 6.9 per cent for extended wear and 1.4 per cent for daily wear. Half of these clinically significant events were diagnosed as CLARE. The incidence of 'non-clinically significant' events was 5.9 per cent for extended wear and 7.2 per cent for daily wear.

In a 1 year clinical trial, Brennan et al.[16] observed that 6.7 per cent of eyes wearing silicone hydrogel lenses and 3.6 per cent of eyes wearing low Dk hydrogel lenses developed sterile keratitis. Three separate 4 month clinical trials generated reported cases of corneal infiltrates in patients wearing silicone hydrogel lenses:

- Morgan and Efron[17] reported that one out of 30 subjects (3.3 per cent) developed CLARE;
- Fonn et al.[18] noted that three out of 24 patients (12.5 per cent) developed small non-staining corneal infiltrates;
- Malet et al.[19] reported that five out of 134 subjects (3.7 per cent) developed infiltrates.

Skotnitsky et al.[20] reported three atypical IK events in patients who had successfully worn silicone hydrogel lenses on an extended wear schedule for at least 15 months with monthly replacement. Each patient presented with severe pain, redness and photophobia. The events were characterized by focal infiltrates with an overlying epithelial defect in the superior periphery to mid-periphery of the cornea and extensive diffuse infiltration. The signs and symptoms of each case were more severe than is typically associated with the forms of sterile keratitis described above. The slow progression of signs and relatively fast resolution meant, however, that the cases could not be diagnosed as being MK. These cases may indicate a material dependency of sterile keratitis.

Gleason et al.[21] reported that the annualized incidence of infiltrative events in patients wearing super-permeable rigid lenses (Dk = 163) was 0.1 per cent for daily wear and 0.2 per cent for extended wear, and Stapleton et al.[22] established the following estimates of relative risk of developing sterile keratitis with different lens types and modalities:

- Daily wear rigid lenses (referent), 1.0;
- PMMA lenses ,1.0;
- Daily wear hydrogel lenses ,2.1;
- Extended wear hydrogel lenses, 2.4.

The incidence of CLARE in patients wearing non-replacement extended wear soft lenses was found by Grant[23] to be 30 per cent per patient year for hydrogel lenses with high water content and 15 per cent per patient year for those with low water. The incidence reduced to about 6 per cent when lenses were replaced regularly. The incidence of CLPU is approximately 3 per cent per patient year among hydrogel extended wear patients.[24]

Pathology

The hazy region of infiltration observed clinically is presumed to comprise primarily inflammatory cells, but it may also include bacterial toxins (often the cause of the problem; see 'Etiology'), serum, proteins and lipid that may leak from the limbal vessels. Sankaridurg et al.[25] developed an animal model (guinea pig) of endotoxin-mediated stromal infiltration. Histopathologic examination of the affected regions of the stroma revealed focal or diffuse infiltration of polymorphonuclear leukocytes.

In an extraordinary study, Holden et al.[26] obtained a biopsy of the cornea and conjunctiva of three patients who suffered from CLPU. All three patients were wearing extended wear soft contact lenses. The diameter of the three infiltrates ranged from 0.3 to 0.6 mm. Histopathologic examination of the corneal sections revealed a focal area of epithelial loss surrounded by a severely attenuated epithelium in all three patients (*Figure 22.9a*). Bowman's layer appeared to be intact and of normal thickness in two patients, but there was a localized area of loss in the other patient (*Figure 22.9b*). The anterior corneal stroma was infiltrated with numerous polymorphonuclear leukocytes beneath the area of epithelial compromise (*Figure 22.9c*). The conjunctival epithelium appeared normal and diffuse inflammatory cell infiltration, predominantly with mononuclear cells, was observed in the conjunctival stroma.

Holden et al.[26] attach great significance to the extent of damage to Bowman's layer. They suggest that the event process could have more severe

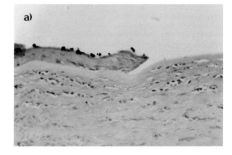

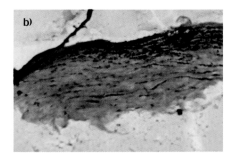

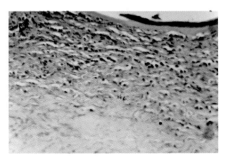

Figure 22.9

Histologic sections from patients who suffer from CLPU. (a) Marked thinning of the epithelium. (b) Loss of Bowman's layer in the center. (c) Infiltration of polymorphonuclear leukocytes into the stroma. (All hematoxylin and eosin stain)

and damaging effects in the event of involvement of Bowman's layer because:

- Injury to this layer may allow rapid spread of the stimulus – for example, toxins – from the superficial layers to the more vulnerable deeper layers of the cornea;
- An intact Bowman's layer may prevent the diffusion of substances or toxins into the underlying stroma or may decrease the rate of flow or penetration, and thus enable the normal defense mechanisms to prepare and cope with the invasion.

This theory assumes that Bowman's layer possesses certain 'barrier properties'.

Etiology

General considerations

It is recognized that in sterile keratitis there is no direct bacterial infection; that is, bacteria do not enter and replicate within the cornea. Instead, bacteria can indirectly exert a pathogenic effect on tissue through toxin or enzyme production, which can activate the immune system, which leads to an inflammatory tissue response. Dead or dying bacteria can also release endotoxins and/or exotoxins that have been implicated as a major cause of tissue damage. Endotoxin comprises lipopolysaccharide. It is a component of the outer membrane of bacteria and imparts its pathogenicity by causing antibody and cytokine production, neutrophil migration and complement activation.[27] Exotoxins are excreted by microorganisms. These toxins can cause inflammatory cells – typically polymorphonuclear leukocytes – to migrate from the limbal vessels to the site of the injury (*Figure 22.10*), creating the infiltration that appears as a stromal haze.

Although there is physiologic evidence that hypoxia is a significant factor in the etiology of MK,[28] the apparent similarity of the incidence of sterile keratitis in low *Dk* hydrogel lenses versus hyper-*Dk* silicone hydrogel lenses[16] suggests that hypoxia is not a significant factor in the etiology of such conditions. As is discussed below, sleeping in lenses is highly significant,[29] but this is probably related to the sub-clinical pro-inflammatory status of the closed lid environment rather than hypoxia beneath the closed lid.

Contact lens induced peripheral ulcer

No microorganisms were recovered by Grant *et al.*[30] from scrapings of the corneas in patients suffering from CLPU, and Holden *et al.*[26] found no evidence of microorganisms in the corneal biopsies of patients with this condition. However, Suchecki *et al.*[4] reported that eight of the 16 patients who had corneal cultures performed, from a cohort of 52 patients suffering from CLPU, had positive cultures. Notwithstanding these differences, it appears from the self-limiting and relatively benign nature of CLPU that this is a non-infectious event.

Although there appears to be no direct bacterial invasion of corneal tissue in CLPU, researchers have observed grampositive colonization of soft contact lenses worn by patients with this condition.[31–33] These observations, coupled with the self-limiting nature of the condition, suggest that CLPU occurs in response to products from remotely sited gram-positive bacteria, such as toxins.[8] All the cases of CLPU observed by Sweeney *et al.*[8] occurred in association with extended lens wear, which suggests that the closed eye environment[34,35] is also of etiologic significance.

Contact lens induced acute red eye

The sub-clinical inflammatory status of the closed eye environment[34,35] is thought to be of etiologic significance in CLARE as well as in CLPU. Furthermore, the level of oxygen beneath contact lenses under the closed eyelid is generally very low,[36] and blood vessels tend to dilate under the influence of hypoxia. Since infiltrates are derived from the limbal vasculature, hypoxia-induced vasodilatation under closed eye conditions could be viewed as a potentially significant predisposing factor. That is, inflammatory cells are able to escape more easily through the wall of a dilated vessel should a suitable additional stimulus present itself.

Holden *et al.*[37] found that 36 per cent of lenses taken from asymptomatic patients versus 100 per cent of lenses taken from patients suffering from CLARE were contaminated with gramnegative bacteria; this and other clinical studies[38] implicate such bacteria in the etiology of CLARE. The etiologic role of gram-negative bacteria in CLARE is further reinforced by a study that used an animal eye model (guinea pig).[39] Single or multiple small focal corneal infiltrates could be induced within 24 hours by inserting lenses contaminated with live gram-negative bacteria into guinea pig eyes. Furthermore, Sankaridurg *et al.*[40] described 10 episodes of CLARE in which *Haemophilus influenzae* was isolated from contact lenses and/or from one of the external ocular sites at the time of the event.

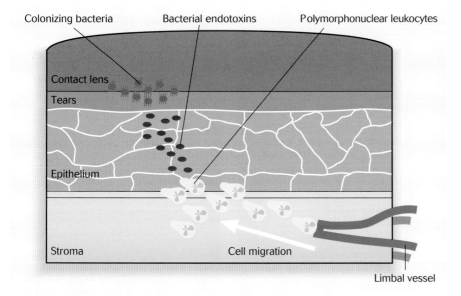

Figure 22.10

Etiology of infiltrates caused by endotoxins released from bacteria that colonize the posterior surface of a contact lens

A range of gram-negative bacteria, including *P. aeruginosa*, that were isolated from the contact lenses of patients with CLARE were unable to infect the mouse cornea.[41] Therefore, it appears that CLARE is an inflammatory reaction that is not caused by direct bacterial invasion of the cornea; rather, this condition is likely to be caused by an accumulation of toxins and other products that are released from gram-negative bacteria adherent to the lens surface, combined with the pro-inflammatory state of the closed eye during lens wear.[8]

Infiltrative keratitis

No published reports relate directly to the etiology of IK, so this must be inferred from the clinical presentation of the condition. The key factor that differentiates IK from CLPU and CLARE is that this condition occurs during the day; that is, closed eye lens wear is not a pre-requisite for the development of IK. Also, the infiltrates take on a characteristic appearance; they are small in number, focal in nature and irregular in shape, with sectorial or circumferential diffuse infiltrative patterns. Again, it appears likely that IK is an inflammatory reaction caused by toxins of unknown origin released from bacteria adherent to the contact lens surface.

Asymptomatic infiltrative keratitis

The etiology of AIK is unclear, although Sankaridurg et al.[38,42] implicated gram-negative bacteria in the etiology of this condition. Sweeney et al.[8] suggest that the mild infiltrates seen in this condition indicate that AIK is a normal protective cellular response of the cornea.

Asymptomatic infiltrates

Asymptomatic infiltrates are characterized by mild stromal infiltrates in the absence of epithelial compromise. It is unclear whether this condition genuinely represents part of the spectrum of infiltrative events related to contact lenses. If the cornea is examined carefully with high magnification on a slit-lamp biomicroscope, mild disturbances to corneal transparency, which could reasonably be interpreted as mild stromal infiltration, are observed frequently in non-lens wearers,[43] although most of these occurrences are clinically insignificant. Hickson and Papas[44] reported the presence of 'subepithelial microinfil-trates' in 4 per cent of normal, asymptomatic subjects who did not wear contact lenses. They also noted a day-to-day variation in the number of infiltrates observed within individual subjects. Certainly, these appearances, which occur coincidentally in contact lens wearers – and which could easily be recorded as AI – may explain the high relative frequency of reports of this condition in the study of Sweeney et al.[8]

Other forms of sterile keratitis
Limbal inflammation

Two non-infectious, inflammatory diseases of the limbus associated with contact lenses can also be associated with the appearance of infiltrates – vascularized limbal keratitis (see Chapter 12) and superior limbic keratoconjunctivitis (see Chapter 13). *Figure 22.11* shows focal infiltrates near the superior limbus in a patient with superior limbic keratoconjunctivitis; the appearance is similar to the type of infiltrative response seen in IK.

Neovascularization

Stromal infiltrates are often seen near the advancing edges of vessels that grow into the cornea in advanced cases of lens-induced neovascularization. In *Figure 22.12*, at least three focal infiltrates (arrows) can be seen at the advancing edge of a plexus of vessels in a soft lens wearer.

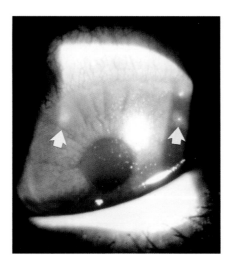

Figure 22.11

Infiltrates (arrows) near a region of limbal redness in the case of a patient who suffered from superior limbic keratoconjunctivitis

Tight lens

A tight, non-moving lens is problematic because potentially pathogenic agents, such as intrinsic cellular debris, can become trapped beneath the lens. The potentially noxious agents are held in close and constant apposition with a fixed location on the corneal surface, and can act as a stimulus for the formation of infiltrates at the location of the insult. With a mobile lens, the probability of compromise is minimized because the pathogenic agents are constantly moved around and dispersed beneath the lens. Early clinical reports of 'acute red eye reaction'[3,45,46] and 'tight lens syndrome'[47,48] strongly concur with contemporary reports of CLARE, which suggests that an immobile lens can induce a CLARE-like reaction.

Mechanical trauma

Two cases of peripheral infiltrates were observed by Efron and Veys[49] in the eyes of patients wearing lenses that contained edge defects. The likely mode of pathogenesis is that the defective lens edge abrades the epithelium. Enzymes, released from decaying epithelial cells act as a chemotaxic stimulus to inflammatory cell migration from the limbal capillaries. It is possible that trauma induced by defective lens edges could be partly responsible for infiltrates observed in patients wearing certain types of molded lenses with imperfect edges.[6]

Lens deposits

Contact lenses are known to coat with proteins, lipids, calcium and other forms of organic and inorganic matter.[50] If such substances denature and are interpreted as being foreign by the immune system

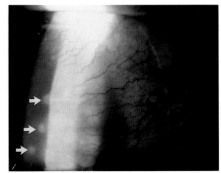

Figure 22.12

Infiltrates in the corneal mid-periphery (arrows) in association with stromal revascularization induced by a soft lens

of the body, they can act as a direct antigenic stimulus to recruitment in the cornea of tissue antibodies, such as polymorphonuclear leukocytes – hence an infiltrative response. Lens deposits may also be implicated in the development of infiltrates by their direct mechanical abrasion of the corneal surface (see 'Mechanical trauma' above).

Indirect evidence that lens deposits are involved in the formation of infiltrates comes from clinical studies that show that the incidence of CLARE in patients who wear conventional extended wear lenses can be reduced from between 15 to 30 per cent per patient year to less than 6 per cent per patient year by changing to frequent replacement or disposable lenses.[23] The reduced incidence of CLARE with regular lens replacement could result from a combination of avoiding the direct stimulus of the denatured deposits and/or obviating the deposits as an additional vehicle for bacterial attachment and subsequent bacterial toxin release.

Solution toxicity

Focal or diffuse infiltrates near the limbus are a classic sign of solution toxicity and/or hypersensitivity.[51] A toxic or allergic reaction can occur from exposure to preservatives, buffers, enzymes, chelating agents or other chemical agents incorporated into contact lens solutions. In the past, solutions that contained thimerosal and chlorhexidine could induce severe toxic reactions characterized by the appearance of infiltrates (*Figure 22.13*). Such substances became absorbed into the lens matrix during lens storage, and later diffused back into the eye in toxic concentrations.

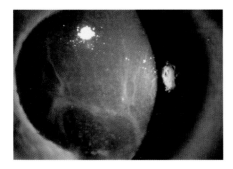

Figure 22.13
A severe case of sterile keratitis caused by solution toxicity. In this case, the patient was wearing soft lenses in association with solutions that contained thimerosal and chlorhexidine

Risk factors

Naduvilath[52] demonstrated an association between the appearance of mucin balls (see Chapter 7) and the development of CLPU. Specifically, CLPU is 1.6 times more likely to occur in patients who display mucin balls than in patients who do not display them.

Socio-economic class has been identified by Stapleton *et al.*[53] as a risk factor for sterile keratitis. Classifications that represent lower management and/or supervisory to semi-skilled and manual workers have a higher risk of developing sterile keratitis compared with classifications that represent professional and managerial occupations This finding may be related to unintelligent non-compliance.[54]

Other factors identified by Stapleton *et al.*[53] as constituting an increased risk for developing sterile keratitis include:
- Infrequent peroxide use;
- Infrequent cold chemical soak;
- Use of chlorine disinfecting solutions;
- Use of heat disinfection systems;
- No use of lens disinfection.

McNally *et al.*[55] attempted to identify risk factors for corneal infiltrative events from a 1 year, randomized clinical trial of 659 patients wearing silicone hydrogel lenses. Significant risk factors included:
- Subject age 18–29 years;
- Smoking;
- Smoking and young age combined;
- History of corneal scar.

Factors examined by McNally *et al.*[55] that were *not* found to be associated with events were:
- Male gender;
- History of extended or daily lens wear;
- Refractive error;
- Neovascularization;
- Assessment of lens fit.

Suchecki *et al.*[4] failed to find an association between smoking and the occurrence of sterile keratitis, although this negative result could be attributed to the fact that they analyzed a much smaller sample (52 patients) than that of McNally *et al.*[55] (659 patients).

Poor hygiene has been indirectly implicated as a significant risk factor for the development of sterile keratitis. The finding of Vajdic *et al.*[15] of a higher incidence of sterile keratitis in patients who wear disposable daily wear soft lenses (15 per cent) versus those who wear disposable extended wear soft lenses (7 per cent) suggests that lens handling and/or the characteristics of lens care products is implicated in the etiology of infiltrative conditions. Furthermore, Bates *et al.*[56]

reported a significant association between the occurrence of sterile keratitis and the level of contact lens hygiene and case contamination in patients who use daily wear hydrogel contact lenses. The above findings concur with the established link (discussed previously) between the development of CLARE and CLPU with the bacterial contamination of lenses.

Management

The management strategy adopted for a patient suffering from an episode of sterile keratitis depends upon the way in which the condition presents clinically.

General advice

All contact lens patients, in particular those who use lenses on an extended wear basis, should be advised that sleeping in lenses carries a greater risk of developing an adverse reaction compared with daily lens wear. Furthermore, patients should be advised to remove their lenses if they develop eye redness and/or discomfort. They should be advised to consult their eyecare practitioner if the redness and discomfort are noticed upon awakening.

Lens removal

In all cases of sterile keratitis, no matter how mild, lens wear should be suspended for at least 1 week. Severe ocular discomfort is alleviated immediately upon lens removal, although photophobia may persist for some hours. Infiltrates remain for weeks or months (see 'Prognosis'). The patient should be examined as a matter of urgency and a tentative diagnosis needs to be made as to whether the keratitis is sterile or infectious. One or more of the following signs and/or symptoms suggests MK:
- Severe ocular pain that persists or worsens following lens removal;
- Extensive and/or intensive epithelial staining overlying the infiltrates;
- Focal infiltrate(s) greater than 1.5 mm in diameter;
- Extensive anterior chamber flare;
- Extreme conjunctival redness that persists following lens removal;
- Significant loss of vision.

In mild cases of sterile keratitis, in which none of the above criteria for a tentative diagnosis of MK are met, the patient must cease lens wear and be examined later the same day and daily thereafter for at least a week to verify that all signs and symptoms are resolving. During this period, the patient may notice a continuance of mild irritation, photophobia and excess tearing.

If the signs and symptoms do not appear to be resolving after 3 or 4 days, or if there is a worsening of any aspect of the condition, it is likely to be MK, and intensive therapy must be applied (see Chapter 23). If there is progressive recovery, lens wear should not be resumed until there has been a 75 per cent resolution of infiltrates and a complete resolution of all other signs and symptoms.

Therapeutic applications

Sweeney et al.[8] suggest that, as a prophylactic measure in more severe cases of sterile keratitis, fluoroquinolones be prescribed for use during the waking hours, combined with antibiotic ointment at night. Unit dose unpreserved saline applied 4–5 times per day or cold compresses and analgesics can help alleviate symptoms. In the case of CLARE, if there is no improvement after adopting these measures, or the condition worsens, corticosteroid eye drops 4–5 times per day can be prescribed and tapered, depending on the clinical response.[8,57] In their series of 52 patients with CLPU, Suchecki et al.[4] prescribed antibiotics for 75 per cent of patients, antibiotic steroids for 23 per cent of patients and topical steroids for 2 per cent of patients.

In cases of suspected MK, a corneal scraping should be performed to determine if the condition is infectious and possibly to identify the offending microorganism. Antibiotics should then be instilled, pending the result of the corneal scraping, because such suspected cases are best presumed to be infectious unless proved otherwise. Corticosteroids may be prescribed subsequently if the result is culture-negative and the epithelium is more or less intact.[57] If the scraping result is culture-positive and the condition continues to worsen, the tentative diagnosis of MK is confirmed and more intensive therapy must begin (see Chapter 23).

Robboy et al.[58] suggest that the design of preventive measures for sterile keratitis should focus on the approaches that use molecular intervention of the inflammatory cascade initiated by the stimuli.

Fit disposable lenses

As revealed earlier, regular lens replacement lessens the risk of developing sterile keratitis. This is primarily attributable to a reduction in lens deposition and consequent inability of bacteria to colonize on the lens and adversely affect the cornea through toxin release. Daily disposable lenses are indicated for patients deemed to be susceptible to repeated episodes of sterile keratitis; however, sterile keratitis can still occur with this modality of lens wear[59] (*Figure 22.14*).

Alleviate mechanical trauma

If the source of the trauma is lens deposits, regular lens replacement should solve the problem. If certain features of the lens – such as a disagreeable physical design or a poor edge finish – are thought to be the cause of sterile keratitis, a different lens type should be prescribed.

Improve care system

A bilateral occurrence of sterile keratitis soon after commencing the use of a new care solution generally indicates a toxic or immediate hypersensitivity reaction to one or more of the components of that solution. As stated previously, the preservatives thimerosal and chlorhexidine have, in the past, been connected with such episodes. Changing to care solutions that contain high molecular weight preservatives, or non-preserved hydrogen peroxide disinfection solutions, usually solves the problem.

Improve hygiene

It is vital to stress to all patients, and in particular to extended wear patients, the importance of strict attention to all aspects of hygiene. Thorough hand washing prior to lens handling and scrupulous attention to lens-case care are key aspects to reinforce.

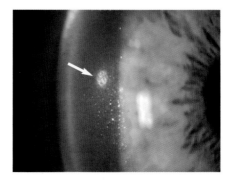

Figure 22.14

Healing ulcer (arrow) in a patient who developed CLPU 5 days after commencing a trial of daily disposable contact lenses

Avoid tight lens fit

Most disposable lenses are available in a choice of base curves. As a general rule, the flattest base curve should be prescribed unless, of course, the lens fit and vision are unacceptable. A loose fit facilitates a more effective exchange of debris and allows some degree of tear mixing beneath the lens and so avoids prolonged apposition of colonizing bacteria against a fixed location on the cornea.

Cease extended wear

If a patient who wears contact lenses on an extended wear basis experiences repeated episodes of sterile keratitis, changing to daily lens wear significantly reduces the risk of further infiltrative events.

Fit rigid lenses

It is now well established that the incidence of virtually all forms of adverse physiologic event is lower in rigid lenses than in soft lenses.[22] Certainly, this is the case in respect of sterile keratitis.[14,15,22] The reasons for the relative safety of rigid lenses are inert materials (generally resistant to long-term deposit build up), small size (not covering the limbus), greater lens movement and consequent tear exchange and mixing, and greater post-lens tear film. Suchecki et al.[4] recommend refitting with rigid lenses as a strategy for patients who have experienced a CLPU.

Fit low water content lenses

According to Swarbrick and Holden,[24] the incidence of CLARE is generally greater with higher water content lenses. This may result from the greater capacity of such lenses to absorb and re-release contaminants into the eye, the more rapid aging of such lenses and the greater propensity for spoilation compared with lower water content lenses.

Alter lens material

Ionic hydrogel materials tend to attract high levels of proteins and low levels of lipids, whereas the opposite is true for non-ionic hydrogel lenses.[50] Thus, practitioners have some control over the extent and type of lens deposits that may form, although considerable intersubject variability in deposition characteristics may, in reality, preclude material type as a variable in attempting to avoid or minimize the occurrence of sterile keratitis.[60]

Anti-fouling lens surfaces

In view of the evidence that bacterial colonization on lens surfaces plays a significant role in the pathogenesis of clinically significant forms of sterile keratitis, attention is being directed to the development of contact lens materials that prevent coating and resist bacterial attachment.

It has been shown that some of the non-steroidal anti-inflammatory agents (NSAIDs) have biofilm-inhibiting properties. Sankaridurg et al.[61] investigated the effect of three common NSAIDs – salicylic acid, sodium diclofenac and ketorolac trimethamine – for their ability to interfere with biofilm formation of a range of microorganisms on disposable soft contact lenses. It was found that NSAIDs can interfere with bacterial colonization on contact lenses, whereby the degree of inhibition of bacterial colonization varies with the type of NSAID and the virulence of strains. Of the compounds tested, salicylic acid proved to be the most effective inhibitor of bacterial colonization. Other strategies include adding compounds such as silver and furanones[62] to the lens surface.

It is likely that contact lenses – especially those designed for extended wear – will eventually be marketed with antibacterial coatings, with the expectation that the incidence of sterile keratitis will fall as a result.

Prognosis

In general, the prognosis for recovery from episodes of sterile keratitis is excellent. The rates of recovery from the three symptomatic forms of sterile keratitis are as follows:
- CLPU – 21 per cent of episodes resolve within 7 days, and the majority of all events completely resolve within 2–3 weeks.[8] Suchecki et al.[4] reported that the mean time to resolution for all infiltrates in cases of CLPU was about 12 days.
- CLARE – redness resolves within 3 days and infiltrates clear within 7–14 days.[8] Sweeney et al.[8] observed that 70 per cent of events resolved within 2 weeks, and all events completely resolved within 6 weeks. If vision is affected adversely (say during the acute phase of a serious event that affects the central cornea), it recovers within 2 days.[8]
- IK – resolves within 14 days.[8]

Figure 22.15a shows a cornea with AI. A single infiltrate can be seen next to the limbus (arrow), and there is increased redness of the adjacent conjunctiva. The patient ceased lens wear, but was not given any form of medication. After 2 weeks the conjunctival redness had subsided and the infiltrate had resolved (*Figure 22.15b*).

Although Sweeney et al.[8] did not document the rate of recovery from asymptomatic forms of sterile keratitis, it is likely that these conditions resolve over a similar time course as that for IK – that is, within about 14 days of lens removal, assuming that the condition was induced by lens wear.

As a general rule, Josephson and Caffery[1] noted that the greater the severity of infiltrates, the longer is the time course of recovery. In the most severe cases they recorded, infiltrates fully resolved within 3 months.

Of the five forms of sterile keratitis, only CLPU resolves to leave a scar (*Figure 22.16*). Indeed, all of the cases of CLPU documented by Sweeney et al.[8] resolved to leave a dense, circumscribed scar that corresponded to the area of the focal infiltrates. The appearance was described as a 'bull's eye' because of the characteristic concentric pattern of the scar formation (*Figure 22.17*). However, there was no loss of vision in any of the cases. The scar is an important 'marker' for CLPU, because in many cases – especially mild events in which the patient chooses not to seek attention – the detection of such a scar on routine examination signals that the patient has suffered from a previous episode of this condition.

Sweeney et al.[9] reported that patients who have experienced CLARE have as much as a 50 per cent chance of recurrence if they continue to wear extended wear lenses. After an initial occurrence, the mean time to the second occurrence is 12.0 ± 11.9 months. The mean time to a third occurrence is 16.5 ± 16.4 months. In the series of sterile infiltrative events surveyed by Sweeney et al.,[8] the number of recurrent events was: CLPU, three out of 24

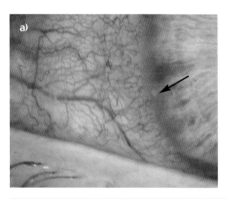
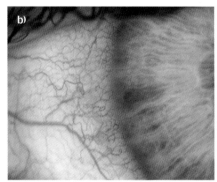

Figure 22.15
(a) Asymptomatic infiltrate (arrow) with adjacent conjunctival redness. (b) After ceasing lens wear for 2 weeks, the infiltrate completely resolved and corneal redness subsided

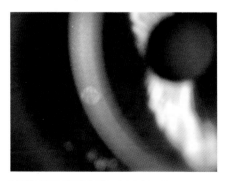

Figure 22.16
Residual scar from a CLPU

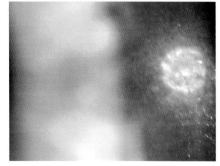

Figure 22.17
'Bull's eye' appearance of a CLPU scar viewed at high magnification

events; CLARE, 10 out of 56 events; IK, six out of 46 events; AIK, four out of 41 events; and AI, 37 out of 102 events.

Differential Diagnosis

Microbial keratitis versus contact lens induced peripheral ulcer

The most critical diagnoses when evaluating a case of stromal infiltrates is to determine whether the condition is infectious or sterile. General guidelines can be applied, such as those outlined in 'Lens removal' above. Of the five forms of sterile keratitis, CLPU is closest to MK in terms of clinical presentation. Indeed, Sweeney et al.[8] give an account of a case of MK that was initially misdiagnosed as CLPU, which highlights the importance of careful patient monitoring during the course of an episode of this condition. Aasuri et al.[63] (see below) reported that eight of the 50 cases of infiltrative events were difficult to diagnose as either CLPU or MK (referring to these cases as 'atypical CLPU with a high index of suspicion of MK').

Aasuri et al.[63] have provided a useful scheme for the differential diagnosis of MK from CLPU. The scheme, which is presented in the form of a table of relevant signs and symptoms (*Table 22.2*), is simple to apply and has considerable clinical utility. A score between 0 and 3, indicated along the top row of *Table 22.2*, is assigned for each of the 10 signs and/or symptoms listed in the first column of *Table 22.2*. These 10 individual scores are tallied to give a total score between 0 and 22, the meaning of which is indicated in *Table 22.3*.

As an example of this scheme, consider a patient wearing contact lenses who presents with the following signs and symptoms and is suspected to have CLPU (the score from *Table 22.2* is given in brackets following each sign and/or symptom):

- Mild discomfort (1);
- No lid swelling (0);
- Localized conjunctival redness (2);
- Round infiltrate (1);
- About 0.7 mm in diameter (1);
- No fluorescein staining (0);
- Slight haze in surrounding cornea (1);
- No endothelial debris (0);
- No hypopyon (0);
- Condition resolving after cessation of lens wear (0).

Table 22.2
Scoring system for infiltrative events (after Aasuri et al.[63])

Parameter	Score			
	0	1	2	3
Symptoms	None	Mild	Moderate	Severe
Lid swelling	Absent		Present	
Conjunctival redness	Absent	Localized	Generalized	
Infiltrate shape		Round		Irregular
Infiltrate size (largest diameter)		<1.0 mm	1.0–2.0 mm	>2.0 mm
Fluorescein staining	Absent	Present		
Surrounding cornea	Clear	Slight haze	Severe haze	
Endothelial debris	Absent	Present		
Hypopyon	Absent		Present	
Effect of lens discontinuation	Resolving	No change	Slight worsening	Significant worsening

Table 22.3
Scoring outcome for infiltrative events (after Aasuri et al.[63])

Total score	Clinical interpretation
0–7	CLPU
8–11	Atypical CLPU; suspected MK
12–22	MK

The total score is 6, which from *Table 22.3* confirms that the patient has CLPU.

Sterile keratitis versus epidemic keratoconjunctivitis

Epidemic keratoconjunctivitis can take on a similar appearance to sterile keratitis – with eye redness, foreign body sensation, tearing and photophobia.[64] This condition is usually bilateral and associated with the formation of focal subepithelial infiltrates scattered over the whole cornea. Tiny pits in the overlying epithelium stain with fluorescein. The infiltrates typically have a distinctive appearance of 'fluffy' edges (*Figure 22.18*), and take much longer to resolve than infiltrates seen in sterile keratitis. In addition, patients who suffer from epidemic keratoconjunctivitis may have an associated upper respiratory tract infection, regional lymphadenopathy and follicular conjunctivitis.

Opacities and scars

It is sometimes difficult to differentiate stromal infiltrates from stromal opacities. A variety of conditions that could be confused with sterile keratitis, such

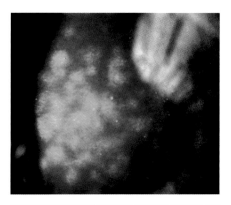

Figure 22.18
Focal infiltrates with characteristic 'fluffy' edges in a patient suffering from epidemic keratoconjunctivitis.

as deep stromal opacities, are discussed in Chapter 20.

Stromal scars are usually whiter in color compared with the typical dull gray appearance of actively forming infiltrates. Stromal scars are also more dense than infiltrates. The key feature that distinguishes scars from infiltrates is that scars are usually observed in an otherwise completely quiet eye without any associated pathology, and they do not resolve over time.

REFERENCES

1 Josephson JE and Caffery BE (1979). Infiltrative keratitis in hydrogel lens wearers. *Int Contact Lens Clin.* **6**, 223–228.
2 Anderson DM (2003). *Dorland's Illustrated Medical Dictionary*, 30th Edition. (Philadelphia: Saunders).

3 Zantos SG (1984). Management of corneal infiltrates in extended-wear contact lens patients. *Int Contact Lens Clin.* **11**, 604–612.

4 Suchecki JK, Ehlers WH and Donshik PC (1996). Peripheral corneal infiltrates associated with contact lens wear. *CLAO J.* **22**, 41–46.

5 Stein RM, Clinch TE, Cohen EJ, *et al.* (1988). Infected vs sterile corneal infiltrates in contact lens wearers. *Am J Ophthalmol.* **105**, 632–636.

6 Mertz PH, Bouchard CS, Mathers WD, *et al.* (1990). Corneal infiltrates associated with disposable extended wear soft contact lenses: A report of nine cases. *CLAO J.* **16**, 269–272.

7 Guillon M, Guillon JP, Bansal M, *et al.* (1994). Incidence of ulcers with conventional and disposable daily wear soft contact lenses. *J Br Contact Lens Assoc.* **17**, 69–76.

8 Sweeney DF, Jalbert I, Covey M, *et al.* (2003). Clinical characterization of corneal infiltrative events observed with soft contact lens wear. *Cornea* **22**, 435–442.

9 Sweeney DF, Grant T, Chong MS, *et al.* (1993). Recurrence of acute inflammatory conditions with hydrogel extended wear. *Invest Ophthalmol Vis Sci.* **34S**, 1008.

10 Martin DK and Holden BA (1982). A new method for measuring the diameter of the *in vivo* human cornea. *Am J Optom Physiol Opt.* **59**, 436–441.

11 Guillon M, Lydon DP and Wilson C (1986). Corneal topography: A clinical model. *Ophthalmic Physiol Opt.* **6**, 47–56.

12 Zantos SG (1981). *The Ocular Response to Continuous Wear of Contact Lenses*, PhD Thesis. (Sydney: The University of New South Wales).

13 Gordon A and Kracher GP (1985). Corneal infiltrates and extended-wear contact lenses. *J Am Optom Assoc.* **56**, 198–201.

14 Hamano H, Watanabe K, Hamano T, *et al.* (1994). A study of the complications induced by conventional and disposable contact lenses. *CLAO J.* **20**, 103–108.

15 Vajdic CM, Sweeney DF, Cornish R, *et al.* (1995). The incidence of idiopathic corneal infiltrates with disposable and rigid gas permeable daily and extended wear. *Invest Ophthalmol Vis Sci.* **36S**, 151.

16 Brennan NA, Coles ML, Comstock TL and Levy B (2002). A 1-year prospective clinical trial of balafilcon a (PureVision) silicone-hydrogel contact lenses used on a 30-day continuous wear schedule. *Ophthalmology* **109**, 1172–1177.

17 Morgan PB and Efron N (2002). Comparative clinical performance of two silicone hydrogel contact lenses for continuous wear. *Clin Exp Optom.* **85**, 183–192.

18 Fonn D, MacDonald KE, Richter D and Pritchard N (2002). The ocular response to extended wear of a high *Dk* silicone hydrogel contact lens. *Clin Exp Optom.* **85**, 176–182.

19 Malet F, Pagot R, Peyre C, *et al.* (2003). Clinical results comparing high-oxygen and low-oxygen permeable soft contact lenses in France. *Eye Contact Lens* **29**, 50–54.

20 Skotnitsky C, Jalbert I, O'Hare N, *et al.* (2002). Case reports of three atypical infiltrative keratitis events with high *Dk* soft contact lens wear. *Cornea* **21**, 318–324.

21 Gleason W, Tanaka H, Albright RA and Cavanagh HD (2003). A 1-year prospective clinical trial of Menicon Z (tisilfocon A) rigid gas-permeable contact lenses worn on a 30-day continuous wear schedule. *Eye Contact Lens* **29**, 2–9.

22 Stapleton F, Dart J and Minassian D (1992). Nonulcerative complications of contact lens wear. Relative risks for different lens types. *Arch Ophthalmol.* **110**, 1601–1606.

23 Grant T (1991). Clinical aspects of planned replacement and disposable lenses. In: *The Contact Lens Yearbook 1991*, p. 7–11, Ed. Kerr C. (Saltwood: Medical and Scientific Publishing Ltd).

24 Swarbrick HA and Holden BA (1997). Extended wear lenses. In: *Contact Lenses*, Fourth Edition, p. 494–539, Eds Phillips AJ and Speedwell L. (Oxford: Butterworth–Heinemann).

25 Sankaridurg PR, Sharma S, Rajeev B, *et al.* (1996). An animal model for contact lens induced corneal inflammation. *Invest Ophthalmol Vis Sci.* **37S**, 872.

26 Holden BA, Reddy MK, Sankaridurg PR, *et al.* (1999). Contact lens-induced peripheral ulcers with extended wear of disposable hydrogel lenses: Histopathologic observations on the nature and type of corneal infiltrate. *Cornea* **18**, 538–543.

27 Stapleton FS, Phillips AJ and Hopkins GA (1997). Drugs and solutions in contact lens practice and related microbiology. In: *Contact Lenses*, p. 93–153, Ed. Phillips AJ and Speedwell L. (Oxford: Butterworth–Heinemann).

28 Solomon OD (1994). Extended wear, corneal hypoxia, and corneal ulcers. *CLAO J.* **20**, 218–219.

29 Levy B, McNamara N, Corzine J and Abbott RL (1997). Prospective trial of daily and extended wear disposable contact lenses. *Cornea* **16**, 274–276.

30 Grant T, Chong MS, Vajdic C, *et al.* (1998). Contact lens induced peripheral ulcers during hydrogel contact lens wear. *CLAO J.* **24**, 145–151.

31 Wilcox MDP, Sweeney DF, Sharma S, *et al.* (1995). Culture negative peripheral ulcers are associated with bacterial contamination of contact lenses. *Invest Ophthalmol Vis Sci.* **36S**, 152.

32 Jalbert I, Willcox MD and Sweeney DF (2000). Isolation of *Staphylococcus aureus* from a contact lens at the time of a contact lens-induced peripheral ulcer: Case report. *Cornea* **19**, 116–120.

33 Wu P, Stapleton F and Willcox MD (2003). The causes of and cures for contact lens-induced peripheral ulcer. *Eye Contact Lens* **29S**, 63–66.

34 Tan KO, Sack RA, Holden BA and Swarbrick HA (1993). Temporal sequence of changes in tear film composition during sleep. *Curr Eye Res.* **12**, 1001–1007.

35 Thakur A and Willcox MD (2000). Contact lens wear alters the production of certain inflammatory mediators in tears. *Exp Eye Res.* **70**, 255–259.

36 Ang JH and Efron N (1990). Corneal hypoxia and hypercapnia during contact lens wear. *Optom Vis Sci.* **67**, 512–521.

37 Holden BA, La Hood D, Grant T, *et al.* (1996). Gram-negative bacteria can induce contact lens related acute red eye (CLARE) responses. *CLAO J.* **22**, 47–52.

38 Sankaridurg PR, Sharma S, Willcox M, *et al.* (2000). Bacterial colonization of disposable soft contact lenses is greater during corneal infiltrative events than during asymptomatic extended lens wear. *J Clin Microbiol.* **38**, 4420–4424.

39 Sankaridurg PR, Rao GN, Sharma S, *et al.* (1997). Production of corneal infiltrates in a guinea pig model using contact lenses soaked in live gram negative bacteria. *Invest Ophthalmol Vis Sci.* **38S**, 137.

40 Sankaridurg PR, Willcox MD, Sharma S, *et al.* (1996). *Haemophilus influenzae* adherent to contact lenses associated with production of acute ocular inflammation. *J Clin Microbiol.* **34**, 2426–2431.

41 Willcox MD and Hume EB (1999). Differences in the pathogenesis of bacteria isolated from contact-lens-induced infiltrative conditions. *Aust NZ J Ophthalmol.* **27**, 231–233.

42 Sankaridurg PR, Sharma S, Willcox M, *et al.* (1999). Colonization of hydrogel lenses with *Streptococcus pneumoniae*: Risk of development of corneal infiltrates. *Cornea* **18**, 289–295.

43 Sweeney DF, Terry RL, Papas E, *et al.* (1996). The prevalence of 'infiltrates' in a non contact lens wearing population. *Invest Ophthalmol Vis Sci.* **37S**, 71.

44 Hickson S and Papas E (1997). Prevalence of idiopathic corneal anomalies in a non contact lens-wearing population. *Optom Vis Sci.* **74**, 293–297.

45 Zantos SG and Holden BA (1978). Ocular changes associated with continuous wear of contact lenses. *Aust J Optom.* **61**, 418–426.

46 Binder PS (1980). The physiologic effects of extended wear soft contact lenses. *Ophthalmology* **87**, 745–749.

47 Netland PA (1990). Tight lens syndrome with extended wear contact lenses. *CLAO J.* **16**, 308.

48 Bouchard CS and Lemp MA (1991). Tight lens syndrome associated with a 24-hour disposable collagen lens: A case report. *CLAO J.* **17**, 141–142.

49 Efron N and Veys J (1992). Defects in disposable contact lenses can compromise ocular integrity. *Int Contact Lens Clin.* **19**, 8–18.

50 Jones L, Evans K, Sariri R, *et al.* (1997). Lipid and protein deposition of *N*-vinyl pyrrolidone-containing group II and group IV frequent replacement contact lenses. *CLAO J.* **23**, 122–126.

51 Binder PS, Rasmussen DM and Gordon M (1981). Keratoconjunctivitis and soft contact lens solutions. *Arch Ophthalmol.* **99**, 87–90.

52 Naduvilath TJ (2003). *Statistical Modelling of Risk Factors Associated with Soft Contact Lens-Related Corneal Infiltrative Events*, PhD Thesis. (Newcastle, Australia: University of Newcastle).

53 Stapleton F, Dart JK and Minassian D (1993). Risk factors with contact lens related suppurative keratitis. *CLAO J.* **19**, 204–210.

54 Efron N (1997). The truth about compliance. *Contact Lens Ant Eye* **20**, 79–86.

55 McNally JJ, Chalmers RL, McKenney CD and Robirds S (2003). Risk factors for corneal infiltrative events with 30-night continuous wear of silicone hydrogel lenses. *Eye Contact Lens* **29S**, 153–156.

56 Bates AK, Morris RJ, Stapleton F, *et al.* (1989). 'Sterile' corneal infiltrates in contact lens wearers. *Eye* **3**, 803–810.

57 Baum J and Dabezies OH Jr (2000). Pathogenesis and treatment of 'sterile' mid-peripheral corneal infiltrates associated with soft contact lens use. *Cornea* **19**, 777–781.

58 Robboy MW, Comstock TL and Kalsow CM (2003). Contact lens-associated corneal infiltrates. *Eye Contact Lens* **29**, 146–154.

59 Hingorani M, Christie C and Buckley RJ (1995). Ulcerative keratitis in a person wearing daily disposable contact lenses. *Br J Ophthalmol.* **79**, 1138.

60 Tighe B (1997). Patient-dependence and material-dependence in contact lens deposition. Annual Clinical Conference and Exhibition of the British Contact Lens Association. Bournemouth, June 6–8, 1997.

61 Sankaridurg PR, Bandara BMK and Willcox MDP (2003). Non-steroidal anti-inflammatory drugs inhibit bacterial colonisation to soft contact lenses. *Invest Ophthalmol Vis Sci.* **44S**, 459.

62 Baveja JK, Willcox MDP, Hume EBH, *et al.* (2004). Furanones as potential anti-bacterial coatings on biomaterials. *Biomaterials* (in press).

63 Aasuri MK, Venkata N and Kumar VM (2003). Differential diagnosis of microbial keratitis and contact lens-induced peripheral ulcer. *Eye Contact Lens* **29S**, 60–62.

64 Kaufman HE, Barron BA and McDonald MB (1998). *The Cornea*, Second Edition (Boston: Butterworth–Heinemann).

MICROBIAL KERATITIS

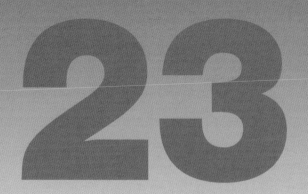

Microbial keratitis is progressive and potentially devastating to the cornea, and is the most severe reaction that can occur in response to contact lens wear. At best, the patient suffers from considerable pain and must incur the discomfort, cost and inconvenience associated with the acute management of this condition. At worst, the patient may suffer from a partial or complete loss of sight. In perhaps the most severe case of microbial keratitis ever recorded,[1] the patient ended up with bilateral large deep corneal ulcers and hypopyon. The right eye perforated spontaneously and the patient developed secondary glaucoma and bilateral optic atrophy. All of this resulted in total bilateral blindness[1] (*Figure 23.1*). Cooper and Constable[2] reported two cases of microbial keratitis leading to blindness that resulted from continuous lens wear.

Microbial keratitis is defined as an inflammation of corneal tissue through direct infection by a microbial agent, such as a bacteria, virus, fungus or protozoa; the term 'infectious keratitis' is essentially synonymous with this. The term 'ulcerative keratitis' has also been used as a synonym for microbial keratitis, but this usage is not always correct because a given case of microbial keratitis may not necessarily be ulcerative, and an ulcerative keratitis may not necessarily be microbial.

Incidence

Contact lens wear is a risk factor for microbial keratitis in general. Estimates of the number of cases of microbial keratitis induced by contact lenses that present at hospital clinics range from 12 per cent[3] to 50 per cent[4] of all presenting cases of microbial keratitis.

Numerous articles have been published that have attempted to define the incidence of microbial keratitis, and the relative risk associated with various types of lenses and modalities of lens wear. It is pertinent that the results of these studies are generally in good agreement.[5]

Determination of the incidence of microbial keratitis among contact lens wearers is problematic for a number of reasons:

- The total number of lens wearers in the population from which patients who suffer from microbial keratitis are derived is difficult to determine;
- It is not always clear as to whether the reported keratitis cases were microbial or sterile;
- It is difficult logistically to identify all cases of microbial keratitis that occur within a defined population.[5]

Notwithstanding these difficulties, Poggio et al.[6] conducted a large prospective study in the New England area of the USA and were able to determine the incidence of microbial keratitis to be 4.1 per 10,000 patients per year for daily hydrogel lens wear and 20.9 per 10,000 patients per year for extended hydrogel lens wear. Studies conducted by numerous authors since then[7–11] have arrived at almost identical results.

Estimates of the incidence of microbial keratitis for daily wear of rigid lenses range from 0.4 to 4.0 per 10,000 patients per year.[6–8,10,11] MacRae et al.[7] reported an incidence of microbial keratitis of 0.2 per 10,000 patients per year with extended wear of rigid lenses.

Holden et al.[12] estimated the incidence of microbial keratitis in patients who use silicone hydrogel lenses on an extended wear basis to be 0.53 per 10,000 patients per year. This value is 40 times less than that reported for the extended wear of hydrogel lenses and eight times less than that reported for the daily wear of hydrogel lenses,[6–11] as discussed above. Holden et al.[12] point out that this is an approximate determination based on a number of assumptions relating, for example, to the number of silicone hydrogel lens wearers worldwide; nevertheless, this early estimate gives rise to the expectation that silicone hydrogel lenses will be associated with a low incidence of microbial keratitis. Carefully controlled, large-scale epidemiologic studies are required to confirm this expectation.

It is interesting that Guillon et al.[13] found a much higher incidence of microbial keratitis per 10,000 daily soft lens wearers in the UK – 39 for conventional lenses and 18 for disposable lenses. The authors attributed these higher incidence figures to the fact that their study gath-

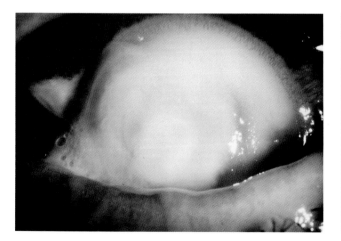

Figure 23.1
Severe case of microbial keratitis that eventually resulted in perforation, optic atrophy and permanent blindness

ered data from primary care settings that utilized a more encompassing definition of microbial keratitis, whereas other studies focused on medically diagnosed cases of confirmed and often severe keratitis.

The data of Guillon *et al.*[13] indicate the likely frequency of all symptomatic forms of infiltrative keratitis cases that present to primary care contact lens practitioners in the UK. Simple calculation reveals that a practitioner who sees 10 patients per week who use conventional daily wear lenses should see approximately two cases of suspected infiltrative keratitis per year. In his analysis of all the data on 'ulcerative keratitis' induced by contact lenses in the USA published up to 1992 – which probably includes cases of sterile keratitis – Benjamin[14] demonstrated that contact lens practitioners in the USA should each expect to see about 1.7 cases of infiltrative keratitis per year – about the same as their British counterparts.

Relative Risk

An alternative approach to determining the incidence of microbial keratitis is to establish the relative risk of developing the condition in response to different combinations of lens type and modality of wear. This form of analysis does not require knowledge of the total population of lens wearers; instead, the number of contact lens wearers with and without microbial keratitis who present to a given clinic over a defined time period needs to be determined.

Using this approach, Matthews *et al.*[15] at Moorfields Eye Hospital in the UK found that, relative to daily rigid lenses wear (the 'referent', which is arbitrarily assigned a risk of 1.0 for developing microbial keratitis), the risk of developing microbial keratitis with other types and modalities of lens wear is:

- Daily wear conventional hydrogel lenses, 1.1;
- Extended wear conventional hydrogel lenses, 2.6;
- Daily wear disposable hydrogel lenses, 4.1;
- Extended wear disposable hydrogel lenses, 8.1.

In a similar study at the John Hopkins Clinic in the USA, Buehler *et al.*[16] reported the risk of developing microbial keratitis to be:

- Daily wear conventional soft lenses, 1.0;
- Extended wear conventional soft lenses, 2.8;

- Extended wear disposable soft lenses, 3.9.

Thus, both of these contemporaneous studies,[15,16] conducted by different researchers on opposite sides of the Atlantic Ocean, confirmed a greater risk of developing microbial keratitis when lenses are worn on an extended wear basis compared with daily lens wear. Other studies of relative risk[8,17–19] support these findings.

The data of Matthews *et al.*[15] also suggest a greater risk associated with the wear of disposable lenses – a notion that is highly controversial since the raison d'être of disposability is that disposable contact lens wear is associated with enhanced safety, not greater risk. Possible explanations for these findings are discussed under 'Etiology'.

Signs and Symptoms

An early symptom of microbial keratitis is a foreign body sensation in the eye associated with an increasing desire to remove the lenses. In the case of an actual foreign body, or with other causes of lens-related ocular discomfort, lens removal leads to immediate relief. Continuing or worsening discomfort after lens removal should lead a clinician to suspect microbial keratitis. Associated symptoms include pain, eye redness, swollen lids, increased lacrimation, photophobia, discharge and loss of vision[20] (*Figure 23.2*).

Aside from the obvious signs of eye redness and lacrimation, typically an area of infiltration is observed at the site of infection[20] (*Figure 23.3*). In the early stages, infiltrates may be confined primarily to

the epithelium. As the disease progresses, the stroma becomes increasingly hazy and the epithelium above the infiltration begins to break down, which leads to staining of the ulcer and surrounding cornea (*Figure 23.4*). The appearance of microbial keratitis in the early stages (*Figures 23.3* and *23.4*) is almost indistinguishable from that of a contact lens peripheral ulcer (CLPU; see Chapter 22).

Conjunctival redness may be confined initially to the limbal and bulbar region adjacent to the field of infection, and thus provides an important clue to the clinician as to its location. This clue is soon lost as the condition advances and the eye becomes more inflamed with circumlimbal conjunctival redness (*Figure 23.5*).

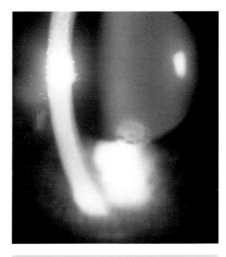

Figure 23.3

Slit-lamp photograph of the corneal ulcer depicted in *Figure 23.2*

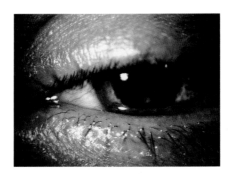

Figure 23.2

Early stages of *Pseudomonas* keratitis, with limbal redness, increased lacrimation and swollen eyelids. A small white ulcer can be seen near the inferior pupil margin

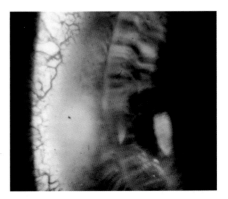

Figure 23.4

Peripheral corneal ulcer in the early stages showing fluorescein staining of the ulcer and background fluorescence, which indicates diffusion of fluorescein into the stroma

Bacterial keratitis can have a rapid and devastating time course. The initial focal ulcer (as in *Figures 23.3* and *23.4*) can progress to form a swirling, circular, milky white infiltrate (*Figure 23.6*). Worsening of the condition leads to the formation of a creamy, pussy ulcer (*Figure 23.7*), anterior chamber flare, iritis and hypopyon. A mucopurulent discharge is evident, although the discharge can sometimes be serous. If not properly treated, the stroma can melt away and lead to corneal perforation in a matter of days (*Figure 23.1*). A grading scale for microbial keratitis is displayed in Appendix A; the sequence of grades also provides an illustration of the sequence of events as the keratitis increases in severity.

The time course of *Acanthamoeba* keratitis is not as rapid; typical signs include corneal staining, pseudodendrites, epithelial and anterior stromal infiltrates, which may be focal or diffuse, and a classic radial keratoneuritis (*Figure 23.8*) – the last being a circular formation of opacification that becomes apparent relatively early in the disease process. A fully developed corneal ulcer may take weeks to form. The pain associated with *Acanthamoeba* keratitis is so severe that it has been described as being almost suicidal.

Pathology

The sight-threatening nature of microbial keratitis has lead to a keen interest in the pathology of this condition and the mode of infection with various microorganisms is now understood more fully. The two microorganisms implicated in the vast majority of cases of microbial keratitis are *Pseudomonas aeruginosa*, a gramnegative bacteria, and *Acanthamoeba*, a free-living amoeba. Other gram-negative bacteria have been cultured from infected corneas at the same time, such as *Serratia, Enterobacter, Escherichia coli* and *Klebsiella*. Gram-positive organisms such as *Staphylococcus aureus* and *S. epidermis* have been isolated less frequently from corneal ulcers in patients with microbial keratitis.

Fungi are known to be capable of invading contact lens materials, but there is no evidence that contact lenses wear is a risk factor for fungal eye infection. Isolated cases of corneal fungal infection caused by *Fusarium*,[21–23] *Curvularia*[21] and *Metarrhizium anisopliae*[24] have been

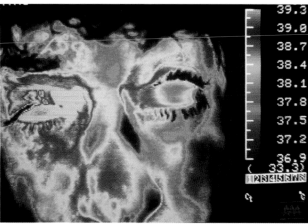
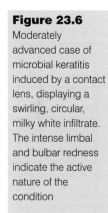

Figure 23.5
Ocular thermogram of a patient with *Acanthamoeba* keratitis of the right eye, showing the increased temperature of the affected eye

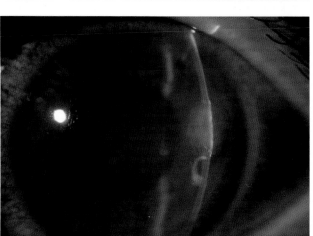

Figure 23.6
Moderately advanced case of microbial keratitis induced by a contact lens, displaying a swirling, circular, milky white infiltrate. The intense limbal and bulbar redness indicate the active nature of the condition

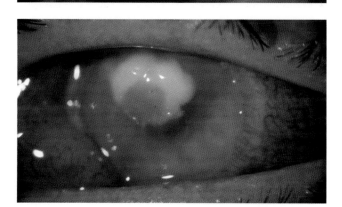

Figure 23.7
Creamy, pussy ulcer in the advanced stage of a microbial ulcer induced by a contact lens

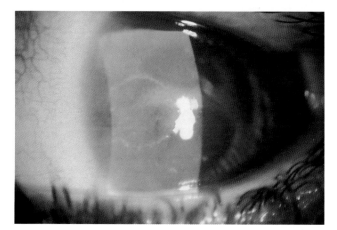

Figure 23.8
Breakdown of the epithelium in the classic pattern of radial keratoneuritis in a patient with *Acanthamoeba* keratitis

reported in contact lens wearers, although this association appears to be casual rather than causal. Similarly, contact lens wearers may coincidentally contract viral infections, such as epidemic keratoconjunctivitis (which is non-ulcerative)[25] or herpes simplex keratitis (which is ulcerative),[26] but again there is no reason to believe that contact lens wear itself is a contributing factor to the development of the infection.

Contact lens wear can alter the flora of certain groups of contact lens wearers – including those who have used certain chemical disinfection systems, elderly contact lens wearers and those who have discontinued contact lens wear.[27,28] However, studies of the microbiological environment of the eyes of contact lens wearers suggest that there is little correlation between the types of bacteria that contaminate lens-care paraphernalia and ocular flora in corresponding patients. Thus, contamination alone cannot explain changes to ocular flora that occur during contact lens wear.

For infection to occur, contact lens wear must somehow compromise corneal defenses against infection.[29,30] Research has focused on the reasons that this compromise favors infection with *Pseudomonas*, and hence the following discussion focuses on this particular pathogen. Consideration is also given to *Acanthamoeba* – the key protozoon implicated in lens-induced microbial keratitis.

Pseudomonas aeruginosa

Using cells removed from corneas by irrigation, Fleiszig *et al.*[31] found that extended wear of hydrogel lenses increases *Pseudomonas* adherence to human corneal epithelial cells (*Figure 23.9*). It has also been demonstrated that *Pseudomonas* lipopolysaccharide is a major factor contributing to the ability of *Pseudomonas* to adhere to the cornea and to contact lenses,[32] and that bacterial pili, which were previously reported to be major factors in *Pseudomonas* adherence, play only a minor role.[33]

A key to understanding the pathology of *Pseudomonas* infection is to understand why this bacterium does *not* adhere to the healthy cornea, whereas it is known to adhere readily to most surfaces, including inert surfaces, without the necessity for specific receptors. The answer lies in the natural protective layers of the corneal surface; specifically, the mucus layer of the tear film and the epithelial cell surface glycocalyx (which also contains mucin molecules and fibronectin) inhibit *Pseudomonas* adherence to the intact healthy corneal surface[34,35] (*Figure 23.10*). The precise mechanism involves *Pseudomonas* binding to mucin molecules and competitive inhibition of bacterial adherence to the cornea. As well, certain tear film components can bind *Pseudomonas*,[36] and the whole human tear fluid can protect the corneal epithelium against *Pseudomonas* virulence mechanisms.[37,38]

Epithelial cell polarity determines the susceptibility of epithelial cells to *Pseudomonas* invasion and cytotoxicity.[39] Specifically, the basolateral cell surfaces (the sides and the bottoms of cells) are much more susceptible to infection than the apical cell membrane (the top surface of cells). This research indicates another way that the intact healthy cornea is able to resist infection and why corneal surface injury predisposes to infection.

It is now known that some strains of *Pseudomonas* invade corneal epithelial cells during corneal infection.[40] Previously, it was thought that this bacterium was an extracellular pathogen (i.e., *Pseudomonas* resided only in extracellular compartments during disease). The significance of bacterial invasion of epithelial cells is that once the bacterium is inside a cell it has the potential to alter host cell function internally. Meanwhile it is protected from factors of the host immune system and from most forms of antibiotic therapy – neither of which can enter epithelial cells. This finding has led to a flurry of new research in the ophthalmic field, as well as in research related to cystic fibrosis and other lung infections caused by *Pseudomonas*.[41] [*Pseudomonas* pneumonia is the leading cause of death in cystic fibrosis, and has become one of the leading causes of death in acquired immunodeficiency syndrome (AIDS) patients.]

In vitro systems have been used to study *Pseudomonas* invasion of corneal epithelial cells, using whole cornea, cultured

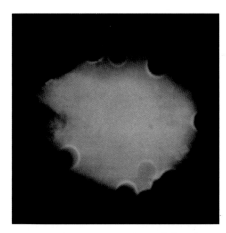

Figure 23.9

In vitro preparation showing *Pseudomonas* bacteria (small orange rods) adherent to a human epithelial cell (orange). The semi-circles at the edge of the cells are an artifact of the preparation mount

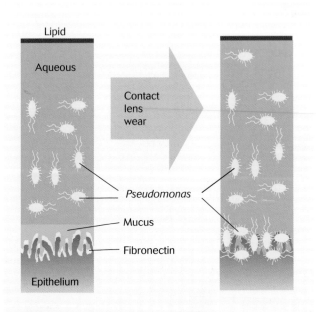

Lipid

Aqueous

Contact lens wear

Pseudomonas

Mucus

Fibronectin

Epithelium

Figure 23.10

The corneal surface. Left: *Pseudomonas* bacteria in the tear film are unable to attach to the epithelial surface because of the mucus and fibronectin layers. Right: contact lens wear depletes the protective layers and *Pseudomonas* attaches to the epithelium

corneal cells and epithelial cells washed from human corneas by irrigation.[42] Using these systems it has been demonstrated that bacterial uptake by cells is an active process that involves the host-cell cytoskeleton, that a host-cell signal transduction mechanisms is involved and that there is rapid replication of bacteria inside host cells. The lipopolysaccharide outer core has been found to be a major bacterial factor in the *Pseudomonas* invasion of epithelial cells.[43]

Another important discovery is that *two* types of *Pseudomonas* cause clinical disease, and that the pathogenesis of the two types is entirely different.[44] One type invades corneal epithelial cells without killing the host cell, and probably causes disease largely via the host immune response (invasive strains). The other type is cytotoxic for corneal and other epithelial cells; that is, these bacteria kill the host cell (cytotoxic strains).[45]

Genetic differences between these two types of *Pseudomonas* explain their different behavior, and these differences lie in the *exsA* regulated pathway of the bacterial chromosome.[46] Using mutants that lack this pathway, it has been demonstrated that strains that were previously cytotoxic changed to the invasive phenotype.[47,48] These results probably explain much of the contradictory information in the previous literature that relates to pathogenesis and the treatment of *Pseudomonas* eye infections. Clearly, these findings also relate to the development of new strategies to reduce the risk of infections related to contact lenses, and to the development of new forms of drug therapy.

Acanthamoeba

Acanthamoeba has chameleon-like tendencies in that it is able to transform from a chemotherapeutically susceptible trophozoite to a resistant cystic form. The trophozoites are polygonal and can be up to 45 μm in diameter. The cysts are double-walled and up to 16 μm in length. *Acanthamoeba* species are distributed widely in the natural environment and have been isolated from swimming pools, hot tubs, soil, dust, reservoirs, under ice, the nasopharyngeal mucosa in healthy humans and even the air we breathe.[49]

Etiology and Risk Factors

The question as to why a given patient develops microbial keratitis is multifactorial, complex and controversial. The various factors that have been proposed as significant in the etiology of microbial keratitis are discussed below. Factors thought to incur an increased risk of developing microbial keratitis are also considered.

Adherence of microorganisms to lenses

If microorganisms can adhere to, and colonize on, the surface of a contact lens, that lens becomes a vector for ocular contamination when the lens is transferred to and from the storage medium, notwithstanding the antimicrobial efficacy of the storage solution, which is discussed separately.

The strength with which microorganisms adhere to lens surfaces depends on the lens material and whether or not the lens has been worn. For example, Beattie *et al.*[50] suggest that *Acanthamoeba* readily attach to silicone hydrogel lenses, which may present an increased risk of infection. In the case of unworn lenses, ionicity, hydrophobicity and water content are the key determinants of adherence; however, adherence is also probably species-dependent – a factor that may explain apparently contradictory published data on the subject.

Microorganisms adhere to worn lenses in accordance with the type of deposit on the lens. The general notion that a worn lens adheres more microorganisms is not always true. For example, ionic lenses of mid-water content have a propensity for depositing charged protein, such as lysozyme. Paradoxically, lysozyme acts as a natural antibacterial agent in the eye. If the lysozyme does not become denatured on the lens surface, it can retain this antibacterial capacity and thus prevent adherence of live bacteria.[51]

Solution inefficacy

It is generally believed that all contact lens disinfection systems on the market provide adequate antimicrobial efficacy during lens storage, provided that the patient is totally compliant.[52] However, this notion has been challenged by Lakkis and Fleiszig,[53] who showed that the more cytotoxic strains of *Pseudomonas* display higher levels of resistance to disinfecting solutions. Also, numerous studies of compliance[54] (see below) demonstrate that only 10–60 per cent of patients can be categorized as fully compliant. It is important, therefore, that a

sufficient 'safety margin' be built into contact lens disinfection systems to allow for a degree of expected non-compliance.

History has taught us that the use of inefficacious disinfecting solutions can increase the risk of microbial keratitis. For example, Efron *et al.*[55] identified a high incidence of microbial keratitis in a cohort of patients who used chlorine-based disinfecting systems. These systems displayed only marginal efficacy.[52] Radford *et al.*[56] went on to demonstrate that, in patients with daily wear disposable lenses, the risk of *Acanthamoeba* keratitis when using a chlorine-based disinfection system was 15 times greater compared with the use of a hydrogen peroxide disinfection system (the referent). As a result of this research, chlorine-based disinfecting systems have been withdrawn from almost all world markets.

Patient non-compliance

Patient non-compliance obviously can contribute to the development of microbial keratitis, but there has been a tendency for its relative importance to be overstated. Matthews *et al.*[15] reported cases of patients who used surfactant cleaning solutions alone (i.e., without disinfecting solutions), and saline solution alone (i.e., without any form of cleaning and disinfection). In many cases these patients were being fully compliant with instructions provided by their practitioners. Radford *et al.*[56] demonstrated that, in patients who used daily wear disposable lenses, the risk of *Acanthamoeba* keratitis when using a now-discontinued chlorine-based disinfection system increased 41 times with non-compliant patients and 56 times when patients used no disinfection system.

There are countless ways in which patients can be erroneous or non-compliant in the execution of their lens care regimes[54] and attempts to enhance compliance by better education are largely unsuccessful.[57] A pragmatic approach to the question of patient non-compliance is to assume that all patients are potentially non-compliant to some degree; consequently, lens care systems should be designed with sufficient redundancy or safety margin to allow for this.[58]

Lens case care

It seems obvious that lens case cleanliness is a key prerequisite to reducing the possibility of ocular contamination and thus the risk of microbial keratitis; however, the proof of such an association is weak. Many patients with soiled lens cases have not suffered microbial keratitis, and numerous patients who develop microbial keratitis have been found to be scrupulous in their lens and case care. Fleiszig and Efron[28] found little correlation between the type and number of microorganisms in the eye and in the lens case of soft lens wearers, which indicates that in uncomplicated lens wear the eye is highly efficient at eradicating microorganisms introduced into it.

Patient hygiene

A fundamental source of lens contamination prior to insertion is the cleanliness or otherwise of the finger used to insert the lens. This raises the issue of personal hygiene. Compliance studies have shown that 16–50 per cent of patients do not pay proper attention to hand washing prior to lens insertion.[59]

Most patients execute their lens care routine in the bathroom, often adjacent to a toilet, which is perhaps not the most sterile environment available, but the most convenient. In the UK, the cold water supply to bathrooms is normally via a storage tank in the roof, which is known to be common breeding environment for *Acanthamoeba*.

The closed eye environment

Overnight wear of lenses is known to be a major risk factor for microbial keratitis.[60] The greater levels of hypoxia and hypercapnia compared with open-eye levels[61] coupled with tear stagnation beneath the lenses in a closed lid environment are factors that could lead to epithelial compromise. Organic debris, such as desquamated epithelial cells, tear film debris and bacteria trapped beneath the lens, and the general sub-clinical inflammatory state under the closed lid[62] physically and metabolically compromise the epithelium and interfere with the defense mechanisms.

Hypoxia

Prolonged hypoxia is known to have a number of adverse effects on the epithelium,[63] such as loss of sensitivity, development of epithelial microcysts, reduced oxygen uptake rate, thinning, glycogen depletion, reduced mitosis, increased fragility and weakened attachments to the underlying stroma. It is not surprising, therefore, that Solomon et al.[64] demonstrated a link between the

level of hypoxia-induced corneal swelling (a good indication of the level of epithelial hypoxia) and the development of microbial keratitis in the rabbit eye. Edema of 20 per cent resulted in microbial keratitis in half the corneas tested and edema of 43 per cent resulted in all the corneas tested developing microbial keratitis.

Various studies have demonstrated the role of hypoxia in binding of *Pseudomonas* to corneal epithelial cells, which is critical because binding is a pre-requisite for corneal infection. Nilsson[65] demonstrated that receptors for lectins (and, presumably, for bacteria, such as *P. aeruginosa*) on the surface of the corneal epithelium are exposed in significantly higher numbers after wear of low *Dk/t* contact lenses than after wear of higher *Dk/t* lenses, and binding of *P. aeruginosa* follows the same pattern. Fleiszig et al.[31] showed that overnight lens wear enhances the binding of *Pseudomonas* to human epithelial calls, and Ren et al.[66] demonstrated that this phenomenon is inversely related to lens oxygen transmissibility.

That microbial keratitis can occur with hyperpermeable silicone hydrogel lenses[12,67] (*Figure 23.11*) indicates that this complication can still occur when there is negligible hypoxia.

Swimming

There is strong anecdotal evidence of *Acanthamoeba* keratitis associated with swimming.[68,69] In three of the four cases of microbial keratitis associated with silicone hydrogel lenses reported by Lim et al.,[67] the patients reported that they had

been swimming prior to developing symptoms.

Continuous overnight use

The risk of microbial keratitis increases with longer periods of continuous overnight use of hydrogel lenses.[17–19] Compared with six nights of continuous use, there is about a 3.3 times greater risk if lenses are worn for between seven and 12 nights continuously, and a 5.6 times greater risk if lenses are worn for more than 13 nights continuously.

Overnight orthokeratology

Overnight orthokeratology refers to the practice of wearing reverse-geometry rigid lenses overnight to mold the cornea in such a way as to reduce the amount of myopia (see Chapter 24). Despite the relative safety of overnight orthokeratology with respect to reversible and non-sight threatening adverse events, a number of reports[70–73] have detailed the occurrence of microbial keratitis during overnight lens wear with reverse-geometry lenses. In view of this strong anecdotal evidence, overnight orthokeratology must be considered a risk factor for microbial keratitis.

Mechanical trauma

Animal models of corneal infectivity have been used to demonstrate that a physical breakdown of the epithelial surface is a precursor to microbial keratitis. Adherence of *P. aeruginosa* is greater to traumatized corneas than to non-traumatized corneas[32,74] (*Figure 23.12*). Furthermore, van Klink et al.[75] concluded that "corneal abrasion was

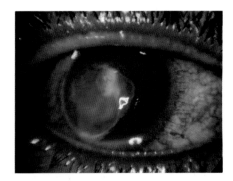

Figure 23.11
Ulcerative microbial keratitis in a patient who had been swimming while wearing his silicone hydrogel lenses (for extended wear) and who had just returned home from a holiday in a hot climate

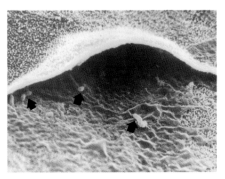

Figure 23.12
Scanning electron micrograph of the cornea showing *Pseudomonas* bacteria (arrows) about to enter beneath an epithelial cell that has partially sloughed off

absolutely necessary for the induction of *Acanthamoeba* keratitis in hamsters infected with contaminated lenses".

Although more subtle forms of epithelial compromise, such as metabolic disturbance, may predispose the development of microbial keratitis, the studies described above confirm that overt, clinically detectable epithelial trauma is a precursor to the development of microbial keratitis. It is for this reason that lens-induced epithelial trauma – which can be caused by excessive lens deposition, poor insertion technique, poor lens designs, ill-fitting lenses, lens defects or foreign bodies – must be minimized in contact lens patients.

Lens deposits

As discussed previously, the nature of deposition governs the degree to which microorganisms attach to the lens surface. A fresh coating of biologically active lysozyme is considered to be an advantage in that it is naturally antimicrobial. Other deposits may provide a nutrient-rich breeding ground for microorganisms, which may form a glycocalyx and eventually a complete biofilm. Future research may be directed to developing strategies to encourage selective deposition from the tear film of components that inhibit biofilm formation and microbial colonization.

Smoking

The finding of Schein et al.[17] and Lam et al.[11] that there is a higher incidence of microbial keratitis in patients who smoke may relate more to the poor hygiene naturally associated with smokers rather than to the systemic or topical ocular pathophysiologic effects of nicotine.

Diabetes

Schein et al.[17] demonstrated that diabetic patients are at greater risk of developing microbial keratitis than are non-diabetic patients, although they did not state the magnitude of this increased risk. The known compromises in the diabetic patient in terms of corneal structure and function, such as altered metabolism and weakened epithelial attachments to the underlying basement membrane, are the probable cause of the increased risk.

Warm climate

Many cases of microbial keratitis are documented in which climate appears to have been a contributing factor;[76] specifically, patients who live in, or travel to, warmer climates seem to have a greater risk of developing microbial keratitis, presumably because of the more favorable living conditions for microorganisms. Living in remote locations, especially in hot climates, is an added complicating factor.[2] This link has not been proved, but is worthy of note. Katz et al.[77] reported a higher incidence of microbial keratitis in the summer months. The relatively low incidence of microbial keratitis in Sweden[9] could be attributed, in part, to the colder climate there.

Gender

For daily wear of hydrogel lenses, males have a 0.45 times higher risk of developing microbial keratitis than females.[18] The reason for this association is not obvious, but may be related to perceived health risks.[78] Males have different attitudes and perceptions relating to health risks than do females, whereby they perceive risks as much smaller and much more acceptable.[78]

Socioeconomic status

Socioeconomic class is a risk factor for microbial keratitis. Classifications that represent lower management and/or supervisory to semi-skilled and manual workers have a 3.3 times higher risk of developing microbial keratitis compared with classifications that represent professional and managerial occupations.[18] This finding may be related to a greater tendency toward unintelligent noncompliant behavior[58] among the lower socioeconomic classes.

Disposable lens use

Radford et al.[56] reported that a relatively small excess risk of developing microbial keratitis is associated with the use of disposable lenses, independent of other risk factors; that is, in apparently compliant patients using efficacious care systems. These authors proposed a number of possible reasons for this increased risk related to the lenses used:
- Rapid *in vivo* lens dehydration;
- High levels of protein absorption;
- Manufacturing imperfection in mass-produced lenses.

An alternative explanation is that the apparently greater risk of microbial keratitis relates to the way in which the lenses were prescribed at the time of the study of Radford et al.[56] Many practitioners in the UK were using disposable lenses to solve intractable problems; thus, it is possible that disposable lenses were being worn by a cohort of patients who were already suffering from significant ocular compromise and were thus more likely to develop microbial keratitis.

There have been reports of both *Pseudomonas*[79] and *Acanthamoeba*[80,81] keratitis occurring in association with daily disposable lens wear.

Management

General advice

As discussed above, abundant evidence is now available as to the various risk factors that relate to the development of microbial keratitis. The key risk factor is overnight lens wear. Patients should be advised that, although sleeping in lenses carries a far greater risk of developing microbial keratitis compared with daily wear, the incidence is still very small. It is up to the patient to weigh up the risk verses the benefits of extended lens wear. As a comparator, Holden et al.[12] point out that the incidence of vision loss of two or more lines of best-corrected visual acuity is between 306 and 871 cases per 10,000 patients per year for laser *in situ* keratomileusis, versus only 0.8 cases per 10,000 patients per year for extended wear hydrogel contact lenses.

The potentially devastating effects of microbial keratitis mean that any case of ocular pain related to contact lenses that persists after lens removal should be treated with grave suspicion. Certainly, all patients should be advised to remove their lenses if they have a sore red eye and to see their practitioner or seek medical attention if the pain persists or worsens in the first few hours after lens removal.

Patients who travel to warm environments should be warned of the possible increased risk of developing microbial keratitis. The importance of compliance with a full care regimen must be emphasized. It may be advisable to warn patients who use extended wear lenses that goggles should be worn when swimming because of the possible increased risk of developing microbial keratitis.

Diabetic patients should be warned of the increased risk of infection as a result of their metabolic condition,[17] but at the same time they should be advised that the incidence of microbial keratitis among diabetic contact lens wearers is still very low.

Ocular examination

A contact lens patient who presents with a sore red eye should be examined as a matter of urgency and a tentative diagnosis must be made as to whether the condition is likely to be microbial keratitis. One or more of the following signs and/or symptoms is strongly suggestive of microbial keratitis:

- Severe ocular pain that persists after lens removal;
- Extensive and/or intensive epithelial staining that overlies the infiltrates;
- Extensive anterior chamber flare;
- Hypopyon;
- Extreme conjunctival redness that persists after lens removal;
- Significant loss of vision.

Medical treatment

For a suspected or confirmed microbial keratitis, a corneal scraping should be performed to determine if the condition is infectious and possibly to identify the offending microorganism. If *Acanthamoeba* keratitis is suspected, confocal microscopy confirms the presence of the trophozoites or cysts (*Figure 23.13*).

Bacterial keratitis

Broad-spectrum antibiotics should be instilled pending the result of the corneal scraping because such episodes are best presumed to be infectious unless proved otherwise. Two approaches can be adopted:

- Dual therapy – involves a combination of two fortified antibiotics to cover common gram-positive and gram-negative pathogens, in the form of an aminoglycoside and a cephalosporin;
- Monotherapy – with a fluoroquinolone, such as ciprofloxacin 0.3% or ofloxacin 0.3%.[82]

Unfortunately, the results of scrapings are often equivocal because antibiotics may have been instilled as a necessary precautionary measure prior to hospitalization, numerous microorganisms may be isolated (which makes it difficult to identify the true culprit) and the result may be falsely culture-negative by chance. Martins *et al.*[83] claim that contact lens cultures may identify the causative organisms in most cases of contact lens-related microbial keratitis.

Specific fortified topical antibiotics, such as gentamicin and cefazolin, may be prescribed if the causative organism is identified positively. These are initially instilled at hourly intervals around the clock. The frequency can be reduced to 2-hourly during the waking hours if the response is favorable. Continuing improvement should allow fortified drops to be substituted for weaker commercial preparations, which are tapered and eventually discontinued. Oral ciprofloxacin may also be indicated to prevent contiguous spread to the sclera.[82] Antibiotics can be delivered by subconjunctival injection or even intravenously if corneal perforation is a possibility.

During the early phase of bacterial keratitis, corticosteroids are generally not prescribed (especially if the ulcer is culture positive) because these drugs inhibit epithelial metabolism and retard the re-epithelialization and other tissue-repair activity. Corticosteroids may be prescribed with extreme caution in the late healing phase to dampen the host response.

Protozoal keratitis

A combination of propamidine isetionate 0.1% (Brolene) and polyhexamethylene biguanide 0.02% drops is well tolerated, non-toxic and largely effective against *Acanthamoeba* species. Alternatively, a combination of Brolene and neomycin or a fluoroquinolone with chlorhexidine may give good results.[84] Topical corticosteroids can be used to control persistent inflammation, but should be terminated before cessation of anti-amoebal therapy.[82]

Kumar and Lloyd[84] point out that the encysted stage in the life cycle of *Acanthamoeba* species appears to cause the intractable problems, and that many biocides are ineffective in killing the highly resistant cysts. Immunologic methods are being investigated as a form of prevention, and oral immunization of animals has been successful in the prevention of *Acanthamoeba* keratitis by inducing immunity before infection occurs.[84] However, it is unlikely that immunization will be used to reduce the incidence of *Acanthamoeba* infection induced by contact lenses in humans.

Additional medical strategies

Numerous other medical strategies may be utilized, depending on circumstances; in summary, these are:

- Mydriatics – (e.g., atropine) to prevent posterior synechia;
- Cycloplegics – to reduce pain from ciliary spasm (atropine also has a cycloplegic effect);
- Collagenase inhibitors – to minimize stromal melting;
- Non-steroidal anti-inflammatory agents – to reduce inflammation and limit the infiltrative response;
- Analgesics – to alleviate pain;
- Tissue adhesives – are applied when the stroma has become extremely thin or perforated;
- Debridement – to enhance the penetration of drugs into the eye;
- Bandage lens – to assist in re-epithelialization;
- Collagen shield – can be soaked in therapeutic drugs, which are slowly released back into the eye during wear.

Surgical interventions include penetrating graft, which may need to be performed in the case of large perforations or non-healing deep central ulceration, or possibly lamellar graft.

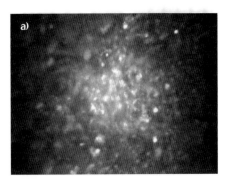
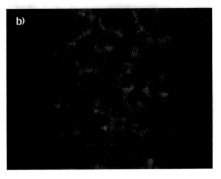

Figure 23.13

Confocal microscopic images. (a) In a patient suffering from *Acanthamoeba* keratitis, showing a mass of *Acanthamoeba* cysts (bright white spots). (b) In a normal patient (shown here for comparison); the irregular shaped objects are stromal keratocytes.

Alleviate mechanical trauma

The clinical strategies that can be adopted to minimize the possibility of mechanical trauma are self-evident. The causes, and their solutions, include:

- Lens deposits – use a more effective care system, have the patient adopt more effective care procedures and/or replace lenses more regularly;
- Poor insertion technique – re-educate the patient on insertion techniques and consider alternative methods of lens insertion;
- Poorly designed lenses – choose an alternative design, or change from soft to rigid lenses or visa versa;
- Ill-fitting lenses – alter lens fit as appropriate;
- Lens defects[85] – advise patients to study lenses carefully for the presence of defects and/or prescribe a lens type known to be of high cosmetic quality;
- Foreign body induced trauma – locate and remove the foreign body, and replace the lens if it has become damaged.

Improve care system

Lens care systems known to be efficacious against the key offending microorganisms should be prescribed.[52] Whatever system is used, it is vital that the patient adheres to the full care regimen specified by the manufacturer (and moderated by the clinician), including the use of separate surfactant cleaners and protein removal systems if these are deemed necessary. This entails giving appropriate advice in the first instance, monitoring patient compliance with this advice at subsequent aftercare visits and taking remedial action if required.

Better hygiene

All patients, and in particular extended wear patients, must be advised of the importance of strict attention to all aspects of hygiene. Thorough hand washing prior to lens handling or in-eye lens manipulation, and scrupulous attention to lens case care are key aspects to reinforce.

Avoid tap water

The risk of developing *Acanthamoeba* keratitis is greatly reduced by avoiding the use of tap water and home-made saline, as *Acanthamoeba* is ubiquitous in water supplies and thrives in saline solution in the absence of preservatives.[86]

Change to daily wear

Available epidemiologic evidence suggests that the risk of developing microbial keratitis is greater when patients sleep in lenses. Changing from extended wear to daily wear therefore represents a safer option.

Fit rigid lenses

Epidemiologic evidence suggests that the risk of developing microbial keratitis is lowest with rigid lens wear. This is attributed to superior tear exchange,[87] greater post-lens tear film thickness, small lens size (not impinging on the limbus) and generally lower levels of problematic deposition on such lenses. Fitting patients with rigid lenses therefore represents a low-risk option for microbial keratitis.

Increase oxygen performance

In view of the link between hypoxia and the induction of microbial keratitis,[64] any measure to increase corneal oxygen availability during lens wear lessens the risk of developing microbial keratitis. In the case of soft lenses, this generally means fitting lenses made out of silicone hydrogel materials.

Prognosis

The prognosis for recovery from microbial keratitis is variable and depends largely on the speed and efficacy of treatment. If lenses are removed by the patient as soon as there is a problem, immediate advice is sought, a correct diagnosis is made and prompt, appropriate and aggressive therapeutic measures are enforced, the prognosis is good and the patient may ultimately be left with only a minor scar that does not interfere with vision. A delay in treatment and the use of inappropriate medication can result in total vision loss.[1,2]

Bourcier *et al.*[4] noted that, out of 300 cases of microbial keratitis induced by contact lenses, 99 per cent of cases resolved with treatment, but only 60 per cent of patients had visual acuity better than the level at admission and 5 per cent had a very poor visual outcome.

In the case of *Staphylococcus* and *Streptococcus*, improvement in the condition may not be apparent until 24–48 hours after therapy has commenced. The microorganisms are generally eradicated from the cornea within 7–10 days.

Pseudomonas infections may appear to worsen slightly during the first 24 hours after medication has commenced. The condition gradually improves thereafter, with the microorganism persisting for 14 days or longer.

Acanthamoeba keratitis has a slow time course of recovery. The condition may progress over many months, with periods of apparent improvement followed by regression. Patients are inevitably left with superficial nebulae that correspond to the site of infection (*Figure 23.14*). Recurrence is common if treatment is stopped prematurely.[84]

Differential Diagnosis

An important diagnosis to be made in the early stages of a suspected microbial keratitis is the differentiation between a sterile keratitis (especially CLPU) versus infective keratitis; a simple scoring scheme[88] to make this determination is discussed in Chapter 22. As Stein *et al.*[89] have pointed out, the key difference between sterile versus microbial keratitis is the severity of the signs and

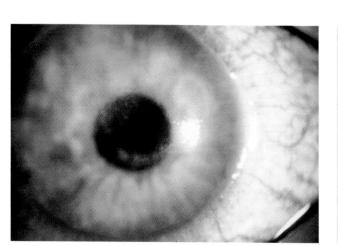

Figure 23.14

Residual scar formation during the late-healing phase of a patient who suffered from *Acanthamoeba* keratitis.

symptoms. Microbial keratitis produces moderate-to-severe pain, unilateral discharge, photophobia, a large area of infiltration, epithelial breakdown and an anterior chamber reaction. Sterile keratitis is associated with smaller regions of infiltration, no discharge, less likelihood of epithelial disruption, mild or absent pain, mild photophobia and no anterior chamber flare. However, these are only general guidelines and there is considerable overlap between the two conditions. In view of the potentially serious consequences of infectious corneal disease, practitioners are advised to consider cases of infiltrative keratitis to be microbial until proved otherwise.

Acanthamoeba keratitis can take on a similar clinical appearance to herpetic keratitis[90] and, to a lesser extent, to *Pseudomonas* keratitis. In advanced stages of these conditions, the clinical geographic distribution of the ulcers across the corneas indicates the likely cause; a classic dendritic form of ulceration is evident in herpetic keratitis (*Figure 23.15*), whereas in *Acanthamoeba* the ulcer takes on a circular pattern.

The ultimate differential diagnosis is provided by the results of cultures, smear tests, tissue staining and confocal microscopy, whereby the offending organism can be identified; however, the results of such tests cannot always be relied upon, for reasons explained earlier. Judgments must often, therefore, be based on clinical evaluation of the presenting signs and symptoms, the pattern of disease progression and the responsiveness of the condition to various treatment alternatives.

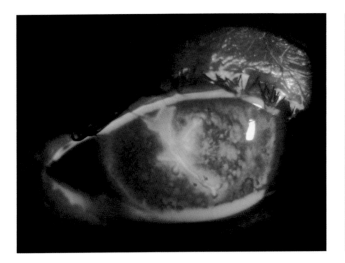

Figure 23.15
Dendritic pattern of corneal ulceration in a contact lens wearer who had contracted herpes keratitis. The patient was an AIDS carrier

REFERENCES

1 Chalupa E, Swarbrick HA, Holden BA and Sjostrand J (1987). Severe corneal infections associated with contact lens wear. *Ophthalmology* **94**, 17–22.

2 Cooper RL and Constable IJ (1977). Infective keratitis in soft contact lens wearers. *Br J Ophthalmol.* **61**, 250–254.

3 Rattanatam T, Heng WJ, Rapuano CJ, *et al.* (2001). Trends in contact lens-related corneal ulcers. *Cornea* **20**, 290–294.

4 Bourcier T, Thomas F, Borderie V, *et al.* (2003). Bacterial keratitis: predisposing factors, clinical and microbiological review of 300 cases. *Br J Ophthalmol.* **87**, 834–838.

5 Stapleton F (2003). Contact lens-related microbial keratitis: What can epidemiologic studies tell us? *Eye Contact Lens* **29S**, 85–89.

6 Poggio EC, Glynn RJ, Schein OD, *et al.* (1989). The incidence of ulcerative keratitis among users of daily-wear and extended-wear soft contact lenses. *N Engl J Med.* **321**, 779–783.

7 MacRae S, Herman C, Stulting RD, *et al.* (1991). Corneal ulcer and adverse reaction rates in premarket contact lens studies. *Am J Ophthalmol.* **111**, 457–465.

8 Cheng KH, Leung SL, Hoekman HW, *et al.* (1999). Incidence of contact-lens-associated microbial keratitis and its related morbidity. *Lancet* **354**, 181–185.

9 Nilsson SE and Montan PG (1994). The annualized incidence of contact lens induced keratitis in Sweden and its relation to lens type and wear schedule: Results of a 3-month prospective study. *CLAO J.* **20**, 225–230.

10 Seal DV, Kirkness CM, Bennett HGB and Peterson M (1999). Population-based cohort study of microbial keratitis in Scotland: Incidence and features. *Contact Lens Ant Eye* **22**, 49–57.

11 Lam DS, Houang E, Fan DS, *et al.* (2002). Incidence and risk factors for microbial keratitis in Hong Kong: Comparison with Europe and North America. *Eye* **16**, 608–618.

12 Holden BA, Sweeney DF, Sankaridurg PR, *et al.* (2003). Microbial keratitis and vision loss with contact lenses. *Eye Contact Lens* **29**S, 131–134.

13 Guillon M, Guillon JP, Bansal M, *et al.* (1994). Incidence of ulcers with conventional and disposable daily wear soft contact lenses. *J Br Contact Lens Assoc.* **17**, 69–76.

14 Benjamin WJ (1992). Risks and incidences of 'ulcerative keratitis'. *J Br Contact Lens Assoc.* **15**, 143–144.

15 Matthews TD, Frazer DG, Minassian DC, *et al.* (1992). Risks of keratitis and patterns of use with disposable contact lenses. *Arch Ophthalmol.* **110**, 1559–1562.

16 Buehler PO, Schein OD, Stamler JF, *et al.* (1992). The increased risk of ulcerative keratitis among disposable soft contact lens users. *Arch Ophthalmol.* **110**, 1555–1558.

17 Schein OD, Glynn RJ, Poggio EC, *et al.* (1989). The relative risk of ulcerative keratitis among users of daily-wear and extended-wear soft contact lenses. A case-control study. Microbial Keratitis Study Group. *N Engl J Med.* **321**, 773–778.

18 Dart JK, Stapleton F and Minassian D (1991). Contact lenses and other risk factors in microbial keratitis. *Lancet* **338**, 650–653.

19 Stapleton F, Dart JK and Minassian D (1993). Risk factors with contact lens related suppurative keratitis. *CLAO J.* **19**, 204–210.

20 Sweeney DF, Jalbert I, Covey M, *et al.* (2003). Clinical characterization of corneal infiltrative events observed with soft contact lens wear. *Cornea* **22**, 435–442.

21 Wilson LA and Ahearn DG (1986). Association of fungi with extended-wear soft contact lenses. *Am J Ophthalmol.* **101**, 434–436.

22 Foroozan R, Eagle RC Jr and Cohen EJ (2000). Fungal keratitis in a soft contact lens wearer. *CLAO J.* **26**, 166–168.

23 Choi DM, Goldstein MH, Salierno A and Driebe WT (2001). Fungal keratitis in a daily disposable soft contact lens wearer. *CLAO J.* **27**, 111–112.

24 Jani BR, Rinaldi MG and Reinhart WJ (2001). An unusual case of fungal keratitis: *Metarrhizium anisopliae. Cornea* **20**, 765–768.

25 Mueller AJ and Klauss V (1993). Main sources of infection in 145 cases of epidemic keratoconjunctivitis. *Ger J Ophthalmol.* **2**, 224–227.

26 Athmanathan S, Pranesh VM, Pasricha G, *et al.* (2001). Atypical *Herpes simplex* keratitis (HSK) presenting as a perforated corneal ulcer with a large infiltrate in a contact lens wearer: Multinucleated giant cells in the Giemsa smear offered a clue to the diagnosis. *BMC Ophthalmol.* **1**, 1.

27 Fleiszig SM and Efron N (1992). Conjunctival flora in extended wear of rigid gas permeable contact lenses. *Optom Vis Sci.* **69**, 354–357.

28 Fleiszig SM and Efron N (1992). Microbial flora in eyes of current and former contact lens wearers. *J Clin Microbiol.* **30**, 1156–1161.

29 Fleiszig SMJ and Efron N (1988). Pathogenesis of contact lens induced bacterial corneal ulcers – a review and an hypothesis. *Clin Exp Optom.* **71**, 147–157.

30 Fleiszig SM and Evans DJ (2002). The pathogenesis of bacterial keratitis: Studies with *Pseudomonas aeruginosa. Clin Exp Optom.* **85**, 271–278.

31 Fleiszig SM, Efron N and Pier GB (1992). Extended contact lens wear enhances *Pseudomonas aeruginosa* adherence to human corneal epithelium. *Invest Ophthalmol Vis Sci.* **33**, 2908–2916.

32 Fletcher EL, Fleiszig SM and Brennan NA (1993). Lipopolysaccharide in adherence of *Pseudomonas aeruginosa* to the cornea and contact lenses. *Invest Ophthalmol Vis Sci.* **34**, 1930–1936.

33 Fletcher EL, Weissman BA, Efron N, *et al.* (1993). The role of pili in the attachment of *Pseudomonas aeruginosa* to unworn hydrogel contact lenses. *Curr Eye Res.* **12**, 1067–1071.

34 Fleiszig SM, Zaidi TS and Pier GB (1994). Mucus and *Pseudomonas aeruginosa* adherence to the cornea. *Adv Exp Med Biol.* **350**, 359–362.

35 Fleiszig SM, Zaidi TS, Ramphal R and Pier GB (1994). Modulation of *Pseudomonas aeruginosa* adherence to the corneal surface by mucus. *Infect Immun.* **62**, 1799–1804.

36 McNamara NA and Fleiszig SM (1998). Human tear film components bind *Pseudomonas aeruginosa. Adv Exp Med Biol.* **438**, 653–658.

37 Fleiszig SM, McNamara NA and Evans DJ (2002). The tear film and defense against infection. *Adv Exp Med Biol.* **506**, 523–530.

38 Fleiszig SM, Kwong MS and Evans DJ (2003). Modification of *Pseudomonas aeruginosa* interactions with corneal epithelial cells by human tear fluid. *Infect Immun.* **71**, 3866–3874.

39 Fleiszig SM, Evans DJ, Do N, *et al.* (1997). Epithelial cell polarity affects susceptibility to *Pseudomonas aeruginosa* invasion and cytotoxicity. *Infect Immun.* **65**, 2861–2867.

40 Fleiszig SM, Zaidi TS, Fletcher EL, *et al.* (1994). *Pseudomonas aeruginosa* invades corneal epithelial cells during experimental infection. *Infect Immun.* **62**, 3485–3493.

41 Lee A, Chow D, Haus B, *et al.* (1999). Airway epithelial tight junctions and binding and cytotoxicity of *Pseudomonas aeruginosa. Am J Physiol.* **277**, L204–L217.

42 Fleiszig SM, Zaidi TS and Pier GB (1995). *Pseudomonas aeruginosa* invasion of and multiplication within corneal epithelial cells *in vitro. Infect Immun.* **63**, 4072–4077.

43 Zaidi TS, Fleiszig SM, Preston MJ, *et al.* (1996). Lipopolysaccharide outer core is a ligand for corneal cell binding and ingestion of *Pseudomonas aeruginosa. Invest Ophthalmol Vis Sci.* **37**, 976–986.

44 Fleiszig SM, Zaidi TS, Preston MJ, *et al.* (1996). Relationship between cytotoxicity and corneal epithelial cell invasion by clinical isolates of *Pseudomonas aeruginosa. Infect Immun.* **64**, 2288–2294.

45 Cowell BA, Weissman BA, Yeung KK, *et al.* (2003). Phenotype of *Pseudomonas aeruginosa* isolates causing corneal infection between 1997 and 2000. *Cornea* **22**, 131–134.

46 Fleiszig SM, Wiener-Kronish JP, Miyazaki H, *et al.* (1997). *Pseudomonas aeruginosa*-mediated cytotoxicity and invasion correlate with distinct genotypes at the loci encoding exoenzyme S. *Infect Immun.* **65**, 579–586.

47 Evans DJ, Kuo TC, Kwong M, *et al.* (2002). Mutation of csk, encoding the C-terminal Src kinase, reduces *Pseudomonas aeruginosa* internalization by mammalian cells and enhances bacterial cytotoxicity. *Microb Pathog.* **33**, 135–143.

48 Cowell BA, Twining SS, Hobden JA, *et al.* (2003). Mutation of lasA and lasB reduces *Pseudomonas aeruginosa* invasion of epithelial cells. *Microbiology* **149**, 2291–2299.

49 Khan NA (2003). Pathogenesis of *Acanthamoeba* infections. *Microb Pathog.* **34**, 277–285.

50 Beattie TK, Tomlinson A, McFadyen AK, *et al.* (2003). Enhanced attachment of *Acanthamoeba* to extended-wear silicone hydrogel contact lenses: A new risk factor for infection? *Ophthalmology* **110**, 765–771.

51 Lawin-Brussel CA, Refojo MF, Leong FL and Kenyon KR (1991). *Pseudomonas* attachment to low-water and high-water, ionic and nonionic, new and rabbit-worn soft contact lenses. *Invest Ophthalmol Vis Sci.* **32**, 657–662.

52 Lowe R, Vallas V and Brennan NA (1992). Comparative efficacy of contact lens disinfection solutions. *CLAO J.* **18**, 34–40.

53 Lakkis C and Fleiszig SM (2001). Resistance of *Pseudomonas aeruginosa* isolates to hydrogel contact lens disinfection correlates with cytotoxic activity. *J Clin Microbiol.* **39**, 1477–1486.

54 Claydon BE and Efron N (1994). Non-compliance in contact lens wear. *Ophthalmic Physiol Opt.* **14**, 356–364.

55 Efron N, Wohl A, Toma N, *et al.* (1991). Corneal ulcers associated with daily wear of disposable hydrogel contact lenses. *Trans Br Contact Lens Assoc.* **14**, 149–154.

56 Radford CF, Bacon AS, Dart JK and Minassian DC (1995). Risk factors for *Acanthamoeba* keratitis in contact lens users: A case-control study. *BMJ* **310**, 1567–1570.

57 Claydon BE, Efron N and Woods C (1997). A prospective study of the effect of education on non-compliant behaviour in contact lens wear. *Ophthalmic Physiol Opt.* **17**, 137–146.

58 Efron N (1997). The truth about compliance. *Contact Lens Ant Eye* **20**, 79–86.

59 Claydon BE, Efron N and Woods C (1996). A prospective study of non-compliance in contact lens wear. *J Br Contact Lens Assoc.* **19**, 133–140.

60 Schein OD, Buehler PO, Stamler JF, *et al.* (1994). The impact of overnight wear on the risk of contact lens-associated ulcerative keratitis. *Arch Ophthalmol.* **112**, 186–190.

61 Ang JH and Efron N (1990). Corneal hypoxia and hypercapnia during contact lens wear. *Optom Vis Sci.* **67**, 512–521.

62 Tan KO, Sack RA, Holden BA and Swarbrick HA (1993). Temporal sequence of changes in tear film composition during sleep. *Curr Eye Res.* **12**, 1001–1007.

63 Holden BA, Sweeney DF, Vannas A, *et al.* (1985). Effects of long-term extended contact lens wear on the human cornea. *Invest Ophthalmol Vis Sci.* **26**, 1489–1501.

64 Solomon OD, Loff H, Perla B, *et al.* (1994). Testing hypotheses for risk factors for contact lens-associated infectious keratitis in an animal model. *CLAO J.* **20**, 109–113.

65 Nilsson SE (2002). Bacterial keratitis and inflammatory corneal reactions: Possible relations to contact lens oxygen transmissibility: the Harold A. Stein Lectureship 2001. *CLAO J.* **28**, 62–65.

66 Ren DH, Petroll WM, Jester JV, *et al.* (1999). The relationship between contact lens oxygen permeability and binding of *Pseudomonas aeruginosa* to human corneal epithelial cells after overnight and extended wear. *CLAO J.* **25**, 80–100.

67 Lim L, Loughnan MS and Sullivan LJ (2002). Microbial keratitis associated with extended wear of silicone hydrogel contact lenses. *Br J Ophthalmol.* **86**, 355–357.

68 Tay-Kearney ML, McGhee CN, Crawford GJ and Trown K (1993). *Acanthamoeba* keratitis. A masquerade of presentation in six cases. *Aust NZ J Ophthalmol.* **21**, 237–245.

69 Radford CF, Minassian DC and Dart JK (2002). *Acanthamoeba* keratitis in England and Wales: Incidence, outcome, and risk factors. *Br J Ophthalmol.* **86**, 536–542.

70 Chen KH, Kuang TM and Hsu WM (2001). *Serratia marcescens* corneal ulcer as a complication of orthokeratology. *Am J Ophthalmol.* **132**, 257–258.

71 Lau LI, Wu CC, Lee SM and Hsu WM (2003). *Pseudomonas* corneal ulcer related to overnight orthokeratology. *Cornea* **22**, 262–264.

72 Wang JC and Lim L (2003). Unusual morphology in orthokeratology contact lens-related cornea ulcer. *Eye Contact Lens* **29**, 190–192.

73 Young AL, Leung AT, Cheung EY, *et al.* (2003). Orthokeratology lens-related *Pseudomonas aeruginosa* infectious keratitis. *Cornea* **22**, 265–266.

74 Klotz SA, Au YK and Misra RP (1989). A partial-thickness epithelial defect increases the adherence of *Pseudomonas aeruginosa* to the cornea. *Invest Ophthalmol Vis Sci.* **30**, 1069–1074.

75 van Klink F, Alizadeh H, He Y, *et al.* (1993). The role of contact lenses, trauma, and Langerhans cells in a Chinese hamster model of *Acanthamoeba* keratitis. *Invest Ophthalmol Vis Sci.* **34**, 1937–1944.

76 Houang E, Lam D, Fan D and Seal D (2001). Microbial keratitis in Hong Kong: Relationship to climate, environment and contact-lens disinfection. *Trans R Soc Trop Med Hyg.* **95**, 361–367.

77 Katz HR, LaBorwit SE and Hirschbein MJ (1997). A retrospective study of seasonal influence on ulcerative keratitis. *Invest Ophthalmol Vis Sci.* **38S**, 136.

78 Flynn J, Slovic P and Mertz CK (1994). Gender, race, and perception of environmental health risks. *Risk Anal.* **14**, 1101–1108.

79 Su DH, Chan TK and Lim L (2003). Infectious keratitis associated with daily disposable contact lenses. *Eye Contact Lens* **29**, 185–186.

80 Blades KJ, Tomlinson A and Seal D (2000). *Acanthamoeba* keratitis occurring with daily disposable contact lens wear. *Br J Ophthalmol.* **84**, 805.

81 Woodruff SA and Dart JK (1999). *Acanthamoeba* keratitis occurring with daily disposable contact lens wear. *Br J Ophthalmol.* **83**, 1088–1089.

82 Kanski JJ (2003). *Clinical Ophthalmology*, Fifth Edition. (Oxford: Butterworth–Heinemann).

83 Martins EN, Farah ME, Alvarenga LS, *et al.* (2002). Infectious keratitis: Correlation between corneal and contact lens cultures. *CLAO J.* **28**, 146–148.

84 Kumar R and Lloyd D (2002). Recent advances in the treatment of *Acanthamoeba* keratitis. *Clin Infect Dis.* **35**, 434–441.

85 Efron N and Veys J (1992). Defects in disposable contact lenses can compromise ocular integrity. *Int Contact Lens Clin.* **19**, 8–18.

86 Moore MB, McCulley JP, Luckenbach M, *et al.* (1985). *Acanthamoeba* keratitis associated with soft contact lenses. *Am J Ophthalmol.* **100**, 396–403.

87 Efron N (1991). Understanding oxygen: *Dk/L*, EOP, oedema. *Trans Br Contact Lens Assoc.* **14**, 65–69.

88 Aasuri MK, Venkata N and Kumar VM (2003). Differential diagnosis of microbial keratitis and contact lens-induced peripheral ulcer. *Eye Contact Lens* **29S**, 60–62.

89 Stein RM, Clinch TE, Cohen EJ, *et al.* (1988). Infected vs sterile corneal infiltrates in contact lens wearers. *Am J Ophthalmol.* **105**, 632–636.

90 Yeung EY, Huang SC and Tsai RJ (2002). *Acanthamoeba* keratitis presenting as dendritic keratitis in a soft contact lens wearer. *Chang Gung Med J.* **25**, 201–206.

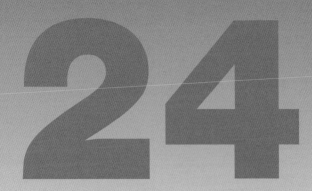

CORNEAL WARPAGE

24

Contact lenses are in direct contact with the eye, so clearly physical forces can act to change the shape of both the lens and the eye. Indeed, both types of change have been documented and both can have important clinical sequelae. This chapter concentrates on changes in ocular shape induced by contact lens wear. Primary consideration is given to *corneal* shape change because this is critical to vision and lens-fitting techniques. However, it is true that contact lenses can also alter the surface topography of the conjunctiva (e.g., indentation rings) and the form of the upper lid (e.g., rigid lens-induced ptosis).

Consideration is given to the various manifestations of changes induced by contact lenses in corneal topography. The chapter title 'Corneal warpage' is adopted because this term has been used consistently in the literature for the past 40 years[1–4] to infer shape change induced by contact lenses. The term 'warpage' has the connotation of gross distortion, which was no doubt deliberately chosen by the early workers in this field[1] to describe the gross changes in corneal topography that could be induced by scleral or polymethyl methacrylate (PMMA) lenses. Interestingly, Schornack[5] used the term 'warpage' to describe corneal shape changes in hydrogel lens wearers. A severe case of rigid lens corneal warpage is shown in *Figure 24.1*.

A myriad of terms have been coined by various authors to describe different phenomena that relate to lens-induced corneal shape change; these include deformation, distortion, warpage, indentation, steepening, flattening, sphericalization, imprinting and wrinkling. These terms are generally self-explanatory and are used when discussing specific forms of corneal shape change. Wrinkling is a change that seems to occur in the epithelium and anterior stroma, and as such is dealt with in Chapter 17 ('Epithelial wrinkling') of Part VI, 'Corneal epithelium'.

While most corneal shape changes induced by contact lenses are unintentional, it must not be overlooked that some clinicians have fitted lenses with the deliberate intention to induce or arrest corneal shape change; the three best-known practices, which have attracted considerable controversy, are:

- Cone compression in keratoconus – with the aim of flattening the cone with an apical bearing to halt or slow its progression;
- Orthokeratology – with the aim of flattening the cornea to reduce myopia;
- Myopia control – with the aim of preventing the development of myopia or arresting the progression of myopia.

These concepts are also reviewed briefly toward the end of this chapter.

Incidence

The incidence of corneal shape change as a result of various categories of lens wear is well known. Finnemore and Korb[6] reported that 98 per cent of PMMA lens wearers develop central corneal clouding (CCC), which inevitably causes some

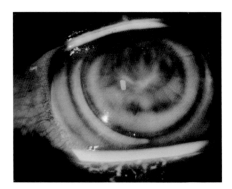

Figure 24.1

Severe case of corneal warpage in a keratoconic eye seen here with the aid of fluorescein after removal of an ill-fitting hybrid rigid-center soft-surround lens

degree of corneal steepening. More generalized distortion, or 'warpage', was noted in 30 per cent of PMMA lens wearers by Rengstorff.[7]

When assessed using conventional keratometric techniques, current generation rigid lenses of low-to-medium oxygen transmissibility (*Dk/t*) induce little or no change in overall corneal shape during daily wear[8] or extended wear.[9,10] Similarly, keratometry fails to highlight significant corneal shape changes in daily[11,12] and extended wear[13] of hydrogel lenses.

Modern videokeratographic corneal mapping techniques reveal that all forms of contact lens wear are able to induce small, but statistically significant, changes in corneal topography.[14–17] Ruiz-Montenegro *et al.*[14] reported the prevalence of abnormalities in corneal shape to be 8 per cent in a control group not wearing contact lenses versus 75 per cent in PMMA lens wearers, 57 per cent in daily rigid lens wearers, 31 per cent in daily soft lens wearers and 23 per cent in extended hydrogel lens wearers. These authors attached some clinical significance to their findings because

- Decreases in best spectacle-corrected visual acuities of up to one line of Snellen acuity were noted in many of the PMMA and rigid lens wearers;
- Correlations were noted between lens decentration and corneal shape change.

Wang *et al.*[17] prospectively studied the eyes of 165 consecutive patients wearing contact lenses evaluated for keratorefractive surgery. Significant corneal warpage induced by contact lenses was detected by corneal topography in 20 eyes of 11 patients, which represented an overall prevalence of corneal warpage of 12 per cent among this cohort contact lens wearers.

Dumbleton *et al.*[18] observed a small degree of central corneal flattening in both major meridians of 0.35D in patients who wore silicone hydrogel lenses over a 9 month period. Gonzalez-Meijome et al.[15] noted a similar phenomenon in silicone hydrogel lens wearers; specifically, they observed an almost homogeneous increase in corneal radius of curvature for all corneal locations, being statistically significant for the 4 mm cord diameter area.

Lens binding is known to occur with daily and extended wear of rigid lenses, the clinical evidence for which is an indentation of the cornea that can be seen in white light and with the aid of fluorescein. Based on subject reports, lens binding occurred in 29 per cent of daily wear[8] and 50 per cent of extended wear[9] rigid lens patients.

Most other forms of lens-induced corneal shape change are either rare or are known to be associated with specific types of poorly designed or ill-fitting lenses.[19] Phillips[20] suggests that some patients may be prone to corneal warpage because of previous adverse lens-wearing experiences or because of a hereditary predisposition to keratoconus. It is not possible to assign specific incidence figures to such rare phenomena.

Signs and Symptoms

The clinical presentation of lens-induced corneal shape change – characterized by time course and precise topographic alterations – can manifest in a variety of forms and depend primarily upon the material, design and fit of the lens. In general, adverse signs and symptoms of corneal shape change include reduced and variable vision, changes in refraction and monocular diplopia.[21] The specific effects of lens-induced shape change are considered in the context of the various forms of topographic alterations that have been described.

Change in overall curvature
Much of the earlier literature concentrated on overall changes in curvature; that is, steepening or flattening of the anterior corneal surface as measured by keratometry. Results have been expressed as changes in either corneal curvature (in millimeters), surface corneal power (in diopters) or refraction (in diopters).

CCC often occurred during the initial period of adaptation to PMMA lens wear and was generally associated with a myopic shift (see Etiology). Thus, newly fitted PMMA patients would complain of hazy vision because of the excess edema and the resultant reduced vision upon removing their lenses and putting on spectacles. Some patients would complain of mild ocular discomfort, but this probably related more to the underlying cause (excessive edema) than to the actual change in corneal shape.

This problem of blurred vision with spectacles after contact lens wear was termed 'spectacle blur',[22] which posed a significant clinical problem because many patients could wear PMMA lenses for a limited period of time only, and needed to wear spectacles at the end of the wearing period.

As the patient adapted and the central corneal edema subsided, a reversal of the induced myopia occurred and the corneal curvature and refraction returned to pre-fitting levels. After 12 months of PMMA lens wear, the cornea often displayed central flattening, which resulted in a hyperopic creep, or reduction in myopia.

Rigid lenses can also induce changes in overall curvature, whereby the extent of change is inversely proportional to the Dk/t and flexibility of the lens. The higher the Dk/t and the more flexible the lens, the less likelihood there is of lens-induced changes, assuming a well-fitting lens. Changes of corneal curvature of more than 0.25D are rare with flexible, rigid lenses and hydrogel lenses.

Clinical evaluation of corneal curvature has traditionally been achieved using the optical keratometer. This instrument is still invaluable and can generally be relied upon to detect overall compromise to corneal shape. The difficulty arises when attempting to assess asymmetric or localized regions of corneal distortion, because most keratometers are based upon an optical configuration that relies upon corneal reflections emanating from a 3 mm diameter circle on the corneal surface. Thus, localized swelling entirely within or outside this 'circle' goes undetected.

Change in corneal symmetry
Numerous videokeratoscopes are currently available and all have computerized algorithms to quantify the degree of irregularity of corneal surface shape. Ruiz-Montenegro et al.[14] used a computerized videokeratoscope that computed a function known as the Surface Asymmetry Index (SAI). Specifically, the SAI provides a quantitative measure of the radial symmetry of the four central videokeratoscope mires surrounding the vertex of the cornea. The higher the degree of central corneal symmetry, the lower the SAI. A high degree of central radial symmetry is characteristic of normal corneas.

Ruiz-Montenegro et al.[14] reported SAI mean values (± standard error of mean) associated with the following forms of lens wear:
- controls not wearing lenses, 0.35 ± 0.03;
- PMMA, 0.86 ± 0.22;
- Daily wear rigid, 0.48 ± 0.09;
- Daily wear hydrogel, 0.48 ± 0.11;
- Extended wear hydrogel, 0.46 ± 0.08.

The SAI was statistically significantly greater than that of the control group for all forms of lens wear, except for daily wear hydrogel lenses.

The clinical significance of this finding was highlighted because the authors observed a correlation between the nature of corneal deformation and the fit of the lens. For example, a superior riding rigid lens was associated with superior flattening, which thus explained the increase in SAI in that case. Such correlations were only observed in PMMA and rigid lens wearers, and an example is depicted in *Figure 24.2*.

Obvious corneal asymmetry can be detected using a keratometer, whereby the mires are not perfectly circular; that is, they may take on an elliptical, pear- or egg-shaped appearance. A sequence of progressively increasing levels of keratometer mire distortion is shown in Appendix A; this can be used as a grading scale to record the level of severity of lens-induced corneal distortion when using a keratometer.

Change in corneal regularity
In addition to SAI, the instrument used by Ruiz-Montenegro et al.[14] also computed a function known as the Surface Regularity Index (SRI). The SRI is a quantitative measure of central and paracentral corneal irregularity derived from the summation of fluctuations in corneal power that occur along semi-meridians of the 10 central photokeratoscope mires. The more regular the anterior surface of the central cornea the lower the SRI. The SRI is highly correlated with best spectacle-corrected visual acuity.

Ruiz-Montenegro et al.[14] reported SRI mean values (± standard error of mean) associated with the following forms of lens wear:

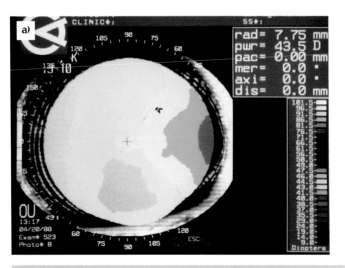
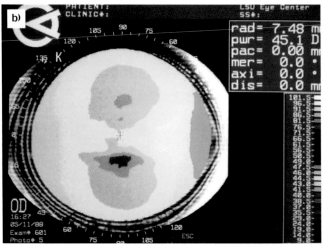

Figure 24.2

(a) Videokeratogram of cornea immediately after removal of a high-riding PMMA lens. Note the superior corneal flattening. (b) Same cornea depicted in (a) 3 weeks after lens removal. The cornea has recovered normal with-the-rule astigmatism

- Non-lens wearing controls, 0.41 ± 0.04;
- PMMA, 1.17 ± 0.34;
- Daily wear rigid, 0.93 ± 0.18;
- Daily wear hydrogel, 0.52 ± 0.08;
- Extended wear hydrogel, 0.51 ± 0.06.

The SRI was statistically significantly greater than that of the control group for PMMA and daily rigid lens wear, but not for daily or extended soft lens wear.

The clinical significance of changes in SRI was confirmed by the observation of the authors of an association in PMMA and rigid lens wearers whereby a decrease in best spectacle-corrected visual acuity occurred in patients who displayed an increased SRI. The patients did not suffer significant discomfort.

A keratometer can detect gross corneal irregularity in the form of lack of clarity of the mires; that is, various sections of the mires appear to be more in focus than others, and the circular mire lines may not appear to be perfectly smooth. Of course, such an assessment only relates to the 3 mm diameter ring of corneal surface that a keratometer samples optically. Other inexpensive instruments, such as the Placido disc and Klein keratoscope, can provide a similar assessment to that offered by the keratometer, but over a wider expanse of cornea. Needless to say, modern videokeratoscopes offer distinct advantages over traditional instruments in terms of the extent of corneal coverage, sensitivity, accuracy, objectivity, computational power and data presentation.

Change in corneal asphericity

Maeda et al.[23] used a computer-based videokeratoscope to develop an indicator of the asphericity of the central cornea, which they termed the 'corneal asphericity index' (CAI). These authors[23] used the CAI to evaluate both normal corneas and corneas with warpage induced by rigid lenses. The CAI (mean ± standard deviation) for the 22 control corneas was 0.33 ± 0.26, which indicates that the normal central cornea has a prolate shape. The average CAI for the 24 corneas with warpage induced by rigid lenses was significantly lower (–0.15 ± 0.36). These data suggest that some corneas have abnormal asphericity in the central cornea when warpage occurs with rigid lenses.

Lens-induced warpage in keratoconus

Szczotka et al.[24] evaluated 205 keratoconus patients using computerized videokeratography for both qualitative corneal topographic patterns and quantitative indices. Of these patients, 56 did not wear contact lenses, 130 wore PMMA or rigid lenses and 19 wore hydrogel lenses. Data from the keratoconus patients were also compared with a control group that comprised normal patients with no history of contact lens wear.

All three keratoconus groups had a significantly increased frequency of an asymmetric bowtie/skewed radial axes (AB/SRAX) pattern compared with normals. Differences among the videokeratography patterns for the keratoconus

patients included a significant shift from the AB/SRAX videokeratographic pattern to the irregular videokeratographic pattern in the PMMA and rigid lens subgroup, as well as an increased frequency of the irregular pattern in the hydrogel lens group versus the no contact lens group. Additional differences between the PMMA and rigid contact lens and no contact lens keratoconus groups included increased values for the quantitative indices of SAI, SRI, SIM-K and central K in the PMMA and rigid lens group.

Corneal indentation

Rigid lenses can adhere to the cornea during open-eye[8] or closed eye[9,25] wear. Adherence can occur at any time of the day in open-eye wear, but is characteristically noticed immediately upon eye opening after overnight wear. In the latter case, the lens usually begins to move freely after a few blinks; persistent binding for more than a few minutes is considered to be problematic. Indentation rings can also be caused by silicone elastomer lenses.[26]

Upon removal of a bound lens, an impression of the lens edge is usually evident on the cornea. Slit-lamp examination with fluorescein reveals the presence of an annular indentation in the cornea (*Figure 24.3a*), mild punctate keratitis primarily outside the lens edge and dense corneal desiccation inside the lens edge. An imprint from the bound edge after lens removal is clearly visible in *Figure 24.3b*, which is an unprocessed

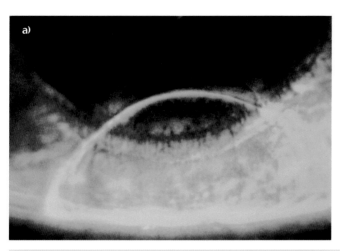
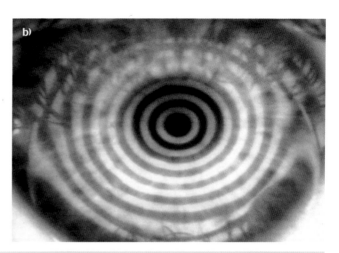

Figure 24.3

(a) Corneal and conjunctival imprint of an inferiorly mislocated bound rigid lens viewed with fluorescein immediately after lens removal. (b) Superior arcuate imprint observed in unprocessed mires of the videokeratoscope after lens removal

image of videokeratoscope rings. Lens binding is usually asymptomatic, but can be mildly uncomfortable.

Pathology

All known forms of changes to corneal topography induced by contact lenses can be explained in terms of three underlying pathologic mechanisms:

• Physical pressure on the cornea exerted either by the lens and/or eyelids;
• Edema induced by contact lenses;
• Mucus binding beneath rigid lenses.

The relative contributions of these factors vary in accordance with the type of topographic alteration.

Change in overall curvature

A comprehensive explanation of corneal shape change during PMMA lens wear was provided by the classic analysis of Carney[27]– an analysis that can be extrapolated from PMMA lens wear to explain virtually all cases of overall corneal shape change with rigid and soft lens wear.

Carney[27] observed corneal shape changes induced by PMMA lenses in normal atmospheric conditions (21 per cent oxygen) and in artificial conditions that ranged from 0 per cent oxygen (anoxia) to 100 per cent oxygen. He demonstrated convincingly that corneal shape change during PMMA lens wear could be attributed to a combination of lens-induced edema through hypoxia and physical pressure from the lens. The precise distribution of these two influences can explain the various forms of

topographic changes observed with all forms of lens wear (see Etiology).

Change in SAI, SRI and CAI

The pathologic processes that explain corneal shape changes characterized by SAI, SRI and CAI are difficult to elucidate because research has not been conducted to differentiate mechanisms that underlie changes in corneal symmetry, regularity and asphericity. In the absence of other explanatory mechanisms, one can only conclude that surface asymmetry, irregularity and asphericity are caused by differing contributions of the two key factors identified earlier – physical pressure by the lens and/or lids and lens-induced hypoxia.

It may also be true that individual differences in corneal rigidity may be a governing factor.[20] Ruiz-Montenegro *et al.*[14] noted that much of the variance in their data could be attributed to a small number of patients who displayed large alterations in SAI and SRI. The implication here is that some patients who have 'softer' or more pliable corneas, or who have an hereditary predisposition to keratoconus,[20] are more susceptible to lens-induced shape changes, and that such patients are slower to recover.

Lens-induced warpage in keratoconus

The mechanical stability of the cornea is compromised in keratoconus.[28] The biomechanical alterations may be introduced by increased sliding of collagen fibers as a result of reduced attachment to Bowman's layer and altered synthesis

of the matrix substance.[29] Biochemical studies of keratoconic corneas have shown an increase in collagenolysis, an increase in the number of reducible collagen cross-links, the formation of proteoglycan bridges along and between corneal collagen fibrils and an apparent loss of keratan sulfate. All of these changes could interfere with corneal strength,[30] and thus render the keratoconic cornea more susceptible to warpage induced by contact lenses.

Corneal indentation

Indentation associated with lens binding appears to be related more to physical pressure and less to the effects of hypoxia. For overnight wear, mucus accumulation beneath the lens is a feature of lens binding (*Figure 24.4*), the etiologic significance of which is considered below.[31]

Etiology

Theoretical and experimental analyses have been undertaken to explain the etiology of lens-induced corneal shape changes. These are considered with respect to the various forms of shape changes described earlier.

Change in overall curvature

The typical pattern of refractive change during PMMA lens wear – an initial myopic shift during adaptation followed by a recovery over 3–6 months and subsequent myopia reduction – can be explained using the model of Carney.[27]

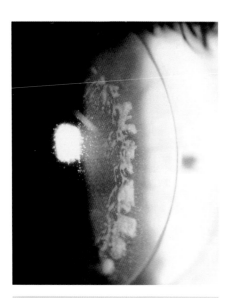

Figure 24.4

Build-up of mucus and debris beneath a bound rigid lens pictured here 2.5 hours after waking

A centrally fitting PMMA lens induces hypoxia beneath the lens, which results in edema in the corresponding central region of the cornea. This phenomenon, known as CCC (see *Figure 18.11*), is characterized by an increased curvature of the central cornea as the stroma in that region thickens, which results in a myopic shift. A moderate increase in corneal thickness of 2 per cent over a 4 mm wide central zone increases corneal surface power by about 1.75D.

After the initial adaptation (subsequent to possible lens refits to provide more movement), the hypoxia is alleviated and the cornea may return to its original shape. Another influence occurs concurrently – a progressive overall flattening of the cornea because of the constant bearing of the lens against the corneal apex. This flattening leads to a hyperopic shift in refraction, which is presumably masked by the initial marked apical steepening caused by hypoxia during the adaptive phase described above.

While the explanation provided above cannot be considered definitive, the following general principles can be applied to explain lens-induced corneal shape change:

- Local lens-induced hypoxia causes localized edema, corneal swelling and myopic shift;
- Overall lens bearing causes corneal flattening and a hyperopic shift.

An additional, but less likely, influence is that a steep lens may mold the cornea into a more curved shape, and thereby induce a myopic shift.

Presumably, rigid lenses of higher oxygen performance influence corneal shape more by way of physical bearing than hypoxic edema. Certainly, there is an increasing shift as rigid lens *Dk/t* increases in favor of physical bearing and against hypoxic edema as etiologic factors in lens-induced shape change. Gleason *et al.*[32] reported that 9.6 per cent of patients wearing hyperpermeable rigid lenses (*Dk* = 163) who successfully completed a 1 year prospective clinical trail demonstrated mean keratometric changes of 0.57D in the horizontal meridian and 0.73D in the vertical meridian.

Modern-generation hydrogel lenses induce minimal levels of edema and contribute little direct tangential physical force to the cornea, so shape changes induced by hydrogel lenses are rarely observed. Hydrogel lenses of lower *Dk/t* can induce low-to-moderate levels of edema across the cornea. An optical analysis of this phenomenon leads to the conclusion that there will be virtually no refractive shift in association with a uniform area of edema greater than 8 mm in diameter.[33]

The slight corneal flattening observed in patients who wear silicone hydrogel lenses[15,18] is associated with a progressive thinning effect of the central cornea, which can remain for up to 3 months after discontinuing lens wear.[15] According to Gonzalez-Meijome *et al.*,[15] mid-peripheral and peripheral areas do not display such a thinning effect during continuous wear. The overall effect seems to be a result of mechanical pressure induced by these silicone hydrogel materials, which are characterized by a relatively high modulus of elasticity.

Change in SAI, SRI and CAI

The data of Ruiz-Montenegro *et al.*[14] provide quantitative proof that rigid lenses disturb corneal symmetry and regularity less than PMMA lenses do, and that hydrogel lenses affect SAI and SRI least. This can only be presumed to be attributed to less physical deformation by softer lenses and less lens-induced hypoxic edema with rigid and soft lenses.

A likely cause of increased SAI in rigid lens wearers could be physical pressure from a lens that constantly tends to decenter in a predictable manner. Ruiz-Montenegro *et al.*[14] and Wilson *et al.*[19] noted a correlation between lens decentration and corneal topographic change.

The precise cause of increased SRI cannot be explained easily in terms of improper lens fitting. Changes in CAI may be related more to a symmetrical lens molding effect.

Further experimentation along the lines of the studies of Carney[27] is required to provide a full explanation of the specific etiology of lens-induced changes to SAI, SRI and CAI.

Lens-induced warpage in keratoconus

Szczotka *et al.*[24] concluded that the increased frequency of qualitative and quantitative corneal irregularity in keratoconus patients who wear rigid lenses may reflect a true mechanical effect of contact lens wear. However, these authors could not reject the possibility that this finding may also reflect an advanced disease state in these patients that limits them to rigid lens wear.

Corneal indentation

Binding of rigid lenses to the cornea during overnight wear has been explained by Swarbrick.[25] Thinning of the post-lens tear film during sleep leaves a very thin, highly viscous layer of mucus-rich tears between the lens and cornea, which acts as a form of glue to bind the lens to the cornea. This tear film thinning is caused by a constant lid pressure against the lens during eye closure.

On eye opening the shear force imparted by the eyelid may be insufficient to initiate lens movement, and the lens remains bound until the mucus film is diluted and thickened by the gradual penetration of aqueous tears. Evidence for this theory comes from clinical observations of fluorescein movement under rigid lenses as the lens becomes unstuck[31] (*Figure 24.5*).

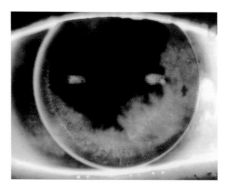

Figure 24.5

Gradual penetration of fluorescein beneath a bound lens as the mucus adhesion breaks down

Rigid lens binding during open-eye lens wear occurs less frequently, and may be explained partially by mucus-mediated adhesion. Another possibility is that, in the course of moving around the cornea and being intermittently compressed by the lids, a rigid lens may assume a position whereby a slight negative pressure is created beneath the lens. This could create a mild suction that temporarily holds the lens in place and results in corneal indentation caused mild the pressure of a static lens edge.

Rae and Huff[26] studied silicone elastomer lens binding *in vitro* to determine what factors may influence its development on the cornea or corneosclera. Lens binding to corneas was not influenced by corneal toricity (0–20D), corneal fitting relationship (2D steep to 4D flat), mucin (2 or 5 per cent) in the tear bath, or transcorneal pressure (11–22 mm/Hg). In isolated corneas or in whole eyes, transient intraocular pressure changes did not influence keratometry readings, ruling these out as potential mechanisms for corneal binding during sleep. Corneoscleral preparations were also examined to simulate a decentered lens. Corneoscleral binding occurred with a significantly greater frequency than corneal binding and was not influenced by corneal toricity, corneal fitting relationship (up to 0.5 mm steeper than K) or mucin concentration. Unlike the final stages of clinical lens adhesion, the binding observed by Rae and Huff[26] permitted lateral lens movement and occurred without leaving an indentation ring. These findings may suggest that the system models the initiation of corneoscleral binding, involving decentration and suction onto the corneoscleral junction. Rae and Huff[26] concluded that corneal binding could not be explained by a chemical attraction between the silicone elastomer lens surface and cornea, with or without mucin interaction, and must be accounted for by other factors found *in vivo*.

Management

As PMMA lenses are rarely fitted today, the difficult fitting problems encountered with such lenses are only of historical interest. However, as has been revealed above, rigid lenses can induce clinically significant changes in corneal topography, which may be especially evident in patients with higher pre-scriptions that require thicker lenses. Such lenses impart greater physical and hypoxic stress on the cornea compared with thinner lenses made of the same material. Of course, in any case of corneal shape change induced by contact lenses, refitting into soft lenses usually provides a cure because soft lenses are known to have little or no effect on corneal topography.

Change in overall curvature

Refractive instability in patients who wear rigid lenses is a possible sign of lens-induced corneal shape change. Of course, other possible causes of refractive instability, such as unstable diabetes or advancing keratoconus, must be ruled out. Once this has been done, the direction of refractive change may provide a clue as to the likely cause. A myopic shift suggests increased corneal curvature, which could result from a steeply fitting lens or central hypoxic edema. A hyperopic shift suggests a flat lens fit and excessive central lens bearing.

Although it is not always possible to determine the precise cause of a shift in refraction, a solution to the problem can be based upon the principle that a well-fitting lens of high oxygen performance induces minimum corneal shape change.

If the clinical decision has been made that the present lens is unacceptable, a new lens must be fitted. Three basic approaches have been suggested for refitting rigid lens wearers who suffer from corneal shape changes:

- Sudden discontinuation – the patient is advised to cease lens wear for an extended period of time (perhaps many weeks). The theory behind this approach is that the cornea is allowed to recover completely in the total absence of the influence of a lens.[34]
- De-adaptation – the patient is advised to continue wearing lenses, but wearing time is gradually reduced to zero. The cornea is then monitored and a lens is refitted when stability has been reached.[35]
- Immediate refit – the patient is immediately refitted with lenses of superior design and higher *Dk/t*, so that recovery occurs more gradually during wear of the replacement lenses.[34,36]

Sudden discontinuation is not considered to be a viable technique for two reasons. First, patients who discontinue in this way, especially after PMMA lens wear, show excessive and unpredictable fluctuations in refractive state and corneal curvature.[37] In addition, permanent corneal distortion has been noted in some patients after sudden discontinuation of PMMA lens wear.[1] Second, this procedure is disconcerting to patients who must endure the wild refractive changes and suffer the inconvenience of not wearing lenses for some time.

De-adaptation is a compromise between the patient management techniques of 'sudden discontinuation' and 'immediate refit'. The preferred technique is 'immediate refit'.[34,36,38] The aim is to refit the patient with a lens of better fit and higher *Dk/t*. It is beyond the scope of this chapter to provide a full set of guidelines to achieve a superior rigid lens fit; suffice to say that a thin, large diameter, aspheric back-surface alignment fit often gives the best results.

Immediate refitting of long-term PMMA contact lens wearers into rigid materials was the aim of a study by Novo *et al.*[39] Six eyes with corneal warpage induced by PMMA contact lenses were assessed. At 6 months after refitting the SRI had diminished by 0.51 ± 0.32 and the SAI improved by 0.32 ± 0.26. The authors[39] concluded that immediate refitting of long-term PMMA contact lens wearers into rigid materials of similar design and fit allows a slightly more regular and symmetric central corneal shape to be attained, which results in improved spectacle visual acuity.

During rigid lens wear, the tear layer may mask any deleterious effects on vision that arise from corneal distortion. Thus, patients are satisfied because they can continue to wear lenses, and vision is adequate. Also, patients should be advised that their new lenses are more flexible and less scratch resistant, and that greater caution is required when cleaning and handling lenses.

If supplementary spectacles are to be prescribed, it is obviously preferable to delay this until the corneal shape has been stabilized. This could take 3 weeks after the lens refit, although a longer period should be allowed if the corneal distortion that prompted the refit was particularly severe.[34]

Changes in SAI, SRI and CAI

Gross changes in corneal asymmetry may be attributed to rigid lens decentration, with corneal flattening in the region of the decentered lens. Refitting a lens with good centration should solve the problem; this may involve fitting a lens of larger diameter and avoiding excessive central bearing. Changes in corneal asphericity are presumably caused by an overall symmetric molding effect.

The exact cause of excessive lens-induced corneal surface irregularity may be difficult to ascertain. If vision has dropped by more than one line of Snellen acuity, refitting with a large diameter lens of high Dk/t may allow the cornea to recover to a more normal topographic form.

Ruiz-Montenegro et al.[14] stated that they do not routinely discontinue contact lens wear in patients who are asymptomatic and have mild alterations to SAI and/or SRI, even if the changes are associated with a small decrease in best spectacle-corrected visual acuity.

Lens-induced warpage in keratoconus

Lens-induced warpage in keratoconus patients can be avoided by fitting lenses with a lower modulus of elasticity and/or adopting an apical clearance fitting philosophy. A potential disbenefit of apical clearance is that the cone may progress more quickly compared with an apical touch fit. Clearly, these competing factors need to be weighed up when deciding on the appropriate strategy for a given patient.

Corneal indentation

Although there is little doubt that mucus adhesion is the principle mechanism for the binding of a rigid lens to the cornea,[31] the literature is full of ambiguous and often contradictory opinions as to lens-fitting strategies to avoid this problem. A review of the pertinent literature by Woods and Efron[40] produced a list of the various opinions that have been suggested, which includes flatten base curve, steepen base curve, increase center thickness, reduce center thickness, reduce back optical zone diameter, reduce total diameter, increase axial edge lift, increase edge band width, use an aspheric design and prescribe lubricants.

It has been suggested that rigid lens binding may be in some way related to long-term deposit formation and lens surface modification. This theory is derived from research that shows the incidence of rigid lens binding in extended wear patients can be reduced by regular lens replacement.[40] Interestingly, lens binding was not alleviated in daily wear rigid lens patients by regularly replacing lenses.[40]

Swarbrick and Holden[41] observed that rigid lens binding is a patient-dependent phenomenon. Their analysis did not reveal patient attributes that would allow a clinician to predict whether a given patient is likely to display binding. Nevertheless, the observation of patient dependence is useful as it serves to alert clinicians that binding is likely to recur in a given patient unless some remedial action is taken.

Significant changes to lens design could be attempted to alleviate further occurrences of binding in a given patient, although it must be recognized that this can only be effected using a systematic 'trial and error' approach in the absence of definitive guidelines in the literature.

As lens binding is a problem that relates specifically to rigid lenses, refitting with soft lenses is an obvious solution.

Prognosis

The prognosis for recovery of normal corneal topography is highly variable and dependent upon the magnitude and duration of the lens-induced deformation forces. While the time course of recovery from physical forces on the cornea may be difficult to predict, recovery from chronic lens-induced edema is known to occur within 7 days of cessation of lens wear.[42]

From a patient-management perspective, knowledge of the rate of recovery from lens-induced shape changes is of particular relevance to patients who are currently wearing rigid contact lenses and are considering either being refitted with soft lenses or undergoing refractive surgery. It is essential that any lens-induced shape change be allowed to subside before refractive surgery is performed.

Change in overall curvature

Dramatic changes in corneal curvature after cessation of long-term PMMA lens wear were documented by Rengstorff.[37] There is an initial reduction in myopia over the first 3 days, averaging 1.32D, followed by a gradual return to baseline over the next 3 weeks. The extent and duration of these changes correlate with the length of time that the PMMA lenses are worn. In general, the refractive changes occur in parallel with corneal shape changes.

Bennett and Tomlinson[34] observed that the pattern of corneal recovery after PMMA lens wear is the same irrespective of whether a 'sudden discontinuation' or 'immediate refit' strategy is adopted. Since vision is better and more stable when adopting the 'immediate refit' strategy, this procedure is favored by the authors.[34]

The prognosis of recovery from severe corneal warpage is not good. Hartstein[1] reported 12 cases of corneal warpage induced by contact lenses that were deemed to be permanent. Morgan[43] reported that in 74 cases of severe PMMA-induced corneal warpage, only half of the corneas displayed satisfactory resolution within 3 months of cessation of lens wear. Wilson et al.[3] advise that corneal warpage induced by rigid lenses can take between 5 and 8 months to recover fully.

Calossi et al.[44] described a case of corneal warpage caused by 14 years of rigid lens wear. The patient was refitted with daily wear soft contact lenses of high water content. Significant changes in both refraction and keratometry were observed after the refit; computerized videokeratography showed that the corneal contour of both eyes had normalized after about 6 months. This case serves to illustrate that it is possible to re-establish a normal cornea without completely suspending contact lens wear by changing from a rigid to a soft material, but the rate of recovery can be protracted.

Wang et al.[17] evaluated the resolution of corneal warpage induced by contact lenses before keratorefractive surgery. In the 12 per cent of patients who demonstrated lens-associated warpage, the mean duration of prior contact lens wear was 21.2 years (range 10–30 years); lens use included daily wear hydrogel ($n = 2$), extended wear hydrogel ($n = 6$), toric ($n = 4$) and rigid lenses ($n = 8$). Up to 3.00D refractive and 2.50D keratometric shifts accompanied by significant topography pattern differences were observed. The average recovery time for stabilization of refraction, keratometry (change within ± 0.5D) and topography pattern was 7.8 ± 6.7 weeks (range 1–20 weeks). Recovery rates differed between the lens types:
- Hydrogel extended wear, 11.6 ± 8.5 weeks;
- Hydrogel toric lens, 5.5 ± 4.9 weeks;
- Hydrogel daily wear, 2.5 ± 2.1 weeks;
- Rigid lens, 8.8 ± 6.8 weeks.

Based on these findings, Wang et al.[17] advise that to optimize the quality and predictability of keratorefractive procedures, an appropriate waiting period is necessary for lens-induced corneal warpage to stabilize. They suggest that the resolution of corneal warpage be documented by stable serial manifested refractions, keratometry and corneal topographic patterns before former lens-wearing patients are scheduled for keratorefractive surgery.

Changes in SAI, SRI and CAI

The patterns of recovery of corneas rendered asymmetric, irregular or aspheric as detected by videokeratoscopy are likely to be similar to those described above for changes in overall curvature; that is, taking the sum of the mean and standard deviation of the data of Wang et al.,[17] recovery is likely to occur within about 16 weeks for rigid lenses, 21 weeks for hydrogel extended wear lenses and 5 weeks for hydrogel daily wear lenses.

Lens-induced warpage in keratoconus

As Szczotka et al.[24] observed, it is difficult to disassociate the warpage effects of rigid lenses from the diseased state of keratoconus; nevertheless, an appreciation of the overall prognosis for keratoconic lens wearers can be gained by considering the success rate of contact lens fitting and rate of progression to keratoplasty. Such a study was undertaken by Smiddy et al.[45] in relation to 115 consecutive patients with keratoconus who had been referred for keratoplasty after previous contact lens fittings were no longer successful. Of 190 non-operated eyes that needed to be fitted with contact lenses, 165 eyes (87 per cent) could be fitted. Of these, 51 eyes (31 per cent) ultimately needed keratoplasty after an average of 38 months of lens wear, and 114 eyes (69 per cent) did not require keratoplasty over an average follow-up interval of 63 months of wearing contact lenses.

Corneal indentation

In relation to a specific binding episode (with associated corneal indentation), prognosis for recovery is good. Swarbrick and Holden[41] reported that 25 per cent of all lenses bound on eye opening were mobile within 10 minutes and 50 per cent were mobile within 30 minutes; however, 40 per cent were still bound

60 minutes later. All lenses could be freed eventually by gentle manipulation of the lens through the lids. In almost two-thirds of cases in which lenses had been assessed as bound on eye opening, clinical signs of binding were apparent 2 hours after eye opening.[41] All signs of binding disappear within 24 hours in the absence of lens wear.

The prognosis for avoiding future episodes of rigid lens binding is not good, given that binding is a patient-dependent phenomenon. A satisfactory prognosis can only be effected in such patients if significant changes are made to lens design or type.

Differential Diagnosis

It is generally possible to differentiate vision loss as a result of corneal shape change from that caused by other factors by reconciling refractive shifts with changes in corneal curvature. Although this relationship generally holds true, it is important to recognize that other factors, such as localized edema, and changes to other refractive components of the eye can alter refractive status.

Corneal warpage induced by contact lenses can take on a very similar clinical appearance to keratoconus (*Figure 24.6*). The key differentiating features of these two conditions in advanced cases are that patients with keratoconus often display corneal thinning, Vogt's striae, Fleischer's ring and progressive corneal steepening (cone development), whereas lens-induced corneal warpage recovers after cessation of lens wear and is not associated with clinically detectable corneal thinning, striae and ring pathology.

In the early stages of keratoconus, however, differentiation from mild lens-induced corneal warpage can be difficult. Lebow and Grohe[46] point out that superior corneal flattening associated with inferior corneal steepening is a videokeratoscopic topography pattern that usually describes both keratoconus and warpage induced by contact lenses. To differentiate these two conditions topographically, these authors[46] analyzed 10 different corneal topographic shape variables and found that three unique measurements of corneal geometry – shape factor (SF), irregularity (CIM) and apical toricity (TKM) – could be used to differentiate these two conditions with a high degree of accuracy and specificity. A similar approach has been described by Smolek et al.[47]

Suggestions that rigid contact lens wear can induce keratoconus[48] have been dismissed because of the lack of sound evidence. Any association between keratoconus and rigid lens wear is almost certainly coincidental rather than causative.

Intentional Corneal Molding

Brief mention needs to be made of three clinical approaches that attempt to utilize the known corneal molding properties of rigid lenses to reshape the cornea.

Cone compression in keratoconus

Confirmed cases of keratoconus are almost always fitted with rigid lenses so as to neutralize corneal distortions and provide satisfactory vision. A variety of fitting philosophies can be adopted to

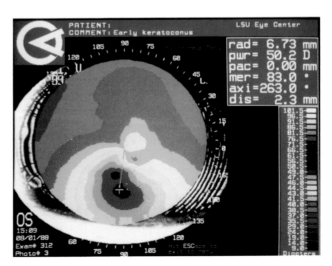

Figure 24.6

Early keratoconus, which takes on a similar appearance to corneal warpage induced by a high-riding rigid lens (compare this image with *Figure 24.2a*)

fit the keratoconic eye, including apical bearing, apical clearance, three-point touch and lid attachment procedures. The theory behind the first of these – apical bearing – is that constant bearing on the cone arrests or slows the progression of the cone. Both scleral and rigid lenses have been used historically for this reason (*Figure 24.7a*).

Korb *et al.*[49] warned that an apical bearing lens fit can result in scarring of the apex of the cone (*Figure 24.7b*) . Furthermore, Ruben and Trodd[50] demonstrated that there was no difference in the rate of progression of keratoconus in lens-wearing groups versus groups not wearing lenses. Despite these observations, the apical bearing technique appears to have been favored by 88 per cent of practitioners, based upon the results of a national USA survey of 1209 keratoconic patients wearing rigid lenses.[51]

Orthokeratology

Orthokeratology is a term used to describe the clinical procedure of deliberately fitting rigid lenses in such a manner that the cornea is molded into a new shape, with the aim of reducing the level of myopia. It is a technique that has been evolving since the 1960s, and the term 'modern orthokeratology' has been coined to distinguish previous approaches from current methods. More specifically, 'modern orthokeratology' refers to the practice of orthokeratology using reverse-geometry lenses, which create heavy central and outer peripheral bearing upon the cornea (*Figure 24.8*). Orthokeratology lenses can be made of high oxygen permeability materials, which enables such lenses to be worn on an overnight basis (i.e., overnight orthokeratology[52]).

The advent and acceptance of keratorefractive surgery for the correction of refractive errors has ensured that interest in other non-surgical approaches, such as orthokeratology, has remained relevant. The resurgence of orthokeratology as a viable alternative to refractive surgery or, indeed, to traditional contact lens or spectacle corrections, is a consequence of three developments:
- Availability of new lens designs, particularly reverse-geometry lenses, and the ability to design and manufacture lenses to produce a specific tear layer thickness profile;
- Availability of videokeratographs to assist with contact lens design and to evaluate corneal shape changes;

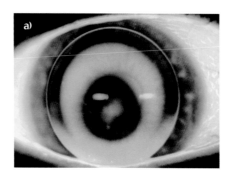
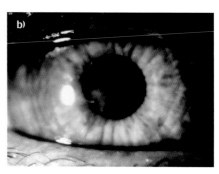

Figure 24.7

(a) Rigid lens fitted to a keratoconic eye, with the fluorescein pattern indicating central and mid-peripheral bearing. (b) Same eye as depicted in (a), pictured here in white light and revealing central corneal scarring induced by the apical lens bearing

- Availability of new materials of high oxygen permeability, which allow overnight lens wear.

The average magnitude of the refractive change using orthokeratology lenses is only about 1.75D,[52,53] and is subject to significant individual variability. The issue of predictability of these changes is still an important and unresolved one. The corneal changes are not permanent, as significant regression occurs over a few hours.[52] Ongoing use of contact lenses (sometimes referred to as 'retainer lenses'), whether for overnight or daily wear, is still needed to sustain the refractive changes. Questions have been raised about the scientific rigor of studies that relate to 'modern orthokeratology' and 'overnight orthokeratology',[54] especially in relation to a lack of appropriate masking, randomization and experimental control.

The corneal curvature changes in orthokeratology appear to result from a combination of short-term corneal molding and a longer term redistribution of anterior corneal tissue.[55,56] It has also been suggested that the tear reservoir generated by the steeper secondary curves leads to pressure changes that are responsible for the corneal tissue redistribution[56,57] (*Figure 24.9*).

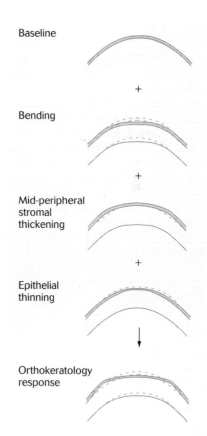

Baseline

Bending

Mid-peripheral stromal thickening

Epithelial thinning

Orthokeratology response

Figure 24.9

The change from baseline corneal shape and thickness produced by a reverse-geometry lens in the process of orthokeratology can be modeled as a result of the composite effects of bending, mid-peripheral stromal thickening and central epithelial thinning

Figure 24.8

Fluorescein pattern for a correctly fitted reverse geometry lens

Despite the relative safety of overnight orthokeratology with respect to reversible and non-sight threatening adverse events, there have been reports of complications, such as recurrent lens binding and central island formation,[58] and there appears to be an increased risk of microbial keratitis during overnight lens wear with reverse-geometry lenses,[59–62] which necessitates a careful risk–benefit analysis for each patient who contemplates this procedure.

Myopia control

It has long been suggested that the progression of myopia can be arrested by fitting rigid lenses instead of soft lenses or spectacles.[63–66] To test this hypothesis, Katz et al.[67] fitted both eyes of 428 Singaporean children aged between 6 and 12 years with either spectacles or rigid lenses. The children had myopia between –1.00D and –4.00D, had not worn contact lenses previously and had no other ocular pathologies. After a 3 month adaptation period, 383 children were followed, and 298 (78 per cent) remained after 24 months. There was an increase in the spherical equivalent of –1.33D and –1.28D, and axial length increased by 0.84 and 0.79 mm over 2 years among children randomized to contact lenses and spectacles, respectively. These findings demonstrate that rigid lenses do not slow the rate of myopia progression. Katz et al.[67] concluded that it is unlikely that this intervention holds promise as a method by which to slow the rate of progression of myopia in children.

REFERENCES

1 Hartstein J (1965). Corneal warping due to wearing of corneal contact lenses. A report of 12 cases. Am J Ophthalmol. **60**, 1103–1104.

2 Mobilia EF and Kenyon KR (1986). Contact lens-induced corneal warpage. Int Ophthalmol Clin. **26**, 43–53.

3 Wilson SE, Lin DT, Klyce SD, et al. (1990). Topographic changes in contact lens-induced corneal warpage. Ophthalmology **97**, 734–744.

4 Asbell PA and Wasserman D (1991). Contact lens-induced corneal warpage. Int Ophthalmol Clin. **31**, 121–126.

5 Schornack M (2003). Hydrogel contact lens-induced corneal warpage. Contact Lens Ant Eye **26**, 153–159.

6 Finnemore VM and Korb JE (1980). Corneal edema with polymethyl methacrylate versus gas-permeable rigid polymer contact lenses of identical design. J Am Optom Assoc. **51**, 271–274.

7 Rengstorff RH (1965). Corneal curvature and astigmatic changes subsequent to contact lens wear. J Am Optom Assoc. **36**, 996–1000.

8 Woods CA and Efron N (1996). Regular replacement of daily-wear rigid gas-permeable contact lenses. J Br Contact Lens Assoc. **19**, 83–89.

9 Woods CA and Efron N (1996). Regular replacement of extended wear rigid gas permeable contact lenses. CLAO J. **22**, 172–178.

10 Polse KA, Rivera RK and Bonanno J (1988). Ocular effects of hard gas-permeable-lens extended wear. Am J Optom Physiol Opt. **65**, 358–364.

11 Baldone JA (1975). Corneal curvature changes secondary to the wearing of hydrophilic gel contact lenses. Contact Intraocul Lens Med J. **1**, 175–179.

12 Tomlinson A (1976). Contact lens and corneal topography with wear of the Soflens. Am J Optom Physiol Opt. **53**, 727–734.

13 Rengstorff RH and Nilsson KT (1985). Long-term effects of extended wear lenses: Changes in refraction, corneal curvature, and visual acuity. Am J Optom Physiol Opt. **62**, 66–68.

14 Ruiz-Montenegro J, Mafra CH, Wilson SE, et al. (1993). Corneal topographic alterations in normal contact lens wearers. Ophthalmology **100**, 128–134.

15 Gonzalez-Meijome JM, Gonzalez-Perez J, Cervino A, et al. (2003). Changes in corneal structure with continuous wear of high-Dk soft contact lenses: A pilot study. Optom Vis Sci. **80**, 440–446.

16 Liu Z and Pflugfelder SC (2000). The effects of long-term contact lens wear on corneal thickness, curvature, and surface regularity. Ophthalmology **107**, 105–111.

17 Wang X, McCulley JP, Bowman RW and Cavanagh HD (2002). Time to resolution of contact lens-induced corneal warpage prior to refractive surgery. CLAO J. **28**, 169–171.

18 Dumbleton KA, Chalmers RL, Richter DB and Fonn D (1999). Changes in myopic refractive error with nine months' extended wear of hydrogel lenses with high and low oxygen permeability. Optom Vis Sci. **76**, 845–849.

19 Wilson SE, Lin DT, Klyce SD, et al. (1990). Rigid contact lens decentration: A risk factor for corneal warpage. CLAO J. **16**, 177–182.

20 Phillips CI (1990). Contact lenses and corneal deformation: Cause, correlate or co-incidence? Acta Ophthalmol (Copenh.) **68**, 661–668.

21 Hostetter TA (1995). Monocular diplopia: Contact lens related warpage? J Ophthalmic Nurs Technol. **14**, 112–117.

22 Brungardt TF and Potter CE (1971). Spectacle blur refraction of long time contact lens wearers. Am J Optom Arch Am Acad Optom. **48**, 418–425.

23 Maeda N, Klyce SD and Hamano H (1994). Alteration of corneal asphericity in rigid gas permeable contact lens induced warpage. CLAO J. **20**, 27–31.

24 Szczotka LB, Rabinowitz YS and Yang H (1996). Influence of contact lens wear on the corneal topography of keratoconus. CLAO J. **22**, 270–273.

25 Swarbrick HA and Holden BA (1987). Rigid gas permeable lens binding: Significance and contributing factors. Am J Optom Physiol Opt. **64**, 815–823.

26 Rae ST and Huff JW (1991). Studies on initiation of silicone elastomer lens adhesion in vitro: Binding before the indentation ring. CLAO J. **17**, 181–186.

27 Carney LG (1975). The basis of corneal shape change during contact lens wear. Am J Optom Arch Am Acad Optom. **52**, 445–453.

28 Andreassen TT, Simonsen AH and Oxlund H (1980). Biomechanical properties of keratoconus and normal corneas. Exp Eye Res. **31**, 435–441.

29 Edmund C (1989). Corneal topography and elasticity in normal and keratoconic eyes. A methodological study concerning the pathogenesis of keratoconus. Acta Ophthalmol. **193S**, 1–36.

30 Bron AJ (1988). Keratoconus. Cornea **7**, 163–169.

31 Swarbrick HA (1988). A possible aetiology for RGP lens binding (adherence). Int Contact Lens Clin. **15**, 13–19.

32 Gleason W, Tanaka H, Albright RA and Cavanagh HD (2003). A 1-year prospective clinical trial of menicon Z (tisilfocon A) rigid gas-permeable contact lenses worn on a 30-day continuous wear schedule. Eye Contact Lens **29**, 2–9.

33 Dixon J (1964). Ocular changes due to contact lenses. Am J Ophthalmol. **58**, 424–433.

34 Bennett ES and Tomlinson A (1983). A controlled comparison of two techniques of refitting long-term PMMA contact lens wearers. Am J Optom Physiol Opt. **60**, 139–147.

35 Arner RS (1977). Corneal deadaptation – the case against abrupt cessation of contact lens wear. J Am Optom Assoc. **48**, 339–341.

36 Bennett ES (1983). Immediate refitting with gas permeable lenses. J Am Optom Assoc. **54**, 239–242.

37 Rengstorff RH (1967). Variations in myopia measurements: An after effect observed with habitual wearers of contact lenses. Am J Optom Arch Am Acad Optom. **44**, 149–161.

38 Rengstorff RH (1979). Refitting long term wearers of hard contact lenses. Rev Optom. **116**, 75–79.

39 Novo AG, Pavlopoulos G and Feldman ST (1995). Corneal topographic changes after refitting polymethyl methacrylate contact lens wearers into rigid gas permeable materials. CLAO J. **21**, 47–51.

40 Woods CA and Efron N (1996). Regular replacement of rigid contact lenses alleviates binding to the cornea. Int Contact Lens Clin. **23**, 13–18.

41 Swarbrick HA and Holden BA (1989). Rigid gas-permeable lens adherence: A patient-dependent phenomenon. Optom Vis Sci. **66**, 269–275.

42. Holden BA, Sweeney DF, Vannas A, et al. (1985). Effects of long-term extended contact lens wear on the human cornea. Invest Ophthalmol Vis Sci. **26**, 1489–1501.

43 Morgan JF (1982). For keratoconus diagnosis: 'Qualitative' ophthalmometry. Ophthalmol Times **7**, 33–36.

44 Calossi A, Verzella F and Zanella SG (1996). Corneal warpage resolution after refitting an RGP contact lens wearer into hydrophilic high water content material. *CLAO J.* **22**, 242–244.

45 Smiddy WE, Hamburg TR, Kracher GP and Stark WJ (1988). Keratoconus. Contact lens or keratoplasty? *Ophthalmology* **95**, 487–492.

46 Lebow KA and Grohe RM (1999). Differentiating contact lens induced warpage from true keratoconus using corneal topography. *CLAO J.* **25**, 114–122.

47 Smolek MK, Klyce SD and Maeda N (1994). Keratoconus and contact lens-induced corneal warpage analysis using the keratomorphic diagram. *Invest Ophthalmol Vis Sci.* **35**, 4192–4204.

48 Gasset AR, Houde WL and Garcia-Bengochea M (1978). Hard contact lens wear as an environmental risk in keratoconus. *Am J Ophthalmol.* **85**, 339–346.

49 Korb DR, Finnemore VM and Herman JP (1982). Apical changes and scarring in keratoconus as related to contact lens fitting techniques. *J Am Optom Assoc.* **53**, 199–205.

50 Ruben M and Trodd C (1976). Scleral lenses in keratoconus. *Contact Interocul Lens Med J.* **2**, 18–24.

51 Edrington TB, Szczotka LB, Barr JT, *et al.* (1999). Rigid contact lens fitting relationships in keratoconus. Collaborative Longitudinal Evaluation of Keratoconus (CLEK) Study Group. *Optom Vis Sci.* **76**, 692–699.

52 Nichols JJ, Marsich MM, Nguyen M, *et al.* (2000). Overnight orthokeratology. *Optom Vis Sci.* **77**, 252–259.

53 Lui W-O and Edwards MH (2000). Orthokeratology in low myopia. Part 1. Efficacy and predictability. *Contact Lens Ant Eye* **23**, 77–89.

54 Efron N (2000). Overnight orthokeratology. *Optom Vis Sci.* **77**, 627–629.

55 Swarbrick HA, Wong G and O'Leary DJ (1998). Corneal response to orthokeratology. *Optom Vis Sci.* **75**, 791–799.

56 Alharbi A and Swarbrick HA (2003). The effects of overnight orthokeratology lens wear on corneal thickness. *Invest Ophthalmol Vis Sci.* **44**, 2518–2523.

57 Sridharan R and Swarbrick H (2003). Corneal response to short-term orthokeratology lens wear. *Optom Vis Sci.* **80**, 200–206.

58 Chui WS and Cho P (2003). Recurrent lens binding and central island formations in a fast-responding orthokeratology lens wearer. *Optom Vis Sci.* **80**, 490–494.

59 Chen KH, Kuang TM and Hsu WM (2001). *Serratia marcescens* corneal ulcer as a complication of orthokeratology. *Am J Ophthalmol.* **132**, 257–258.

60 Lau LI, Wu CC, Lee SM and Hsu WM (2003). *Pseudomonas* corneal ulcer related to overnight orthokeratology. *Cornea* **22**, 262–264.

61 Wang JC and Lim L (2003). Unusual morphology in orthokeratology contact lens-related cornea ulcer. *Eye Contact Lens* **29**, 190–192.

62 Young AL, Leung AT, Cheung EY, *et al.* (2003). Orthokeratology lens-related *Pseudomonas aeruginosa* infectious keratitis. *Cornea* **22**, 265–266.

63 Jessen GN (1964). Contact lenses as a therapeutic device. *Am J Optom Arch Am Acad Optom.* **41**, 429–435.

64 Stone J and Powell-Cullingford G (1974). Myopia control after contact lens wear. *Br J Physiol Opt.* **29**, 93–108.

65 Kelly TS, Chatfield C and Tustin G (1975). Clinical assessment of the arrest of myopia. *Br J Ophthalmol.* **59**, 529–538.

66 Perrigin J, Perrigin D, Quintero S and Grosvenor T (1990). Silicone-acrylate contact lenses for myopia control: 3-year results. *Optom Vis Sci.* **67**, 764–769.

67 Katz J, Schein OD, Levy B, *et al.* (2003). A randomized trial of rigid gas permeable contact lenses to reduce progression of children's myopia. *Am J Ophthalmol.* **136**, 82–90.

PART VIII CORNEAL ENDOTHELIUM

ENDOTHELIAL BEDEWING

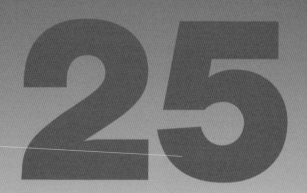

Eye care practitioners from time to time observe deposits such as keratic precipitates on the endothelial surface. These may be benign or may be associated with a broad range of uveal responses. In 1979, McMonnies and Zantos[1] described the appearance of endothelial deposits of uncertain origin in patients who were intolerant to contact lens wear (*Figure 25.1*). They described this condition as 'endothelial bedewing'. This condition was further discussed soon thereafter by Zantos and Holden;[2] however, since then, this topic has received little attention in the literature.

As discussed in this chapter, it is not at all clear that endothelial bedewing is *induced* by contact lens wear; however, there appears to be an *association* between lens wear and endothelial bedewing. This association is worth considering because specific management strategies need to be employed to solve the problem.

Incidence

The appearance of deposits or pigment spots on the endothelium (or on the anterior lens capsule) is commonly encountered during routine slit-lamp examination of all patients. These deposits are often benign and do not affect vision, except in rare cases.[3]

Hickson and Papas[4] conducted an extensive biomicroscopic examination on 70 normal, asymptomatic, consecutively presenting, non-wearers of contact lens and found that 20 per cent of the sample displayed endothelial bedewing. The authors concluded that endothelial bedewing can occur idiopathically in non-wearing eyes.

McMonnies and Zantos[1] reported seeing 25 patients with endothelial bedewing associated with contact lens intolerance over a 9 month period, and

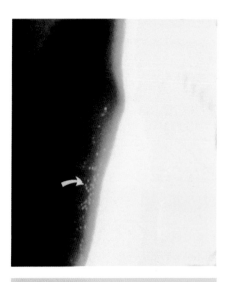

Figure 25.1
Endothelial bedewing observed using marginal retroillumination (arrow)

suggested that this condition is not uncommon. However, it is important to recognize that these observations were made some time ago, when the contact lens market was dominated by soft contact lenses which were replaced infrequently, made of materials (primarily hydroxyethyl methacrylate, HEMA) of low oxygen transmissibility and maintained using relatively unsophisticated lens care systems. At that time, contact lenses in general were associated with a higher prevalence of adverse reactions – relating to spoiled lenses and mildly toxic solution preservatives – compared with the present-day situation.

Extensive surveys of adverse responses to contact lenses have failed to document the prevalence of endothelial dysfunction of any kind.[5-7] It is therefore not possible to deduce the prevalence of endothelial bedewing associated with contact lenses in modern contact lens practice.

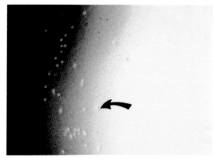

Figure 25.2
Endothelial bedewing observed at high magnification. In this case the individual cells are displaying 'reversed illumination' (arrow).

Signs and Symptoms

Endothelial bedewing associated with contact lenses is characterized by the appearance of small inclusions in the region of the inferior central cornea near to or immediately below the inferior pupil margin. They appear at the level of the endothelium. The area of bedewing can vary in shape. For example, endothelial bedewing may appear as an oval cluster of inclusions or as a less discrete dispersed formation. The condition is usually bilateral.[1]

The preferred slit-lamp observation technique is marginal retroillumination, in which the attention of the observer is directed to the region of the cornea in front of the border between the brightly illuminated iris and the dark pupil. Using this technique, the particles or inclusions appear as small discrete circular optically translucent entities. Most cells appear to display an optical phenomenon known as 'reversed illumination', whereby the distribution of light within the cell is the opposite of the background distribution of light (*Figure 25.2*). However, in some cases of endothelial bedewing the inclusions can also display reversed illumination. The optical basis for these characteristic forms of illumination are discussed in Chapter 15.

When viewed in direct illumination, endothelial bedewing can appear as fine white precipitates or as an orange–brown dusting of cells. Colored particles are likely to be cellular debris (see Pathology), and their actual color can give a clue to the length of time they have been present. Newly deposited cells are often whitish in color, but these become pigmented over time.

Figure 25.3 is a slit-lamp photograph taken of the right eye of a 35-year-old man referred for assessment of suitability for contact lenses to correct myopia. An extensive 'dusting' of brown pigment can be observed in a spindle shape characteristic of pigment dispersion syndrome (the so-called Krukenberg spindle).

There appears to be no fixed pattern of associated signs. Among their detailed case reports of three patients, McMonnies and Zantos[1] noted the following signs (in addition to bedewing): conjunctival redness, epithelial erosion, epithelial edema and reduced corneal transparency. There were no cases of flare in the anterior chamber.

The main associated feature of endothelial bedewing is either total or partial intolerance to lens wear. Some patients may present after having recently abandoned lens wear. Patients may also complain of 'fogging' of vision or stinging. Note, however, that the association between bedewing and lens intolerance is not obligatory; McMonnies and Zantos[1] observed two cases of endothelial bedewing in successful lens wearers.

Mackie[8] described a condition that he named 'total endothelial bedewing'. According to Mackie, this is an acute phenomenon that occurs in soft lens wearers. Patients usually present complaining of blurred vision. The condition resolves rapidly (within 2 days of lens removal) and does not recur. It is unclear whether Mackie was observing the same phenomenon as that reported by McMonnies and Zantos.[1]

Pathology

McMonnies and Zantos[1] originally surmised that the bedewing particles were either droplets of clear fluid (edema) within the endothelial cells or inflammatory cells, such as leukocytes or macrophages, resting on the posterior surface of the endothelium. Particles that display a 'reversed illumination' optical appearance are likely to be inflammatory cells. The reason is that 'reversed illumination' indicates the presence of material of higher refractive index within the entity that displays this appearance compared with the refractive index of the medium around that entity. The material of higher refractive index acts as a converging refractor, which causes a crossing over of the light rays. The cytoplasm, organelles and nucleus of an inflammatory cell resting on the endothelial surface are of a higher refractive index than that of the surrounding clear aqueous humor, and thus the reversed illumination. An inflammatory cell embedded within the endothelium probably does not display reversed illumination because the difference in refractive index between the inflammatory cell and the surrounding endothelial cell(s) is not significant enough.

Fluid droplets that lie within the endothelium are of a lower refractive index than the surrounding cytoplasm, organelles and nucleus of an endothelial cell and are therefore expected to display 'unreversed illumination', whereby the distribution of light within the particles is the same as the background distribution of light. Fluid drops on the surface of the endothelium are surrounded by aqueous humor and thus are unlikely to display such optical characteristics because of the lack of refractive index difference between the fluid drop and aqueous.

Bergmanson and Weissman[9] described an additional feature of endothelial bedewing – that inflammatory cells start off on the endothelial surface, but eventually become subsumed or engulfed by the endothelium and end up residing between adjacent endothelial cells and sealed off from the anterior chamber by zonula occludens. These authors produced convincing electron micrographs to support this hypothesis. As described above, such engulfed inflammatory cells are expected to produce a less pronounced appearance of reversed illumination because of the lower refractive index difference between the contents of the engulfed cell and those of the surrounding endothelial cells. It is likely that inflammatory cells observed in endothelial bedewing lie on the endothelium in the first instance, and some may become subsumed into the endothelium later.

Bergmanson[10] also provided evidence of fluid drops that form within the endothelium. *Figure 25.4* is an electron micrograph of the endothelium after

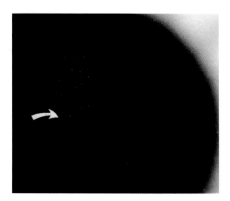

Figure 25.3
Pigment dispersion observed using indirect retroillumination (arrow)

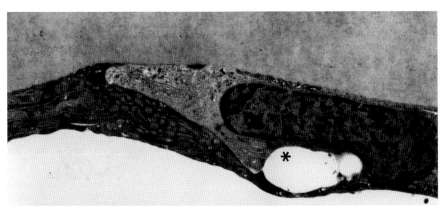

Figure 25.4
Electron micrograph of fluid inclusion (asterisk) between adjacent endothelial cells.

daily wear of an aphakic hydrogel lens in a 66-year-old person. In this instance, an intercellular edematous space (indicated by the asterisk) formed *between* adjacent endothelial cells.

Whatever the location of the bedewing (on or within the endothelium), that most inclusions display reversed illumination suggests these are of inflammatory origin, which in turn suggests that some forms of endothelial bedewing may have an inflammatory basis (see 'Etiology'). *Figure 25.5* illustrates endothelial bedewing.

On the assumption that endothelial bedewing can represent a mild inflammatory uveal response, the origin of the inflammatory cells is likely to be the iris and/or ciliary body. During inflammation, vascular permeability is increased and inflammatory cells leave vessels in the iris and ciliary body and float around in the aqueous until they come to rest on the endothelial surface. One would therefore expect occasionally to observe mild aqueous flare in patients with endothelial bedewing, but this does not appear to have been reported.

Etiology

The appearance and characteristic distribution of endothelial bedewing, and the associated signs and symptoms of eye redness, stinging and blurred vision (aside from lens intolerance), strongly suggest that the syndrome of endothelial bedewing can represent a mild anterior uveal inflammation. Although it is clear that contact lenses can induce a variety of inflammatory responses of the ocular surface tissues, it is less certain that contact lenses can induce a uveal inflammation.

Theoretically, contact lenses could induce an inflammatory response. In most body tissues, hypoxia can lead to the release of inflammatory mediators, such as prostaglandins, which can in turn cause inflammation. One possible mechanism is depicted in *Figure 25.6*. In this model, hypoxia induces the release from corneal tissue of prostaglandins, which diffuse into the aqueous humor and eventually enter iris tissue. A mild inflammatory response is initiated and inflammatory cells are released into the aqueous; these eventually come to rest on the endothelial surface.

Efron *et al.*[11] examined whether corneal edema induced by contact lenses was at least part inflammatory by measuring the

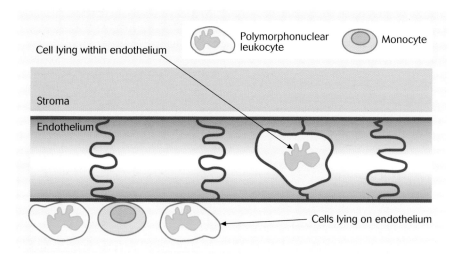

Figure 25.5
Endothelial bedewing in the form of inflammatory cells

level of edema in response to contact lens wear in a group of human subjects who took prostaglandin inhibitor drugs prior to lens wear. There was no difference between the level of edema in this group of subjects versus that in a control group who did not take prostaglandin inhibitor drugs, which led to rejection of the hypothesis that corneal edema induced by contact lenses has an inflammatory component. Nevertheless, a sequelae of events similar to that depicted in *Figure 25.6* and described above is possible, perhaps with a family of inflammatory mediators other than prostaglandins.

It may well be that, instead of contact lenses inducing a mild uveal response of which endothelial bedewing is a sign, the converse is true. That is, a patient may develop a mild anterior uveal response for reasons unrelated to lens wear, but the mild inflammatory status of the eye *causes* lens intolerance. Indeed, the latter explanation is the more likely scenario. Whatever the cause, it is important that clinicians be aware of the association so that appropriate management strategies can be put in place.

Management

As alluded to above, patients who suffer from endothelial bedewing will have already devised strategies to alleviate the symptoms before they present to the

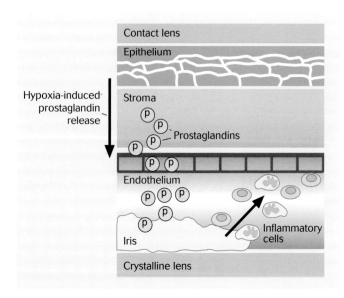

Figure 25.6
Possible etiology of endothelial bedewing

clinic – namely, reducing wearing time or ceasing lens wear. Simply put, this is a condition that is managed by symptomatology rather than signs. Wearing time should be reduced to a level that represents the balance between the needs of the patient to wear lenses for a desired length of time each day versus the level of discomfort that can be tolerated.

The presence of inflammatory cells on the endothelial surface should be viewed with great caution by clinicians, who need to consider a variety of possible causes. Certainly, all forms of uveitis should be considered as a possibility and tests should be conducted to exclude such possibilities (see 'Differential diagnosis').

In all cases of endothelial bedewing, intraocular pressures should be measured as there is a possibility that some inflammatory cells may have migrated into the anterior angle and created a blockage of aqueous outflow. Gonioscopy is also indicated, especially if intraocular pressure is elevated.

Prognosis

The pattern of recovery from endothelial bedewing is variable. McMonnies and Zantos[1] reported that in some cases the bedewing completely disappeared within 4 months, and in other cases it changed little over many months. These authors[1] also reported that lens intolerance persisted for many months in some patients, even after the bedewing had disappeared.

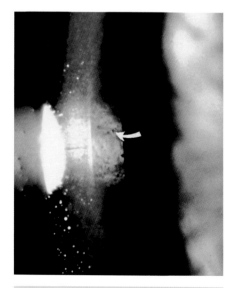

Figure 25.7
Contact lens induced endothelial blebs (arrow)

Differential Diagnosis

Various anomalies of the endothelium can potentially be confused with endothelial bedewing. Corneal guttata are focal accumulations of collagen on the posterior surface of Descemet's membrane, which lead to localized bulging of the endothelial surface. This in turn leads to the appearance of dark spots in the endothelial mosaic when viewed using specular reflection. Endothelial blebs (from localized endothelial cell edema) induced by contact lenses can take on an identical appearance (*Figure 25.7*; see Chapter 26). Differential diagnosis is effected by viewing the cornea using marginal retroillumination, which confirms the presence of the reversed or unreversed illumination appearance of bedewing. Guttata and blebs do not display these optical phenomena.

When the cornea is viewed using marginal retroillumination, bedewing can take on an appearance that is identical to either epithelial microcysts or vacuoles/bullae (see *Figure 15.3*). The procedure to differentiate between these two conditions is to view the cornea using a fine optical section at high magnification. At the very least, the depth of the pathology in the cornea can be determined (i.e., at the level of the epithelium or endothelium). If the endothelial bedewing has taken the form of cells resting on the surface of the endothelium, these are observed as fine spots on the posterior corneal surface. If the bedewing cells have been engulfed into the endothelium, they may not be visible. Similarly, epithelial microcysts are not observed in optic section. Thus, the appearance of spots on the endothelium when observed in optic section confirms the diagnosis of a cellular form of endothelial bedewing, whereas the absence of spots does not assist in differential diagnosis.

The associated signs assist in the differential diagnosis of endothelial bedewing versus epithelial microcysts. The latter are typically associated with extended lens wear and symptoms are minimal or absent. However, endothelial bedewing is associated with stinging, eye redness, corneal clouding and lens intolerance.

The possibility that the patient suffers from a form of uveitis that has occurred coincidentally with lens wear must be considered. The signs and symptoms associated with endothelial bedewing can closely mimic some of the mild manifestations of uveitis, such as Fuch's heterochromatic cyclitis. *Table 25.1* compares the signs and symptoms of endothelial bedewing and Fuch's heterochromatic cyclitis as a guide to differential diagnosis.

If a uveitis of any sort is suspected – including an intractable case of endothelial bedewing associated with indicators

---

Table 25.1
Comparison of endothelial bedewing associated with contact lenses and Fuch's heterochromatic cyclitis

Feature	Contact lens associated endothelial bedewing	Fuch's heterochromatic cyclitis
Age of onset	Any age	<45 years
Sex	No preference	No preference
Associated factors	Contact lens wear	Vitreous opacities 'Smudging' of iris crypts Iris pigment loss Iris atrophy
Symptoms	Intolerance to lens wear 'Fogging' of vision Stinging	Blurred vision
Signs	Conjunctival redness Epithelial erosion Epithelial edema Reduced corneal transparency	Faint anterior chamber flare
Cells	White or pigmented precipitates Form at inferior cornea	Only white precipitates Scattered diffusely over cornea
Laterality	Usually bilateral	Usually unilateral
Secondary complications	Glaucoma	Glaucoma Cataract

of active pathology, such as a red irritable eye and/or anterior chamber flare – therapeutic interventions may be required, such as the prescription of corticosteroids to dampen the inflammatory response, mydriatics to prevent the formation of posterior synechiae and analgesics to reduce the pain. If uveitis is confirmed in a contact lens wearer, lens wear should be ceased until the condition has resolved fully.

REFERENCES

1 McMonnies CW and Zantos SG (1979). Endothelial bedewing of the cornea in association with contact lens wear. *Br J Ophthalmol.* **63**, 478–481.

2 Zantos SG and Holden BA (1981). Guttate endothelial changes with anterior eye inflammation. *Br J Ophthalmol* **65**, 101–103.

3 Efron N and Collin HB (1979). Epicapsular stars with visual loss. *Am J Optom Physiol Opt.* **56**, 441–445.

4 Hickson S and Papas E (1997). Prevalence of idiopathic corneal anomalies in a non contact lens-wearing population. *Optom Vis Sci.* **74**, 293–297.

5 Stapleton F, Dart J and Minassian D (1992). Nonulcerative complications of contact lens wear. Relative risks for different lens types. *Arch Ophthalmol.* **110**, 1601–1606.

6 Hamano H, Watanabe K, Hamano T, *et al.* (1994). A study of the complications induced by conventional and disposable contact lenses. *CLAO J.* **20**, 103–108.

7 Sankaridurg PR, Sweeney DF, Sharma S, *et al.* (1999). Adverse events with extended wear of disposable hydrogels: Results for the first 13 months of lens wear. *Ophthalmology* **106**, 1671–1680.

8 Mackie IA (1993). Adverse reactions to soft contact lenses. In: *Medical Contact Lens Practice. A Systematic Approach*, p. 142–145, Ed. Mackie IA (Oxford: Butterworth–Heinemann).

9 Bergmanson JPG and Weissman BA (1992). Hypoxic changes in corneal endothelium. In: *Complications of Contact Lens Wear*, p. 37–68, Ed. Tomlinson A. (St Louis: Mosby–Year Book).

10 Bergmanson JPG (2001). Light and electron microscopy. In: *The Cornea. Its Examination in Contact Lens Practice*, p. 136–177, Ed. Efron N. (Oxford: Butterworth–Heinemann).

11 Efron N, Holden BA and Vannas A (1984). Effect of prostaglandin-inhibitor naproxen on the corneal swelling response to hydrogel contact lens wear. *Acta Ophthalmol (Copenh.)* **62**, 746–752.

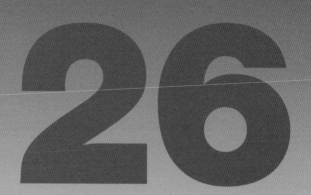

ENDOTHELIAL BLEBS

Prior to 1977, it was thought that contact lenses could only affect the cornea by direct mechanical influence or oxygen deprivation. As the endothelium is located on the posterior surface of the cornea and is known to obtain all of its required oxygen from that dissolved in the aqueous humor,[1] this tissue layer was thought to be immune from the effects of contact lenses.

The first clue that contact lenses could alter the corneal endothelium came from Zantos and Holden,[2] who noted that the endothelial mosaic undergoes a dramatic alteration in appearance within minutes of inserting a contact lens. Specifically, they reported observing a number of black, non-reflecting areas in the endothelial mosaic – which they called blebs – and an apparent increase in the separation between cells. These changes can be observed under high magnification (×40) using the slit-lamp biomicroscope (*Figure 26.1*).

The contact lens fraternity remained skeptical for some time, and it was not until both the appearance of blebs was verified independently[3] and reports of endothelial polymegethism induced by contact lenses were published by Schoessler and Woloschak[4,5] in the early 1980s that serious research commenced into understanding the endothelial response to lens wear.

Prevalence

The prevalence of endothelial blebs is thought to be essentially 100 per cent among contact lens wearers.[2] That is, blebs can be observed in all patients within 10 minutes of lens insertion. There is a large variation in the intensity of the response between patients.[2,6,7] Asian subjects have a significantly higher degree of endothelial bleb formation than the non-Asian population for closed eye lens wear.[8]

Signs and Symptoms

The black, non-reflecting areas observed in the endothelial mosaic correspond with the position of individual cells or groups of cells. The initial impression one gains is that cells have 'fallen off' the posterior surface of the cornea, to leave behind gaps or black holes.[2] In corneas that display a marked blebbing response, it also seems as if all the endothelial cells throughout the field of view have become separated further and the endothelial surface takes on a more textured and three-dimensional appearance.[2]

The 'bleb response' displays a characteristic time course (*Figure 26.2*). Blebs can be observed within 10 minutes of lens insertion. The number of blebs peaks in 20–30 minutes, then subsides to a low level after about 45–60 minutes. A low-level bleb response can be observed throughout the remainder of the wearing period.[2]

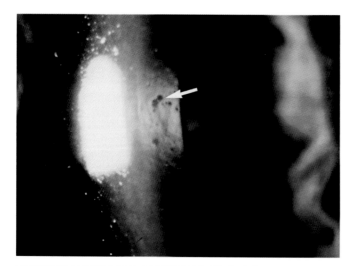

Figure 26.1

Blebs (arrow) induced by a contact lens in the endothelial mosaic observed in specular reflection with the slit-lamp biomicroscope

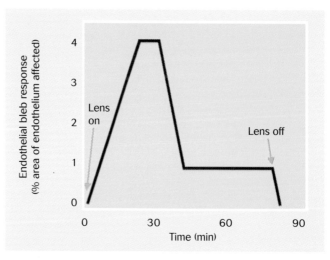

Figure 26.2

Time course of appearance and resolution of endothelial blebs induced by contact lenses.

Hydrogel lenses cause a greater bleb response than well-fitting rigid lenses, and hydrogel lenses of greater average thickness also induce a greater response than thinner lenses. However, the design and fit of hydrogel lenses have little effect on the bleb response.[6] Ohya *et al.*[7] observed that blebs are confined to the central regions of the cornea beneath rigid lenses, but occur throughout the cornea with soft lenses; that is, blebs are seen in all corneal areas covered by contact lenses.

Williams and Holden[9] observed two additional phenomena in patients who wear soft lenses on an extended wear basis. First, there appears to be an increase in the number of blebs in the late evening, prior to going to sleep. Second, the overall magnitude of the bleb response can be seen to decrease over the initial 8 days of extended wear. Furthermore, Bruce and Brennan[10] noted that the overall bleb response was reduced by approximately 50 per cent after 4 months of soft lens extended wear compared with baseline values. These observations suggest that some form of short-term[9] and long-term[9,10] adaptation of the endothelium is taking place.

Despite their stunning clinical appearance, blebs are asymptomatic and thought to be of little clinical significance. They are, however, of great interest to physiologists endeavoring to understand the workings of the cornea.

Pathology

Electron microscopy

Histologic studies of the endothelial bleb response were conducted by Vannas *et al.*[11] using both corneas from eyes that were enucleated (because of melanomas) and corneas of beating-heart, brain-death cadavers. The 'blebbed' endothelium displayed edema of the nuclear area of cells, intracellular fluid vacuoles and fluid spaces between cells. Thus, endothelial blebs appear to be the result of a local edema phenomenon, whereby the posterior surface of the 'blebbed' endothelial cell is bulged toward the aqueous. The endothelial cell bulges in the posterior direction because this represents the path of least resistance; that is, the posterior stromal surface (Descemet's membrane) provides much greater resistance to endothelial cell swelling than does the aqueous humor.

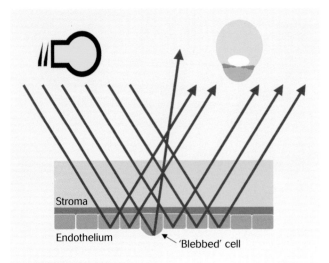

Figure 26.3
Optical theory to explain the appearance of endothelial blebs induced by contact lenses when viewed in specular reflection with the slit-lamp biomicroscope

Slit-lamp biomicroscopy

A simple optical model can be constructed to explain the appearance of blebs as seen with the slit-lamp biomicroscope (*Figure 26.3*). When the endothelium is viewed using specular reflection, light rays reflect from the tissue plane that corresponds to the interface between the posterior surface of the endothelium and the aqueous humor. This interface acts as a reflective surface because it represents a significant change in tissue refractive index. The light rays that are reflected from this interface give rise to an observed image of an essentially flat (or slightly undulating) and featureless endothelial cell mosaic.

Light rays that strike 'blebbed' endothelial cells are deflected away from the observation path, to leave a corresponding area of darkness. Thus, an endothelial bleb is simply an individual endothelial cell (or group of adjacent cells) that has become swollen and bulged in the direction of the aqueous humor, which gives rise to the compelling optical illusion that the cell (or cells) has disappeared.

Confocal microscopy

The confocal microscope has been used to observe the endothelial bleb response at very high magnification (×680).[12,13] Kaufman *et al.*[12] observed the corneas of three patients wearing hydrogel contact lenses of high water content for the first time. In one patient, endothelial changes that consisted of irregularly shaped (round or oval) dark regions were observed within the endothelial mosaic. These changes were most evi-

dent 20 minutes after lens insertion, and by 30 minutes the changes were fewer and less prominent. Kaufman *et al.*[12] suggested that their results confirmed the 'localized edema' theory of endothelial bleb formation.

Efron *et al.*[13] obtained images from each eye of 15 normal subjects (age range 19–36 years, mean 26 ± 6 years) before and after 20 minutes wear of a +5.50D 58 per cent water content hydrogel lens in one eye. The extent of the bleb response was graded using the grading scales shown in Appendix A of this book (also see 'Observation and grading'); the images were also assessed qualitatively. After 20 minutes of lens wear, the mean bleb response in the lens-wearing eye was grade 1.0 (range 0.0 to 3.2). Two subjects did not display blebs. No blebs were observed in the non-lens wearing eyes. Individual blebbed cells that comprised a bright central spot, surrounded by a darker annulus, were observed in the endothelium of most subjects.

In one subject, the endothelium was imaged at baseline and over a time sequence of 5, 10, 15 and 20 minutes of lens wear (*Figure 26.4*). The time sequence reveals the initial appearance of a dark border, which broadens into a thick, dark annulus after 15–20 minutes of lens wear (*Figure 26.5*).

An optical model is used to illustrate the appearance of endothelial blebs under confocal microscopy (*Figure 26.6*). This model employs normal light reflection because light rays pass to and from the endothelium through the confocal microscope objective lens via a pathway of light directly toward and away from the

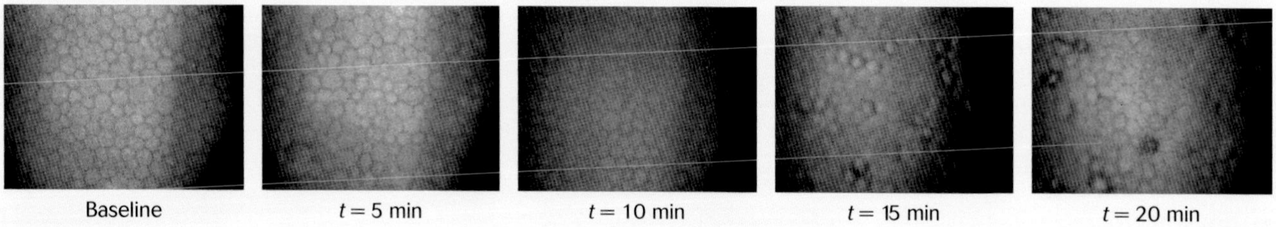

| Baseline | $t = 5$ min | $t = 10$ min | $t = 15$ min | $t = 20$ min |

Figure 26.4

Confocal microscope images of the development of endothelial blebs over a 20 minute period

cornea, perpendicular to its surface. This is different from specular microscopy on the slit-lamp biomicroscope, whereby angular light reflection is employed to observe the endothelium (*Figure 26.3*).

The model illustrates a single 'blebbed' cell flanked on either side by a normal 'non-blebbed' cell. It can be seen from the confocal model that light is normally reflected from the flat surface of the 'non-blebbed' cells and the apex of the blebbed endothelial cell, all of which appear bright. The sloping sides of the blebbed cell reflect light away from the objective and thus appear dark. This model therefore explains the confocal appearance of a blebbed cell as having a dark annulus that surrounds a bright central spot (*Figure 26.5*). These observations are consistent with the prevailing theory that blebs represent swelling of individual endothelial cells in the posterior (aqueous) direction.

Etiology

The etiology of endothelial blebs has been explained by Holden *et al.*[14] These authors attempted to induce blebs using a variety of stimulus conditions, and concluded that one physiologic factor common to all successful attempts to form blebs was a local acidic pH change at the endothelium.

Two separate factors induce an acidic shift in the cornea during contact lens wear:

- An increase in carbonic acid caused by the retardation of carbon dioxide efflux (hypercapnia)[15] by a contact lens;
- Increased levels of lactic acid as a result of lens-induced oxygen deprivation (hypoxia)[15] and the consequent increase in anaerobic metabolism (*Figure 26.7*).

When silicone elastomer contact lenses are worn, such metabolic changes do not

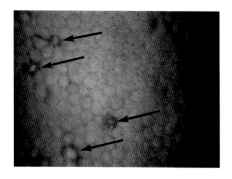

Figure 26.5

Enlargement of a confocal microscope image of blebs (arrows), each showing a bright center surrounded by a thick dark annulus. The surrounding unaffected endothelium reflects brightly

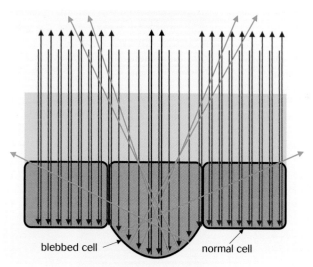

blebbed cell — normal cell

Figure 26.6

Optical theory to explain the appearance of endothelial blebs induced by contact lenses when viewed in normal reflection with the confocal microscope

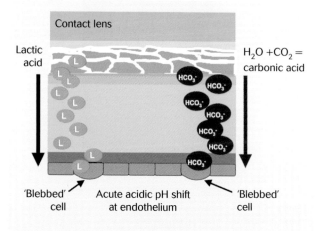

Contact lens

Lactic acid

$H_2O + CO_2 =$ carbonic acid

'Blebbed' cell   Acute acidic pH shift at endothelium   'Blebbed' cell

Figure 26.7

Etiology of endothelial blebs induced by contact lenses

take place because of the extremely high oxygen permeability of such lenses.

Endothelial blebs are not observed in the contralateral eye when induced by lens wear in the ipsilateral eye,[16] and they are observed in graft corneas,[17] which thus precludes the possibility of central neural control of this phenomenon. Also, endothelial blebs induced by contact lenses are unaffected by prostaglandin-inhibitor drugs, which precludes an inflammatory basis for the response.[18]

Bonanno and Polse[19] confirmed by direct measurement that hypoxia and hypercapnia induced by contact lenses result in an acidic shift in the cornea, and these authors noted that the extent of acidosis they measured is in the range in which endothelial function may be affected. Furthermore, the time course of the appearance of blebs after lens insertion and of the resolution after lens removal is consistent with the time course of corneal pH change as measured by Bonanno and Polse.[19]

The cornea becomes hypoxic and hypercapnic during sleep so it is expected that the consequent acidic changes induce blebs. Various authors[6,20] have, indeed, confirmed that there is a diurnal variation in the endothelial bleb response, whereby more blebs can be observed immediately upon awakening from sleep.

The question arises as to the precise mechanism by which acidosis causes endothelial cells to swell. All cells in the human body function optimally when surrounded by extracellular fluid maintained within an acceptable range of pH, temperature, tonicity, ion balance, etc. Carbonic acid and lactic acid may alter the physiologic status of the environment that surrounds the endothelial cells by shifting pH in the acidic direction. This may induce changes in membrane permeability and/or membrane pump activity, which results in a net movement of water into endothelial cells. The resultant cellular edema is observed as 'blebbing'.

Observation and Grading

The corneal endothelium can be viewed by specular reflection using a slit-lamp biomicroscope at ×40 magnification. To observe the endothelium using this technique, the angle between the illumination and observation systems must be symmetric about a plane that extends normally from the cornea, and is typically between 75° and 90°. The endothelial mosaic can be seen adjacent to a bright reflex from the corneal surface (*Figure 26.1*). Using this technique, only the mid-peripheral nasal or temporal endothelium are viewed; this does not pose a problem because changes in these regions are representative of changes elsewhere in the cornea.[9]

Although individual endothelial cells can only just be resolved at ×40 magnification, blebs have a stark appearance and are easily recognizable. A variety of sophisticated automated specular endothelial microscopes can be used to view the endothelium;[21] these instruments offer higher magnification and superior resolution compared with slit-lamp observation. As discussed previously, the confocal microscope provides an even higher level of magnification that allows detailed examination of individual cells. Endothelial specular microscopes[7,8] and confocal microscopes[12,13] are invaluable as research tools when it is necessary to quantify endothelial changes and understand the pathology of this phenomenon; however, a general appraisal of the endothelial bleb response can still be obtained satisfactorily with a good quality, high magnification slit lamp.[2]

The extent of endothelial bleb formation can be graded using the grading scale for this response provided in Appendix A; however, the usual connotation associated with contact lens grading scales concerning the urgency for clinical action

(see Chapter 29) does not apply here because endothelial blebs induced by contact lenses are thought to be innocuous, irrespective of the level of severity of blebbing. The 0 to 4 scale of the bleb response shown in Appendix A can be considered as being approximately linear. High magnification slit-lamp photographs of endothelial blebbing of grades 0 (normal), 2 (slight) and 4 (severe) are shown in *Figure 26.8*.

Management

While the phenomenon of endothelial blebs is of immense interest from a physiologic standpoint, there are no readily apparent clinical ramifications. The bleb response occurs to a greater or lesser degree in most patients, and displays a characteristic time course. It is not known whether a propensity for the endothelium of a patient to exhibit blebbing is a positive or negative attribute. Williams[6] surmises that the severity of an endothelial bleb response is reduced in patients who display increased levels of endothelial polymegethism, which could partially explain the apparent long-term adaptation of the bleb response. Specifically, a low-level bleb response has been interpreted as an indication that the endothelium has lost its capacity to respond to changes in its immediate environment; that is, the endothelium has become 'exhausted'.

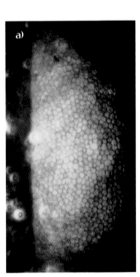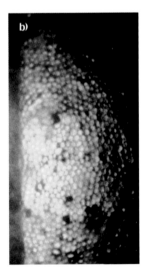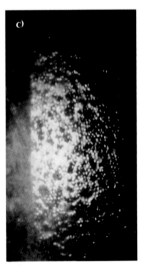

Figure 26.8
High magnification slit-lamp photographs of contact lens-induced endothelial blebs: (a) grade 0, (b) grade 2 and (c) grade 4

Theoretically, the bleb response can be used as a relative measure of the combined impact on the cornea of a given patient of hypoxia and hypercapnia induced by contact lenses. That is to say, in a given patient, a lens with lower average oxygen transmissibility induces a more severe bleb response.[6] This concept has been explored experimentally.[7,8] Ohya et al.[7] observed the time course, frequency and location of endothelial blebs in 11 eyes of nine patients who wore contact lenses. Eight types of contact lenses with various oxygen transmissibilities (Dk/t) were used. The authors demonstrated an inverse correlation between the number of blebs and the Dk/t of the contact lens. In addition, Hamano et al.[8] demonstrated a significantly higher degree of bleb formation with lenses of lower Dk/t values.

The above results imply that a comparison of the severity of the bleb response could have clinical utility in selecting lenses of optimal gas transmission characteristics. However, Bruce and Brennan[22] suggest that the bleb response is of little use for the longitudinal monitoring of patients wearing a given lens type, in view of the lack of variability in the magnitude of its response relative to its test–retest reliability.

Prognosis

The prognosis for recovery from endothelial blebs is excellent. After removal of a contact lens, blebs disappear within minutes.[2,7] They will continue to recur when lens wear is reintroduced and resolve when lenses are removed, but in any event, blebs are harmless.

Differential Diagnosis

Primary chronic corneal disorders such as Fuch's endothelial dystrophy are often characterized by the presence of guttata, which appear as small shallow depressions in the endothelial mosaic in the early stages of the disease process and as distinct black holes in advanced cases.[23] In the case of guttae caused by dystrophy, extensive confluent areas of blebbing may be apparent (*Figure 26.9*); such confluence is not observed in blebbing induced by contact lenses. The key distinction between guttae related to corneal dystrophy and blebs induced by

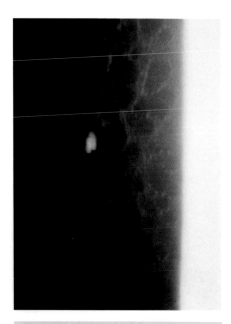

Figure 26.9
Corneal dystrophy depicting severe guttate changes

contact lenses is simply the permanence of guttae and the transience of blebs.

Brooks et al.[24] point out that, in addition to being an effect induced by contact lenses, blebs may also be seen in a wide variety of pathologic conditions, which include superficial keratopathies, deep keratopathies, anterior uveitis and contusion injury. These blebs vary in size in different conditions and are often transient.[25] They also have a different appearance from those induced by contact lenses in that the areas of darkness are more diffuse and there is no apparent separation of cells throughout the field.[25]

Interestingly, transient phenomena that closely resemble endothelial blebs are observed in patients with acute superficial eye disorders. Specifically, Zantos and Holden[26] noted such transient changes in cases of acute 'red eye' associated with extended contact lens wear; these formations have exactly the same appearance as blebs induced by contact lenses, but are different in that they persist for many days after cessation of lens wear.

REFERENCES

1 Fatt I and Bieber MT (1968). The steady-state distribution of oxygen and carbon dioxide in the *in vivo* cornea. I. The open eye in air and the closed eye. *Exp Eye Res.* **7**, 103–112.

2 Zantos SG and Holden BA (1977). Transient endothelial changes soon after wearing soft contact lenses. *Am J Optom Physiol Opt.* **54**, 856–858.

3 Vannas A, Makitie J, Sulonen J, et al. (1981). Contact lens induced transient changes in corneal endothelium. *Acta Ophthalmol (Copenh.)* **59**, 552–559.

4 Schoessler JP and Woloschak MJ (1981). Corneal endothelium in veteran PMMA contact lens wearers. *Int Contact Lens Clin.* **8**, 19–25.

5 Schoessler JP (1983). Corneal endothelial polymegethism associated with extended wear. *Int Contact Lens Clin.* **10**, 144–156.

6 Williams L (1986). *Transient Endothelial Changes in the* in vivo *Human Cornea*, PhD Thesis. (Sydney: University of New South Wales).

7 Ohya S, Nishimaki K, Nakayasu K and Kanai A (1996). Non-contact specular microscopic observation for early response of corneal endothelium after contact lens wear. *CLAO J.* **22**, 122–126.

8 Hamano H, Jacob JT, Senft CJ, et al. (2002). Differences in contact lens-induced responses in the corneas of Asian and non-Asian subjects. *CLAO J.* **28**, 101–104.

9 Williams L and Holden BA (1986). The bleb response of the endothelium decreases with extended wear of contact lenses. *Clin Exp Optom.* **69**, 90–92.

10 Bruce AS and Brennan NA (1993). Epithelial, stromal, and endothelial responses to hydrogel extended wear. *CLAO J.* **19**, 211–216.

11 Vannas A, Holden BA and Makitie J (1984). The ultrastructure of contact lens induced changes. *Acta Ophthalmol (Copenh.)* **62**, 320–333.

12 Kaufman SC, Hamano H, Beuerman RW, et al. (1996). Transient corneal stromal and endothelial changes following soft contact lens wear: A study with confocal microscopy. *CLAO J.* **22**, 127–132.

13 Efron N, Hollingsworth J, Koh HH, et al. (2001). Confocal microscopy. In: *The Cornea: Its Examination in Contact Lens Practice*. p. 86–135, Ed. Efron N. (Oxford: Butterworth–Heinemann).

14 Holden BA, Williams L and Zantos SG (1985). The etiology of transient endothelial changes in the human cornea. *Invest Ophthalmol Vis Sci.* **26**, 1354–1359.

15 Ang JH and Efron N (1990). Corneal hypoxia and hypercapnia during contact lens wear. *Optom Vis Sci.* **67**, 512–521.

16 Efron N, Kotow M, Martin DK and Holden BA (1984). Physiological response of the contralateral cornea to monocular hydrogel contact lens wear. *Am J Optom Physiol Opt.* **61**, 517–522.

17 Marechal-Courtois C, Lamalle D, Libert D and Delcourt JC (1987). Endothelial blebs in clear corneal grafts fitted with soft contact lenses. *CLAO J.* **13**, 231–234.

18 Efron N, Holden BA and Vannas A (1984). Prostaglandin-inhibitor naproxen does not affect contact lens-induced changes in the human corneal endothelium. *Am J Optom Physiol Opt.* **61**, 741–744.

19 Bonanno JA and Polse KA (1987). Corneal acidosis during contact lens wear: Effects of hypoxia and CO_2. *Invest Ophthalmol Vis Sci.* **28**, 1514–1520.

20 Khodadoust AA and Hirst LW (1984). Diurnal variation in corneal endothelial morphology. *Ophthalmology* **91**, 1125–1128.

21 Stevenson RW (1994). Non-contact specular microscopy of the corneal endothelium. *Optician* **208**(5460), 22–26.

22 Bruce AS and Brennan NA (1994). Comparison of clinical diagnostic tests in hydrogel extended wear. *Optom Vis Sci.* **71**, 98–103.

23 Kaufman HE, Barron BA and McDonald MB (1998). *The Cornea*, Second Edition. (Boston: Butterworth–Heinemann).

24 Brooks AM, Grant G and Gillies WE (1988). The use of specular microscopy to investigate unusual findings in the corneal endothelium and its adjacent structures. *Aust NZ J Ophthalmol.* **16**, 235–243.

25 Brooks AM, Grant G and Gillies WE (1989). The influence of superficial epithelial keratopathy on the corneal endothelium. *Ophthalmology* **96**, 704–708.

26 Zantos SG and Holden BA (1981). Guttate endothelial changes with anterior eye inflammation. *Br J Ophthalmol.* **65**, 101–103.

ENDOTHELIAL CELL LOSS

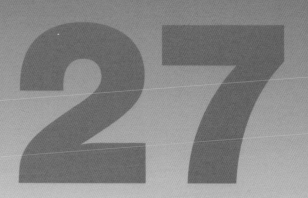

Concern that contact lenses may affect the corneal endothelium *adversely* has resulted in endothelial examination becoming a routine procedure during biomicroscopic examination of the cornea of contact lens wearers (*Figure 27.1*). This concern can be traced back to the original observation by Zantos and Holden[1] in 1979 of acute transient changes ('blebs') in the corneal endothelium associated with contact lens wear (see Chapter 26). This discovery gave the first clue to researchers and clinicians that the corneal endothelium was susceptible to short-term alterations in the physiologic environment at the ocular surface.

Attention has also been directed toward the chronic endothelial changes induced by contact lenses; these include an *apparent* endothelial cell loss and changes in cell size and/or shape. This chapter addresses the controversial question as to whether contact lens wear results in endothelial cell loss (*Figure 27.2*). The

issue of alterations to cell shape and size induced by contact lenses is dealt with in Chapter 28.

Opinions differ as to whether observable changes in the endothelium are of any real clinical significance; nevertheless, practitioners ought to be able to examine and assess the integrity of the endothelium, and should be prepared to interpret any changes observed in the context of the various theories concerning corneal endothelial structure and function.

Normal Endothelial Cell Density

The corneal endothelium is a monolayer of approximately half a million cells (at birth) that constitutes the posterior corneal surface. Anteriorly, the endothelium is in apposition with a basement membrane formed by secretions from

the endothelium itself. The basement membrane is known as the posterior limiting lamina (or Descemet's membrane). The anterior surface of the endothelial cell is known as the basal surface. The posterior (apical) surface of the endothelium is in direct contact with the aqueous humor.

On examination with the slit-lamp biomicroscope, the endothelium can be observed using specular reflection. In the normal endothelium of an infant, all cells are approximately the same size and have a characteristic hexagonal shape. These features can only just be resolved using a good quality slit-lamp biomicroscope at the highest magnification (×40; *Figure 27.1*).

The convention that has been adopted universally to denote the number of endothelial cells in the human cornea is to present the *endothelial cell density*, expressed as the number of cells per square millimeter. In the normal eye,

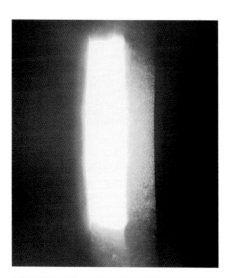

Figure 27.1
High magnification slit-lamp biomicroscope photograph of a normal corneal endothelium seen in specular reflection

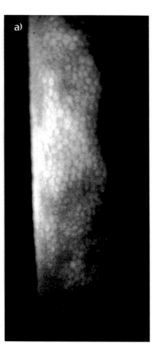
a)

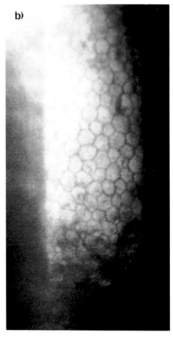
b)

Figure 27.2
Very high magnification slit-lamp biomicroscope photographs of (a) high and (b) low endothelial cell density

endothelial cell density decreases from approximately 4400 cells/mm^2 at birth to 2200 cells/mm^2 at 80 years of age[2,3] (*Figure 27.3*). Obviously, any change in cell density thought to be attributed to contact lens wear must be considered in the context of this normal age change.

Signs and Symptoms

Early studies by Hirst *et al.*,[4] Holden *et al.*[5] and MacRae *et al.*,[6] all using different experimental methodologies, observed various degrees of endothelial polymegethism (see Chapter 28) in long-term contact lens wearers, but failed to find evidence of a loss of endothelial cells. However, subsequent studies have challenged this notion.

Dada *et al.*[7] examined the effects of long-term daily wear of polymethyl methacrylate (PMMA) lenses on the corneal endothelium in eight patients who had been prescribed lenses in one eye only. A significant reduction in cell density was observed in the lens-wearing eyes.

MacRae *et al.*[8] examined 162 PMMA contact lens wearers and age-matched controls; 81 subjects had worn contact lenses for more than 20 years. These authors[8] found that, although the mean endothelial cell density in the PMMA lens-wearing group was not different from that of controls, a significantly greater percentage of lens wearers (11 per cent, 9 of 81 patients) had cell densities less than 2000 cells/mm^2 compared with controls (2.5 per cent, two of 81 patients). That is, these authors noted a subgroup of PMMA contact lens wearers who were more susceptible to reduced endothelial cell densities with long-term contact lens use.

Setala *et al.*[9] made similar observations to MacRae *et al.*[8] These authors[9] used a specular microscope to examine the endothelia of 101 subjects with 10 years or more experience of wearing soft and PMMA lenses, and 50 matched control subjects. The mean corneal endothelial cell density of the lens wearers (2846 cells/mm^2) was statistically significantly less than that of the control eyes (2940 cells/mm^2). The mean endothelial cell density of the eyes exposed to lens wear for more than 25 years (30 eyes) was 2575 cells/mm^2, and very low densities (<2000 cells/mm^2) were observed in 16 eyes of the lens wearing group (8 per cent). Cell densities less than 2500 cells/mm^2 were observed in a total of

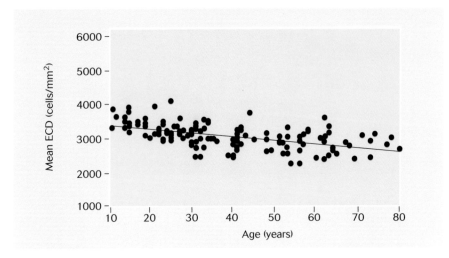

Figure 27.3
Relation between endothelial cell density (ECD) and age

41 eyes (20 per cent) in the lens-wearing group, whereas in the control group (100 eyes) all of the subjects, except one, had cell densities of more than 2500 cells/mm^2 in both eyes.

McMahon *et al.*[10] reported that a group of 16 long-term PMMA lens wearers had an endothelial cell density (2147 cells/mm^2) that was statistically significantly less than that of a matched control group of non-lens wearers (2865 cells/mm^2).

The effect on endothelial cell density of the duration of wearing periods of soft contact lenses was explored by Lee *et al.*[11]. These authors divided 90 soft contact lens wearers into three equal groups: short-term users (<5 years lens wear), intermediate-term users (6–10 years lens war) and long-term users (>10 years lens wear). The control group comprised 30 non-wearers of contact lenses. All eyes were examined with a specular microscope. The authors found that soft contact lens wear correlated significantly with decreasing corneal endothelial cell densities with time.

Sanchis-Gimeno *et al.*[12] studied differences in endothelial cell density in a pair of 31-year-old monozygotic female twins; one had been wearing contact lenses for the previous 15 years and the other had not worn contact lenses. Lower central corneal endothelial cell densities were found in both eyes of the monozygotic twin who wore contact lenses.

None of the reports highlighted above listed any adverse effects of reduced endothelial cell density in lens wearers.

Pathology

Perhaps an initial interpretation of a reduced endothelial cell density is that there are fewer cells on the posterior corneal surface, perhaps because cells suffer apoptosis or somehow become dislodged. It is known that intraocular surgery can cause endothelial cells to dislodge as a result of direct trauma to the endothelium,[13,14] but this effect could not be happening with soft lenses.

One possible explanation for the apparent endothelial cell loss induced by contact lenses is provided by Wiffen *et al.*,[15] who compared central and peripheral corneal endothelial cell densities in normal subjects and long-term contact lens wearers. Specifically, endothelial cell density was measured by contact specular microscopy in the corneal center and temporal periphery of both eyes of 43 long-term contact lens wearers and in 84 normal subjects who had not worn contact lenses. The latter group included 43 age- and sex-matched controls for the contact lens wearers. Central cell density (2723 ± 366 cells/mm^2) was significantly higher than peripheral cell density (2646 ± 394 cells/mm^2) for the normal group, but not for the contact lens wear group (2855 ± 428 cells/mm^2 central; 2844 ± 494 cells/mm^2 peripheral). Based on their results, Wiffen *et al.*[15] suggested that contact lens wear causes a mild redistribution of endothelial cells from the central to the peripheral cornea.

This observation of Wiffen *et al.*[15] of cell redistribution from the center to periphery of the cornea could explain the apparent loss of cells reported elsewhere. Invariably, those who have reported lens-induced endothelial cell loss would have examined the central corneal endothelium only, and would have been unaware of any *increase* in cell density in the corneal mid-periphery through endothelial cell redistribution. That is, while there is no actual endothelial cell loss, there is a reduction in endothelial cell density in the central region of the cornea, which is counterbalanced by a commensurate increase in cell density in the corneal mid-periphery. The overall endothelial cell population of the cornea is therefore unaffected by contact lens wear.

Figure 27.4 illustrates the endothelial cell redistribution theory of Wiffen *et al.*[15] Since gaps are not observed between the cells in endothelia with reduced cell densities, the cell redistribution must involve a spreading out and perhaps thinning of central cells, and a 'bunching up' of more peripheral cells.

Etiology

The reason why endothelial cells apparently redistribute from the center to the periphery of the cornea is unclear. It may represent some form of physiologic adaptation to lens wear. Wiffen *et al.*[15] suggest that central lens-induced hypoxia may be the driving force. If this phenomenon is linked to polymegethism induced by contact lenses, the corneal acidosis – which is thought to be responsible for that effect (see Chapter 28) – may also play a role in endothelial cell redistribution.

Observation and Grading

The corneal endothelium can be viewed by specular reflection using a variety of instruments, such as contact or non-contact specular microscopes, confocal microscopes or slit-lamp biomicroscopes. To observe the endothelium using the slit-lamp biomicroscope, a magnification of at least ×40 must be used and the angle between the illumination and observation systems should be symmetric about a plane that extends normally from the cornea, and is typically between 75° and 90°. The endothelial mosaic can be seen adjacent to a bright reflex from the corneal surface (see *Figure 27.1*). Using this technique, only

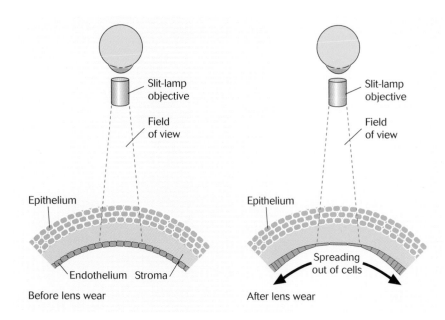

Figure 27.4

Cell redistribution theory to explain the reduction in endothelial cell density of the central cornea induced by contact lenses

the mid-peripheral nasal or temporal endothelium is viewed; this does not pose a problem if the same approximate area is observed each time for comparative purposes (e.g., to assess changes in a patient over time).

The observation of individual endothelial cells is at the very limit of resolution when using a slit-lamp biomicroscope at the typical maximum ×40 magnification. Even with the assistance of a graduated eyepiece graticule or a reference grading scale, endothelial cell density is difficult to estimate, and often impossible to determine in the presence of normal involuntary micronystagmoid and vibratory eye movement.

The endothelium can be examined effectively in the clinic with the aid of an automatic non-contact endothelial camera. Such instruments incorporate sophisticated digital video-image capture and computer image-analysis technology.[16] For example, the Topcon Specular Microscope SP2000 provides a photographic printout of the endothelium, a printout that includes a five-point scale for grading endothelial cell density within the range 1000–3000 cells/mm^2 (*Figure 27.5*). Endothelial cameras offer higher magnification and superior resolution than slit-lamp observation, and are essential if endothelial cell density is to be determined.

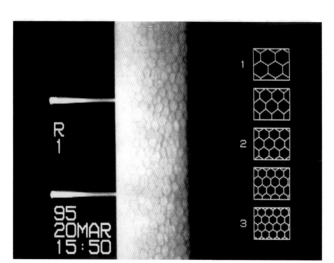

Figure 27.5

Printout from a Topcon Specular Microscope that shows the corneal endothelial mosaic and the accompanying cell density grading scale. In this case, it can be seen that endothelial cell density is about 2800 cells/mm^2

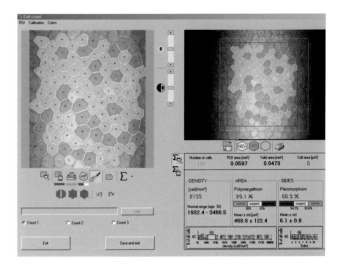

Figure 27.6
Automated analysis of endothelial morphology using the image analysis software of the Nidek Confoscan 3 Corneal Confocal Microscope

Modern confocal microscopes also come equipped with automated endothelial analysis software. A suitable image of the endothelium is captured and digitized. A region of interest is then defined by electronically interposing a square border onto the image displayed on a computer screen. The image is automatically enhanced to sharpen the cell borders and the cells are automatically traced. Any gaps can be closed manually. Various parameters can then be calculated and presented graphically (*Figure 27.6*).

Management

Studies of changes in endothelial cell density in response to ophthalmic surgery suggest that a lower limit of 400-700 cells/mm[2] is required to maintain corneal health and transparency;[17] below this value, the endothelium decompensates and the cornea becomes edematous. Such low endothelial cell densities are rarely, if ever, seen among contact lens wearers. For example, only 11 per cent and 8 per cent of long-term contact lens wearers examined by MacRae *et al.*[8] and Setala *et al.*,[9] respectively, had endothelial cell densities less than 2000 cells/mm[2].

On the assumption that a reduced endothelial cell density in the central cornea results form a mild cell redistribution rather than actual cell loss, this is a phenomenon that may not really need to be managed. However, a more conservative approach can be adopted whereby it is assumed that any change induced by an external influence, such as contact lens wear, is potentially adverse, and preventive or remedial measures should be adopted. By this reasoning, any measures to minimize the known physiologic effects of lens wear, such as fitting lenses of superior gas transmissibility or lenses that have a reduced physical impact on the eye, could be adopted.

Prognosis

Information about the recovery from lens-induced central endothelial cell redistribution has not been reported in the literature. However, Wiffen *et al.*[15] believe that such a redistribution may reverse itself when contact lens wear is discontinued. They base this belief on studies[18,19] that measured central and peripheral cell density in patients who discontinued contact lens wear in conjunction with excimer laser photorefractive keratectomy. Both studies[18,19] found significant increases in central cell density and significant decreases in peripheral cell density. Another investigation[20] showed an increase in central cell density after excimer laser *in situ* keratomileusis in contact lens wearers, but not in patients who had not worn contact lenses. These observations suggest that the prognosis for recovery of lens-induced central endothelial cell redistribution may be reasonably good.

Differential Diagnosis

Any suspected reduction of endothelial cell density must be differentiated from the effects of aging,[2,3] intraocular surgery,[13,14] eye disease[21] or systemic disease.[22] Certainly, these effects were accounted for in the various studies of endothelial cell density that support the notion of cell redistribution[8-11], generally by employing age-matched control groups and by avoiding subjects who suffered from any systemic or eye disease or who had previously undergone ocular surgery.

REFERENCES

1 Zantos SG and Holden BA (1977). Transient endothelial changes soon after wearing soft contact lenses. *Am J Optom Physiol Opt.* **54**, 856–858.
2 Yee RW, Matsuda M, Schultz RO and Edelhauser HF (1985). Changes in the normal corneal endothelial cellular pattern as a function of age. *Curr Eye Res.* **4**, 671–678.
3 Hollingsworth J, Perez-Gomez I, Mutalib HA and Efron N (2001). A population study of the normal cornea using an *in vivo*, slit-scanning confocal microscope. *Optom Vis Sci.* **78**, 706–711.
4 Hirst LW, Auer C, Cohn J, *et al.* (1984). Specular microscopy of hard contact lens wearers. *Ophthalmology* **91**, 1147–1153.
5 Holden BA, Sweeney DF, Vannas A, *et al.* (1985). Effects of long-term extended contact lens wear on the human cornea. *Invest Ophthalmol Vis Sci.* **26**, 1489–1501.
6 MacRae SM, Matsuda M, Shellans S and Rich LF (1986). The effects of hard and soft contact lenses on the corneal endothelium. *Am J Ophthalmol.* **102**, 50–57.
7 Dada VK, Jain AK and Mehta MR (1989). Specular microscopy of unilateral hard contact lens wearers. *Indian J Ophthalmol.* **37**, 17–19.
8 MacRae SM, Matsuda M and Phillips DS (1994). The long-term effects of polymethyl methacrylate contact lens wear on the corneal endothelium. *Ophthalmology* **101**, 365–370.
9 Setala K, Vasara K, Vesti E and Ruusuvaara P (1998). Effects of long-term contact lens wear on the corneal endothelium. *Acta Ophthalmol Scand.* **76**, 299–303.
10 McMahon TT, Polse KA, McNamara N and Viana MA (1996). Recovery from induced corneal edema and endothelial morphology after long-term PMMA contact lens wear. *Optom Vis Sci.* **73**, 184–188.
11 Lee JS, Park WS, Lee SH, *et al.* (2001). A comparative study of corneal endothelial changes induced by different durations of soft contact lens wear. *Graefes Arch Clin Exp Ophthalmol.* **239**, 1–4.
12 Sanchis-Gimeno JA, Lleo A, Alonso L, *et al.* (2003). Differences in corneal anatomy in a pair of monozygotic twins due to continuous contact lens wear. *Cornea* **22**, 243–245.
13 Friberg TR, Doran DL and Lazenby FL (1984). The effect of vitreous and retinal surgery on corneal endothelial cell density. *Ophthalmology* **91**, 1166–1169.

14 Brooks AM and Gillies WE (1991). Effect of angle closure glaucoma and surgical intervention on the corneal endothelium. *Cornea* **10**, 489–497.

15 Wiffen SJ, Hodge DO and Bourne WM (2000). The effect of contact lens wear on the central and peripheral corneal endothelium. *Cornea* **19**, 47–51.

16 Stevenson RW (1994). Non-contact specular microscopy of the corneal endothelium. *Optician* **208**(5460), 22–26.

17 Kaufman HE, Barron BA and McDonald MB (1998). *The Cornea*, Second Edition. (Boston: Butterworth–Heinemann).

18 Trocme SD, Mack KA, Gill KS, *et al.* (1996). Central and peripheral endothelial cell changes after excimer laser photorefractive keratectomy for myopia. *Arch Ophthalmol.* **114**, 925–928.

19 Stulting RD, Thompson KP, Waring GO, 3rd and Lynn M (1996). The effect of photorefractive keratectomy on the corneal endothelium. *Ophthalmology* **103**, 1357–1365.

20 Perez-Santonja JJ, Sahla HF and Alio JL (1997). Evaluation of endothelial cell changes 1 year after excimer laser *in situ* keratomileusis. *Arch Ophthalmol.* **115**, 841–846.

21 Liesegang TJ (1991). The response of the corneal endothelium to intraocular surgery. *Refract Corneal Surg.* **7**, 81–86.

22 Roszkowska AM, Tringali CG, Colosi P, *et al.* (1999). Corneal endothelium evaluation in type I and type II diabetes mellitus. *Ophthalmologica* **213**, 258–261.

ENDOTHELIAL POLYMEGETHISM

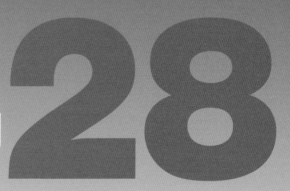

In the early 1980s, a series of articles[1-5] was published that alerted contact lens practitioners to a potentially adverse effect of contact lens wear that could be observed in the cornea – namely, endothelial polymegethism (*Figure 28.1*). These observations were made soon after the reports published by Zantos and Holden[6] of transient changes in the endothelium induced by contact lenses (endothelial blebs; see Chapter 26), so a picture was emerging at that time of previously unknown acute and chronic lens-induced endothelial changes. The critical role of the endothelium in maintaining corneal health was well known, so reports of endothelial compromise were of considerable concern to the profession.

A considerable number of clinical studies and much laboratory research has been undertaken over the past two decades in an attempt to gain an appreciation of the nature and magnitude of the endothelial response to contact lens wear and the possible ramifications of these changes. As is often the case with scientific enquiry, differences of opinion have emerged and some issues are still unresolved. This chapter examines the phenomenon of endothelial polymegethism induced by contact lenses from a clinical and scientific perspective and considers the debate as to whether these changes are of any real clinical significance.

Normal Endothelial Cell Morphology

The variation in apparent size of cells in the endothelium (or in any other tissue layer) is expressed as the *coefficient of variation of cell size* (COV); this dimensionless ratio is calculated by dividing the standard deviation of the cell areas in a defined field by the arithmetic mean area of all cells in that field. The COV is a measure of the degree of *endothelial polymegethism*. ('Polymegethism' is derived from the Greek word 'megethos' meaning 'size'; 'poly' means 'many'.)

Endothelial cells can also vary in shape. The term *endothelial polymorphism* means 'many shapes' and the term *pleomorphism* means 'different shapes'. Individual endothelial cells can have anything from three to nine sides, although the majority of cells in a normal endothelium have six sides.

In the normal eye, the COV increases throughout life. Thus, any changes thought to be attributed to contact lens wear should be referenced against these normal age changes. Consequently, the term *endothelial polymegethism*, when discussed in this chapter in the context of an induced change, should generally be taken to mean a degree of change in excess of that expected for a given age.

Signs and Symptoms

Reports of endothelial polymegethism induced by contact lenses were first published by Schoessler and Woloschak in the early 1980s.[1,2] These authors provided a convincing anecdotal demonstration of endothelial polymegethism in 10 patients who had worn polymethyl methacrylate (PMMA) lenses for at least 5 years. Subsequent research by Hirst *et al.*,[3] Holden *et al.*[4] and MacRae *et al.*[5] provided statistical validation of this phenomenon. *Figure 28.2* is a compelling illustration of the effect of contact lens

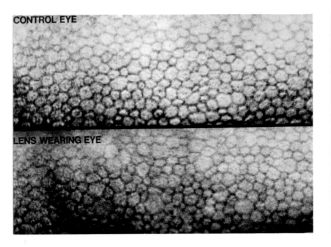

CONTROL EYE

LENS WEARING EYE

Figure 28.1
High magnification slit-lamp biomicroscope photograph of a corneal endothelium that displays extensive polymegethism induced by contact lenses

Figure 28.2
Polymegethous corneal endothelium of the eye of a patient who wore an extended wear lens in one eye only (bottom frame) for 5 years because of uniocular myopia. The endothelium of the fellow control eye (not lens-wearing) is shown in the top frame

wear on the corneal endothelium; illustrated is a pair of endothelial photomicrographs of a patient who wore an extended wear lens for 5 years in one eye only because of uniocular myopia. The bottom frame is the endothelium of the lens-wearing eye and the top frame is that of the fellow eye (not lens-wearing). A greater variation in endothelial cell size (polymegethism) is clearly evident in the lens-wearing eye.

Hirst *et al.*[3] also reported a substantially lower percentage of hexagonal cells in patients wearing PMMA contact lenses compared with matched control eyes not wearing lenses. Such polymorphic changes are generally associated with changes in polymegethism.

As discussed in Chapter 27, a number of authors[7–13] subsequently described an apparent reduction in central endothelial cell density as well as polymegethism in long-term contact lens wearers. Wiffen *et al.*[10] went on to explain that there is no actual loss of cells; rather, there is a redistribution of cells from the center to the mid-periphery of the cornea, which results in a decrease in endothelial cell density of the central cornea and an increase in cell density of the mid-peripheral cornea, with no presumed net change of the endothelial cell density of the entire cornea. As becomes evident later in this chapter, the cell redistribution theory is an important consideration in the construction of models of the etiopathology of age-related versus lens-induced polymegethism.

Prevalence

Endothelial polymegethism is a natural age change that occurs in all humans[14,15] (*Figure 28.3*). Contact lenses essentially have the effect of accelerating such changes. Although such accelerated changes are not observed when lenses of extremely high oxygen transmissibility are worn (such as silicone elastomer,[16] silicone hydrogel[17] and hyperpermeable rigid[18] lenses), virtually all other lens types that induce some measure of chronic hypoxic stress induce a degree of endothelial polymegethism and polymorphism.[7–13,19]

General appearance

The endothelium of a new-born baby has a very regular and uniform appearance, in which all cells are almost exactly the same size and display classic hexagonality. In, say, a 25 year old – that is, at an age when contact lens wear might begin –

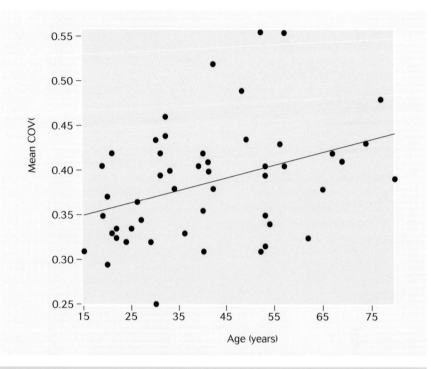

Figure 28.3

Relation between percentage increase in coefficient of variation (COV) of endothelial cell size (polymegethism) and age

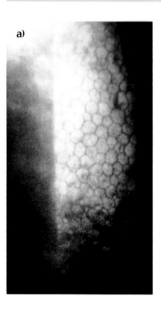
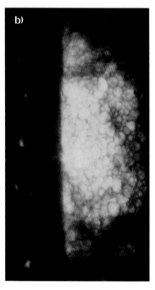

Figure 28.4

Very high magnification slit-lamp biomicroscope photographs of (a) low grade and (b) high grade corneal endothelial polymegethism induced by contact lenses

the endothelium typically displays a low degree of polymegethism. The ratio of the diameter of the smallest cell to the largest cell that can be seen could be 1:5. In advanced cases of polymegethism, the ratio of smallest to largest cell can be as great as 1:20 (*Figure 28.4*). It is possible to make a qualitative assessment of the extent of polymegethism based on observation of the endothelial mosaic; techniques for assessing endothelial polymegeth-

ism are described under 'Observation and Grading'.

Corneal exhaustion syndrome

Sweeney[20] has drawn an anecdotal association between endothelial polymegethism and a condition that she termed 'corneal exhaustion syndrome'. This is a condition in which patients who have worn contact lenses for many years suddenly develop a severe intolerance to lens wear characterized by ocular discomfort, reduced vision, photophobia and an excessive edema response. These patients also displayed a distorted endothelial mosaic and moderate-to-severe polymegethism.

Although the link between endothelial polymegethism and corneal exhaustion syndrome is not proved, it is plausible that chronic lens-induced hypoxia results in a number of pathologic tissue changes (endothelial polymegethism being one of these) that can result in intolerance to lens wear.

Aside from the possibility of corneal exhaustion syndrome, no other symptoms are associated with endothelial polymegethism.

Pathology

To understand precisely what happens to endothelial cells when polymegethism develops, it is important to understand how the classic appearance of the endothelium as viewed by specular reflection relates to the overall three-dimensional structure of endothelial cells. When the endothelium is viewed using specular reflection, light rays reflect from the tissue plane that corresponds to the interface between the apical surface of the endothelium and the aqueous humor. This interface acts as the main reflective surface because it represents a significant change in tissue refractive index; that is, the difference in refractive index between the apical surface of the endothelial cell and the aqueous humor is greater than that between the basal surface of the endothelial cell and posterior-limiting lamina of the stroma. The light rays that are reflected from the apical endothelium–aqueous interface give rise to an observed image of the endothelial mosaic. Light rays that strike the junction between endothelial cells are deflected away from the observation path, which leaves corresponding dark lines that are observed as cell borders.

Assuming no change in central endothelial cell density, the specular appearance of polymegethism suggests that some cells are becoming smaller and some are becoming larger. However, according to the theory of Wiffen et al.,[10] endothelial cell redistribution away from the center of the cornea leads to a reduced central endothelial cell density. On the basis that this does occur, then the appearance of polymegethism suggests that some cells remain the same size and some become larger. Irrespective of the assumption made concerning changes in central endothelial cell density, a disparity in cell size is apparent. However, this disparity is evident only at the apical endothelium–aqueous interface, and does not necessarily relate to volumetric changes in the cytoplasmic mass of endothelial cells anterior to this interface.

A true appreciation of the morphologic changes that constitute polymegethism can be gained by considering the theoretical analysis of Bergmanson,[21] who conducted an ultrastructural study of the corneas of six long-term contact lens wearers. He observed that the lateral cell walls, which are normally extremely interdigitated, but essentially oriented normal to the endothelial surface, had straightened out and oriented obliquely. The interpretation of this observation in terms of the three-dimensional structure of the endothelium is that endothelial cells have changed shape, but the volume of each cell has remained constant. Thus, by observing only the apical surface of the endothelium on specular reflection, one is presented with the compelling illusion that a disparity in cell size has developed. In reality, the cells have merely become reoriented in three-dimensional space (*Figure 28.5*).

A further observation of Bergmanson[21] of equal significance is that, although the endothelium of contact lens wearers showed some inter- and intra-cellular edema, the cells were otherwise of a healthy appearance and contained normal, undamaged organelles. This raises the interesting and controversial possibility that, rather than representing an adverse effect, endothelial polymegethism is a non-problematic adaptation to chronic metabolic stress.

The suggestion that endothelial polymegethism is a benign tissue change has been challenged by researchers who have demonstrated a link between endothelial polymegethism and corneal hydration control.[11,22] In these studies the effect of contact lens wear on corneal hydration control was measured by inducing corneal edema and then recording the exponential rate of corneal deswelling. Recovery from edema is significantly slower in the corneas of contact lens wearers (versus matched controls), a deficit that is dose-related (i.e., the effect is more pronounced the longer lenses have been worn). *Figure 28.6* is a re-representation of the data of McMahon et al.,[11] which demonstrate

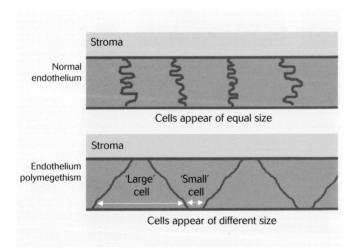

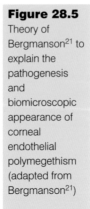

Figure 28.5 Theory of Bergmanson[21] to explain the pathogenesis and biomicroscopic appearance of corneal endothelial polymegethism (adapted from Bergmanson[21])

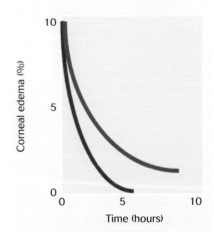

Figure 28.6
Corneal deswelling after induced edema in PMMA lens wearers (blue) vs. non-wearers (red; adapted from McMahon et al.[11])

that corneal deswelling after induced edema in PMMA lens wearers is considerable slower than that in non-wearers. Such observations must be considered in the context of a loss of corneal hydration control being a normal age-related change in the human population; typically, the cornea of a 65-year-old person takes 10 per cent longer to recover from stromal swelling compared with that of a 20-year-old person.[23]

An unfortunate conundrum in science is that correlation does not prove causation. Thus, it cannot be concluded with absolute certainty that the loss of corneal hydration control in contact lens wearers results from lens-induced endothelial polymegethism. However, it is not unreasonable to postulate such a causal relationship in view of the critical role of the endothelium in corneal hydration control.

The corneal hydration control process – known as the 'pump-leak' mechanism[24] – comprises, as the name suggests, two critical components, both of which are located in the endothelium. The *leak* refers to the constant tendency for water to move from the aqueous humor into the stroma through gaps between endothelial cells, and the *pump* refers to an active mechanism whereby endothelial cells pump bicarbonate ions into the aqueous, to create an osmotic force that draws water out of the stroma (*Figure 28.7*).[25] These counteracting forces are metabolically controlled so as to maintain a constant level of stromal hydration, while at the same time affording a mechanism of nutrient and waste exchange between the cornea and aqueous humor.

The suggestion that endothelial damage induced by contact lenses results in either an increased leak or a reduction in pump efficiency, or both, is confounded by the failure of Bergmanson[21] to detect such damage upon ultrastructural examination of the organelles of endothelial cells of long-term contact lens wearers.

Etiology

It is likely that the etiology of endothelial polymegethism is precisely the same as the etiology of endothelial blebs, whereby the former represents a chronic response and the latter represents an acute response to the same stimuli.

The etiology of endothelial blebs – or acute localized endothelial edema – is reviewed in Chapter 26. The key evidence comes from Holden *et al.*,[26] who attempted to induce blebs using a variety of stimulus conditions, and concluded that one physiologic factor common to all successful attempts to form blebs was a local acidic pH change at the endothelium. It is likely that polymegethism in contact lens wearers also results from lens-induced endothelial acidosis, for the simple reason that the extent of polymegethism is apparently governed by the same dose–hypoxic response as blebs, albeit on a different time scale.

Two separate factors induce an acidic shift in the cornea during contact lens wear:
- An increase in carbonic acid caused by retardation of the carbon dioxide efflux (hypercapnia)[27] by a contact lens;
- Increased levels of lactic acid as a result of lens-induced oxygen deprivation (hypoxia)[27] and the consequent increase in anaerobic metabolism (*Figure 28.8*).

When silicone elastomer contact lenses are worn, such metabolic changes do not take place because of the extremely high oxygen permeability of these lenses. No evidence of endothelial polymegethism could be found by Schoessler *et al.*[16] in the corneas of patients who wore silicone elastomer lenses.

Bonanno and Polse[28] confirmed by direct measurement that hypoxia and hypercapnia induced by contact lenses result in an acidic shift in the cornea, and these authors noted that the extent of acidosis measured is in the range in which endothelial function may be affected.

The cornea becomes hypoxic and hypercapnic during sleep, so it is expected that the consequent acidic changes should induce endothelial polymegethism, which is known to be age related.[14,15] Schoessler and Orsborn[29] published a case report of extreme endothelial polymegethism in the right eye (compared with the left eye) of a 23-year-old woman after 4 years of unilateral ptosis in the right eye.

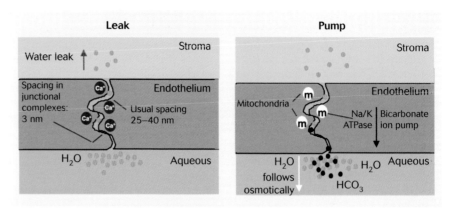

Figure 28.7

The pump–leak process of corneal hydration control encompasses a 'leaky' endothelium (left) and an endothelial bicarbonate pump (right)

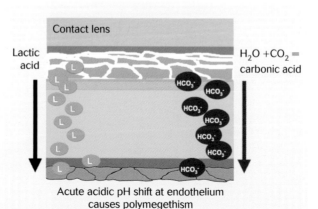

Acute acidic pH shift at endothelium causes polymegethism

Figure 28.8

Etiology of corneal endothelial polymegethism induced by contact lenses

Consideration needs to be given to the mechanism by which acidosis causes changes to the three-dimensional shape of endothelial cells, which in turn gives rise to the appearance of polymegethism when viewed by specular reflection. All cells in the human body function optimally when surrounded by extracellular fluid maintained within an acceptable range of pH, temperature, tonicity, ion balance, etc. The increased carbonic acid and lactic acid may cause an acidic pH shift in the extracellular fluid that surrounds endothelial cells. This may induce changes in membrane permeability and/or membrane pump activity that result in water movement that acts to elongate endothelial cell walls.[21] A reconfiguration of cell shape then occurs to preserve cell volume, which results in the appearance of polymegethism at the apical surface of the endothelium.

Observation and Grading

Techniques that can be used to examine the corneal endothelium include slit-lamp biomicroscopy, specular microscopy and confocal microscopy. The clinical application of these techniques is reviewed in Chapter 27. Basically, the slit-lamp biomicroscope does not have sufficient magnification or resolution to enable an assessment of the degree of endothelial polymegethism. Such an assessment can be achieved only by capturing an image of the endothelium using one of the instruments described above and either subjecting the image to computer-assisted image analysis (whereby the COV and other cell population characteristics can be calculated), or comparing the image with a grading scale for polymegethism, such as that presented in Appendix A.

Figure 28.1 is an enlarged view of the slit-lamp biomicroscopic appearance of the endothelium of a young woman who had been wearing a soft lens of low oxygen transmissibility (38 per cent water content hydroxyethyl methacrylate, HEMA) for 10 years. Considerable variation in the size of individual endothelial cells (polymegethism) is clearly evident.

Doughty[30] outlined the following limitations with respect to quantification of the degree of polymegethism in terms of the COV:

- The coefficient is valid only for the individual from whom it was obtained, and so cannot be used for intersubject comparison;

- COV can be ambiguous in that it does not indicate whether there is an overall increase or decrease in mean cell area (the COV can be the same in either case);
- The error associated with calculation of COV, typically by measuring up to 200 cells, is too great (analysis of 3000 cells is required for good accuracy, which is generally precluded because of time and cost constraints).

Despite this critical analysis, evaluation of the degree of endothelial polymegethism against grading scales is a valuable technique upon which clinically relevant differences can be detected and management decisions can be based.

Management

Figure 28.9 is a construction of the approximate relationship between COV and oxygen transmissibility, which indicates that lenses of lower oxygen performance induce higher levels of polymegethism. Although this relationship provides a clear indication as to how to minimize or prevent polymegethism induced by contact lenses, it is unclear if there is a need to take any measures to reverse or prevent this process because of the uncertainty as to whether endothelial polymegethism is an unwanted pathologic change or a harmless physiologic adaptation.

Whether or not one would wish to reverse or prevent endothelial polymegethism from the perspective of the health of the endothelium itself is an interesting, but secondary, consideration. What is certain is that endothelial polymegethism provides an indication that the cornea has been subjected to

prolonged metabolic stress. The source of this stress is probably chronic tissue acidosis, which in turn can be caused by chronic hypoxia and hypercapnia induced by contact lenses. Clinicians have long recognized the importance of minimizing lens-induced hypoxia and hypercapnia because these changes are known to induce a wide variety of adverse affects to all layers of the cornea and conjunctiva.[4]

Thus, from a clinical perspective, it is essential to take note of the presence of significant endothelial polymegethism and to take action to minimize the metabolic stress to the cornea known to be associated with this change. Strategies to alleviate hypoxia and hypercapnia induced by contact lenses include:

- Fitting soft or rigid lenses made from materials of higher oxygen permeability;
- Reducing lens thickness;
- Sleeping in extended wear lenses less frequently;
- Changing from extended lens wear to daily lens wear;
- Reducing lens wearing time;
- Fitting rigid lenses with more movement and edge lift (to enhance oxygen-enriching tear exchange).

The real battle against endothelial polymegethism induced by contact lenses and, indeed, all chronic lens-induced changes is being fought in the polymer laboratories and lens design studios of the major contact lens manufacturers. Although practitioners will always have a choice to make concerning the best lens for a given patient, such decisions can only be made within an envelope of available lens designs and materials. As time goes on, this envelope will shift to

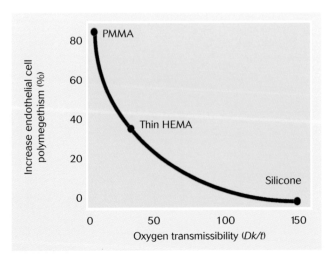

Figure 28.9

Relation between percentage increase in coefficient of variation (COV) of endothelial cell size (polymegethism) versus lens oxygen transmissibility (*Dk/t*). Units of *Dk/t* are [×10⁻⁹ (cm × mlO₂)/(sec × ml × mmHg)].

encompass more and more sophisticated and highly permeable polymers, such as silicone hydrogels. Such trends are already becoming apparent; for example, the prescribing rate of very low *Dk* HEMA in the UK dropped from 40 per cent in 1996[31] to 2 per cent in 2001,[32] and has remained at this low level since then.[33] The natural outcome of such trends will be an overall lowering of the degree of polymegethism and related chronic tissue changes in the worldwide population of lens wearers.

Prognosis

The prognosis for recovery from endothelial polymegethism is poor. After removal and cessation of wear of high water content contact lenses that had been worn on an extended wear basis for an average of 5 years, Holden *et al.*[34] were unable to detect a recovery from endothelial polymegethism during an observation period of 6 months (*Figure 28.10*).

MacRae *et al.*[5] examined the extent of endothelial polymegethism in a group of former users of PMMA contact lenses, who had worn them for an average of 9.6 years, but who had discontinued them for an average of 4.3 years. When compared with age-matched controls, these patients demonstrated significant increases in polymegethism and differences in pleomorphism. They concluded that endothelial polymegethism induced by PMMA lenses is not completely reversible.

McLaughlin and Schoessler[35] were unable to demonstrate a significant improvement in endothelial morphology 4 months after re-fitting patients who had been wearing PMMA lenses with rigid lenses of high oxygen transmissibility. Thus, all the available evidence suggests that endothelial polymegethism induced by contact lenses is essentially a permanent change; if there is any recovery back to age-related normality, this is likely to take many years.

The prognosis for overall corneal health based upon action taken as a result of observed endothelial polymegethism may be excellent, even though the endothelium may remain polymegethous for a considerable period of time, perhaps until death. The reason is that many other changes induced by chronic hypoxia and hypercapnia, such as reduced epithelial thickness, reduced oxygen consumption, epithelial microcysts and stromal edema,[4] dissipate in a matter of weeks or months after cessation of lens wear.[4,34] These changes can be minimized subsequently by adopting strategies to optimize corneal oxygen availability during lens wear, such as those outlined above.

Notwithstanding the good prognosis for corneal health described above, it has been suggested that the existence of endothelial polymegethism in itself may represent a continuing liability in view of the finding of Rao *et al.*[36] that corneal edema induced by cataract surgery takes much longer to recover in patients who display pre-operative corneal endothelial polymegethism. Although this observation has been challenged subsequently,[37] the possibility that endothelial polymegethism may compromise corneal health if surgical intervention of the eye is required later in life should not be discounted.

Differential Diagnosis

A variety of degenerative (acquired) and dystrophic (hereditary) changes in the endothelium have been described, but a detailed account of these is beyond the scope of this book. These conditions are characterized by opacities, lesions or bleb-like formations (as in the case of Fuch's endothelial dystrophy), which generally cannot be confused with endothelial polymegethism.

What is more important in the context of differential diagnosis is the capacity to distinguish between the etiologies of any observed endothelial changes. As well as being a natural age change,[14,15] endothelial polymegethism can occur as a result of, or in association with, both ocular insult (such as injury,[38] chronic solar radiation,[39] ptosis,[29] endothelial guttatae,[40] intraocular surgery[41] and keratoconus[42]) and systemic disease (diabetes mellitus[43] and cystic fibrosis[43]). Practitioners should therefore be alert to the fact that endothelial polymegethism observed in the eyes of contact lens wearers may be caused by factors or conditions other than contact lens wear.

REFERENCES

1 Schoessler JP and Woloschak MJ (1981). Corneal endothelium in veteran PMMA contact lens wearers. *Int Contact Lens Clin.* **8**, 19–25.
2 Schoessler JP (1983). Corneal endothelial polymegethism associated with extended wear. *Int Contact Lens Clin.* **10**, 144–156.
3 Hirst LW, Auer C, Cohn J, *et al* (1984). Specular microscopy of hard contact lens wearers. *Ophthalmology* **91**, 1147–1153.
4 Holden BA, Sweeney DF, Vannas A, *et al.* (1985). Effects of long-term extended contact lens wear on the human cornea. *Invest Ophthalmol Vis Sci.* **26**, 1489–1501.
5 MacRae SM, Matsuda M, Shellans S and Rich LF (1986). The effects of hard and soft contact lenses on the corneal endothelium. *Am J Ophthalmol.* **102**, 50–57.
6 Zantos SG and Holden BA (1977). Transient endothelial changes soon after wearing soft contact lenses. *Am J Optom Physiol Opt.* **54**, 856–858.
7 Dada VK, Jain AK and Mehta MR (1989). Specular microscopy of unilateral hard contact lens wearers. *Indian J Ophthalmol.* **37**, 17–19.
8 MacRae SM, Matsuda M and Phillips DS (1994). The long-term effects of polymethyl methacrylate contact lens wear on the corneal endothelium. *Ophthalmology* **101**, 365–370.
9 Setala K, Vasara K, Vesti E and Ruusuvaara P (1998). Effects of long-term contact lens wear on the corneal endothelium. *Acta Ophthalmol Scand.* **76**, 299–303.

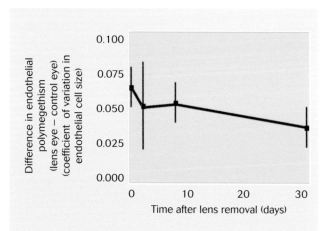

Figure 28.10

Degree of polymegethism plotted for 30 days after cessation of lens wear (relative to control eyes not wearing lenses). The apparent trend toward recovery is not statistically significant (adapted from Holden *et al.*[4])

10 Wiffen SJ, Hodge DO and Bourne WM (2000). The effect of contact lens wear on the central and peripheral corneal endothelium. *Cornea* **19**, 47–51.

11 McMahon TT, Polse KA, McNamara N and Viana MA (1996). Recovery from induced corneal edema and endothelial morphology after long-term PMMA contact lens wear. *Optom Vis Sci.* **73**, 184–188.

12 Lee JS, Park WS, Lee SH, *et al.* (2001). A comparative study of corneal endothelial changes induced by different durations of soft contact lens wear. *Graefes Arch Clin Exp Ophthalmol.* **239**, 1–4.

13 Sanchis-Gimeno JA, Lleo A, Alonso L, *et al.* (2003). Differences in corneal anatomy in a pair of monozygotic twins due to continuous contact lens wear. *Cornea* **22**, 243–245.

14 Yee RW, Matsuda M, Schultz RO and Edelhauser HF (1985). Changes in the normal corneal endothelial cellular pattern as a function of age. *Curr Eye Res.* **4**, 671–678.

15 Hollingsworth J, Perez-Gomez I, Mutalib HA and Efron N (2001). A population study of the normal cornea using an *in vivo*, slit-scanning confocal microscope. *Optom Vis Sci.* **78**, 706–711.

16 Schoessler JP, Barr JT and Fresen DR (1984). Corneal endothelial observations of silicone elastomer contact lens wearers. *Int Contact Lens Clin.* **11**, 337–341.

17 Covey M, Sweeney DF, Terry R, *et al.* (2001). Hypoxic effects on the anterior eye of high-*Dk* soft contact lens wearers are negligible. *Optom Vis Sci.* **78**, 95–99.

18 Barr JT, Pall B, Szczotka LB, *et al.* (2003). Corneal endothelial morphology results in the Menicon Z 30-day continuous-wear contact lens clinical trial. *Eye Contact Lens* **29**, 14–16.

19 Esgin H and Erda N (2002). Corneal endothelial polymegethism and pleomorphism induced by daily-wear rigid gas-permeable contact lenses. *CLAO J.* **28**, 40–43.

20 Sweeney DF (1992). Corneal exhaustion syndrome with long-term wear of contact lenses. *Optom Vis Sci.* **69**, 601–608.

21 Bergmanson JP (1992). Histopathological analysis of corneal endothelial polymegethism. *Cornea* **11**, 133–142.

22 Nieuwendaal CP, Odenthal MT, Kok JH, *et al.* (1994). Morphology and function of the corneal endothelium after long-term contact lens wear. *Invest Ophthalmol Vis Sci.* **35**, 3071–3077.

23 O'Neal MR and Polse KA (1986). Decreased endothelial pump function with aging. *Invest Ophthalmol Vis Sci.* **27**, 457–463.

24 Maurice DM (1972). The location of the fluid pump in the cornea. *J Physiol.* **221**, 43–54.

25 Hodson S and Miller F (1976). The bicarbonate ion pump in the endothelium which regulates the hydration of rabbit cornea. *J Physiol.* **263**, 563–577.

26 Holden BA, Williams L and Zantos SG (1985). The etiology of transient endothelial changes in the human cornea. *Invest Ophthalmol Vis Sci.* **26**, 1354–1359.

27 Ang JH and Efron N (1990). Corneal hypoxia and hypercapnia during contact lens wear. *Optom Vis Sci.* **67**, 512–521.

28 Bonanno JA and Polse KA (1987). Corneal acidosis during contact lens wear: Effects of hypoxia and CO_2. *Invest Ophthalmol Vis Sci.* **28**, 1514–1520.

29 Schoessler JP and Orsborn GN (1987). A theory of corneal endothelial polymegethism and aging. *Curr Eye Res.* **6**, 301–306.

30 Doughty MJ (1990). The ambiguous coefficient of variation: Polymegethism of the corneal endothelium and central corneal thickness. *Int Contact Lens Clin.* **17**, 240–248.

31 Morgan PB, Ramsdale C and Efron N (1997). Trends in UK contact lens prescribing 1996. *Optician* **213**(5583), 35.

32 Morgan PB and Efron N (2001). Trends in UK contact lens prescribing 2001. *Optician* **221**(5803), 38–39.

33 Morgan PB and Efron N (2003). Trends in UK contact lens prescribing 2003. *Optician* **225**(5904), 34–35.

34 Holden BA, Vannas A, Nilsson K *et al.* (1985). Epithelial and endothelial effects from the extended wear of contact lenses. *Curr Eye Res.* **4**, 739–742.

35 McLaughlin R and Schoessler J (1990). Corneal endothelial response to refitting polymethyl methacrylate wearers with rigid gas-permeable lenses. *Optom Vis Sci.* **67**, 346–351.

36 Rao GN, Aquavella JV, Goldberg SH and Berk SL (1984). Pseudophakic bullous keratopathy. Relationship to preoperative corneal endothelial status. *Ophthalmology* **91**, 1135–1140.

37 Bates AK and Cheng H (1988). Bullous keratopathy: A study of endothelial cell morphology in patients undergoing cataract surgery. *Br J Ophthalmol.* **72**, 409–412.

38 Ling TL, Vannas A and Holden BA (1988). Long-term changes in corneal endothelial morphology following wounding in the cat. *Invest Ophthalmol Vis Sci.* **29**, 1407–1412.

39 Good GW and Schoessler JP (1988). Chronic solar radiation exposure and endothelial polymegethism. *Curr Eye Res.* **7**, 157–162.

40 Burns RR, Bourne WM and Brubaker RF (1981). Endothelial function in patients with cornea guttata. *Invest Ophthalmol Vis Sci.* **20**, 77–85.

41 Matsuda M, Suda T and Manabe R (1984). Serial alterations in endothelial cell shape and pattern after intraocular surgery. *Am J Ophthalmol.* **98**, 313–319.

42 Matsuda M, Suda T and Manabe R (1984). Quantitative analysis of endothelial mosaic pattern changes in anterior keratoconus. *Am J Ophthalmol.* **98**, 43–49.

43 Lass JH, Spurney RV, Dutt RM, *et al.* (1985). A morphologic and fluorophotometric analysis of the corneal endothelium in type I diabetes mellitus and cystic fibrosis. *Am J Ophthalmol.* **100**, 783–788.

PART IX GRADING SYSTEMS

GRADING SCALES

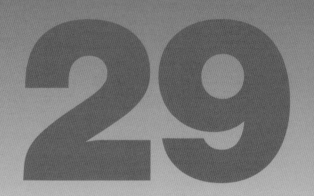

In all health care disciplines, it is important to record as accurately as possible the clinical signs observed in patients. Classically, this has involved a discursive account of the condition being entered onto a record card. The severity of the condition would be recorded using wording that offers a general connotation of the level of severity, such as 'mild' or 'severe'. A potential problem with this approach is that these terms are somewhat general and have been used in the absence of any form of standardization; that is, what appears to be 'mild' to one clinician may seem to be 'severe' to another.

As an aid to accurate record keeping, health care practitioners of all disciplines have become accustomed to using standardized grading scales of various functions and qualities. A grading scale may be defined as: "A tool that enables quantification of the severity of a condition with reference to a set of standardized descriptions or illustrations". In essence, grading scales offer clinicians a 'common language' to describe clinical phenomena.

In the contact lens literature, descriptive grading scales[1–3] have take the form of an agreed series of numbers or letters, each of which corresponds to a written account of the severity of a condition. The clinician makes a judgment of the severity of a condition that is being observed with reference to the descriptive grading scale and records the appropriate number or letter.

Illustrative grading scales represent a more advanced form to denote the severity of a clinical condition (*Figure 29.1*). A series of photographs, paintings or drawings that depict a given condition in various stages of severity offers the clinician a visual reference against which the severity of a condition can be assessed and future changes in severity may be judged. A number of *ad hoc* photographic grading scales have been

published in the contact lens literature that relate to specific conditions, such as corneal staining,[4] conjunctival redness[5] and papillary conjunctivitis.[6,7]

A number of authors have developed systematic sets of grading scales for a representative range of the most frequently viewed and clinically relevant conditions encountered in contact lens practice. This chapter reviews the various grading scales that have been produced, and explains in detail the clinical application of the Efron Grading Scales, which are presented in Appendix A.

Illustrative Grading Scales

Five sets of illustrative grading scales have been developed for use in contact lens practice. For any given complication, a typical grading scale comprises a series of five images, from grade 0 (normal) to grade 5 (severe). These are discussed below in chronologic order of publication.

Koch grading scales

These grading scales were published in 1984 as an appendix entitled 'Atlas of Illustrations' in an A5-sized soft-cover textbook published by Koch *et al*.[8] The

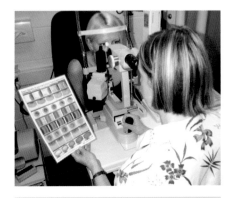

Figure 29.1
Grading scales (A4 card version) in use

grading scales were prepared by a medical artist named Perrin Sparks Smith, and are in the form of line sketches. Most of the sketches are white on black or black on white, with some use of red, green or gray block color. Many of the illustrations are supplemented by a written description.

Annunziato grading scales

In about 1992, Annunziato *et al*.[9] published an atlas that comprised 130 A4-sized loose-leaf pages secured in a three-ringed binder. This work was sponsored by Alcon Ltd and was conducted under the auspices of the Southwest Independent Institutional Review Board (an ophthalmic clinical trials research group) in Fort Worth, Texas, USA. The grading scales were in the form of full-color paintings and the ophthalmic artist was Monte Lay. Most of the paintings are accompanied by a brief description of the condition and salient features are highlighted with the aid of a black-and-white line diagram.

Vistakon grading scales

An A5-sized spiral-bound handbook of contact lens management was published by Vistakon (a Johnson and Johnson company) in 1996, under the authorship of Andersen *et al*.[10] All of the illustrations are slit-lamp photographs. Although this book was primarily intended as a guide to the management of contact lens complications, most of the conditions are presented in the form of a series of numbered photographs in varying degrees of severity, and as such essentially constitutes a series of grading scales. The photographs are accompanied by explanatory text.

CCLRU grading scales

The Cornea and Contact Lens Research Unit (CCLRU) grading scales were first formally published in 1997,[11] although they were released prior to this and distributed initially as an A2-sized poster, and subsequently in the form of an A4-sized plasticized card. There is no specific author attribution, as the production of these scales was apparently the result of a 'team effort' of staff at the Cornea and Contact Lens Research Unit (CCLRU) in the School of Optometry at the University of New South Wales in Sydney, Australia. All of the conditions are depicted in the form of slit-lamp photographs without accompanying text. Guidance is also given to grade certain conditions, for which a series of graded photographs is not provided. The development of the scales was sponsored by an educational grant from Johnson and Johnson Vision Products, Inc.

Efron grading scales

The first edition of these grading scales was published in the first edition of this book in 1999,[12] although they were released prior to this and distributed simultaneously in the form of an A1-sized poster and an A4-sized plasticized card in a protective slit case that contained instructions for use. These grading scales were all painted by the ophthalmic artist Terry Tarrant, and the development of the scales was sponsored by Hydron UK, Ltd (now CooperVision Ltd). The first edition of the grading scales depicted eight complications of contact lens wear, whereas the second edition in Appendix A of this book depicts 16 complications.

The second edition was officially released as the 'Millennium Edition' in 2000, and has been available in card and poster form since January 1 2000. A handy plastic-coated A4-sized version of these grading scales, which comes in a handsome protective slip case with comprehensive instructions for use, is available free from CooperVision. Simply send a request, with your full postal address, to gradingscales@coopervision.co.uk.

Comparison of Grading Scale Designs

Contact lens practitioners may come across clinical notes that have recorded the severity of a given complication with reference to any of the five sets of grading scales described above (a coherent set of grading scales is sometimes referred to as a 'grading system'). For this reason, practitioners need to be aware of the characteristics of these scales and the way in which they compare.

Grades depicted

The Koch and CCLRU scales only depict grades 1–4 (not grade 0). Grade 0 is depicted for some of the complications in the Vistakon system. The Annunziato and Efron systems display grades 0–5 for all complications. Depictions of grade 0 are often useful as a baseline reference when grading complications of low severity.

Severity descriptors

The descriptions attached to the five grades of severity differ slightly between grading systems (cited in *Table 29.1*). Severity descriptors are not assigned to the grades in the Koch system. In the other four systems, grades 0–2 have slightly different meanings, whereas grades 3 and 4 are described as 'moderate' and 'severe', respectively. Thus, allowing for subtle differences in nomenclature, all five systems have the same five-point grading system and have adopted remarkably similar descriptors for these grades.

Sub-classifications

In the Koch and Efron systems, a single grading scale that comprises five images is used to depict different levels of severity of each complication. However, in the Annunziato, CCLRU and Vistakon systems, a single complication can be 'sub-classified' and depicted in the form of a number of grading scales so that different manifestations of that complication can be graded. For example, in the CCLRU system, three grading scales are employed to facilitate an independent assessment of the severity of corneal staining in terms of type, depth and extent.

Conditions depicted

Putting aside sub-classifications, the number of primary conditions depicted varies markedly between grading systems, from six sets of primary grading scales in the CCLRU system to 16 in the Efron system. The primary condi-

tions depicted in each of the five grading systems are presented in *Table 29.2*. A number of interesting observations can be made from *Table 29.2*:

- A total of 21 complications are depicted in all of the grading systems combined;
- A grand total of 53 grading scales have been developed in all of the grading systems combined;
- Only three conditions are depicted in all five grading systems (conjunctival redness, corneal staining and papillary conjunctivitis);
- Eight conditions are found only in one or other of the grading systems;
- Three conditions are found only in the Efron system (corneal ulcer, endothelial blebs and superior limbic keratoconjunctivitis).

Photographic versus painted grading scales
Problems with photographic scales
The advantage of photographic grading scales is that photographs of actual conditions are depicted. However, certain difficulties are encountered when compiling photographic grading scales. An immense slide library is required – but even if such a resource is available, a number of compromises are necessary. For example, a given condition such as neovascularization can present in many different forms, and it is generally not possible to identify a series of photographs that display precisely the same manifestation of that condition at various levels of severity.

The clinical utility of series of photographs of a given condition at varying levels of severity may be confounded by the fact that the photographs are invariably of different patients who have different ocular characteristics, such as iris color, conjunctival vasculature, pupil size and lid anatomy. Furthermore, photographs are taken from various angles, at different magnifications, with various

Table 29.1
Severity descriptors used in various grading scales

Grade	Grading system				
	Koch	Annunziato	CCLRU	Vistakon	Efron
0	Not stated	None	Absent	None	Normal
1	Not stated	Trace	Very slight	Slight	Trace
2	Not stated	Mild	Slight	Mild	Mild
3	Not stated	Moderate	Moderate	Moderate	Moderate
4	Not stated	Severe	Severe	Severe	Severe

Table 29.2
Complications depicted in various grading scales

Complication	Grading system					
	Koch	Annunziato	CCLRU	Vistakon	Efron	Total
Blepharitis				✓	✓	2
Conjunctival redness	✓	✓	✓	✓	✓	5
Conjunctival staining			✓	✓	✓	3
Corneal distortion	✓	✓			✓	3
Corneal infiltrates		✓		✓	✓	3
Corneal neovascularization	✓	✓*		✓	✓	4
Corneal edema	✓	✓†		✓	✓	4
Corneal staining	✓	✓†	✓‡	✓*	✓	5
Corneal ulcer					✓	1
Endothelial blebs					✓	1
Endothelial polymegethism			✓		✓	2
Epithelial microcysts	✓	✓			✓	3
Epithelial edema	✓					1
Iritis		✓				1
Limbal redness		✓	✓	✓	✓	4
Limbal staining				✓		1
Meibomian gland dysfunction				✓	✓	2
Papillary conjunctivitis	✓	✓	✓‡	✓	✓	5
Pinguecula				✓		1
Pterygium				✓		1
Superior limbic keratoconjunctivitis					✓	1
Total (21)	8	10	6	13	16	53

*Two sub-classification grading scales are presented.
†Four sub-classification grading scales are presented.
‡Three sub-classification grading scales are presented.

illumination conditions, using different levels of staining, etc. Inconsistencies in color rendering of sequential images can occur as a result of the use of different types of photographic film and variations in photographic processing techniques, or of the use of different electronic settings with digital photography. The precise level of severity of a condition may not be available from the slide library, which leads to further compromise.

Some complications, such as epithelial microcysts or stromal striae and folds, are extremely difficult to photograph; indeed, few photographs of such conditions exist. This artificially constrains the range of complications from which a series of graded photographic images can be compiled.

Advantages of painted scales
The advantages of using artist-rendered (painted) versus photographic grading scales are as follows:
- The desired level of severity of a given condition can be depicted;
- Any chosen manifestation of a given condition can be illustrated;
- The severity of the manifestation of a given condition can be systematically advanced through the image set;
- All images of a given complication can be painted using precisely the same color scheme, and can be standardized with respect to angle of view, magnification and associated ocular features (such as iris color);
- Confounding artifacts unrelated to the complication being depicted (such as associated or secondary complications) can be avoided;
- Ancillary clues can be introduced to reinforce the notion of increasing severity (such as increasing light scatter of the slit-lamp illumination reflex or increasing limbal redness);
- Artistic license can be adopted to embellish certain features or obscure others for clarity.

Many of the design features described above can be seen, for example, in the grading scale sequence for corneal neovascularization in Appendix A. The key pathologic change is obvious – vessels of a given type (superficial plexus) progressively encroach onto the cornea from the

6 o'clock location. Associated subtle pathologic signs are deliberately painted in to reinforce the notion of a worsening condition: the limbus becomes progressively more engorged, the corneal slit-lamp reflex becomes progressively more diffuse and the central cornea becomes progressively more hazy. All other factors are kept constant: the full cornea is depicted from the same angle ('front on') in each case, iris size is constant and the iris detail and color is identical in each of the five frames. All of these features combine to form a powerful, self-evident and unambiguous sequence of progressive corneal neovascularization.

Efron Grading Scales: Design and Application

Since the Efron Grading Scales are featured in Appendix A of this book, detailed consideration is given to the design principles that underpinned their development, and the appropriate techniques for their clinical application are described.

Design features
The primary design criteria upon which the Efron Grading Scales are based are simplicity, convenience and ease of use by clinicians. A total of 16 sets of grading images are depicted in two panels, each of which comprises eight complications. Each complication has a banner heading. These 16 grading scales cover the key anterior ocular complications of contact lens wear. Those shown on the panel beginning with 'conjunctival redness' are frequently encountered; those in the other panels are less common and thus are less likely to be graded routinely. On each panel, complications are depicted in the approximate order (from top to bottom) that they would be encountered in the course of a typical slit-lamp examination of the eye.

As noted above, each complication is illustrated in a row of five images that depict progressively increasing severity, from grade 0 on the left to grade 4 on the right. 'Traffic light' coloring from green (normal) to red (severe) is used to border the images to facilitate ready association of any image with its intended level of severity, without the need to cross-reference the image against the grade numbers and descriptors at the top of each panel. The gradation of severity of the complications and the maximum level of severity depicted are based on an appraisal of evidence in the literature and accumulated clinical experience.

Image size

Each complication has been painted to an equivalent level of magnification that addresses the compromise between, first, being large enough to depict the key features of the tissue changes and, second, being low enough to relate to what practitioners can observe with the available clinical techniques. The approximate magnification of each complication (relative to a whole cornea depicted as ×1) is given in *Table 29.3*. *Figure 29.2* shows the 16 complications at grade 4 severity (each of which is identified by a letter code in *Table 29.3*), and indicates the approximate magnification of the images with a series of size boxes.

Table 29.3
Magnification of complications (relative to a whole cornea being ×1) depicted in the Efron Grading Scales

Complication	Magnification	Image depicted in Figure 29.2
Corneal staining	×1	A
Corneal ulcer	×1	B
Corneal infiltrates	×1	C
Corneal neovascularization	×1	D
Papillary conjunctivitis	×1	E
Meibomian gland dysfunction	×1	F
Blepharitis	×1	G
Superior limbic keratoconjunctivitis	×2	H
Limbal redness	×2	I
Conjunctival staining	×2	J
Conjunctival redness	×2	K
Corneal distortion	×2	L
Corneal edema	×40	M
Epithelial microcysts	×100	N
Endothelial blebs	×200	O
Endothelial polymegethism	×600	P

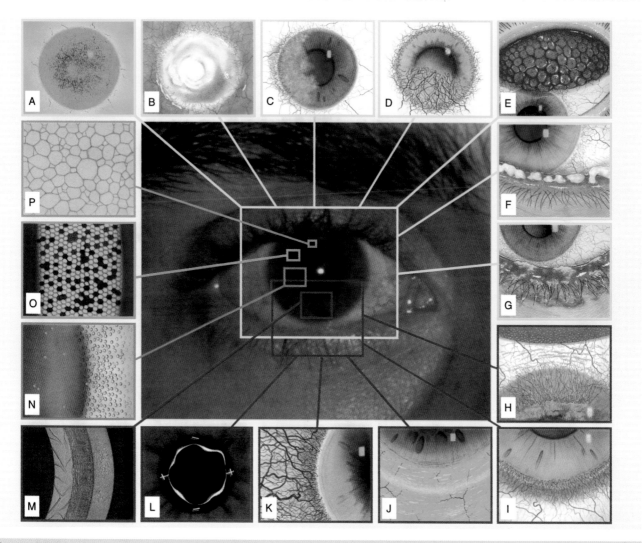

Figure 29.2
The 16 complications represented in the Efron Grading Scales (presented in full in Appendix A), depicted here at grade 4 severity. The approximate magnification of each complication (relative to the whole cornea being ×1 magnification) is indicated by colored boxes interposed over the image of the eye. The 16 complications are labelled with a letter code and are identified in *Table 29.3*.

As a consequence of the magnification levels at which these complications are depicted, some exceptions that relate to grading technique are:

- Epithelial microcysts and endothelial blebs cannot be viewed at the resolution depicted, although they can be detected and graded at ×40 magnification on a slit-lamp biomicroscope;
- Endothelial polymegethism can only be assessed with the aid of an endothelial or confocal microscope.

All other complications can be viewed at the resolution depicted and are capable of being graded by direct observation and/or using a slit-lamp biomicroscope at magnifications up to ×40.

How to grade

Observe the tissue change of interest directly or with the aid of a slit-lamp biomicroscope, under low and/or high magnification as required, and estimate the level of severity with reference to the appropriate grading scale to the nearest 0.1 scale unit. For example, a tissue change that is judged to be considerably more severe than grade 2, but not quite as severe as grade 3, may be assigned a grade of 2.8 or 2.9. Although this procedure can sometimes be difficult, grading to the nearest 0.1 scale unit (rather than simply assigning a whole-digit grade of 0, 1, 2, 3 or 4) affords much greater grading performance and increases the sensitivity of the grading scale to detect real changes or differences in severity.[13]

How to record grading

As various grading scales are available, it is important to designate clearly the grading system used and the specific tissue change being graded. A more expedient approach might be to print or stamp the 16 tissue changes onto a record card, each with an accompanying box in which to enter the assigned grade. It may be necessary to make additional annotations on an accompanying set of printed sketches of the eye to describe the condition more fully – for example, to indicate the location of the pathology (*Figure 29.3*).

Interpretation of grading

The five-stage 0 to 4 grading scale is based on a universally accepted concept whereby a higher numeric grade denotes a greater clinical severity. In general, a level of severity of more than grade 2 is considered to be clinically meaningful. This schema can be applied to any tissue change, even those not depicted on any given grading scale. Severity descriptors, color code and clinical interpretation of the grades illustrated in the Efron Grading Scales are shown in *Table 29.4*; it must be recognized that the clinical interpretations are only very general guidelines, and are not intended to replace sound professional judgment. There are two exceptions with respect to the interpretations described in *Table 29.4*. Corneal ulceration may require urgent action when detected or even suspected at any level of severity. Endothelial blebs require no clinical action, even at grade 4.

Grading Performance

Despite the apparent consistency in the construct of the five grading systems for contact lens complications, the various grading scales were developed independently and take on different appearances; therefore, grading estimates of the severity of a specific condition derived using the different systems cannot necessarily be expected to be identical. For example, inspection of grading scales that relate to papillary conjunctivitis (*Figure 29.4*) in the five systems reveals clear differences between the ranges of severity depicted for like conditions.

Statistical descriptors

The classic approach to assessing grading performance is to have a clinician grade the severity of a large number of images of contact lens complications of differing severity presented in a random sequence ('test'), and then to have the same clinician repeat this exercise some time later with the same images presented in a different ran-

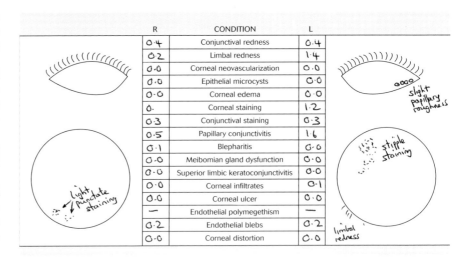

Figure 29.3

Suggested design of record card for use in conjunction with the Efron Grading Scales

Table 29.4
Severity descriptor, color code and clinical interpretation of the grades illustrated in the Efron Grading Scales

Grade	Severity descriptor	Color code	Clinical interpretation
0	Normal	Green	Clinical action not required
1	Trace	Lime	Clinical action rarely required
2	Mild	Yellow	Clinical action possibly required
3	Moderate	Orange	Clinical action usually required
4	Severe	Red	Clinical action certainly required

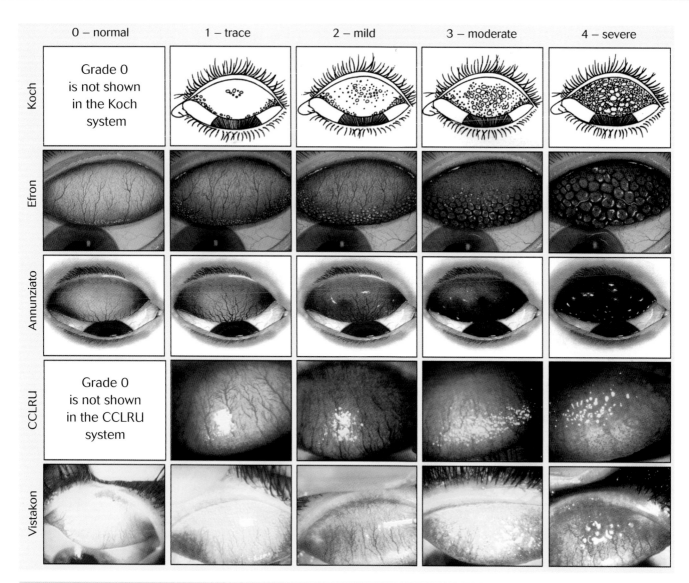

	0 – normal	1 – trace	2 – mild	3 – moderate	4 – severe
Koch	Grade 0 is not shown in the Koch system				
Efron					
Annunziato					
CCLRU	Grade 0 is not shown in the CCLRU system				
Vistakon					

Figure 29.4

Grading scales for papillary conjunctivitis

domized sequence ('retest'). The clinician must grade to the nearest 0.1 grading scale unit, and the assumption is made that the clinician does not remember the grades assigned at the first attempt when making the second attempt; that is, the grading attempts are independent. Having done this, the data can be used to derive various useful indices of grading performance, as follows.

Concordance

Concordance is the frequency of perfect agreement between grades assigned. For example, if 100 images were independently graded on two occasions, and there was perfect agreement on 12 occasions, there would be 12% concordance. The issue addressed here is: how often do your repeated grading estimates agree?

Sensitivity

'Sensitivity' is more a characteristic of the grading scale rather than the observer. A grading scale can be said to have 'fine' or 'coarse' sensitivity. A grading scale that accords fine sensitivity results in a superior grading performance; that is, better reliability, consistency and confidence (see below). The converse is true of a grading scale that accords coarse sensitivity. The issue addressed here is: what is the capability of the grading scale to facilitate the detection of a change or difference in severity of an observed condition?

Precision

Precision is the difference between grading estimates among colleagues. The issue addressed here is: do you grade high or low compared with colleagues?

Accuracy

Accuracy is the difference between grading estimates and a 'gold standard'. The issue addressed here is: do you grade high or low compared with the gold standard ('the truth')?

Reliability

Reliability is mathematically defined as a ±1 standard deviation of test–retest distribution. The issue addressed here is: how tightly clustered are your repeated grading estimates?

Consistency

Consistency is mathematically defined as (1.96 × reliability), and is also termed the 'coefficient of repeatability' or '95% confidence limits'. The issue addressed here is: what is the range within which your grading estimates cannot be considered to differ or change? Or, putting it another way: what is your 'level of sloppiness' when grading?

Confidence

Confidence is the extent to which grading is executed in fine increments. The issue addressed here is: to what extent do you have the confidence to grade to the nearest 0.1 grading scale unit?

Bias

Bias is defined mathematically as the mean of the test–retest discrepancies. The issue addressed here is: has there been a shift in your grading criteria between the first and second testing sessions?

Research studies

The grading performance of a group of clinicians using two artist-rendered (Annunziato and Efron) and two photographic (Vistakon and CCLRU) grading systems was assessed in terms of precision and reliability by Efron *et al.*[14] Specifically, 13 clinicians each graded 30 images – by interpolation or extrapolation to the nearest 0.1 increment – of each of the three contact lens complications common to all four grading systems; namely, corneal staining, conjunctival redness and papillary conjunctivitis. This entire procedure was repeated approximately 2 weeks later, to yield a total database that comprised 9360 individual grading estimates.

Analysis of variance revealed statistically significant differences in both precision and reliability between systems, observers and conditions. The artist-rendered systems generally afforded lower grading estimates than the photographic systems. The reason for this becomes readily apparent upon inspection of *Figure 29.4*. It is clear that the higher grades of papillary conjunctivitis depicted in the painted grading scales (Annunziato and Efron) represent greater levels of severity than those depicted in the photographic grading scales (CCLRU and Vistakon). For example, the grade 4 image in the CCLRU scale is, perhaps, equivalent to about grade 2.5 on the Efron scale. It is unlikely that the narrow severity range of the photographic sys-

tems is a deliberate design strategy, but instead arises from a lack of suitable photographs of severe conditions. In view of these significant between-system differences in grading performance, it is advisable to use the same grading system consistently.

Complications can be graded more reliably using the artist-rendered systems than with the photographic systems. This finding may be related to the greater control over the progression of severity that an artist can depict, compared with the situation for photographic grading scales, in which the selection of images designed to represent a systematic progression of severity is constrained by the availability of suitable images.

Conjunctival redness and papillary conjunctivitis could be graded more reliably than corneal staining. This may be because of the greater variability in the manifestations of corneal staining patterns that can be observed, versus the more characteristic and predictable clinical presentations of conjunctival redness and papillary conjunctivitis. Grading reliability generally was unaffected by the *severity* of the condition being assessed.

Efron *et al.*[14] concluded that, notwithstanding the above differences, all four grading systems are validated for clinical use. It was determined that practitioners can initially expect to use these systems with an average reliability of ±0.6 grading scale units. The estimates of grading reliability reported by Efron *et al.*[14] were somewhat inferior than those reported elsewhere (*Table 29.5*) and may be related to the level of experience and/or training of the subjects used in their experiments (see below).

Perhaps one way to interpret the data in *Table 29.5* is that, when using grading scales for the first time, a confidence range of about 1.2 is to be expected; however, with experience, this confidence range may reduce to 0.7 grading scale units. Rounding this value upward for a conservative estimate, it can be considered that, in general, a change or difference in grading scale unit of more than about 1.0 is clinically meaningful. This conclusion was also reached by Efron[21] in an experiment conducted on over 400 observers who all performed the same grading exercise. Practitioners can determine their own grading precision using The Efron Grading Tutor (see Chapter 30).

Efron *et al.*[14] reported that they were disappointed, but not surprised, to

observe that the experimental subjects tended to grade to the nearest whole-digit or half-digit grading scores, as evidenced from inspection of the frequency distribution of all grading estimates made during the experiment (*Figure 29.5*). This occurred despite constant encouragement to the subjects to grade to the nearest 0.1 grading scale increment. This observation highlights the natural reluctance of clinicians to grade using fine increments.[13]

Influence of knowledge, training and experience

A number of factors are likely to influence the accuracy and reliability of grading estimates when using clinical grading tools, including the design and presentation of the grading tool, the complexity and/or severity of the condition being graded and the time constraints within which grading must be executed (or other extraneous pressures on performance). A number of attributes of the person who executes the grading are also likely to influence grading performance; these attributes can be defined broadly as a 'clinical skills set', the components of which fall into the three categories of knowledge, training and experience.

Knowledge

The attribute knowledge refers to the relevant knowledge of the person who executes the grading.[22,23] Specifically, it relates to the broad knowledge base that underpins the particular clinical task under consideration, which in this case is the use of clinical grading scales for contact lens complications. The 'knowledge base' that underpins this clinical task is acquired by a broad education in ophthalmic science and clinical practice, and a specific education in the field of contact lenses and related ophthalmic pathology, such as would be gained after having trained as an optometrist or ophthalmologist.

Training

Training refers to the extent of instruction and/or learning with the specific grading tool. This attribute is concerned with dedicated instruction and training in the theoretical development and clinical application of grading scales for contact lens complications. Such training could occur in the form of lectures, tutorials or clinical workshops, or via the use of purpose-designed training packages such as The Efron Grading Tutor (see Chapter 30).

Table 29.5
Grading reliability and subject experience and/or training reported in various studies

Author	Number of subjects	Level of experience/ training of subjects	Grading tool	Condition		
				Corneal staining	Conjunctival redness	Papillary conjunctivitis
Chong et al.[15]	5	"Highly experienced in using clinical grading systems"	Photographic* Verbal† Morphs‡	±0.25 ±0.20 ±0.25	±0.19 ±0.21 ±0.16	±0.20 ±0.21 ±0.19
Dundas et al.[16]	2	"Trainee optometrists"	CCLRU*	±0.18		
Papas[17]	7	"Highly trained and accustomed to using the grading scale for over 1 year"	CCLRU*		±0.40	
Twelker and Bailey[18]	2	"Experienced"	Efron§		±0.30	
Efron et al.[14]	13	"Minimal experience in using grading scales"	Efron§ Annunziato§ CCLRU* Vistakon*	±0.67 ±0.61 ±0.76 ±0.76	±0.55 ±0.58 ±0.53 ±0.59	±0.54 ±0.60 ±0.64 ±0.63
MacKinven et al.[19]	2	"Trainee optometrists"	CCLRU*			±0.12
Efron et al.[20]	9	"Experienced users of grading scales"	Efron§ Morphs¶	±0.34 ±0.48	±0.38 ±0.49	±0.56 ±0.36

*Printed grading scales based on photographs.
†Verbal descriptor grading scales.
‡Computer-generated grading morphs based on photographs.

§Printed grading scales based on artist-rendered paintings.
¶Computer-generated grading morphs based on artist-rendered paintings.

Experience

Experience is the accumulated amount of time spent using the grading tool. This attribute relates to the repeated use of a grading scale, whereby grading performance might be expected to improve over time as a result of accumulated experience and ongoing learning by 'trial and error'.

Research studies

It might be supposed that a professional with the above-defined clinical skills set would demonstrate a superior grading performance compared with that of a person who does not possesses this clinical skills set. However, it could be argued that clinical grading using a pictorial grading scale is a simple visual matching task and that such a clinical skills set is not necessarily required for good accuracy and reliability.

Efron et al.[24] conducted a study to investigate the combined influence of knowledge, training and experience (i.e., the possession of a clinical skills set) on various aspects of grading performance (i.e., accuracy, reliability, bias and confidence) when assessing the severity of contact lens complications.

Nine optometrists (who were in possession of a relevant clinical skills set) and nine 'non-optometrists' (management and engineering university students who were, by definition, without the relevant clinical skills set) were each

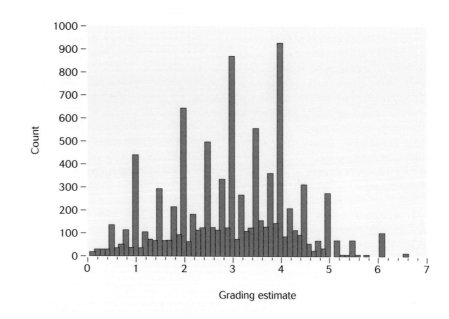

Figure 29.5
Frequency distribution of all grading estimates of the severity of a range of contact lens complications (n = 9360)

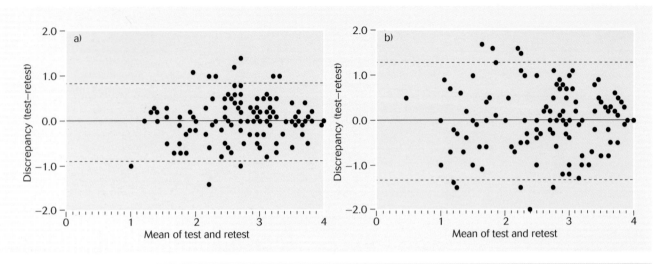

Figure 29.6

Plot of test–retest grading discrepancies versus mean of the test–retest grading estimates of the severity of a range of contact lens complications, for (a) optometrists and (b) 'non-optometrists'. The solid line in each graph represents the mean of the test–retest discrepancies and the dotted lines represent the 95% confidence limits of the test–retest discrepancies ($n = 144$ for each graph)

invited to grade – to the nearest 0.1 increment – an image of each of 16 contact lens complications using Efron Grading Scales. This procedure was repeated 2 weeks later, to yield a total database that comprised 576 individual grading estimates. The mean of the test and retest grading estimates was the same for the optometrists (2.8 ± 0.7) and the non-optometrists (2.6 ± 0.9); that is, non-optometrists can grade accurately. The median grading reliability of the optometrists (±0.41) was statistically significantly lower (i.e., superior) than that of the non-optometrists (±0.67; *Figure 29.6*). Non-optometrists tended to display a reluctance to grade by interpolation and to grade subtle clinical signs less reliably.

Efron et al.[24] concluded that, when averaged over several attempts, non-optometrists arrive at similar estimates of severity as do optometrists when grading ocular complications of contact lens wear; however, they do so less reliably. Thus, possession of the clinical skills set is not required to grade accurately, but at least certain elements of the clinical skills set are required for reliable grading.

Effect of training and experience on grading performance

The experiment described above did not address the question of the *relative*

contributions of the three attributes of the clinical skills set to grading reliability. To examine this, Efron et al.[25] conducted a further experiment whereby the influence of training and experience on grading reliability was assessed in a group of subjects with a common knowledge base.

A group (23) of optometry students who were unfamiliar with the use of grading scales each used The Efron Grading Tutor computer program (described in Chapter 30) to ascertain grading reliability at an 'initial' experimental session and a 'final' session 3 weeks later. Of these subjects, 12 were given a tutorial on grading techniques and were asked to complete two grading exercises between the initial and final sessions; this was designated as the 'trained' group. The other 11 subjects (the 'untrained' group) received no such training between the two sessions. Differences in grading reliability between the initial and final grading sessions were evaluated for both groups.

Grading reliability was superior (lower) for the combined subject cohort at the final visit (mean ± standard deviation, 0.33 ± 0.12) compared with the initial visit (0.46 ± 0.25). However, there was no difference in the improvement in grading reliability between the two groups. From this, Efron et al.[25] concluded that grading reliability improves statistically with some experience,

although perhaps not to a clinically meaningful extent. No added benefit can be derived from supplemental training in terms of grading reliability.

Conclusions

The grading scales presented in Appendix A were devised as a clinical aid to accurate record keeping. These grading scales provide a practitioner-friendly means to record adverse responses to contact lens wear and to monitor changes in severity over time. The assignment of general guidelines that relate to the necessity for clinical action with respect to each level of severity can be of assistance to clinicians in formulating a general framework for patient management. The grading scales also nurture a common language that can assist practitioners to communicate clinical information within and beyond the confines of contact lens practice.

Clinicians are encouraged to use grading scales as part of their routine contact lens practice so as to foster a disciplined and consistent approach to clinical decision making, which ultimately will be to the benefit of our patients. As a general rule, a change or difference of more than about 1.0 grading scale unit, or an absolute level of severity of more than grade 2, is considered to be clinically meaningful.

REFERENCES

1　Davies M (1978). Safety evaluation of new soft lens materials. In: *Soft Contact Lenses. Clinical and Applied Technology*, p. 378–379, Ed. Ruben M. (London: Bailliere Tindall).

2　Mandell RB (1987). Slit lamp classification system. *J Am Optom Assoc.* **58**, 198–201.

3　Woods RL (1989). Quantitative slit lamp observations in contact lens practice. *J Br Contact Lens Assoc.* Scientific Meetings, 42–45.

4　Courtney RC and Lee JM (1982). Predicting ocular intolerance of a contact lens solution by use of a filter system enhancing fluorescein staining detection. *Int Contact Lens Clin.* **9**, 302–310.

5　McMonnies CW and Chapman-Davies A (1987). Assessment of conjunctival hyperemia in contact lens wearers. Part I. *Am J Optom Physiol Opt.* **64**, 246–250.

6　Begley CG (1992). Giant papillary conjunctivitis. In: *Complications of Contact Lens Wear*, p. 237–252, Ed. Tomlinson A. (St. Louis: Mosby).

7　Lofstrom T, Anderson JS and Kruse A (1998). Tarsal abnormalities: A new grading system. *CLAO J.* **24**, 210–215.

8　Koch DD, de Sanabria MC, Sanning FB and Soper JW (1984). Atlas of illustrations. In: *Adverse Effects of Contact Lens Wear. An Atlas for the Ophthalmic Practitioner*, p. 41–57. (Thorofare: Slack).

9　Annunziato T, Davidson RG, Christensen MT, *et al.* (1992). *Atlas of Slit Lamp Findings and Contact Lens-Related Anomalies.* (Fort Worth: Southwest Independent Institutional Review Board).

10　Andersen JS, Davies IP, Kruse, A *et al.* (1996). *Handbook of Contact Lens Management.* (Jacksonville: Vistakon).

11　CCLRU (1997). CCLRU grading scales (Appendix D). In: *Contact Lenses*, Fourth Edition, p. 863–867, Eds Phillips AJ and Speedwell L. (Oxford: Butterworth–Heinemann).

12　Efron N (1999). Grading scales for contact lens complications. Appendix A. In: *Contact Lens Complications*, First Edition, p. 171–179. (Oxford: Butterworth–Heinemann).

13　Bailey IL, Bullimore MA, Raasch TW and Taylor HR (1991). Clinical grading and the effects of scaling. *Invest Ophthalmol Vis Sci.* **32**, 422–432.

14　Efron N, Morgan PB and Katsara SS (2001). Validation of grading scales for contact lens complications. *Ophthalmic Physiol Opt.* **21**, 17–29.

15　Chong E, Simpson T and Fonn D (2000). The repeatability of discrete and continuous anterior segment grading scales. *Optom Vis Sci.* **77**, 244–251.

16　Dundas M, Walker A and Woods RL (2001). Clinical grading of corneal staining of non-contact lens wearers. *Ophthalmic Physiol Opt.* **21**, 30–35.

17　Papas EB (2000). Key factors in the subjective and objective assessment of conjunctival erythema. *Invest Ophthalmol Vis Sci.* **41**, 687–691.

18　Twelker JD and Bailey IL (2000). Grading conjunctival hyperaemia using a photography-based method. *Invest Ophthalmol Vis Sci.* **41S**, 927.

19　MacKinven J, McGuinness CL, Pascal E and Woods RL (2001). Clinical grading of the upper palpebral conjunctiva of non-contact lens wearers. *Optom Vis Sci.* **78**, 13–18.

20　Efron N, Morgan PB and Jagpal R (2002). Validation of computer morphs for grading contact lens complications. *Ophthalmic Physiol Opt.* **22**, 341–349.

21　Efron N (1998). Grading scales for contact lens complications. *Ophthalmic Physiol Opt.* **18**, 182–186.

22　Quigley HA, Reacher M, Katz J, *et al.* (1993). Quantitative grading of nerve fiber layer photographs. *Ophthalmology* **100**, 1800–1807.

23　Wallace DE, McGreal GT, O'Toole G, *et al.* (2000). The influence of experience and specialisation on the reliability of a common clinical sign. *Ann R Coll Surg Engl.* **82**, 336–338.

24　Efron N, Morgan PB and Jagpal R (2003). The combined influence of knowledge, training and experience when grading contact lens complications. *Ophthalmic Physiol Opt.* **23**, 79–85.

25　Efron N, Morgan PB, Farmer C, *et al.* (2003). Experience and training as determinants of grading reliability when assessing the severity of contact lens complications. *Ophthalmic Physiol Opt.* **23**, 119–124.

GRADING MORPHS

Although grading performance can be enhanced by interpolation to the nearest 0.1 grade unit,[1] most practitioners find the process of mental interpolation between two discrete grading steps to be quite difficult, notwithstanding that this task becomes easier with practice. One way of partially overcoming this difficulty is to re-engineer the grading scales into a continuous movie sequence, progress through which can be controlled by the clinician attempting to decide upon a grade. Modern computer software technology is available to undertake such tasks; the process of merging discrete images into a continuous movie sequence is known as 'morphing'. The results of morphing will be familiar to many readers because this technique is used extensively in the visual arts to change the appearance of an object or person into another – for example, changing the face of a man into an ape.

Morphing is a technique that allows accurate interpolation of numerous progressively changing images between a 'start' and an 'end' image, calculated pixel by pixel. When these images are presented one after the other in rapid succession, a movie or animation results, which allows one to observe the 'start' image being transformed into the 'end' image. The greater the number of interpolated images, the smoother is the movie sequence. If the 'start' and 'end' images are not identical, the morphing technician can program the computer to link common elements in these images that are identified manually. The only limitation to the number of interpolated images is the amount of computer memory available, because a high-resolution image in many colors can be memory intensive.

Efron Grading Morphs

Morphing animation sequences have been developed for each of the 16 complications depicted in Appendix A and have been incorporated into a computer program called 'Efron Grading Morphs'. This program is available on the accompanying CD-ROM.

The 'Efron Grading Morphs' and 'The Efron Grading Tutor' (described below) operate on either IBM-compatible PC platforms (Windows 95 or higher) or Apple Macintosh platforms (Mac OS 7.6 or higher). If using Mac OS X or higher, the programs open in the Classic Environment. The software may also operate on other computer configurations, although full testing has only been performed on the above configurations.

Operation of the 'Efron Grading Morphs' program is described below.

Program operation

When the file 'Efron Grading Morphs' is opened, the program begins to run, and a title page appears. Click on 'View Morphs' (or hit 'Enter' on your keyboard); a second window appears, from which you can choose any one of the 16 available grading morphs shown in the menu along the top and bottom of the window.

A particular grading morph can be selected by clicking on the relevant picture in the menu bar along the top or bottom of the window. When this is done, the selected grading morph is displayed in the centre of the window. The slide bar beneath the grading morph can be adjusted by clicking and holding the small black rectangular slide bar control handle and moving it in the appropriate direction. When the slide bar control handle is moved to the right, the grading morph advances and the level of severity increases. Moving the slide bar control handle to the left reverses the grading morph to a lower level of severity. The slide bar control handle can be moved back and forth in this way until the desired level of severity is achieved.

The numeric grading that indicates the level of severity of the condition being displayed is indicated in the right-hand box as the grading morph is adjusted. This numeric grading is indicated to the nearest 0.1 grading scale unit, within the range from 0.0 (normal) to 4.0 (severe). The slide bar control handle can be released, re-engaged and moved as many times as required, before selecting an alternative grading morph, or quitting.

The Efron Grading Morphs program window is shown in *Figure 30.1*. In this example, papillary conjunctivitis has been selected; this is indicated in the panel on the right-hand side of the window. The slide bar control handle has been advanced to grade 2.7; this numeric grade is also displayed in the right-hand panel.

For masking purposes, the numeric grading can be 'hidden' by clicking on the button 'Hide grade' on the left-hand control panel. The numeric grading can then be revealed by clicking on the 'Show grade' button on the left-hand control panel, and so on.

To view a movie sequence of the selected Morph, click on 'Play movie'. A movie sequence of the morph, which lasts approximately 10 seconds, is shown.

A different grading morph can be selected by clicking on the picture that relates to any one of the other grading morphs shown in the menu bars. The operating procedure as described above is identical for all 16 grading morphs.

Clicking the 'Help' button on the left-hand control panel opens a separate window that pictorially indicates how the program should be used. In this view, clicking on 'Return to morphs' in the lower right corner (or hitting 'Enter' on your keyboard) re-opens the main window platform from which any of the 16 grading morphs can again be selected.

The program can be restarted by clicking the 'Restart' button on the left-hand control panel. Clicking on this button returns the user back to the beginning.

Clicking the 'Quit' button on the left-hand control panel quits the program.

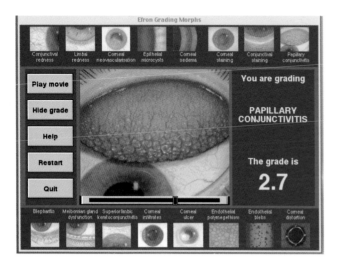

Figure 30.1
Efron Grading
Morphs program
window. In this
example, the
papillary
conjunctivitis morph
is active

of interpolation of grades when using computer morphs, it might be expected that grading can be executed with greater reliability when using this tool versus printed scales.

Efron *et al.*[2] evaluated the performance of the Efron Grading Morphs computer program by:

- Determining grading accuracy when using this program in relation to that obtained using the original five discrete printed images of the Efron Grading Scales (from which the morphs were constructed);
- Comparing grading reliability between these two grading tools.

The aim of these authors[2] was to determine whether computer morphs accord superior grading performance compared with printed scales.

Nine experienced optometrists were each invited to grade – to the nearest 0.1 increment – an image of each of 16 contact lens complications, using printed Efron Grading Scales and the Efron Grading Morphs program. This entire procedure was repeated approximately 2 weeks later, to yield a total database that comprised 576 individual grading estimates. Good accuracy was achieved using computer morphs, as evidenced by the similarity between the mean of the test and retest grading estimates for the printed scales (2.8 ± 0.7) and the computer morphs (2.6 ± 0.8).

There was no difference in median reliability between the printed scales (± 0.41) and the computer morphs (± 0.43). *Figure 30.2* depicts the grading

Grading scales versus morphs
Technical differences

The creation of printed scales involves computer-based scanning of the original artwork and conversion of the RGB (red–green–blue) electronic files used to store and display color images on computers to CMYK (cyan–magenta–yellow–black) electronic files used to control CMYK-colored inks when printing to paper. This conversion alters the stored color information and results in a shift in the hue, saturation and value (brightness) of the colors of the grading scales when they appear in printed form. Computer morphs, on the other hand, are viewed on a display monitor in RGB format.

As a result of the above considerations, printed scales on paper might be expected to look different from computer morphs on a computer screen. Also, the

individual images on the printed scales are relatively small (36×27 mm) and static, whereas the computer morph images on screen are relatively large (97×79 mm on a 15 inch computer screen that displays 1024×768 pixels) and dynamic. In view of the differences described above, computer morphs may or may not be accurate or accord the same reliability as the generally accepted and well-established printed scales. This question was examined by Efron *et al.*[2] (see below).

Performance differences

In contrast with the recommended method of using printed scales – by interpolation of the score to the nearest 0.1 grading scale unit – no such interpolation is required when using continuously variable computer morphs. As there is no 'guesswork' required by way

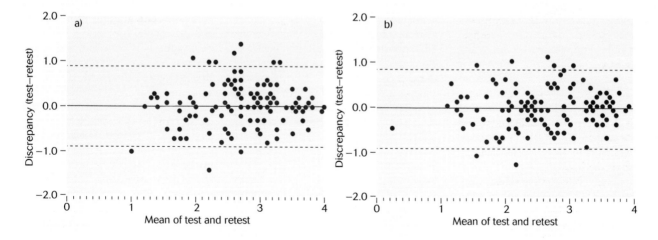

Figure 30.2

Plot of test–retest grading discrepancies versus mean of the test–retest grading scores for all observers and ocular complications, for (a) printed scales and (b) computer morphs. The solid line in each graph represents the mean of the test–retest discrepancies and the dotted lines represent the 95% confidence limits of the test–retest discrepancies ($n = 144$ for each graph)

discrepancies versus the mean of the test and retest grading estimates for the printed scales and computer morphs. It is clear by inspection that there is no general relation between the discrepancies and the means, which indicates that grading reliability is unaffected by the severity of the condition being assessed using either grading tool.

The differences in grading estimates between the two grading tools versus condition severity are presented in *Figure 30.3*. Again, there does not appear to be any relation between these discrepancies and condition severity.

Chong *et al.*[3] reported inferior grading reliability (i.e., higher standard deviations) for grading conjunctival redness and papillary conjunctivitis, and no difference for grading corneal staining, when using printed scales versus computer morphs. However, the differences with respect to grading conjunctival redness and papillary conjunctivitis were small and the authors failed to verify the statistical significance of these differences. The study of Efron *et al.*[2] found no overall statistically significant difference in grading reliability when a broad range of conditions was graded using printed scales versus computer morphs. Computer morphs were thus considered to have been validated in terms of their accuracy and reliability compared with printed scales. The notion that computer morphs offer superior grading reliability compared with printed scales must therefore be rejected.

The Efron Grading Tutor

A Grading Tutor computer program has been developed for use by students, practitioners and researchers, and has a variety of potential applications. This program is available on the accompanying CD-ROM.

An important application of this program is to help practitioners assess, and possibly enhance, their grading performance. Specifically, The Efron Grading Tutor does the following:
- Helps hone your grading skills;
- Identifies if you develop any grading bias;
- Determines your grading consistency;
- Calculates your grading accuracy;
- Compares your performance with that of experts;
- Explains what all this means clinically.

The Efron Grading Tutor has a similar interface to the Efron Grading Morphs

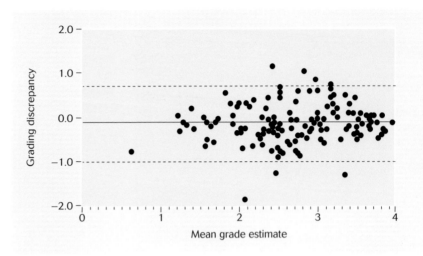

Figure 30.3

Differences in grading estimates when using printed scales and computer morphs versus mean of grading estimates for all observers and ocular complications. The solid line represents the mean of the grading differences and the dotted lines represent the 95% confidence limits of the differences ($n = 144$)

program. It is assumed that the user is familiar with the Efron Grading Morphs program, which provides instructions on the general principles of how to grade the severity of a condition using morphs. The Tutor invites the user to grade the severity of 16 images of contact lens complications, twice in random sequence (a total of 32 gradings is performed). A given complication is graded by adjusting a slide bar until the severity of the condition as depicted in the morph matches that of the image under consideration. Severity is graded on a continuous scale that ranges from 0.0 (normal) to 4.0 (severe). The numeric gradings are revealed to the user only after all 32 gradings have been attempted. On completion of this grading exercise, a series of windows appears that give the user the information listed above.

A supplementary 'Help' window can be called up, which presents further tips on grading and provides other useful information.

Program operation

When the file 'The Efron Grading Tutor' is opened, the program begins to run, and a title page appears with an invitation to enter your name (this is optional). Hit 'Enter' to continue.

You are now presented with the options 'Instructions' and 'Start Tutor'. Clicking on 'Instructions' reveals a series of windows that explains how to use this program. Once the user is familiar

with using The Efron Grading Tutor, viewing the instructions is not necessary. In this case, simply click on 'Start Tutor' (or hit 'Enter' on your keyboard).

When you start the Tutor, the first image to be graded appears, together with the matching morph.

To grade the image, the slide bar beneath the grading morph movie frame is adjusted by clicking and holding the small rectangular slide bar control handle and moving it in the appropriate direction. When the slide bar control handle is moved to the right, the grading morph movie advances and the level of severity increases. Moving the slide bar control handle to the left reverses the grading morph movie to a lower level of severity. The slide bar control handle can be moved back and forth in this way until the level of severity is achieved that matches that of the image under consideration. The slide bar control handle can be released, re-engaged and moved as many times as required before advancing to the next image.

The Efron Grading Tutor program window is shown in *Figure 30.4*. In this example, the user has been invited to grade an image of epithelial microcysts (the left-hand image); the condition being graded (in this case, epithelial microcysts) is indicated on the bottom bar. The top bar indicates that this is the first image being graded. The slide bar control handle beneath the morph on the right-hand side has been adjusted so that the level of severity displayed in the morph matches that of the left-hand image; this numeric grade is deliberately *not* displayed (to avoid observer bias).

When you are satisfied that you have matched the first image as best as possible, click 'Next' (or hit 'Enter' on your keyboard) to advance to the second image. You can keep track of how many images you have graded (up to the maximum 32 images) by referring to the grading instruction along the top of the window.

Click 'Next' again (or hit 'Enter' on your keyboard), and so on, until all 32 images have been graded. After grading the 32nd image, click on the 'Results' button (or hit 'Enter' on your keyboard). You will be led through a series of windows that present you with information concerning your own grading performance. One of these windows presents a detailed analysis whereby the grading estimate you assigned to each image is compared with the mean grading estimate assigned by a panel of 10 'experts' (*Figure 30.5*).

Toward the end of this series of windows, a summary window is presented (*Figure 30.6*). The information given includes:

- Your name;
- Day, date and time the grading exercise was performed;
- All 32 grading estimates (tabulated in non-randomized form);
- Grading bias;
- Grading consistency;
- Grading accuracy (relative to 10 'experts').

The summary window can be printed by clicking on the 'Print' button at the bottom of the window.

Clicking the 'Help' button on the lower menu bar opens a series of windows that offers tips on how to improve your grading technique, defines some of the terms used in this program and advises on where to obtain further information on grading technique, grading scales and contact lens complications. Clicking the 'Return' button (or hitting 'Enter' on your keyboard) re-opens the Tutor window.

The program can be restarted by clicking the 'Restart' button on the lower menu bar. Clicking this button returns the user to the start of the program.

Clicking the 'Quit' button on the lower menu bar quits the program.

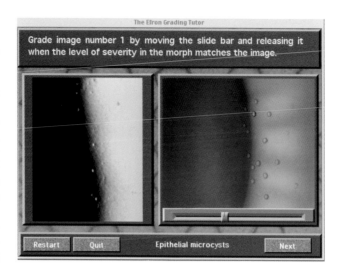

Figure 30.4
The Efron Grading Tutor program window. The operator is invited to grade an image of epithelial microcysts

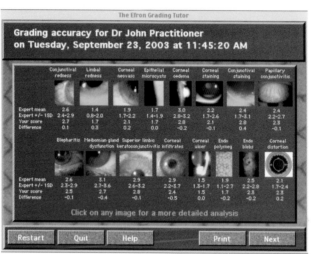

Figure 30.5
The Efron Grading Morphs program window for analyzing grading accuracy

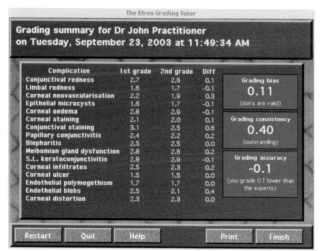

Figure 30.6
The Efron Grading Morphs program summary window

Conclusions

Although there is no difference in grading performance when using printed scales versus computer morphs,[2] there are clearly advantages of using of both tools. Printed scales offer the convenience of being readily accessible, whereby they may be kept next to the slit-lamp biomicroscope. The use of computer morphs ensures that grading estimates are made to the nearest 0.1 grading scale increment, which obviates the tendency observed with printed scales to grade to the nearest whole-digit or half-digit grade.

Computer morphs also offer the opportunity of integration with computer-based record-keeping systems. For example, a grading determined on a morphing tool can be entered automatically into a patient's electronic record. Computer morphs have the advantage of allowing students and practitioners to better conceptualize the continuum and range of severity of various forms of ocular pathology induced by contact lenses, and can be incorporated into self-help grading tutorial programs, such as The Efron Grading Tutor; in this context, computer morphs constitute a valuable learning , teaching and research tool.

REFERENCES

1 Bailey IL, Bullimore MA, Raasch TW and Taylor HR (1991). Clinical grading and the effects of scaling. *Invest Ophthalmol Vis Sci.* **32**, 422–432.
2 Efron N, Morgan PB and Jagpal R (2002). Validation of computer morphs for grading contact lens complications. *Ophthalmic Physiol Opt.* **22**, 341–349.
3 Chong E, Simpson T and Fonn D (2000). The repeatability of discrete and continuous anterior segment grading scales. *Optom Vis Sci.* **77**, 244–251.

APPENDIX A
GRADING SCALES FOR CONTACT LENS COMPLICATIONS

The grading scales presented in this Appendix were devised by Professor Nathan Efron and painted by the ophthalmic artist, Terry R Tarrant.

These grading scales are presented in two panels and are designed to assist practitioners to quantify the level of severity of a variety of contact lens complications. The eight complications on page 240 are those that are more likely to be encountered in contact lens practice. Many of these complications are graded routinely by some practitioners. The eight complications on page 242 are encountered less commonly in contact lens practice, or represent pathology that is rare or unusual. The order of presentation of the complications on each panel, from top to bottom, reflects the likely order in which these complications may be encountered in the course of a systematic examination using the slit-lamp biomicroscope.

Opposite each of the two grading scale panels is a table (set out in the same format as the corresponding panel of complications) that briefly explains the salient features of each image. An explanation as to how to use these grading scales in clinical practice is given in Chapter 29.

The development of these grading scales was kindly sponsored by Hydron Ltd (now CooperVision).

A handy plastic-coated A4-sized version of these grading scales, which comes in a handsome protective slip case with comprehensive instructions for use, is available free from CooperVision. Simply send a request, with your full postal address, to gradingscales@coopervision.co.uk

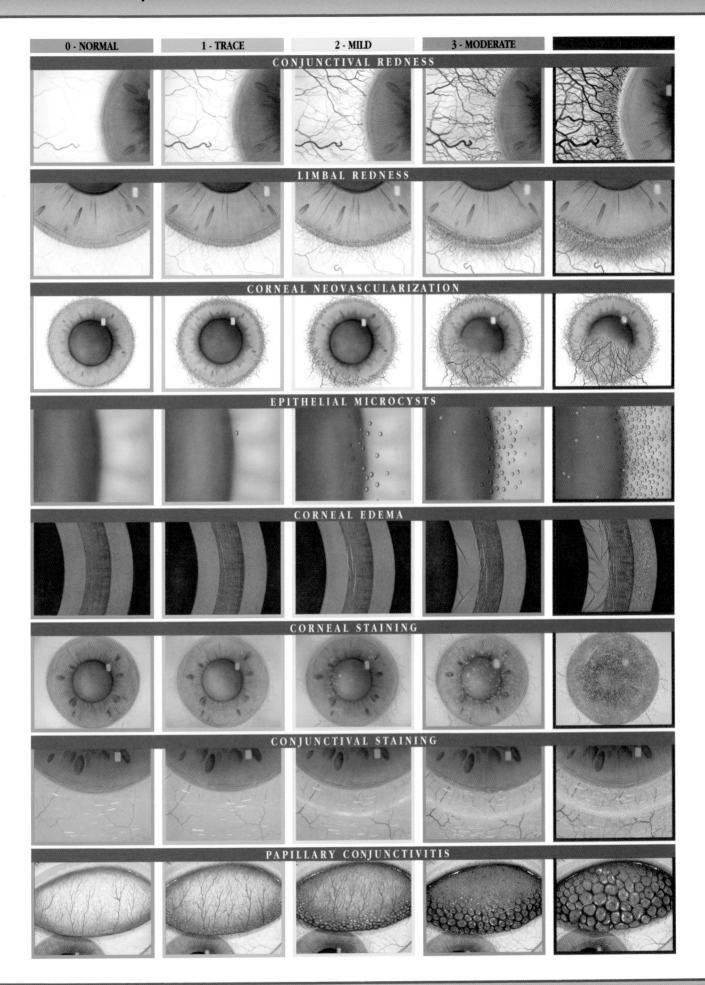

0 - NORMAL	1 - TRACE	2 - MILD	3 - MODERATE	

CONJUNCTIVAL REDNESS

LIMBAL REDNESS

CORNEAL NEOVASCULARIZATION

EPITHELIAL MICROCYSTS

CORNEAL EDEMA

CORNEAL STAINING

CONJUNCTIVAL STAINING

PAPILLARY CONJUNCTIVITIS

0 - NORMAL	1 - TRACE	2 - MILD	3 - MODERATE	4 - SEVERE
CONJUNCTIVAL REDNESS				
'White' bulbar conjunctiva One major vessel Clear cornea	Small increase in conjunctival redness Major vessel more engorged	Further increase in conjunctival redness Limbal redness Slight ciliary flush	Conjunctiva very red Increased limbal redness Ciliary flush	Conjunctiva extremely red Limbus very red Intense ciliary flush Reflex on major vessel
LIMBAL REDNESS				
'White' limbus White corneal reflex	Slightly increased limbal redness White corneal reflex	Increased limbal redness Increased conjunctival redness White corneal reflex	Limbus very red Increased conjunctival redness Speckled corneal reflex	Limbus extremely red Conjunctival redness Hazy corneal reflex
CORNEAL NEOVASCULARIZATION				
Clear cornea White reflex	Vessels encroach <1 mm from lower left quadrant (LLQ)	Vessels encroach 2–3 mm from LLQ Limbal redness Reflex less crisp Central corneal haze	Vessels encroach 4–5 mm from LLQ Corneal haze around vessels Speckled reflex	Vessels encroach 6 mm from LLQ Lipid at leading edge of vessels Very diffuse reflex
EPITHELIAL MICROCYSTS				
High magnification view of pupil margin Clear cornea	Single microcysts at pupillary margin Microcyst displays reversed illumination	16 microcysts Some appear faint (newly formed)	About 70 microcysts Some microcysts at the surface stain with fluorescein	About 180 microcysts Many at the surface stain with fluorescein
CORNEAL EDEMA				
Clear cornea and 3 mm wide parallelepiped Left: endothelium Centre: stroma Right: epithelium	Single vertical stria in posterior cornea	Three vertical striae in posterior cornea	Many vertical striae in posterior cornea Folds in endothelium	Many vertical striae in posterior cornea Many folds in endothelium Epithelial bullae
CORNEAL STAINING				
Clear cornea No staining Fluorescein in eye Cobalt blue reflex	Light punctate staining Slight conjunctival redness	More punctate staining Increased redness	Light pan-corneal punctate staining Diffuse reflex	Heavy pan-corneal punctate staining Very diffuse reflex
CONJUNCTIVAL STAINING				
Clear cornea Fluorescein pooling in some folds Cobalt blue reflex	Increased fluorescein pooling in folds Slight staining at position of lens edge	More fluorescein pooling in folds Interrupted lens edge staining Increased conjunctival redness	Widespread fluorescein pooling in folds Continuous lens edge staining Conjunctival redness	Widespread fluorescein pooling in folds Heavy lens edge staining Conjunctival redness Limbal staining
PAPILLARY CONJUNCTIVITIS				
Pale conjunctiva Vessels clearly visible Slight roughness at tarsal fold	Pink conjunctiva Vessels visible Increased roughness at tarsal fold	Red conjunctiva Vessels less visible Papillae at tarsal fold Reflexes on some papillae	Very red conjunctiva Vessels barely visible Large papillae Bright papillary reflexes Single mucus strand	Extremely red conjunctiva Vessels not visible Very large papillae Bright papillary reflexes More mucus strands

0 - NORMAL	1 - TRACE	2 - MILD	3 - MODERATE	4 - SEVERE

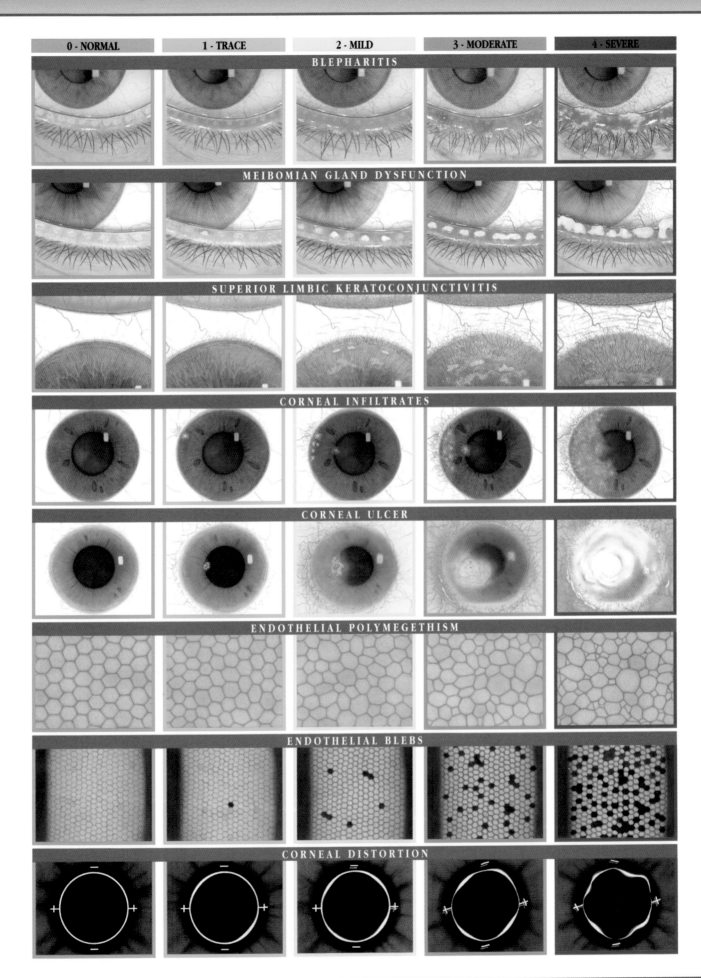

BLEPHARITIS

MEIBOMIAN GLAND DYSFUNCTION

SUPERIOR LIMBIC KERATOCONJUNCTIVITIS

CORNEAL INFILTRATES

CORNEAL ULCER

ENDOTHELIAL POLYMEGETHISM

ENDOTHELIAL BLEBS

CORNEAL DISTORTION

0 - NORMAL	1 - TRACE	2 - MILD	3 - MODERATE	4 - SEVERE
BLEPHARITIS				
Pale lid margin Openings of meibomian glands visible Clean lashes	Pink lid margin Openings of meibomian glands less visible Clean lashes	Red lid margin Openings of meibomian glands barely visible Yellow crust at base of lashes Some lashes stuck together	Telangiectasis of lid margin Increased crusting More lashes stuck together Bulbar conjunctival redness	Severe telangiectasis of lid margin Excess yellow crusting Lashes stuck together Increased bulbar conjunctival redness Skin irritation
MEIBOMIAN GLAND DYSFUNCTION				
Pale lid margin Openings of meibomian glands visible Clean lashes	Pink lid margin Cloudy expression at some gland orifices	Red lid margin Milky expression at most gland orifices Increased tearing	Red lid margin Yellow expression at all gland orifices Expressions becoming continuous	Thick creamy yellow expression at all gland orifices Expressions continuous Bulbar conjunctival redness
SUPERIOR LIMBIC KERATOCONJUNCTIVITIS				
Clear conjunctiva Clear superior limbus Clear cornea Clear reflex	Increased conjunctival redness Slight limbal redness Clear cornea	Conjunctival redness and staining Increased limbal redness Corneal staining and infiltrates	Greater conjunctival redness and staining Increased limbal redness 2–3 mm fibrovascular pannus Greater corneal staining and infiltrates	Severe conjunctival redness and staining Severe limbal redness 5 mm fibrovascular pannus Severe corneal staining and infiltrates
CORNEAL INFILTRATES				
Clear cornea Clear conjunctiva and limbus Clear reflex	Single small gray infiltrate at 10 o'clock near limbus Adjacent limbal redness	Five small gray infiltrates at 9–10 o'clock near limbus Adjacent limbus more red	Numerous small hazy gray infiltrates at 8–10 o'clock in peripheral cornea Adjacent limbus very red	Hazy gray confluent infiltrates that cover left half of cornea Adjacent limbal redness from 5 to 11 o'clock Mild conjunctival redness
CORNEAL ULCER				
Clear cornea Clear conjunctiva and limbus Clear reflex	<1 mm corneal ulcer at left pupil margin Stains with fluorescein Mild limbal redness at 7–11 o'clock	2–3 mm corneal ulcer Haze around ulcer Intense limbal redness at 7–11 o'clock Ciliary flush	6 mm corneal ulcer Haze around ulcer General corneal haze Intense circumlimbal redness Conjunctival redness Increased ciliary flush	White pan-corneal ulcer Cornea opaque Intense circumlimbal and conjunctival redness Intense ciliary flush
ENDOTHELIAL POLYMEGETHISM				
Cells same size Hexagonal shape Coefficient of variation (COV) = 0.15	Small variance in cell size COV = 0.25	Increased variance in cell size COV = 0.35 Some five-, six- and seven-sided cells	Considerable variance in cell size COV = 0.45 Some three-, four-, five-, six- and seven-sided cells	Substantial variance in cell size COV = 0.55 Some three-, four-, five-, seven-, eight- and nine-sided cells
ENDOTHELIAL BLEBS				
Cells same size Hexagonal shape No blebs	One bleb	Three single blebs Two double-cell blebs	Large number of blebs 'Thickened' cell borders	Very large number of blebs Increased spacing between cells
CORNEAL DISTORTION				
Bright, sharp, circular keratometer mire	Slightly distorted keratometer mire Variation in thickness of circle	Distorted keratometer mire Variation in thickness of circle Loss of focus of right and top +/– signs	Very distorted keratometer mire Greater variation in thickness of circle Loss of focus and distortion of all +/– signs	Extremely distorted keratometer mire Greater variation in thickness of circle with some gaps Loss of focus and distortion of all +/– signs

APPENDIX B
GUILLON TEAR FILM CLASSIFICATION SYSTEM

All the pre-ocular and pre-lens tear film patterns depicted in this appendix were imaged and captured photographically using a tearscope. All tear film lipid patterns should be assessed before any other examination and should be judged 2 seconds after the blink when the upward motion of the tear film (a viscosity characteristic) has stopped.

Pre-ocular tear film lipid patterns

	Dark eye	Light eye	
Open meshwork (marmorial)	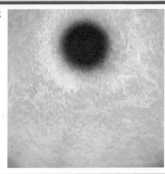	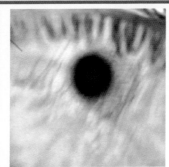	Observed in 21% of the population 13–50 nm thickness Gray appearance of low reflectivity Sparse, open meshwork pattern faintly visible after the blink In the lower thickness range it may not be visible at low magnification Thought to represent a deficient lipid layer
Closed meshwork (marmorial)	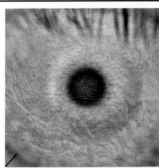	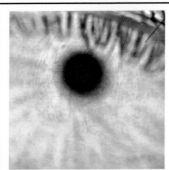	Observed in 10% of the population 30–50 nm thickness Gray appearance of average reflectivity More compact meshwork pattern Thought to represent a normal lipid layer
Wave (flow)	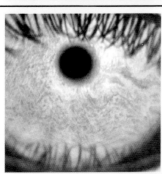	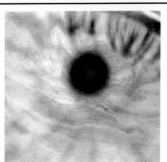	Observed in 23% of the population 50–80 nm thickness Pattern of vertical or horizontal gray waves of good visibility between blinks Most common lipid layer
Amorphous	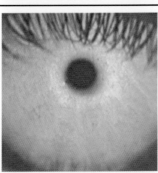	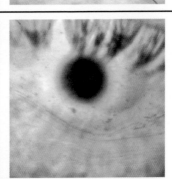	Observed in 24% of the population 80–90 nm thickness Even pattern with whitish highly reflective surface Thought to represent an ideal, well-mixed lipid layer
First-order color fringes	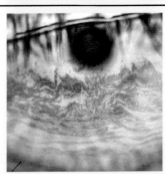	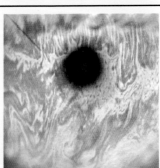	Observed in 10% of the population 90–140 nm thickness Discrete brown and blue well-spread lipid layer interference fringes superimposed on a whitish background Thought to represent a regular, very full lipid layer

Excessive and contaminated lipids

Second-order color fringes

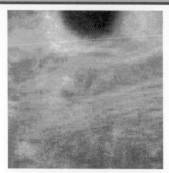

Observed in 5% of the population
140–180 nm thickness
Discrete green and red tightly packed lipid layer interference fringes
   superimposed on a whitish background
Thought to represent an abnormal lipid layer of increased thickness in the
   colored areas

Globular lipid with multiple colors

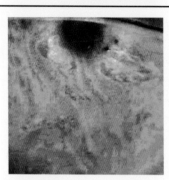

Observed in 7% of the population
>180 nm thickness
Highly variable colors, but typically combinations of brown, blue, green and
   red, irregularly spread
Sometimes globules of intense color appear
Thought to represent an extremely heavy and irregular lipid layer, often
   associated with oversecretion, blepharitis or lipid contamination

Lipid break-up and cosmetics

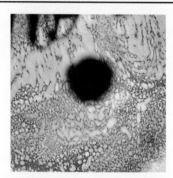

Abnormal lipid pattern
Seen when cosmetic products invade the tear film and break the lipid layer.
   The area devoid of lipid coverage appears dark gray as the light is reflected
   specularly from the bare aqueous phase. The area covered by lipid is highly
   reflective and can be confined to form isolated circular islands

Eye ointments

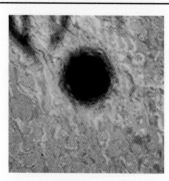

Abnormal appearance
Ointments destroy the normal tear film structure
Heavy striated fringes of yellow, brown, blue, green and purple, which are
   often irregularly distributed, indicating the variable thickness of the ointment

Face cream

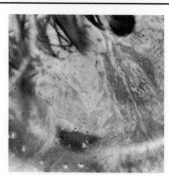

Lipid break-up observed when moisturizers or face creams invade and break
   the lipid layer
Colored fringes on gray background

Pre-soft lens tear film

The following sequence of images can be taken to represent an ideal pre-lens tear film going through the process of thinning caused by drainage and evaporation. Initially, the presence of a superficial lipid layer reduces evaporation and the thick aqueous phase ensures the separation of the lipid and mucus phases. Following thinning of the aqueous phase, some lipid components migrate posteriorly and come into contact with the mucus phase and lens surface, which produces non-wetting patches

An alternative interpretation of this sequence of images is that they represent different tear film structures that appear immediately after eye opening. In this case, the images are arranged from 'best' to 'worst' and can be used to grade the quality of the pre-lens tear film.

Meshwork lipid coverage

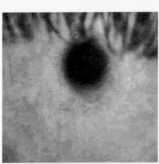

Appearance of a good tear film on the surface of a soft contact lens immediately after eye opening
Thin lipid layer present
Aqueous layer fringes not visible denote an aqueous phase >3.5 μm thick

Lipid with aqueous fringes

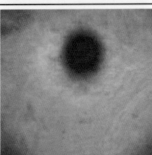

Appearance of tear film on the surface of a soft contact lens 4 seconds after eye opening
Very thin lipid layer of low visibility
Blue, green, yellow and red aqueous interference fringes faintly visible under the lipid layer
Aqueous layer 2–3.5 μm thick

Aqueous fringes

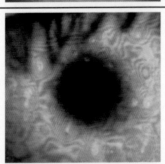

Appearance of tear film on the surface of a soft contact lens 8 seconds after eye opening
Lipid layer virtually absent
Narrow green and red aqueous interference fringes are easily visible
Aqueous layer 2 μm thick

Dry area

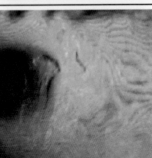

Appearance of tear film on the surface of a soft contact lens 12 seconds after eye opening
Lipid layer absent
Widely spaced, bright green and red aqueous interference fringes visible
Aqueous layer <1 μm thick
Edge of the mucus layer visible
Lens surface visible at the center of the dry spot

Lipid contamination

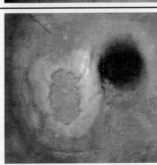

Appearance of tear film on the surface of a soft contact lens contaminated with lipid
Oval non-wetting patch occurs immediately after eye opening
Contaminating lipids highly visible
Blue, green, yellow and red interference fringes visible in a thin aqueous phase

Pre-rigid lens tear film

As for the pre-soft lens tear film, the following sequence of images of the pre-rigid lens tear film can be taken to represent either (a) an ideal pre-lens tear film going through the process of thinning, or (b) different tear film structures immediately after eye opening ranked from 'best' to 'worst'.

Complete lipid cover

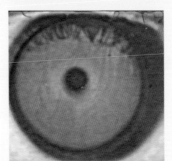

Appearance of an ideal tear film on the surface of a rigid lens immediately after eye opening
Seen in only 5% of cases
Thin and complete lipid cover
Blue, green, yellow and red aqueous layer interference fringes faintly visible

Thick aqueous layer

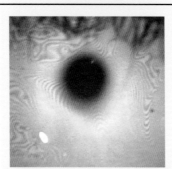

Appearance of tear film on the surface of a rigid lens 4 seconds after eye opening
Very thin lipid layer
Narrow aqueous layer interference fringes denote a thick aqueous phase
Aqueous layer >2 μm thick

Medium aqueous layer

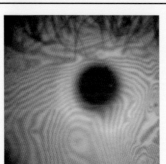

Appearance of tear film on the surface of a rigid lens 8 seconds after eye opening
Lipid layer absent
Well-defined aqueous layer interference fringes
Thinning of aqueous phases superiorly may be induced by the upper tear meniscus
Aqueous layer 1–2 μm thick

Thin aqueous layer

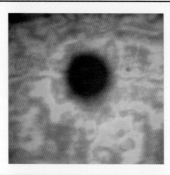

Appearance of tear film on the surface of a rigid lens 12 seconds after eye opening
Lipid layer absent
Broad, bright red and green aqueous layer interference fringes
Aqueous layer <1 μm thick

Drying

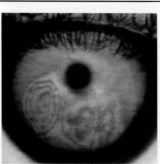

Appearance of tear film on the surface of a rigid lens 16 seconds after eye opening
Lipid layer absent
Irregular broad, bright red and green aqueous layer interference fringes visible, some in a circular pattern, formed by the evaporating tear film
Aqueous layer <0.5 μm thick inferiorly and absent superiorly

INDEX

Single User License Agreement

NOTICE. WE ARE WILLING TO LICENSE THE MULTI-MEDIA PROGRAM PRODUCT TITLED CONTACT LENS COMPLICATIONS 2E ("MULTIMEDIA PROGRAM") TO YOU ONLY ON THE CONDITION THAT YOU ACCEPT ALL OF THE TERMS CONTAINED IN THIS LICENSE AGREEMENT. PLEASE READ THIS LICENSE AGREEMENT CAREFULLY BEFORE OPENING THE SEALED DISK PACKAGE. BY OPENING THAT PACKAGE YOU AGREE TO BE BOUND BY THE TERMS OF THIS AGREEMENT. IF YOU DO NOT AGREE TO THESE TERMS WE ARE UNWILLING TO LICENSE THE MULTIMEDIA PROGRAM TO YOU, AND YOU SHOULD NOT OPEN THE DISK PACKAGE. IN SUCH CASE, PROMPTLY RETURN THE UNOPENED DISK PACKAGE AND ALL OTHER MATERIAL IN THIS PACKAGE, ALONG WITH PROOF OF PAYMENT, TO THE AUTHORIZED DEALER FROM WHOM YOU OBTAINED IT FOR A FULL REFUND OF THE PRICE YOU PAID.

Ownership and License

This is a license agreement and NOT an agreement for sale. It permits you to use one copy of the MULTIMEDIA PROGRAM on a single computer. The MULTIMEDIA PROGRAM and its contents are owned by us or our licensors, and are protected by US and international copyright laws. Your rights to use the MULTIMEDIA PROGRAM are specified in this Agreement, and we retain all rights not expressly granted to you in this Agreement.

- You may use one copy of the MULTIMEDIA PROGRAM on a single computer.
- After you have installed the MULTIMEDIA PROGRAM on your computer, you may use the MULTIMEDIA PROGRAM on a different computer only if you first delete the files installed by the installation program from the first computer.
- You may not copy any portion of the MULTIMEDIA PROGRAM to your computer hard disk or any other media other than printing out or downloading non-substantial portions of the text and images in the MULTIMEDIA PROGRAM for your own internal informational use.
- Your may not copy any of the documentation or other printed materials accompanying the MULTIMEDIA PROGRAM.

Neither concurrent use on two or more computers nor use in a local area network or other network is permitted without separate authorization and the payment of additional license fees.

Transfer and Other Restrictions

You may not rent, lend or lease this MULTIMEDIA PROGRAM. Save as permitted by law, you may not and you may not permit others to (a) disassemble, decompile or otherwise derive source code from the software included in the MULTIMEDIA PROGRAM (the "Software"), (b) reverse engineer the Software, (c) modify or prepare derivative works of the MULTIMEDIA PROGRAM, (d) use the Software in an on-line system or (e) use the MULTIMEDIA PROGRAM in any manner that infringes on the intellectual property or other rights of another party.

However, you may transfer this license to use the MULTIMEDIA PROGRAM to another party on a permanent basis by transferring this copy of the License Agreement, the MULTIMEDIA PROGRAM and all documentation. Such transfer of possession terminates your license from us. Such other party shall be licensed under the terms of this Agreement upon its acceptance of this Agreement by its initial use of the MULTIMEDIA PROGRAM. If you transfer the MULTIMEDIA PROGRAM, you must remove the installation files from your hard disk and you may not retain any copies of those files for your own use.

Limited Warranty and Limitation of Liability

For a period of sixty (60) days from the date you acquired the MULTIMEDIA PROGRAM from us or our authorized dealer, we warrant that the media containing the MULTIMEDIA PROGRAM will be free from defects that prevent you from installing the MULTIMEDIA PROGRAM on your computer. If the disk fails to conform to this warranty you may as your sole and exclusive remedy, obtain a replacement free of charge if you return the defective disk to us with a dated proof of purchase. Otherwise the MULTIMEDIA PROGRAM is licensed to you on an "AS IS" basis without any warranty of any nature.

WE DO NOT WARRANT THAT THE MULTIMEDIA PROGRAM WILL MEET YOUR REQUIREMENTS OR THAT ITS OPERATION WILL BE UNINTERRUPTED OR ERROR-FREE. THE EXPRESS TERMS OF THIS AGREEMENT ARE IN LIEU OF ALL WARRANTIES, CONDITIONS, UNDERTAKINGS, TERMS AND OBLIGATIONS IMPLIED BY STATUTE, COMMON LAW, TRADE USAGE, COURSE OF DEALING OR OTHERWISE ALL OF WHICH ARE HEREBY EXCLUDED TO THE FULLEST EXTENT PERMITTED BY LAW, INCLUDING THE IMPLIED WARRANTIES OF SATISFACTORY QUALITY AND FITNESS FOR A PARTICULAR PURPOSE.

WE SHALL NOT BE LIABLE FOR ANY DAMAGE OR LOSS OF ANY KIND (EXCEPT PERSONAL INJURY OR DEATH RESULTING FROM OUR NEGLIGENCE) ARISING OUT OF OR RESULTING FROM YOUR POSSESSION OR USE OF THE MULTIMEDIA PROGRAM (INCLUDING DATA LOSS OR CORRUPTION), REGARDLESS OF WHETHER SUCH LIABILITY IS BASED IN TORT, CONTRACT OR OTHERWISE AND INCLUDING, BUT NOT LIMITED TO, ACTUAL, SPECIAL, INDIRECT, INCIDENTAL OR CONSEQUENTIAL DAMAGES. IF THE FOREGOING LIMITATION IS HELD TO BE UNENFORCEABLE OUR MAXIMUM LIABILITY TO YOU SHALL NOT EXCEED THE AMOUNT OF THE LICENSE FEE PAID BY YOU FOR THE MULTIMEDIA PROGRAM. THE REMEDIES AVAILABLE TO YOU AGAINST US AND THE LICENSORS OF MATERIALS INCLUDED IN THE MULTIMEDIA PROGRAM ARE EXCLUSIVE.

Termination

This license and your right to use this MULTIMEDIA PROGRAM automatically terminate if you fail to comply with any provisions of this Agreement, destroy the copy of the MULTIMEDIA PROGRAM in your possession or voluntarily return the MULTIMEDIA PROGRAM to us. Upon termination you will destroy all copies of the MULTIMEDIA PROGRAM and documentation.

Miscellaneous Provisions

This Agreement will be governed by and construed in accordance with English law and you hereby submit to the non-exclusive jurisdiction of the English Courts. This is the entire agreement between us relating to the MULTIMEDIA PROGRAM, and supersedes any prior purchase order, communications, advertising or representations concerning the contents of this package, No change or modification of this Agreement will be valid unless it is in writing and is signed by us.